FOOT
AND
ANKLE
TRAUMA

FOOT AND ANKLE TRAUMA

EDITED BY
BARRY L. SCURRAN, D.P.M.

Chief, Department of Podiatric Surgery
Chief, Medical Staff Education
Kaiser Permanente Medical Center
Hayward, California
Clinical Associate Professor
Department of Surgery
California College of Podiatric Medicine
San Francisco, California
Clinical Instructor
Stanford University School of Medicine
Palo Alto, California

CHURCHILL LIVINGSTONE
NEW YORK, EDINBURGH, LONDON, MELBOURNE

Library of Congress Cataloging in Publication Data

Foot and ankle trauma / edited by Barry L. Scurran.
    p. cm.
  Includes bibliographies and index.
  ISBN 0-443-08578-1
  1. Foot—Fractures. 2. Foot—Wounds and injuries. 3. Ankle—Fractures.
4. Ankle—Wounds and injuries. I. Scurran, Barry L.
  [DNLM: 1. Ankle—injuries. 2. Dislocations—therapy. 3. Foot—injuries.
4. Fractures—therapy. 5. Tendon Injuries—therapy.]
RD563.F644 1989
617.5′85—dc20
WE 880 F6862
for Library of Congress
    89-8199
    CIP

Distributed in the United Kingdom by Churchill Livingstone, Robert Stevenson House, 1–3 Baxter's Place, Leith Walk, Edinburgh EH1 3AF, and by associated companies, branches, and representatives throughout the world.

Accurate indications, adverse reactions, and dosage schedules for drugs are provided in this book, but it is possible that they may change. The reader is urged to review the package information data of the manufacturers of the medications mentioned.

The Publishers have made every effort to trace the copyright holders for borrowed material. If they have inadvertently overlooked any, they will be pleased to make the necessary arrangements at the first opportunity.

Acquisitions Editor: *Kim Loretucci*
Assistant Editor: *Nancy Terry*
Copy Editor: *Kamely Dahir*
Production Designer: *Jill Little*
Production Supervisor: *Jocelyn Eckstein*

Printed in the United States of America

First published in 1989

A very special thank you to my loving family, Hope, Erin, and Jamie, who suffered with me through each deadline and yet encouraged me to complete this project.

CONTRIBUTORS

Omar Bayne, M.D.
Department of Orthopedic Surgery, Kaiser Permanente Medical Center, Hayward, California

Marc Bernbach, D.P.M.
Faculty and Lecturer, The Podiatry Institute, Tucker, Georgia; Special Consultant, West Haven Veterans Administration Medical Center, West Haven, Connecticut; Private Practice, Waterbury, Connecticut

Timothy A. Binning, D.P.M.
Department of Podiatric Surgery, Kaiser Permanente Medical Center, Oakland California

Jeffrey S. Boberg, D.P.M.
Visiting Clinician, Department of Podiatric Surgery, Ohio College of Podiatric Medicine and the Cleveland Foot Clinic, Cleveland, Ohio

Timothy R. Buell, D.P.M.
Department of Podiatric Surgery, Kaiser Permanente Medical Center, Sacramento, California

Albert Burns, D.P.M.
Professor and Chairman, Department of Podiatric Surgery, California College of Podiatric Medicine, San Francisco, California

Mark Burton, D.P.M.
Podiatric Staff, Jean's Hospital, Philadelphia, Pennsylvania; Private Practice, Yardley, Pennsylvania

Thomas Cain, D.P.M.
Faculty and Lecturer, The Podiatry Institute, Tucker, Georgia; Private Practice, Lilburn, Georgia

Bradley D. Castellano, D.P.M.
Department of Podiatric Surgery, Northlake Regional Medical Center; Faculty, The Podiatry Institute, Tucker, Georgia

Raymond Cavaliere, D.P.M.

Assistant Professor, Department of Surgery, New York College of Podiatric Medicine, New York, New York

Robert A. Cooke, D.P.M.

Department of Podiatric Surgery, Kaiser Permanente Medical Center, Hayward, California

Stephen V. Corey, D.P.M.

Department of Podiatric Surgery, Northlake Regional Medical Center; Faculty, The Podiatry Institute, Tucker, Georgia

Nicholas Daly, D.P.M., M.S.

Department of Podiatric Surgery, Kaiser Permanente Medical Center, Hayward, California

Steven DeValentine, D.P.M.

Chief, Department of Podiatric Surgery, Kaiser Permanente Medical Center, South Sacramento, California; Assistant Clinical Professor, Department of Podiatric Surgery, California College of Podiatric Medicine, San Francisco, California

Richard DiNapoli, D.P.M.

Lecturer and Faculty, The Podiatry Institute, Tucker, Georgia; Private Practice, Manchester, New Hampshire

Michael S. Downey, D.P.M.

Assistant Professor and Acting Chairman, Department of Surgery, Pennsylvania College of Podiatric Medicine; Member, Podiatric Trauma Team, St. Joseph's Hospital, Philadelphia, Pennsylvania

Douglas H. Elleby, D.P.M.

Department of Surgery, Atlanta Hospital and Medical Center, Atlanta, Georgia; Department of Surgery, Kenestone Hospital, Marietta, Georgia

Michael A. Figura, D.P.M.

Private Practice, Country Podiatrists, Inc., St. Louis, Missouri

Joshua Gerbert, D.P.M.

Former Dean for Academic Affairs, and Professor and Chairman, Department of Podiatric Surgery, California College of Podiatric Medicine, San Francisco, California

Flair Goldman, D.P.M.

Chief, Department of Podiatric Surgery, Kaiser Permanente Medical Center, Santa Clara, California

Donald R. Green, D.P.M.

Clinical Instructor, Department of Orthopedics, University of California, San Diego, School of Medicine, La Jolla, California; Clinical Professor, Department of Surgery, California College of Podiatric Medicine, San Francisco, California; Former Chairman and Professor, Department of Surgery, Pennsylvania College of Podiatric Medicine, Philadelphia, Pennsylvania

George Gumann, D.P.M.

Department of Surgery, Orthopedic Service, Martin Army Community Hospital, Fort Benning, Georgia; Clinical Instructor, Department of Surgery, Pennsylvania College of Podiatric Medicine, Philadelphia, Pennsylvania; Clinical Instructor, Department of Surgery, Dr. William Scholl College of Podiatric Medicine; Clinical Instructor, Department of Surgery, California College of Podiatric Medicine, San Francisco, California

Warren S. Joseph, D.P.M.

Assistant Professor, Department of Medicine, and Chief, Section of Infectious Diseases, Pennsylvania College of Podiatric Medicine; Consultant, Department of Podiatric Infectious Diseases, St. Joseph's Hospital, Philadelphia, Pennsylvania

Jeffrey M. Karlin, D.P.M.

Department of Podiatric Medicine and Surgery, Kaiser Permanente Medical Center, Hayward, California; Director, Residency Training, Kaiser Foundation Hospital, Hayward, California; Assistant Clinical Professor, Department of Podiatric Surgery, California College of Podiatric Medicine, San Francisco, California; Clinical Instructor, Department of Medicine, Stanford University School of Medicine, Palo Alto, California

William W. Kirchwehm, D.P.M.

Private Practice, Lompoc, California

Guido LaPorta, D.P.M., M.S.

Northeast Foot and Ankle Institute, Scranton, Pennsylvania

Stanley B. Leis, D.P.M.

Department of Podiatric Surgery, Kaiser Permanente Medical Center, West Los Angeles, California

Kieran T. Mahan, D.P.M.

Vice President for Academic Affairs and Dean, and Associate Professor, Department of Surgery, Pennsylvania College of Podiatric Medicine, Philadelphia, Pennsylvania

D. Scot Malay, D.P.M.

Assistant Professor, Department of Surgery, Pennsylvania College of Podiatric Medicine, Philadelphia, Pennsylvania; Faculty, Podiatric Education and Research Institute; Attending Podiatric Surgeon, and Member, Resident Training Committee, St. Joseph's Hospital, Philadelphia, Pennsylvania; Attending Podiatric Surgeon, The Graduate Hospital, Philadelphia, Pennsylvania

David E. Marcinko, D.P.M.

Chief and Assistant Residency Director, Department of Podiatric Surgery, Atlanta Hospital and Medical Center; Peachtree Podiatric Group, P.C., Atlanta, Georgia

Lawrence M. Oloff, D.P.M.

Dean for Academic Affairs; Director, Special Problems Clinic; Associate Professor, Department of Surgery, California College of Podiatric Medicine, San Francisco, California; Assistant Clinical Professor, Department of Dermatology, Stanford University School of Medicine, Palo Alto, California

Mark E. Reiner, D.P.M.
Methodist Hospital of Jonesboro, Jonesboro, Arkansas

Elliot H. Rose, M.D.
Clinical Assistant Professor, Division of Plastic and Reconstructive Surgery, Stanford University School of Medicine, Palo Alto, California; Attending Surgeon, Department of Plastic Surgery, Palo Alto Veterans Administration Hospital, Palo Alto, California; Active Staff, Microsurgical and Transplantation Services, Peninsula Hospital, Burlingame, California

John A. Ruch, D.P.M.
Academic Director, The Podiatry Institute; Attending Staff, Northlake Regional Medical Center; Private Practice, Tucker, Georgia

Christina C. Rude, D.P.M.
Chief, Department of Podiatry, Kaiser Permanente Medical Center, San Jose, California

Ross Rudolph, M.D., F.A.C.S.
Head, Division of Plastic and Reconstructive Surgery, Scripps Clinic and Research Foundation; Associate Clinical Professor, Department of Plastic Surgery, University of California, San Diego, School of Medicine, La Jolla, California

Claudia Sands, D.P.M.
Department of Podiatric Surgery, Kaiser Permanente Medical Center, Hayward, California

John M. Schuberth, D.P.M.
Attending Staff, Department of Orthopedics/Podiatry, Kaiser Permanente Medical Center, San Francisco, California; Clinical Instructor, Stanford University School of Medicine, Palo Alto, California; Clinical Faculty, Department of Surgery, California College of Podiatric Medicine, San Francisco, California

Barry L. Scurran, D.P.M.
Chief, Department of Podiatric Surgery, and Chief, Medical Staff Education, Kaiser Permanente Medical Center, Hayward, California; Clinical Associate Professor, Department of Surgery, California College of Podiatric Medicine, San Francisco, California; Clinical Instructor, Stanford University School of Medicine, Palo Alto, California

Robert Sheinberg, D.P.M.
West Broward Foot and Ankle Inc., Fort Lauderdale, Florida

Stephen H. Silvani, D.P.M.
Residency Director of Podiatrics, Department of Orthopedics, Kaiser Permanente Medical Center, Walnut Creek, California; Clinical Instructor, Stanford University School of Medicine, Palo Alto, California; Associate Clinical Professor, Department of Surgery, California College of Podiatric Medicine, San Francisco, California

Thomas F. Smith, D.P.M.
Special Consultant, Veterans Administration Medical Center, Augusta, Georgia; Instructor, Diabetic Foot Clinic, Medical College of Georgia, Augusta, Georgia;

Clinical Instructor, Department of Surgery, Pennsylvania College of Podiatric Medicine, Philadelphia, Pennsylvania; Lecturer and Faculty, The Podiatry Institute, Tucker, Georgia

Daniel Tuerk, M.D.

Subchief, Department of Plastic Surgery, Kaiser Permanente Medical Center, Hayward, California

Robert Tupper, D.P.M.

Department of Podiatry, Veterans Administration Medical Center, Augusta, Georgia

Harold W. Vogler, D.P.M.

Professor, Department of Surgery, Pennsylvania College of Podiatric Medicine; Chairman, Division of Foot and Ankle Surgery; Chief of Traumatology, Director of Four-Year Residency in Reconstructive and Traumatologic Surgery of the Foot and Ankle, St. Joseph's Hospital, Philadelphia, Pennsylvania

John H. Walter, Jr., D.P.M., M.S.

Associate Professor, Department of Podiatric Surgery and Orthopedics, Pennsylvania College of Podiatric Medicine; Director, Foot and Ankle Pain and Fracture Center, Philadelphia, Pennsylvania

Thomas H. Walter, D.P.M.

Associate Professor, Department of Surgery/Trauma Division, New York College of Podiatric Medicine, New York, New York; Clinical Assistant Professor, Department of Surgery, West Haven Veterans Administration Hospital, West Haven, Connecticut

Gerard V. Yu, D.P.M.

Associate Professor and Immediate Past Chairman, and Director of Second Year Residency Training in Podiatric Surgery, Department of Podiatric Surgery, Ohio College of Podiatric Medicine and The Cleveland Foot Clinic; Chairman, Division of Podiatry, Meridia Huron Hospital, Cleveland, Ohio

FOREWORD

The management of traumatic injuries has developed so rapidly in the last decade, making many fairly recent concepts completely obsolete. In particular, the management of injuries to the foot and ankle is finally being approached through the application of scientific principles.

Presently, no single text that adequately addresses the multitude of injuries of the foot and ankle and their appropriate management is available. However, in bringing together *Foot and Ankle Trauma*, editor Barry L. Scurran fills this great void in current therapy.

The book is divided into five sections and thirty-two chapters. The five sections, General Concepts, Soft Tissue and Related Trauma, Fractures and Dislocations, Ankle Trauma, and Complications, cover virtually every type of injury that is seen affecting the foot.

The combined strength of the book is due to the outstanding group of contributing authors, drawing from every facet of podiatric medicine and surgery, plastic surgery, and orthopedics. Additionally, the editor succeeds in providing excellent geographic representation, thus avoiding any regionalization of ideas.

Foot and Ankle Trauma is an outstanding text and should be in the library of every serious student and practitioner who treats lower extremity trauma.

E. Dalton McGlamry, D.P.M., D.Sc.(hon)
The Podiatry Institute
Northlake Regional Medical Center
Tucker, Georgia
Peachtree Podiatric Group, P.C.
Atlanta, Georgia

PREFACE

Foot and Ankle Trauma was created to fill a void. Until now the practitioner who dealt either regularly or infrequently with these localized injuries had no single source for current diagnostic or therapeutic techniques. Likewise, students lacked a reference on which to build an educational foundation with regard to general principles and specific foot and ankle injuries. For these reasons this textbook was conceived.

The organization of the book facilitates easy reference to specific injuries, as well as detailed information on five areas of foot and ankle trauma. The section on general principles focuses on current concepts in wound healing, general fracture management, and complex repair of skin loss. The sections on soft tissue injuries and fractures and dislocations offer a detailed approach to specific injuries, both as a reference source and as a specific guide for effective diagnosis and treatment of injuries—from the nail bed through the rearfoot, in adult and pediatric patients.

The ankle and its complexities are dealt with in a separate, equally detailed section, with emphasis placed on the complexities of differential diagnosis in these often oversimplified injuries.

Complications, a difficult topic in itself, are addressed specifically and separately to allow the student and practitioner alike to delve into these special problems in trauma management.

Authors have been chosen based on their specific expertise, as sound clinical judgment is born of experience. To avoid regional influences, the background and geographic locations of the authors are intentionally diverse. This broad-base experience and knowledge is shared here with you, the reader.

Study of foot and ankle traumatology is a dynamic, progressing field. A very few years ago much of the information offered in this text was not available. Since the principles and treatment offered herein will continue to evolve, it behooves the practitioner and student to be fully informed of the state of the art to be able to critically evaluate the worthiness or applicability of any future developments. *Foot and Ankle Trauma* was structured to be just such a work, no more, no less.

Barry L. Scurran, D.P.M.

ACKNOWLEDGMENTS

This work would not be possible without the foresight of those physicians who believe that skill and training rather than degree alone are more appropriate indicators in determining who shall provide emergency facility care. Such individuals include Physicians-in-Chief Bernard Rhodes, M.D., J. Harper Gaston, M.D., and Paul Jewett, M.D., along with Chiefs of Emergency Services Paul Swinderman, M.D., Caleb Foote, M.D., and David Gallagher, M.D.

A special thank you to my associates, staff, and The Permanente Medical Center—all of whom support our ongoing efforts and quality of care.

CONTENTS

Current Concepts in Wound Healing

Ross Rudolph, M.D.

Healing of traumatic wounds to the foot and ankle is similar to healing occurring elsewhere in the body, although there are certain differences due to regional circulation and increased exposure to injury. An understanding of the normal processes of wound healing is essential for any health care practitioner who treats wounds in the foot and ankle.

CLASSIC PHASES OF WOUND HEALING

The majority of clinical and experimental research in wound healing has been of the classic sutured wound without skin loss. This research has identified three basic phases of wound healing: (1) inflammatory or "lag," (2) fibroblastic, and (3) maturation (Fig. 1-1).[1]

Inflammatory Phase

In the first 2 to 3 days after being wounded, injured tissues undergo a number of simultaneous processes that prepare them for definitive healing.[1] Capillaries dilate and their walls become porous so that fluid exudes into the wounded tissue. Polymorphonuclear leukocytes (white blood cells) are released into the wound. Vasoactive substances such as kinins and prostaglandins are also released; these further contribute to vasodilatation and also cause pain. The typical red appearance of a fresh wound is due to this vasodilatation. Fibrin coagulates and seals the wound edges together like glue. The strength of the wound at this point is due to the fibrin glue, to any sutures that have been placed, and to the epithelium that grows rapidly across the surface if the edges are carefully opposed.

The word *inflammation* is often thought of as connoting undesirable characteristics. Yet, in the normal healing wound, a certain amount of inflammation is essential for the healing process to proceed normally. Studies have shown that both in poorly controlled diabetes[2] and in therapeutic administration of glucocorticoid steroids,[3] the inflammatory process is suppressed, contributing to poor wound healing. Control of diabetes and avoidance of steroids will thus contribute to improved wound healing by allowing a normal inflammatory phase.[4]

Fibroblastic Phase

In the 2 to 3 weeks following injury, the wound enters into a second phase in which rapid gain of strength occurs. Fibroblasts move into the fibrin clot and begin synthesizing large amounts of collagen. The wound itself may visibly become thickened and red because of the exuberant synthesis of new collagen.

Simultaneous collagen degradation occurs at the wound edges but is more than balanced by

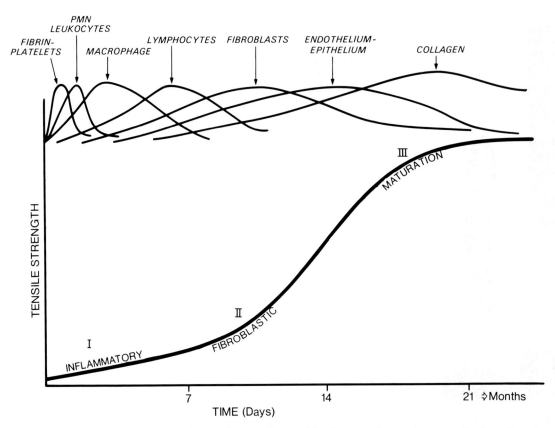

Fig. 1-1. Graph denotes the three classic phases of wound healing, with tensile strength plotted against elapsed time from wounding. (Adapted from Shilling J: Wound healing. Surgical Rounds July: 46, 1983, with permission.)

the increase in new collagen. During this phase, nutrients such as vitamin C and protein are particularly important for collagen synthesis, as is adequate oxygenation of the wound. Trace elements such as zinc are also important during this fibroblastic phase. Owing to the simultaneous degradation and synthesis of collagen, a patient severely lacking in nutrients may undergo wound separation (dehiscence) rather than healing. Optimal wound healing is most likely in a well-nourished patient.

Maturation Phase

The third phase of wound healing takes place over the next 6 to 12 months. Clinically, the nod-

ular, thick scars generated in the second phase of wound healing gradually soften and flatten. This process is due to a continued remolding of the scar tissue as simultaneous collagen synthesis and degradation occur, albeit at a slower rate than during the fibroblastic phase.

Plastic surgical revision of scars is often deferred during this period. The patient seen for facial lacerations at 3 weeks following an automobile accident is counseled to wait at least 6 months for surgical revision as during this time there is continued improvement of scar nodularity. The same process may occur in the foot: nodular, somewhat tender, itchy scars may gradually resolve and flatten over 6 to 12 months (Fig. 1-2), and therefore any surgical revision should be delayed if possible.

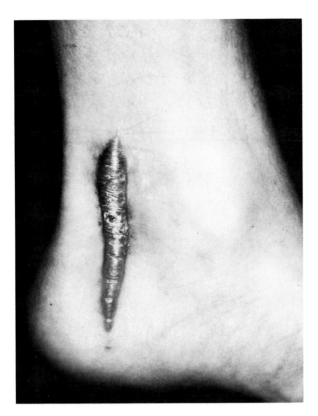

Fig. 1-2. Thick nodular scars, even hypertrophy scars or keloids, are not addressed surgically until after the maturation phase of wound healing is complete.

On occasion, the maturation process may be hastened by judicious intralesional injection of steroids such as Kenalog (triamcinolone acetonide), which causes further flattening of the wound and reduction of itching and pain.[5] However, injection of Kenalog into a maturing wound may produce atrophy once the maturation process has been completed.

HEALING MECHANISMS WITH SKIN LOSS

When a wound has undergone loss of skin so that an open defect occurs, two additional natural healing processes come into play: *wound contraction* and *epithelialization*.[1]

Wound Contraction

Wound contraction draws the edges of a wound toward the center by forces generated within the wound. In the past, this process has been called *granulating in*. This clinical term refers to the filling of the open wound with a reddish, pebbly, cobblestone type of tissue composed of new capillaries, new fibroblasts, and new collagen.[1] After 3 to 4 days, this granulation tissue begins to exert centripetal forces on the edges of the wound.

If adequate tissue mobility exists, wound contraction may be a very effective process and lead to satisfactory closure. In contrast, if the surrounding tissue is relatively rigid and immobile (as in much of the ankle and foot), wound contraction will not be as effective in closing the wound, and epithelialization will play more of a role. In areas such as the thigh or buttock, large wounds will successfully contract, whereas relatively small wounds in the medial malleolus area will not heal with contraction (Fig. 1-3).

As Peacock and Van Winkle have pointed out, the surgeon can determine whether a wound will heal by contraction by seeing whether the wound edges can be manually opposed.[6] If the edges cannot be brought together easily, it is unlikely that wound contraction will produce satisfactory closure.

The mechanism by which wound contraction occurs has been sought for many years. Active living cells are required to produce the active force of contraction, and these cells are most likely of fibroblast origin. In 1972, Gabbiani and associates, using electron microscopy, found cells in contracting wounds that appeared to share characteristics of both fibroblasts and smooth muscle cells.[7] These cells, in addition to having a fibroblastic rough endoplastic reticulum, contained filaments made up of 40 to 80 Å microfilaments in bundles with electron-dense bodies, very similar to filaments found in smooth muscle cells. Strips of granulation tissue containing these cells reacted in vitro as did smooth muscle, contracting with agonists and relaxing with antagonists. Finally, immunofluorescent staining of actin demonstrated that these cells contained considerable actin in the musclelike bundles.

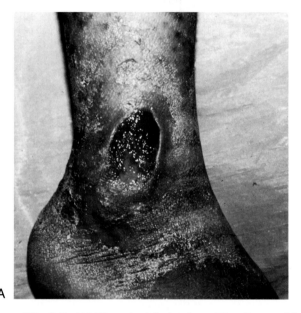

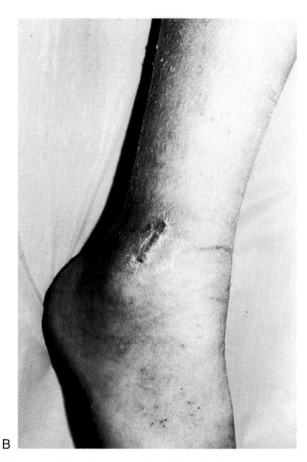

A   B

Fig. 1-3. **(A)** Wound with skin loss. This 7-year-old child avulsed the skin of the lateral malleolus in the spokes of a bicycle wheel. **(B)** The same wound 14 days later has healed by epithelialization. Wound contraction is less effective owing to the relative rigidity and immobility of the malleolar skin.

Myofibroblasts are most prominent in wounds during the active phase of granulation and contraction. If myofibroblast content is compared in wounds covered with split-thickness skin grafts or full-thickness skin grafts, the myofibroblast population disappears faster in those wounds covered with full-thickness grafts; this parallels the reduced contraction of wounds grafted with full-thickness skin.[8]

Myofibroblasts have been identified in the nodules of Dupuytren's contracture, in the contracted capsules around silicone breast implants and around painful pacemaker pockets, in the scar tissue of cirrhosis, and in the contracted scar tissue of breast cancer.[8] Nearly all tissues in the body that undergo scar contraction have been

shown to contain myofibroblasts. Myofibroblasts have been found throughout the substance of granulating wounds, suggesting that the pull is uniform throughout the granulation tissue. In extravasation injury caused by the antitumor drug Adriamycin (doxorubicin hydrochloride), wound contraction is diminished and myofibroblasts are scanty. The same is true in ulcers caused by radiation.[9]

Clinically, wound contraction can be slowed or even stopped by the presence of infection or by large amounts of necrotic eschar (Fig. 1-4). A thick leathery eschar that settles in a wound can prevent the edges from contracting; removal of such an eschar can aid the process of wound contraction.[9]

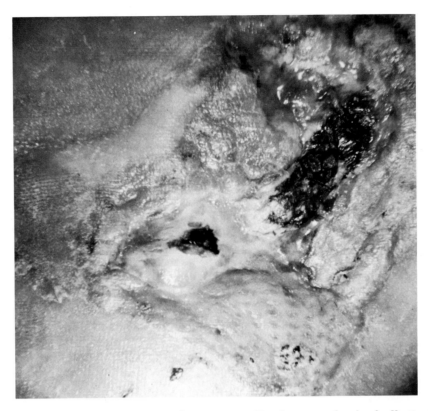

Fig. 1-4. Thick necrotic eschar slows wound contraction. For this wound to heal effectively, debridement is essential.

Epithelialization

The second process that leads to closure of an open wound is the spread of epithelium over the wound surface. Epithelium originates from normal epidermis at the periphery of the wound. In addition, epithelialization develops from epithelial structures within the wound if a partial-thickness loss has occurred. The epithelium grows over the wound surface until it meets other epithelium, at which time it ceases to grow. As it grows across the wound surface, epithelium has an invasive capability and will undermine necrotic or desiccated wound tissue. The epithelium seems to retain an invasive characteristic in some situations. Large wounds that many years before had healed with extensive epithelialization, particularly thermal burns, may develop a slow-growing squamous cell carcinoma known as Marjolin's ulcer. The possibility of carcinoma developing in a chronic wound should always be considered and biopsy done as appropriate if there is a clinical suspicion of carcinoma.[9]

The major disadvantage of wound healing by epithelialization is the unstable quality of the final wound. As the epithelium grows across the underlying tissues, it fails to develop the normal rete pegs that interlock epidermis and dermis. Therefore, a wound healed by epithelialization is often fragile.

Relatively minor trauma can strip the epithelium from the underlying tissue and produce a recurrent wound. In the patient with a venous stasis ulcer of the medial ankle, prolonged bed rest will often allow healing primarily by epithelialization (since wound contraction is ineffective). The shiny, thin, atrophic scar that results has fragile epithelium, and trauma frequently results in recurring ulceration. Even adhesive tape applied to a wound that is healed by epithelization may strip off the fresh epithelium and should be avoided.

USING NATURAL WOUND HEALING

The three phases of wound healing without skin loss and the processes of contraction and epithelialization in wounds with skin loss are nature's way of sealing wounds to protect the wounded organism from the environment. The thoughtful surgeon can often take advantage of these natural healing processes by controlling local and systemic factors.

The Sutured Clean Wound

As previously noted, control of diabetes mellitus and avoidance of glucocorticoids can improve the inflammatory phase of wound healing. Healing in the fibroblastic phase can be promoted by providing adequate protein, vitamins B and C, and zinc. Although there is no evidence that increased vitamin B, C, zinc, or protein will speed wound healing in a normal patient, patients on limited diets, particularly those who are elderly, may be deficient. If there is a clinical suspicion of protein, zinc, or vitamin malnutrition, supplementation with a high-protein, high-calorie diet and with vitamins B, C, and zinc is appropriate, particularly as it is inexpensive and without major side effects.[9]

Protecting the wound against infection, trauma, and external contamination is appropriate to avoid wound disruption. Antibiotics and cleansing of contaminated wounds are helpful, as are protective dressings. Prolonged sutures may be indicated in an area subject to considerable repeated trauma such as the sole of the foot (Fig. 1-5). Thus, foot sutures may be left in place for 2 to 3 weeks in an ambulatory patient, versus 1 week in other body areas such as the trunk.

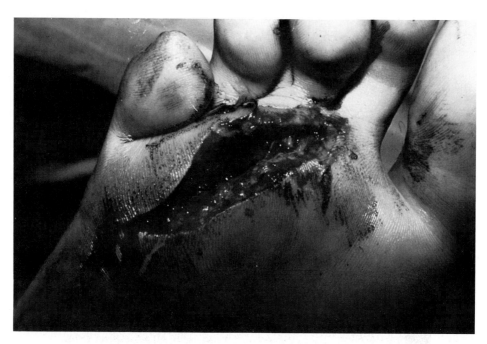

Fig. 1-5. Prolonged sutures are indicated in plantar lacerations that are subject to the repeated microtrauma of weight bearing. The principles of wound healing in the face of contamination, as in this lawnmower laceration, must be strictly adhered to.

Wound Contraction and Epithelialization

Both wound contraction and epithelialization are inhibited by infection and necrotic tissue. Selective surgical debridement will remove most necrotic tissues. Topical treatment with half-strength (0.25 percent) Dakin's hypochlorite solution will reduce the bacterial population and dissolve necrotic tissue further.

The process of epithelialization can be further speeded by the gentle use of local heat and by maintaining a moist hydrated environment. The latter can be achieved by the use of continuously wet dressings or by an occlusive dressing, so long as the underlying serous exudate does not become infected.[10]

Generally, the use of wet-to-dry dressings on open wounds is to be discouraged. In a wound filled with large amounts of necrotic tissue, surgical debridement followed by the use of half-strength Dakin's solution is more effective. If a wound is free of necrotic tissue, is filling with granulation tissue, and has new growth of epithelium around the edges, wet-to-dry dressings cause bleeding and pain and can tear off fresh epithelium. In a wound in which the natural healing processes of contraction and epithelialization are being used, a nonadherent dressing such as Xeroform gauze with an overlying gauze pad and a wrap or tape to hold it in place is much gentler to the wound and more effective in promoting healing.[9]

The surgeon can often use the processes of contraction and epithelialization to good advantage. Thus, in a fresh wound with mobile surrounding tissue, contraction will close the wound and produce a satisfactory result. Examples of this would be a full-thickness small burn on the thigh of an elderly person or a small tissue loss on the dorsal surface of a toe where contraction will pull the normal pulp into a better position. Similarly, superficial abrasions, burns (Fig. 1-6), or split-thickness donor sites (Fig. 1-7) will heal satisfactorily by epithelialization.

In contrast, large tissue losses of a major portion of the dorsum or the sole of the foot will not heal well by contraction, as the contraction will

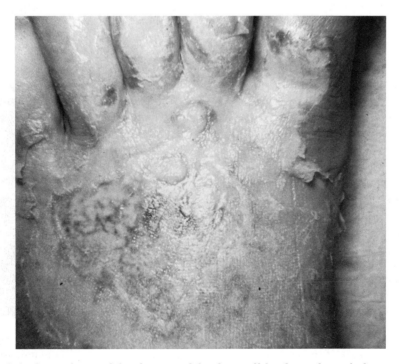

Fig. 1-6. Partial thickness burn of the dorsum of the foot will heal satisfactorily by epithelialization.

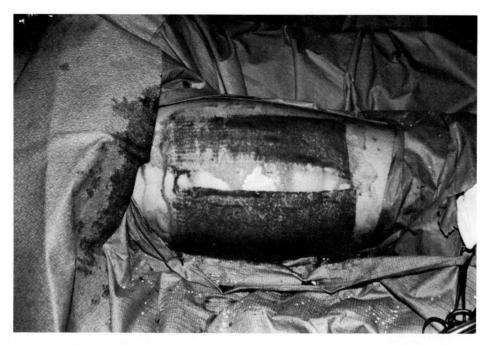

Fig. 1-7. This large donor site used for a split-thickness skin graft generally heals satisfactorily by epithelialization.

tend to pull the tissues into a distorted position. Epithelial growth over an area such as the medial ankle will produce an unstable wound since surrounding tissues are immobile and cannot contract. Where there is large tissue loss, where there is tissue loss across a joint, where contraction will cause deformity, or where epithelialization alone will produce an unstable wound cover, tissue replacement by skin grafts or flaps becomes appropriate (Fig. 1-8).

HEALING IN COMPROMISED TISSUES

The processes described so far assume that healing is taking place in a normal individual under satisfactory local conditions. There are, however, a large number of conditions that can inhibit wound healing. Many of these, if recognized, can be managed to improve the speed and final outcome of wound healing. The foot and ankle are particularly susceptible to many of these tissue-compromised conditions.

Arterial Insufficiency

A major deterrent to healing of wounds in the foot and ankle is arterial insufficiency, which can occur both in wounds without loss of skin that have been sutured, or in wounds with loss of skin and ulceration. Patients who are heavy smokers, who have Buerger's disease or diabetes mellitus, or who have arteriosclerotic cardiovascular disease are particularly prone to arterial occlusion. Commonly, the first sign of leg arterial insufficiency is a nonhealing wound in a foot after minor trauma. Misguided attempts at surgical closure can be disastrous if vascular insufficiency is not first identified.

Nonhealing ulcerations typically occur on the anterior lower leg but can occur elsewhere, especially on the toes (Fig. 1-9). Any patient with ulcers or nonhealing wounds of the foot and ankle should have the blood supply to the foot evaluated.[11] This can be done most simply by palpation of pulses at the groin, knee, dorsalis pedis, and posterior tibial artery areas. If the average trained practitioner does not feel pulses, they are most likely not there. Noninvasive vascular studies can be done at relatively little cost and discomfort to the patient. Arteriography can be done if appropriate.

In the face of major arterial insufficiency, any surgical procedure is contraindicated unless the insufficiency can first be corrected. Femoral by-pass, aortofemoral bypass, or even balloon dilation via angiography are all possible ways of increasing blood supply to the arterially insufficient leg. Correction of arterial insufficiency often leads to spontaneous healing of previously nonhealing wounds on the foot and ankle.

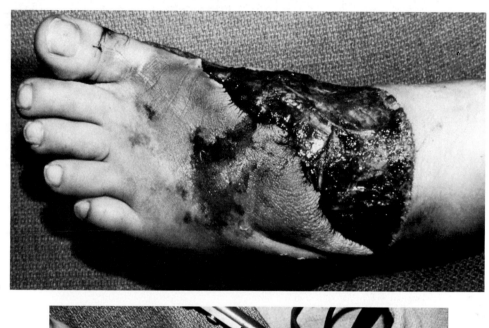

A

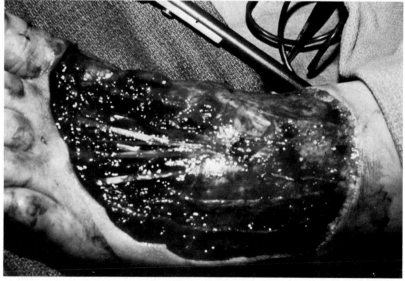

B

Fig. 1-8. (**A–D**) A large soft tissue loss sustained in a motorcycle accident. A wound of this extensive surface area will certainly not heal by contraction. Skin replacement with a meshed split-thickness skin graft was performed, and at 1 year after surgery (**D**) the wound is well healed with a satisfactory cosmetic as well as functional result. On clean, well-vascularized wounds, skin grafts can often be used without meshing, producing a smoother final surface. (*Figure continues.*)

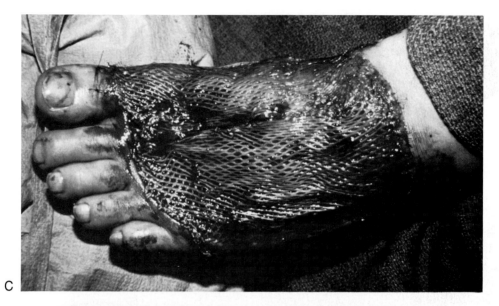

C

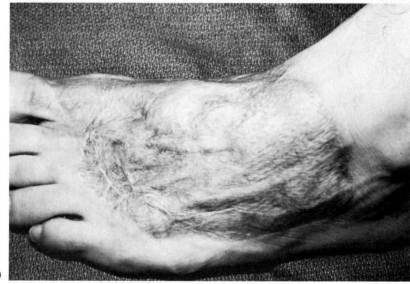

D

Fig. 1-8 *(Continued)*. **(C & D)**

Diabetes Mellitus

In patients with diabetes mellitus, the foot is particularly susceptible to poor healing. This has commonly been ascribed to an occlusion of the microvasculature, thought to be related to the increased thickness of basement membrane, as seen in diabetic kidney capillaries. The theory of microvascular occlusion being responsible for poor wound healing has led to a certain unjustified fatalism concerning healing of foot wounds. In fact, it is not at all clear that microvascular occlusion diminishes blood supply in the extremities. Even if present, basement membrane thickening may not depress circulation below a critical level.[2,12,13]

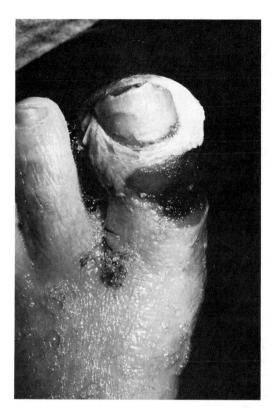

Fig. 1-9. This nonhealing digital ulcer clearly indicates inadequate blood supply. Evaluation is necessary to identify the cause of this vascular compromise.

Diabetic neuropathy often causes numbness in the foot. Therefore, the foot is subject to repeated trauma that can lead either to ulceration or to lack of healing of chronic ulcers.[9] Adequate padding, good foot care, and avoidance of trauma may help to protect the diabetic foot. Diabetic neuropathy is probably a more important factor in poor healing than is microvascular occlusion (Fig. 1-10).

An important factor in poor wound healing in diabetics is the frequent occurrence of arteriosclerotic occlusion of proximal vessels. No surgery should be contemplated on a foot wound in a diabetic patient without first testing for pulses. Should there be a question of vascular insufficiency, noninvasive arterial studies and arteriography, if indicated, should be done.[11] If vascular insufficiency is present and is surgically remedi-

able, wound healing is likely to be significantly improved.

Finally, as noted above, uncontrolled diabetes mellitus interferes with the inflammatory first phase of wound healing and, therefore, will reduce the ability of wounds to heal.[13] Uncontrolled diabetes also leads to reduced function of polymorphonuclear leukocytes in controlling infection in a wound. Thus, ideal control of diabetes will improve the success of wound healing after foot trauma.

In the event that necrotic tissue is present in a foot wound, debridement should be done and infections should be adequately drained to allow natural wound healing processes to take place. Assessment of vascular and sensory status will make foot wound healing in diabetics more successful.

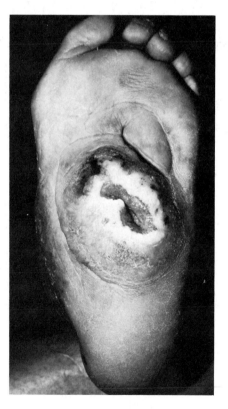

Fig. 1-10. Severe, chronic, nonhealing ulcer in a neuropathic diabetic woman. In general, neuropathy plays a far more significant role in depressing healing in diabetics than does microvascular occlusion.

Venous Stasis

Varicose veins, deep venous occlusion, and venous stasis are major inhibitors of wound healing in the foot and, particularly, the ankle. Venous stasis tissue disease typically develops as a result of incompetent valves in the venous system, creating a long column of deoxygenated blood when the individual is in the standing position. Alternatively, major trauma to the leg such as fractures can interfere with the deep venous system, causing deep venous thrombosis, and thus lead to permanent inhibition of venous return.

When venous compromise is untreated, a typical woody fibrosis develops at the medial ankle with blue-black skin discoloration.[9] Post-traumatic ulcerations in this area are resistant to topical treatment if the patient remains ambulatory. Prophylaxis with compression stockings is helpful but is rarely compulsively used by patients with venous hypertension. Treatment of the venous hypertension ulcer at the medial ankle consists of using compression stockings to reduce venous hypertension as much as possible. In addition, topical cleansing and use of an Unna boot are helpful. If major infection or large ulcerations occur, hospitalization with bed rest is indicated.

Unfortunately, the tissues around the medial ankle are relatively unyielding and become even more so in the face of chronic venous hypertension. Therefore, ulcers tend to heal by epithelialization rather than contraction. This results in a fragile wound cover that is frequently traumatized, leading to recurrent open wounds.

A patient with venous stasis ulcers should first be evaluated for correctable superficial varicosities. If this is the case, appropriate vein stripping or sclerotherapy techniques may bring about significant improvement so long as deep veins are functional. If the deep veins are occluded by deep venous thrombosis, removal of superficial varicosities may not be possible. In the patient who does not have the type of venous lesion amenable to vein stripping or sclerotherapy, treatment is more difficult. Experimental attempts at venous reconstruction have suggested some promise for the future but at present are not useful in the majority of situations.

It is most important for a patient who has venous stasis to wear compression stockings whenever possible and to use good local wound care to prevent infection and trauma.

Smoking

The smoker with a foot or ankle injury may have compromised healing that is largely preventable. Smoking interferes with the healing process in the foot and ankle by two basic processes. One is the generalized potentiation of arteriosclerosis that can occur in smoking patients, particularly those with Buerger's disease. Such patients manifest a rapid arteriosclerotic occlusion of the large vessels feeding the foot and ankle. Even minor trauma can lead to nonhealing wounds and, ultimately, amputation owing to arterial insufficiency. Although this process may not be reversible if smoking is stopped, nevertheless, the acceleration is reduced.

In the patient without accelerated arteriosclerotic vascular occlusive disease, smoking can still be deleterious to wound healing.[4] Nicotine in inhaled cigarette smoke achieves its vasoconstrictive effect primarily via the sympathetic nervous system, and this can lead to diminished blood supply in the extremities. The nicotine effect is relatively transient, lasting in most patients between 30 and 40 minutes. Perhaps of equal importance is the replacement of normal oxygen-carrying hemoglobin with carboxyhemoglobin, owing to the inhaled carbon monoxide in cigarette smoke. Cigarette smoke can contain as much as 1 percent (by volume) of carbon monoxide. In chronic smokers, 5 to 10 percent and perhaps even 20 percent of the hemoglobin may be carboxyhemoglobin.[14] Carboxyhemoglobin reduces oxygen availability and shifts the oxygen hemoglobin curve to the left, requiring a greater decrease in oxygen tension before oxygen can be released.

Clearly, the heavy smoker who sustains foot and ankle trauma would be advised to decrease or stop smoking. Inhalation of oxygen may be of benefit to such patients if they are hospitalized. Oxygen inhalation increases the dissociation of carbon monoxide from hemoglobin, reducing the half-life of carboxyhemoglobin from 250 minutes with air breathing to 40 minutes with inhaled oxygen. An additional advantage of oxygen administration is that it becomes more difficult for the patient to smoke in a hospital setting.[4]

For the ambulatory patient with foot and ankle trauma, advice to decrease smoking is universally given but often ignored. For the patient in whom elective foot and ankle surgery is planned, the question arises as to how long to advise stopping smoking. Ideally, of course, patients should stop permanently. However, the major beneficial effect on wound healing is likely to be achieved by stopping smoking as little as 48 hours before surgery. This certainly will avoid the nicotine effect and remove most of the carbon monoxide. Patients are more likely to cooperate and stop smoking for 1 to 2 days than for 2 to 3 weeks prior to surgery.[4]

Steroids (Glucocorticoids)

Patients receiving long-term glucocorticoid therapy for systemic diseases commonly have poor healing of sutured wounds and slowed epithelialization and contraction of open wounds.[3] Ideally, such steroid medication should be discontinued, but often this is not possible owing to underlying systemic diseases. Extensive studies have shown that steroids interfere with multiple aspects of the three phases of sutured wound healing, as well as with contraction and epithelialization. Particularly in the early phases of inflammation, steroids will interfere with the healing process. In contrast, if steroids are given after the healing process has begun, interference with wound healing is less of a problem.

Post-traumatic ulcerations in the foot, ankle, and lower leg in the patient receiving glucocorticoid therapy can be treated with topical vitamin A and D ointment.[15] Topical vitamin A is a direct antagonist of the local steroid effect. Although vitamin A often cannot be used systemically because of concerns about reversing steroid effect, topical vitamin A and D ointment (available as a nonprescription drug) applied twice a day can be

of benefit. Patients often notice increased redness within a few days of starting the local treatment, secondary to increased inflammation and vascularity.

Contributing to the poor wound healing in patients receiving glucocorticoids is their tendency to have thin, fragile skin. Steroids are commonly being given for diseases that involve vasculitis, which in itself may interfere with wound healing.

A common trauma problem in the patient receiving glucocorticoids is an acute laceration of the lower leg or ankle producing a triangular flap. Suturing with soft silk sutures can be done if there is no excess tension. Often, however, these flaps are exceptionally thin and, even if sutured carefully back into position, will undergo necrosis and slough. It may be better to resect the damaged skin and place an immediate split-thickness skin graft, or to defat the flap and use is as a graft, on such a leg injury in patients receiving high-dose glucocorticoids.

Vasculitis

Trauma in the patient with vasculitis of the lower extremity frequently results in a nonhealing wound. Vasculitis alone may result in tissues being unable to heal normally. The effect of vasculitis may be compounded by the problems of thinned skin and delayed wound healing resulting from the glucocorticoid steroids with which such patients are often treated. In addition, at least in the face, tissues that have been sympathectomized (as treatment for vasospastic disease) may be unusually sensitive to epinephrine-containing anesthetic solutions. Vecchione reported problems with tissue slough when the standard Xylocaine (lidocaine)-epinephrine mixture was used during facelifts in patients who had cervical sympathectomy for Raynaud's disease.[16] Possibly the same effect could occur in the lower extremity if sympathectomy has been done. Normally, epinephrine-containing solutions would not be used in the toes. Theoretically, the use of such solutions would also be best avoided in other parts of the foot and ankle when local anesthetic is being used to repair trauma in patients who have had prior sympathectomies.

Hematoma

A hematoma can occur as a result of trauma. Generally, large hematomas are not a problem in the foot and ankle because of the relatively unyielding tissues, which do not allow accumulation of a large volume. In contrast, the soft tissues of the lower leg and particularly the thigh may develop large amounts of hematoma after injury. In general, hematomas that are diffused through a thigh or lower leg are allowed to resolve spontaneously. Considerable swelling and bruising may persist for weeks and even months. On occasion, a hematoma of the lower extremity will result in a fibrous or fatty nodule that may require later surgical correction.

Of more concern is the development of a hematoma under a flap resulting from surgery or trauma or under a skin graft (Fig. 1-11).[4] The effects of hematomas under flaps and grafts appear to go beyond the mere mechanical blocking of blood vessel return. Extensive studies by Mulliken and Healey[17] and others[18] have suggested that there is a direct toxic effect of the hematoma pigments on the overlying devascularized skin. Often a thin, traumatically caused lower leg flap that is sutured back in position and later found to be necrotic is found, when explored, to have a hematoma underneath.

If hematomas are recognized underneath flaps, whether surgical or traumatic, or under skin grafts, they should be evacuated as soon as possible. Evacuation of a hematoma within 12 hours is likely to lead to survival of the overlying flap.[17]

Radiation

Radiotherapy for malignant disease can inhibit wound healing, either in sutured wounds resulting from surgery or in the more pernicious ulcerations developing after trauma to radiated tissue.[19] Major carcinomas in the foot and ankle often are treated by amputation rather than radia-

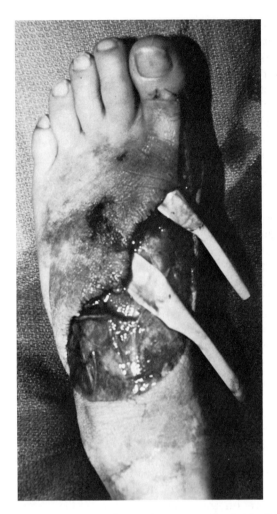

Fig. 1-11. Hematoma beneath a traumatized skin flap. Effects appear to go beyond local mechanical blocking of blood vessel return. Hematoma pigments may be directly toxic to overlying devascularized skin.

tion. However, with increasing use of radiotherapy for both primary treatment and palliation, more disease resulting from radiotherapy will probably be seen by physicians in the future.

The exact etiology of radiation inhibition of wound healing is not clear. Traditionally, this has been ascribed to interference with microcirculation. However, studies in our laboratories[20,21] and others[22] have suggested that permanent inhibition of fibroblasts and fibroblast stem cells is at least as important in radiated wound problems.

Extreme caution should be used in treating an area where there are visible sequelae of radiotherapy. Typical postradiotherapy changes following a usual dose of 5,000 to 6,000 rads include shiny atrophy of the skin, telangiectasia, woody fibrosis, and hyperpigmentation. A history of radiotherapy without obvious changes to the skin suggests a radiation dose of 1,000 to 1,600 rads.[4]

Owing to the hazards of poor healing, extreme caution must be used in performing any surgery in a heavily irradiated field. If a chronic ulcer develops in irradiated tissue after minor trauma, it typically appears as a painful, punched-out ulcer filled with shaggy necrotic tissue. Such ulcers show little or no spontaneous healing by contraction and epithelialization. Conservative debridement and cleansing are appropriate. Skin grafts and local flaps in a heavily irradiated field are almost always doomed to failure.[19] An extensive radiation ulcer often requires myocutaneous or fasciocutaneous flaps and may even require free flap transfer with microvascular techniques to close the wound.

Pressure Ulcers

Ulceration resulting from pressure is a common problem in the lower extremity, particularly on the posterior heel in bedridden patients. However, pressure ulcers caused by ill-fitting shoes or prosthetic appliances can occur anywhere on the insensitive foot (Fig. 1-12). The trauma causing pressure ulcers is not mysterious but rather is a direct consequence of an immobile foot or ankle lying on a hard surface sufficiently long enough for tissue necrosis to occur as a result of capillary occlusion.

All pressure ulcers are preventable if appropriate care is given to avoid pressure.[4] Therefore, the occurrence of pressure-ulcer trauma in a foot or ankle suggests observing the patient's total social milieu to determine what went wrong. If the patient is at home, some modification should be made after appropriate treatment or the ulceration will simply recur. Ulcerations of the heel resulting from prolonged hospitalization in intensive care units are an unfortunate consequence of modern therapy in which skin care of the heel is forgotten in the heat of attending to the patient's more vital systems.

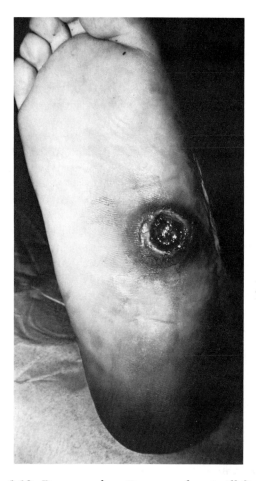

Fig. 1-12. Pressure ulceration secondary to ill-fitting ankle-foot orthosis in a 20-year-old neuropathic patient. This wound is preventable if proper caution and prophylactic care are undertaken.

Management involves standard techniques of wound care. If the eschar, as on the posterior heel, is dry, clean, and relatively small, it can be allowed to separate spontaneously. If the ulceration is large or infected, the wound should be debrided and half-strength Dakin's solution applied. Once the wound is clean and filled with healthy granulation tissue, the ulceration can be closed by split-thickness skin grafting. Local fasciocutaneous flaps may be used on the sole of the foot for small pressure ulcerations as long as care is taken in the postoperative and particularly the home situation to ensure that recurrent pressure does not occur.

Sickle Cell Disease

Sickel cell ulcers are frequently seen in black patients with homozygous sickle cell disease and appear on the anterior and medial lower leg. The presence of hemoglobin S produces red blood cells that lack normal elasticity and, therefore, can reduce capillary blood flow. Even minor trauma can lead to wounds that do not heal and typically develop into larger, quite painful ulcerations.

Therapy of small ulcerations relies on debridement and spontaneous closure. In larger ulceration, skin grafting can be done. The success of such grafting is markedly increased if normal hemoglobin is transfused to allow more normal oxygenation. Regrettably, the healed wounds are subject to recurring breakdown, as high as 94 percent. If feasible, permanent muscle or myocutaneous flaps may provide better wound healing. These flaps carry larger vessels with them and are less dependent for survival on the compromised microcirculation of the ulcer bed.[4]

Factitious Wounds

An unusual but exceedingly troublesome type of trauma that can occur anywhere in the body is factitious, or self-induced, trauma. Self-induced trauma should be suspected in any chronic traumatic wound that does not heal with reasonable wound care.[4] Well-executed flaps and skin grafts that repeatedly break down should raise the suspicion of factitious wounding. Often in a hospital setting, patients who inflict or aggravate their own wounds are seeking a secondary gain of increased attention. For such patients, increased attention outweighs the disadvantages and discomfort of having a wound. Such patients are difficult to deal with as they typically deny self-wounding and are usually not amenable to suggestions of psychiatric referral. Techniques such as painting the wound with tetracycline that is later sought with fluorescence on the patient's hands have been suggested but have been met with mixed success. Direct confrontation of the patient often produces little but mutual anger, and the patient may move on to another physi-cian. Perhaps the most important thing for the practitioner to know about factitious wounding is that it can occur and is a possibility in any otherwise mysterious wound.

CONCLUSIONS

Injuries and surgical incisions on the foot and ankle heal in the same manner as wounds in other areas of the body. They undergo the inflammatory or lag phase, followed by the fibroblastic or collagen synthesis phase, and ending with the maturation phase during which the scar remodels and softens. Wounds with lost skin also undergo the processes of wound contraction and epithelialization.

Natural wound healing can be used under favorable conditions. Healing of sutured traumatic lacerations or surgical incisions is improved by keeping the wound clean and avoiding trauma. Natural healing by epithelialization and wound contraction is speeded by gentle debridement of necrotic tissue and reduction of infection. Local heat and a moist environment speed epithelialization.

Healing by wound contraction is satisfactory when there are small tissue losses and sufficient surrounding tissue mobility to allow the wound to close. Wounds with large tissue losses or smaller losses in a relatively immobile area such as the medial ankle are less able to heal successfully by wound contraction. Epithelialization is a satisfactory process in partial thickness injuries such as second degree burns, abrasions, and split-thickness donor sites. Large wounds or smaller wounds over bony prominences that heal by epithelialization tend to be unstable.

Open wounds should initially be treated by gentle debridement and then with half-strength Dakin's solution. Wet-to-dry dressings should be avoided. Once the wound is clean, filling with granulation tissue, and healing by contraction and epithelialization, applying a nonadherent dressing is appropriate.

A number of conditions affect the success of healing. Anywhere in the body, and particularly in the foot and ankle, these include arterial insufficiency, diabetes mellitus, venous stasis, smoking, systemic steroids, vasculitis, hematoma, radiotherapy, pressure ulcers, sickle cell disease, and factitious wounding. Understanding these specific problems in compromised tissue often allows more rational management of traumatic wounds in the foot and ankle.

REFERENCES

1. Rudolph R, Fisher JC, Ninnemann JL: Skin Grafting. p. 1. Little, Brown, Boston, 1979
2. Goodson WH, III, Hunt TK: Wound healing in well-controlled diabetic men. Surg Forum 35:614, 1984
3. Green JP: Steroid therapy and wound healing in surgical patients. Br J Surg 52:523, 1965
4. Rudolph R, Hunt TK: Healing in compromised tissues. p. 65. In Rudolph R (ed): Problems in Aesthetic Surgery; Biological Causes and Clinical Solutions. Williams & Wilkins, Baltimore, 1987
5. Rudolph R: Wide spread scars, hypertrophic scars, and keloids. Clin Plast Surg 14:253, 1987
6. Peacock EE, Jr., Van Winkle W: Wound Repair. 3rd Ed. WB Saunders, Philadelphia, 1984
7. Gabbiani G, Hirschel BJ, Ryan GB, Statkov PR, Majno G: Granulation tissue as a contractile organ. A study of structure and function. J Exp Med 135:719, 1972
8. Rudolph R: Contraction and the control of contraction. World J Surg 4:279, 1980
9. Rudolph R, Noe JM: Chronic Problem Wounds. Little, Brown, Boston, 1983
10. McGrath M: Healing of the open wound. p. 13. In Rudolph R (ed): Problems in Aesthetic Surgery; Biological Causes and Clinical Solutions. Williams & Wilkins, Baltimore, 1987
11. Rudolph R: Nonhealing leg and foot wounds resulting from correctable arterial occlusion. Plast Reconstr Surg 71:209, 1983
12. Goodson WH, III, Hunt TK: Studies of wound healing in experimental diabetes mellitus. J Surg Res 22:221, 1977
13. Goodson WH, III, Hunt TK: Wound healing and the diabetic patient. Surg Gynecol Obstet 149:600, 1979
14. Astrup P, Kjeldsen K: Carbon monoxide, smoking and atherosclerosis. Med Clin North Am 58:323, 1973
15. Hunt TK, Ehrlich HP, Garcia JA, Dunphy JE: Effect of vitamin A on reversing the inhibitory effect of cortisone on healing of open wounds in animals and man. Ann Surg 170:633, 1969
16. Vecchione TR: Rhytidectomy flap necrosis in Raynaud's disease. Plast Reconstr Surg 72:713, 1983
17. Mulliken JB, Healey NA: Pathogenesis of skin flap necrosis from an underlying hematoma. Plast Reconstr Surg 63:540, 1979
18. Angel MF, Narayanan K, Swartz WM et al: The etiologic role of free radicals in hematoma-induced flap necrosis. Plast Reconstr Surg 77:795, 1986
19. Rudolph R: Complications of surgery for radiotherapy skin damage. Plast Reconstr Surg 70:179, 1982
20. Rudolph R, Arganese T, Woodward M: The ultrastructure and etiology of chronic radiotherapy damage in human skin. Ann Plast Surg 9:282, 1982
21. Rudolph R: Chronic skin ulceration after radiotherapy for cancer. West J Med 126:525, 1982
22. Withers HR, Peters LJ, Kogelnik HD: The pathobiology of late effects of irradiation. p. 439. In Meyn RE, Withers HR (eds): Radiation Biology in Cancer Research. Raven Press, New York, 1980

2

Management of Closed Fractures

Christina C. Rude, D.P.M.

A break in the continuity of the bone that does not communicate with the outside of the body is called a closed fracture. In other words, there is no wound associated with the fracture site caused by an external penetrating object or by the fractured bone ends themselves.

The treatment of patients with closed fractures includes a thorough assessment of the fracture, evaluation of the general condition of the patient, and open or closed reduction as indicated. Following initial treatment, the patient is observed for possible complications. Should problems arise, appropriate action is taken after careful assessment.

EVALUATION OF THE PATIENT

History

The general condition of the patient is stabilized before attention is directed to extremity fractures. On first encounter with the patient, it is important to make a quick assessment of certain aspects of the injury. A rapid inspection should be made to ensure that the position of the fractured or dislocated bones is not causing gross circulatory embarrassment. For example, talar or subtalar joint dislocation can endanger the rest of the foot by impingement on the posterior tibial artery. If possible, this dislocation should be immediately reduced by gentle manual traction. A posterior splint can then be placed to maintain the reduction until definitive treatment is carried out.

If the patient already has had a splinting device placed on the injured part, it is checked at this time. A good splint is well padded and comfortable and provides some stability to the injured area. Any constricting splint, padding, dressing, or clothing is released.

An orderly history and physical examination can now be completed. The time of the injury is important. Swelling of the extremity increases for 6 to 12 hours after the injury.[1] Therefore, the reduction is best accomplished as soon as possible because the swelling greatly decreases the elasticity of the tissues. A description of the nature of the injury helps to determine the direction and strength of the deformity forces. It is often helpful to seek information from an eyewitness, especially if the patient has trouble recalling the details. Different types of problems can be anticipated depending on the cause of the injury. For example, high-velocity impact will more likely result in multiple bone fragments and significant soft tissue injury.

The age of the patient is another determining factor since fractures in children are different in their occurrence and healing from those of adults. The general health of the patient should be assessed. Conditions such as diabetes, rheumatoid arthritis, renal disease, cancer, osteoporosis, and so forth will influence the nature of the fracture and the treatment. Patients with neurologic disease, a history of alcohol abuse, or any type of peripheral neuropathy may sustain complete fracture-disclocation without any recollection of a traumatic event.

Pertinent information regarding allergies, medications, prior hospitalization and surgery, previous fractures, and existing medical conditions should be obtained. If anesthesia will be required for closed or open reduction, a review of the pulmonary, cardiac, hepatic, and renal systems is important as well as a determination of the time of last food intake. The patient's occupation and recreational pursuits are also important factors in the choice of an appropriate treatment plan.

Physical Examination

Examination of the injured area is the first part of the physical assessment. Clinical signs of fracture include local swelling, ecchymosis, deformity, localized bone tenderness, impaired function, abnormal mobility, and crepitus. Some signs may not be present, such as abnormal mobility or dysfunction in a greenstick, fatigue, or impacted fracture. Crepitus, the grating of unstable bone ends on each other, should not be deliberately elicited by the examiner, as it is painful to the patient and may cause additional injury. Localized bone tenderness is probably the most reliable clinical sign of fracture in neurologically intact patients. It may be the only sign of bony injury in certain fractures that are difficult to detect radiographically (e.g., a nondisplaced fracture of the cuneiforms, navicular, or physis or a fatigue fracture). If the injured part is comfortably splinted prior to the examination, it may be possible to confirm the diagnosis without moving the part. However, thorough inspection must be made for the presence of communicating wounds, abrasions, lacerations, burns, or other injuries to surrounding soft tissues.

Assessing soft tissue damage is as important as recognizing the presence of a fracture. Acute compartment syndrome can rapidly develop in a patient with a severe crush injury. The signs of this complication are tense skin over an area that is diffusely tender in its entirety, paresthesias, pallor, and pain with passive motion of the digits. Ischemia results when interstitial pressure rises above the intracapillary pressure, which is somewhat lower than diastolic pressure.[2] Dangerous tissue ischemia can develop, therefore, even in the presence of palpable pedal pulses. Once the problem is recognized, it is treated as soon as possible by fasciotomy of the involved compartment. Permanent damage occurs in tissues that are ischemic for more than 4 to 6 hours.[3] Careful examination for compartment syndrome of the leg should also be included. This has reportedly occurred after pedal fractures.[4]

Besides noting the presence and character of the posterior tibial and dorsalis pedis pulses, the temperature, color, and capillary refill of the toes are also recorded. Normal color is pink, rather than blue or pale. Always compare findings with the other foot. Damage to vessels can occur from the following mechanisms: (1) muscle spasm contusion from bone fragments or external blow, or from the traction of abnormal position; (2) thrombosis or embolus; (3) rupture or perforation of the vessel wall; or (4) pressure occlusion caused by impingement of bone fragments. Vascular injury is frequently encountered in severe midfoot fractures.[5-7] Leakage from vessels can occur several hours later when vasospasm ceases or when increased pressure bursts the thrombus. It is therefore important to make repeated observations of both vascular and neurologic status during initial care of the patient.

Evaluation of damage to nerves is made by noting sensation to pinprick over the dorsum, plantar aspect, and first interspace. Pain or instability from the fracture rather than nerve damage may affect the motor examination. A complete severance of the nerve is unusual in a closed fracture, in which nerve damage is usually caused by contusion from a bone fragment. Loss of sensation to all toes in stocking-type distribution indicates ischemia rather than nerve injury. Careful documentation of neurovascular status before and after reduction should be made.[8]

Once the examination of the injured area is completed, the rest of the patient is thoroughly evaluated. In the trauma patient it is especially important to assess other areas of possible injury that may be overlooked by the patient who has focused on one injured part. No narcotics can be administered until the absence of a head injury is confirmed. Suspect the presence of other fractures, keeping the mechanism of injury in mind. For example, the contralateral heel, spine, and wrists are carefully examined in any patient with a calcaneal fracture.[9]

Radiographic Examination

The injured part is properly splinted before the patient is sent to the radiology department. Splinting provides a more comfortable position for the patient and helps prevent further tissue damage. Gross deformities of angulation or rotation can usually be aligned with gentle traction and maintained in a splint.

Always obtain radiographs if there is any suspicion of bony injury. It is often not possible to differentiate a contusion from a fracture by clinical examination. Certain medical conditions such as diabetes, alcoholism, or any peripheral neuropathy will obscure the diagnosis. Trivial trauma can result in fracture in patients with debilitating or bone-weakening conditions such as rheumatoid arthritis or osteoporosis.

Useful Views

Always order at least two views that are perpendicular to each other. Include the joints above and below the fracture. When no fracture can be found on routine views, do not rule out the possibility of bone injury. The radiograph may need to be repeated until satisfactory resolution of the area is obtained. Special additional views may be necessary to visualize the fracture. Views for calcaneal fracture include dorsoplantar, lateral, calcaneal axial, medial oblique for the anterior process, and an anteroposterior view of the ankle to demonstrate possible lateral ballooning of the calcaneus impinging on the fibula, in addition to possible concomitant ankle injury.[10] Foot films as well as ankle films should be ordered for the patient with a history of ankle sprain. Look for fracture of the midfoot, calcaneus, and fifth metatarsal.[11,12] The plantar axial view is ordered for visualization of the sesamoids. Bilateral views are often helpful in differentiating a fracture from incidental findings, especially for sesamoids, accessory bones, and open epiphyses. Midfoot and

rear-foot fractures can often be appreciated clearly with a tomogram or CT scan. Finally, a technetium scan will indicate the presence of a fatigue fracture weeks before the standard radiograph is positive.

Radiographic Analysis

Once satisfactory films are obtained, they are thoroughly inspected in an orderly fashion. The film is examined for abnormalities in bones, joints, or soft tissues. The entire radiograph is assessed so as not to overlook additional fractures or dislocations. Is there a fracture present? Look for a break in cortical continuity, jagged radiolucent fracture lines, abnormal overlap of cortices, and radiopaque overlap of impacted cancellous bone.[13] There may be spicules or fragments of bone with an irregularity at abutting bone surfaces. It is often helpful to have bilateral films to compare obscured bony outlines of midfoot or rear-foot fracture-dislocations.

An older fracture has smooth, rounded edges and possibly sclerotic bone ends.[14] If the fracture is older, is there evidence of healing, such as trabeculae or callus crossing fracture gaps?

Note the position of the bone fragments. Are they displaced? By how much? Are they angulated or rotated, and in which direction? What is the condition of the bone? Is the fracture associated with osteopenia, tumor, cyst, or congenital disease of bone? Are there multiple lesions? Multiple fractures?

Carefully examine the joints and joint surfaces for dislocation, subluxation, or transchondral fracture. Note the joint space. An increase could indicate intra-articular hemorrhage.

When the information provided by the initial radiographs is unclear, additional views are ordered or further consultation is sought.

CLASSIFICATION OF FRACTURES

A classification system helps the examiner understand the mechanism of injury. This standardizes the approach to the fracture and helps in

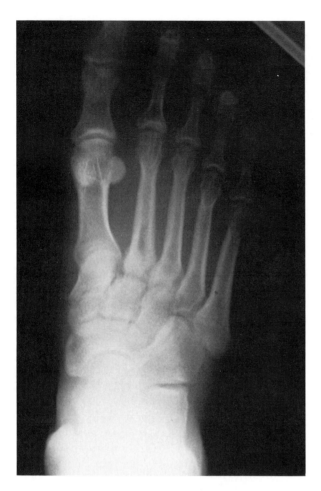

Fig. 2-1. Tapping fracture caused by direct blow to the medial cuneiform.

determining the treatment plan. Rockwood and Green devised a classification system that can be used in fractures of the foot.[1]

Direct Trauma

A blow of varying velocity causes varying degrees of tissue damage. *Tapping fractures* result from a blow of low velocity and cause slight tissue damage. There is no comminution (Fig. 2-1). *Crush fractures* are caused by a high-velocity blow and result in extensive soft tissue damage as well as a comminuted fracture (Fig. 2-2).

Indirect Trauma

Closed fractures caused by indirect trauma result from a force acting at a distance from the fracture site. *Traction forces* cause a transverse fracture line at the site of attachment of ligaments or tendons. These fractures are also called avulsion or pull-off fractures (Fig. 2-3). *Angulation forces* result in a transverse fracture that is not associated with attachment of tendon or liga-

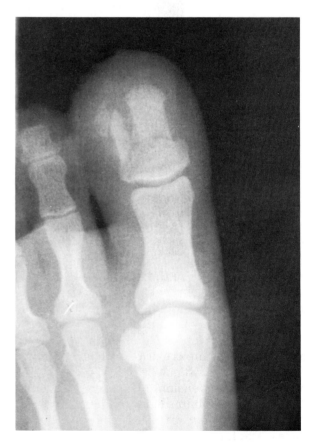

Fig. 2-2. Comminuted fracture of distal phalanx of hallux caused by a horse hoof.

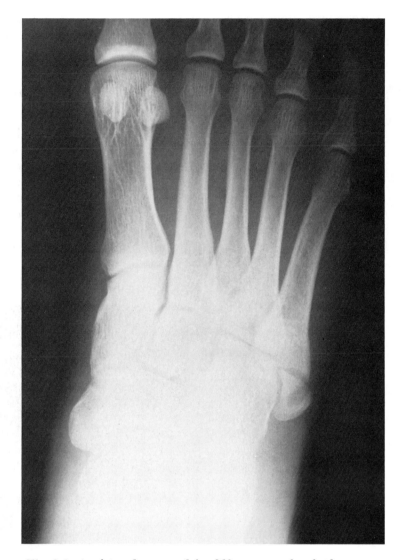

Fig. 2-3. Avulsion fracture of the fifth metatarsal styloid process.

ments. This fracture is caused by a bending force in one plane against a long bone. The bone fails on the convex, or tension side, creating a fracture. The bone may splinter on the concave side (Fig. 2-4). *Spiral fractures* result from rotational forces. The fracture is seen as an oblique line 45 degrees to the long axis of the bone (Fig. 2-5). *Compression forces* cause an impaction fracture of the shaft of a long bone into softer cancellous bone (Fig. 2-6). *Angulations and axial compression forces* cause a transverse fracture line with a butterfly fragment (Fig. 2-7). *Angulation and rotation forces* will result in oblique fracture lines. This is often observed in ankle fractures where supination-external rotation causes oblique fracture at the distal fibula (Fig. 2-8).

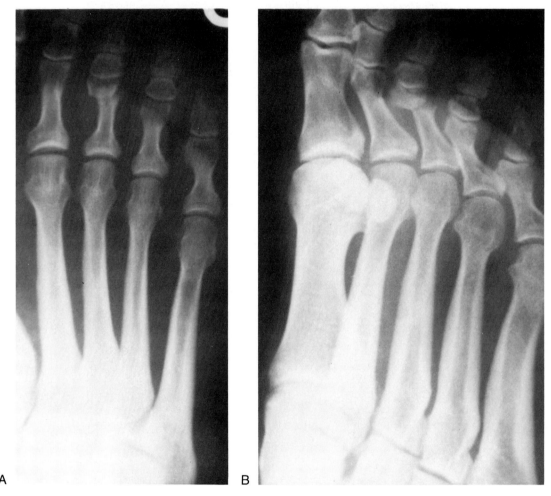

A

B

Fig. 2-4. Transverse fracture at the neck of proximal phalanx in third toe. (**A**) Anteroposterior view. (**B**) Oblique view.

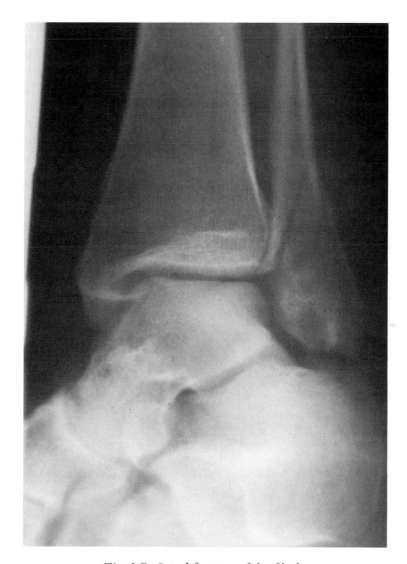

Fig. 2-5. Spiral fracture of the fibula.

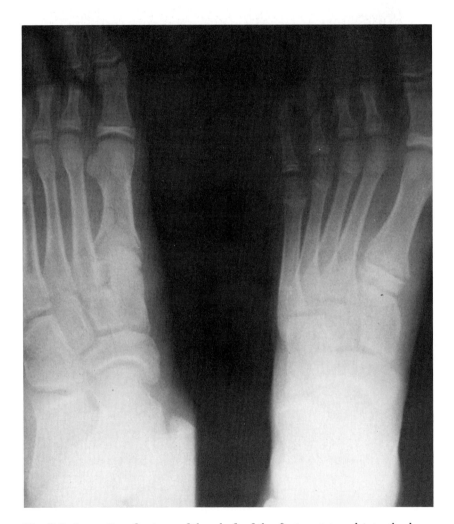

Fig. 2-6. Impaction fracture of the shaft of the first metatarsal into the base.

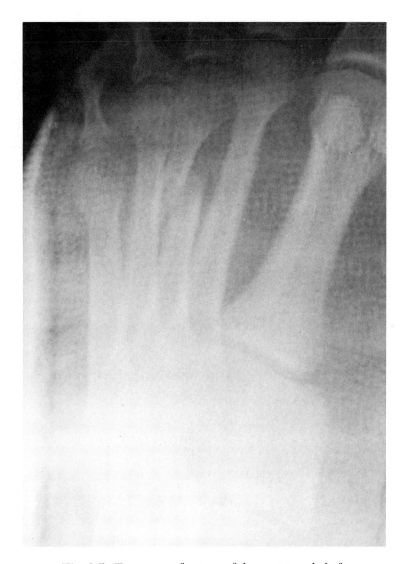

Fig. 2-7. Transverse fracture of the metatarsal shaft.

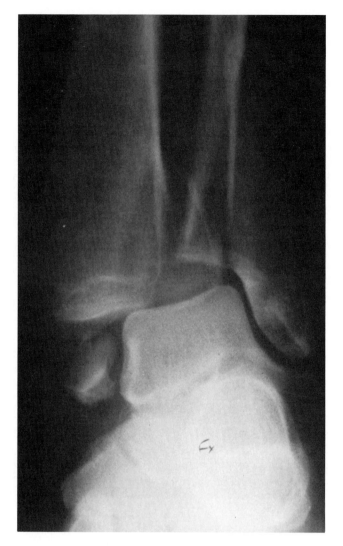

Fig. 2-8. Long spiral fracture of fibula in severe ankle fracture-dislocation.

TREATMENT

After examination of the patient and assessment of the radiographs, the fracture can be described clearly in terms of location, type, direction of angulation or rotation, displacement, joint involvement, and presence of pathology. Decisions regarding the treatment of the fracture can be made according to established guidelines when the fracture is described and understood in these terms. The objectives of fracture treatment are well established: to achieve healing of the fragments in anatomic alignment and to restore normal function in the shortest period of time.

Does the fracture need to be reduced? In the following circumstances closed reduction is not indicated: (1) there is no displacement (e.g., certain cuneiform or cuboid fractures); (2) no reduction is possible, such as in severe comminution; (3) the reduction cannot be held by external immobilization; (4) a strong traction force has produced and maintains the displacement; (5) the fracture is open.[15]

When should the fracture be treated by open reduction? Surgical treatment of the fracture is appropriate in four situations. First, if the fracture cannot be reduced by closed manipulation, or if closed reduction efforts have failed, open reduction is indicated. Second, the fracture should be opened and reduced if it involves a displaced articular surface where anatomic reduction is critical for function and reasonable results are possible with open methods. Third, if the fracture is significantly displaced and resulted from avulsion forces, open reduction is indicated.[16] Fourth, if ischemia of the foot does not resolve after closed manipulation, the fracture should be opened.[5] Also, injuries in which there are multiple adjacent fractures may require open reduction to provide adequate stability.

The patient's age, health, occupation, desires, and recreational pursuits and the surgeon's skill are also important components in the overall development of the treatment plan.

If the fracture does not need open or closed reduction, does it need to be immobilized? Fractures are immobilized (1) to prevent pain, (2) to prevent motion of fragments that interferes with healing, and (3) to prevent displacement or angulation of unstable bone fragments.[17] Certain stable fractures may be treated without immobilization. These include impacted fractures in which displacement does not occur with joint motion, undisplaced fractures of tarsal bones, small chip fractures, and some severely comminuted fractures of the calcaneus.[18,19] The position of the fragments may not be perfectly anatomic, but acceptable. Treatment is directed toward recovering function by early mobilization, which is the central feature of this approach. The fractured bones may not need immobilization, but protection from weight bearing may be indicated, depending on the nature of the fracture.

In any fracture in which severe swelling is a factor, treatment should initially be directed toward controlling the edema. The patient is put to bed rest with the extremity elevated above the heart. A well-padded dressing is made with several layers of cotton wadding secured with elastic wrap or light plaster. Once the swelling has subsided, which may take several days, attention is directed toward open or closed reduction, as the situation dictates.

Closed Reduction

The case that starts botched up, stays botched up.[1]

The success of closed manipulation depends on adequate preparation of the surgeon and patient. Attention given to timing, anesthesia, mechanism of injury, and method of reduction will provide the framework for an optimal result.

Timing
Swelling is maximal 6 to 12 hours after the injury has occurred. The manipulations required to reduce a fracture before swelling has peaked are much less forceful than those required once the soft tissues are distended by edema. If possible, the fracture is best reduced soon after the injury. When the fracture cannot be reduced within this time frame, it is often better to wait a few days for edema to subside. The limb is treated with elevation and compression as above.

Anesthesia
No reduction should be attempted without some form of anesthesia. The forces of pain, muscle spasm, and inelastic soft tissues may be impossible to overcome without the relaxation provided by adequate anesthesia.

Forceful manipulations before the patient is comfortably relaxed are usually not effective and can cause further tissue damage with increased swelling. This situation can result in a failed closed manipulation that would have been successful had the preparation been more careful. The surgeon and anesthesiologist can always find some form of anesthesia appropriate for the patient, depending on location of the fracture, extent of the injury, and medical condition of the patient.

Mechanism of Injury
A thorough understanding of the forces that caused the fracture, maintain the displacement, and could possibly prevent reduction is essential before the reduction is attempted. The nature of

the injury and the radiographic position of the fragments are carefully considered when planning the reduction. Other factors that may frustrate the reduction effort are the presence of loose bone fragments within the fracture site, the strength and direction of muscle pull on tendons attached to each bone fragment, and the interposition of soft tissue.

Reduction Technique

Simply stated, closed reduction consists of traction, manual repositioning of bone fragments, and maintenance of that position in a circular plaster cast. A step-by-step approach is described below. Details of treatment for specific fractures are included in subsequent chapters.

1. The patient is placed in a comfortable position appropriate for reduction. This position is usually supine with the knee flexed 60 to 90 degrees. The knee can be flexed by suspending the thigh in a sling or by hanging the leg over the edge of the table. The patient is anesthetized. The radiographs have been studied and are in easy view of the surgeon and assistant. The manipulative technique has been reviewed.
2. While countertraction is provided by the assistant, the surgeon applies slow, steady traction along the long axis of the bone. Guarded measured strength is more effective than sudden jerky motions. The forces of muscle tone, edema, and interlocked bone fragments may take several minutes to overcome.
3. Once length is obtained, rotatory deformity is corrected just prior to apposition. Correct angulation after apposition. If no bony crepitus is appreciated, soft tissue is probably interposed between the bone fragments. Perfect apposition is not necessary. However, rotation and angulation are not acceptable. If the bone heals in an angulated or rotated position, the normal plane of motion in the joints proximal and distal to the fracture site is disrupted. This may lead to osteoarthritis.
4. A padded circular plaster cast is applied by the assistant while the position is maintained by the surgeon. The plaster is well molded in the arch and at the fracture site, providing three-point pressure to maintain the reduction. Molding pressure is done with the palms and thenar eminence rather than finger tips. Finger dents in the plaster may cause painful pressure points, possibly leading to pressure necrosis. The cast should immobilize the joints proximal and distal to the fracture site. Because of their poor molding characteristics, synthetic casting materials are best left to later stages of fracture care.
5. Postreduction radiographs are always obtained. If the reduction is not satisfactory, another attempt is made. When it is apparent that further attempts will not be fruitful, preparation is made for open reduction.

Certain fractures can be reduced by closed methods and then maintained with percutaneous wires. This is done in the operating room under sterile technique and with the aid of fluoroscopy. The foot is then placed in a plaster cast as above.

Aftercare

Any injured patient who has had a plaster cast placed within the first 8 hours after the injury must be closely monitored. If the patient is allowed to go home, written and oral instructions are reviewed. The patient is told to elevate the extremity above the heart and move the toes, both of which help control the edema. The patient must be informed that pale, blue toes, diffuse pain unrelieved by pain medication, or onset of numbness in the toes are signs that the cast may be too tight. Immediate return to the treatment center is in order. If it has been determined that the cast is tight, it is split along its length and all padding is cut to the skin. The cast is spread wide enough to relieve the constriction, which will be indicated by the return of color and sensation to the toes and relief of the patient's discomfort. The cast can be held in place by an elastic bandage. When the swelling decreases, the cast is rebandaged more securely, or a new cast is applied.

Patients who are allowed to go home should be

checked the following day for comfort and efficiency of the cast. If there is any doubt about the circulatory status, the patient stays overnight in the hospital. A constant, localized, burning pain is usually the sign of a pressure point. These complaints should not be ignored. As pressure ischemia develops into an ulceration, it loses sensation and then is not detected until tissue damage has occurred. Special care must be taken when caring for patients with peripheral neuropathy. For these patients, the cast has extra padding over bony prominences, and is usually changed more frequently.

The patient usually returns to the treatment center in 1 to 3 weeks, depending on the nature of the fracture and initial swelling. At this time, since the swelling will have subsided, the cast no longer fits well, is less comfortable and effective, and is therefore replaced. A radiograph is obtained to ensure proper alignment of the fragments. The first week is the most common time for complications arising from soft tissue and loss of position to occur.

Restoring Function

The rehabilitation program begins as soon as reduction is secured. If plaster immobilization is not employed in the treatment, mobilization of joints and active muscle exercise can begin almost immediately. When a cast is utilized, the principle of treatment is to use the part as much as possible without jeopardizing the healing process. Active exercise of muscles in and out of plaster is encouraged. This means flexing and extending the toes and flexing and extending the knee. A walking cast is used as soon as it is safe for the stability of the fracture. If there is any doubt regarding fracture stability, weight bearing is postponed since the cast does not completely immobilize the foot when walking.[20] Early functional activity facilitates bone repair by maintaining normal circulation. Muscle action assists in edema control and helps preserve tone. Once the cast is removed, physical therapy is frequently helpful in recovering lost joint motion and muscle strength.

Healing

Healing progresses uneventfully when the prerequisites for normal union are present: good blood supply, adequate immobilization, and satisfactory apposition of the fragments. Other factors that favor certain union are fracture in cancellous bone, absence of infection, minimal soft tissue injury, or impacted fracture. Healing time will be prolonged or not occur at all if there is a wide gap between the fragments, severe soft tissue injury, or impaired blood supply.

When can the fracture be considered healed? Depending on the site, type of fracture and treatment, and condition of the patient, the time for normal fracture healing may be 6 to 12 weeks. There are three clinical tests of union: (1) no motion at the fracture site; (2) no tenderness to palpation at the fracture site; (3) no tenderness with angulational stress against the fracture site. In addition, a delayed union or nonunion may have some localized swelling or bogginess, erythema, or redness at the site. Radiographic indicators of bony union are trabeculae that are continuous across the fracture site or uniform uninterrupted callus that unites the fragments and blends with both (Fig. 2-9). Occasionally, it may be difficult to appreciate these signs, especially when internal fixation obscures the view, or when the fracture is difficult to visualize because of bony overlaps. When the union is not stable, deossification will be seen on the radiographs taken 2 weeks after weight bearing is allowed.[20]

COMPLICATIONS

If problems arise, they fall into one of two categories: those related to bone and those related to soft tissue.

Bone

Infection
Bone infection following a closed fracture is an unusual complication. However, it is occasion-

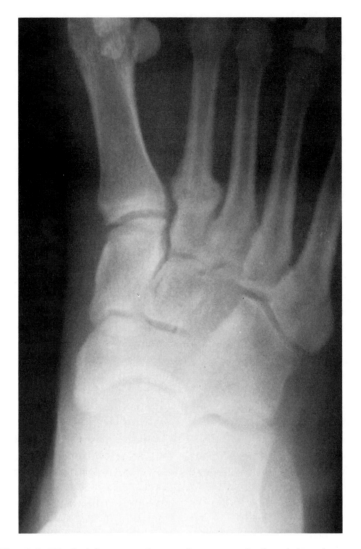

Fig. 2-9. Healed fracture of second metatarsal after delayed union.

ally seen in children[21] and in patients with compromised immune status.[22,23] Signs of hematogenous osteomyelitis may be subtle or obvious. When pain recurs after initial discomfort has subsided, infection may be the cause. The pain is usually progressive and does not respond to the usual measures, such as pain medication, elevation, and immobilization. Other indicators are local erythema, warmth, and fluctuance. The patient may be febrile with leukocytosis and a shift to the left on the differential white blood cell count. Occasionally, the patient exhibits signs of systemic toxicity such as anorexia, malaise, and lethargy. The treatment is appropriate antibiotics and surgical debridement in most cases.

Delayed Union and Nonunion
The rate of bone repair is influenced by several factors: fracture location, type of fracture, age, blood supply, infection, and distracting forces. However, the most important determinant of eventual healing is proper immobilization.[24] The bone ends cannot unite if motion is present between the fragments. Motion must be eliminated

and this condition maintained until healing is accomplished. Some unions may be deemed "slow," taking longer than expected, but exhibiting radiographic evidence of repeated movement of bone fragments. This results in hyperemia, resorbing the bone ends, and the union is labeled "delayed." There is a fuzzy, ill-defined fracture gap and the appearance of a cavity on the radiograph. Granulation tissue fills the gap, and conversion to bone is still possible if the bone is adequately immobilized. However, continued motion will frustrate the process, resulting in a cessation of cellular activity and nonunion. On the film, this is seen as smooth, sclerotic bone ends with a sharp margin at the gap. Evidence of a true nonunion on technetium scan is a photon-deficient gap at the fracture site.[25] Interposed soft tissue between the fracture fragments, if large enough, can also prevent bony union. This is commonly seen in avulsion fractures of the medial malleolus.

Treatment of delayed unions or nonunions depends on assessment of cellular activity at the fracture gap. This is based on evidence found on the radiograph and the technetium bone scan. Once this is determined, simple further immobilization or open reduction, bone grafting, or electrical stimulation is appropriately applied.

Malunion

Malunion results when the bone heals with an angulation or rotation that cannot be compensated for by remodeling of the bone. The deformity may cause degenerative arthritis in the joints influenced by that bone. The complication is best avoided by accurate reduction, proper immobilization, and careful initial radiographic assessment. Sometimes, when the bone is healed, an osteotomy may be indicated to correct severe deformity.

Shortening

Fractures of the talus and calcaneus can result in limb length discrepancy if there is loss of bony substance in a severely comminuted fracture. Fractures of the tibia can result in shortening either from loss of bone or from disturbance of growth when the child's physis is involved. In children's fractures, another cause of length discrepancy is the increased blood supply to healing bone, which enhances the growth rate, making that extremity or bone longer. For this reason, bayonet apposition, that is, side-by-side apposition, is not unacceptable in long bone fractures of children.[21]

Avascular Necrosis

Blood supply to a fracture fragment can be lost by thrombosis of blood vessels or when blood vessels are directly damaged by the injury. Avascular necrosis is a well-known complication of fracture-dislocations of the talus (Fig. 2-10).[26–28] Disruption of the blood supply causes death of cellular elements in the bone. A sequence of events then occurs representing death, repair, and maturation of the new bone. Sclerotic bone on the radiograph signals the first stage. The dead bone casts an opaque shadow in contrast to the adjacent, hyperemic, "washed-out" bone. The second stage begins when capillaries invade the necrotic tissue. It takes many months or even years to replace the dead bone in the regeneration stage. During this period the bone is soft, immature, and easily distorted by loading, which may cause collapse of normal contour. When articular cartilage is damaged, it is replaced by fibrocartilage. The imperfect surface of the fibrocartilage and loss of normal joint contour usually lead to degenerative arthritis. During the final stage, the bone matures to full strength.

Joints

The most common problem following immobilization for an injury is probably joint stiffness. Persistent edema in the injured extremity further increases the likelihood of joint stiffness. Potential causes of excessive edema include inadequate immobilization, insufficient limb elevation following injury, failure to maintain functional activity, infection near joints, including those caused by pin tracts, injury to the joint itself, and systemic causes (congestive heart failure, hypertension, renal disease). As the edema organizes, it binds together connective tissue fibers, causing intra-articular and periarticular adhesions. Further stiffness is caused by muscles or tendons bound down at the fracture site.

To avoid these complications, direct treatment

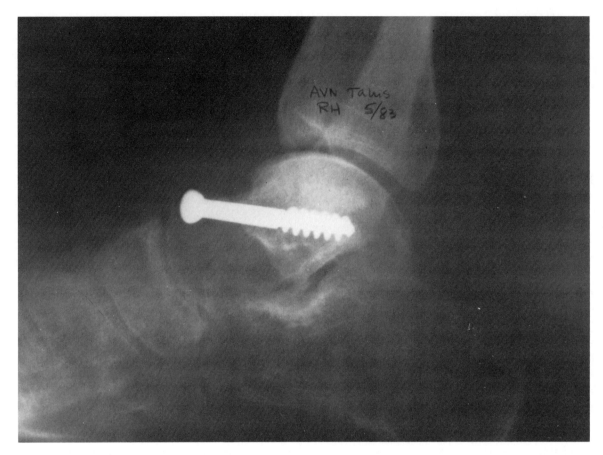

Fig. 2-10. Avascular necrosis of the talus.

toward decreasing edema and mobilizing joints and muscles as much as possible while the fracture heals. Elevation of the limb above the level of the heart is important. Elevation to the level of the thigh with the extremity outstretched on a chair, for example, constricts the saphenous vein at the inguinal ligament and may cause further edema. Only those joints that influence fracture site motion should be immobilized. Encourage active motion of those joints not restricted by the cast. Weight bearing begins as soon as it can safely be tolerated by the healing bone. Use of the muscles helps reduce venous and lymphatic stasis, as well as muscle atrophy. The leg and foot

may become quite edematous immediately after release from plaster support. Wearing an elastic support during this period is recommended. It is applied in the morning before the limb has swollen.

Joint dysfunction can result from the position of the foot and ankle in the cast. The ankle joint is immobilized in neutral position unless the nature of the injury dictates otherwise. The plaster is well molded in the medial arch with dorsal pressure against the metatarsal heads to prevent claw toe deformity.

Degenerative arthritis can be a late complication resulting from avascular necrosis, joint fractures and dislocation, or angular deformity that disrupts joint surface congruity. It is best avoided by adequate initial treatment. However, if the arthritic pain is disabling, selected joint fusions may be indicated as treatment.

Complications Associated with Other Tissues

Injuries to Nerves

Early evaluation of injuries to nerves has been discussed above. Ischemic damage to nerves can be caused by swelling in a tight cast. The cast acts as a venous tourniquet preventing outflow, but not arterial inflow. A compartment-like syndrome develops, in which tissue pressure collapses the capillaries, preventing blood flow. The resultant ischemia can permanently damage nerves and muscle tissue.

Direct trauma to nerves in closed fractures must be carefully assessed. The most common neurologic injury sustained in closed fractures is concussion, contusion, or traction, in which nerve continuity is not affected. Recovery is usually spontaneous. However, it is possible for the nerve to be severed if the fracture occurs in close proximity to the nerve course. When signs of recovery do not occur within a reasonable time, surgical exploration is indicated. The regenerating nerve fiber can be expected to grow at 2 to 3 cm/month.[26] Through generous incision the nerve is identified above and below the level of the injury. Neurolysis or primary repair is performed as necessary.

Secondary nerve injuries become apparent weeks or months after the initial injury. Constant friction or compression can cause nerve damage. Repeated passive motion of the nerve over the roughened bone may result in traumatic neuritis. The nerve is also subject to compression by bony callus, fibrosis, or a poorly padded cast. The peroneal nerve as it passes external to the fibular neck is especially susceptible to this injury, which leads to a footdrop deformity. When crutches are too long, poorly padded, or improperly used, damage to upper extremity nerves can result.

A delayed nerve injury becomes apparent many months or years after the original injury. The nerve can become stretched or compressed by deformity, bone thickening, or osteophyte formation from late arthritis. Tardy posterior tibial nerve palsy can be caused by an ankle fracture that healed in valgus. Damage to planter nerves can be caused by poor reduction or malunion of midfoot fractures.

Injuries to Vessels

The initial examination of vascular injury is of primary importance. Diffuse pain, pallor, pulselessness, paresthesias, cyanosis, and paralysis are signs of injury to vessels. Several types of vascular injury have been described above. The vessel may be in a spasm as a response to contusion, stretch, or laceration. Thrombosis or embolism may obstruct circulation. Finally, the vessel may be damaged by perforation or complete rupture. When findings on examination are unclear, the Doppler ultrasound unit can be a useful adjunctive device to determine the presence of blood flow. When damage to the posterior tibial or dorsalis pedis artery is suspected, surgical exploration is indicated. The damaged artery can safely be ligated, if the other is known to be intact; otherwise, the vessel is repaired. Vascular consultation is sought as needed, especially when the obstruction is proximal to the foot.

It is important to monitor neurovascular status frequently during the initial treatment phase. The trauma of reduction maneuvers or pressure from a cast is often the culprit in vascular injury. Unrecognized vascular injury can result in gangrene, especially in patients with pre-existing peripheral vascular disease. Ischemic damage to muscles from compartment syndrome or a tight cast causes irreversible contracture with fibrosis.

Traumatic aneurysm and arteriovenous fistula are two late sequelae to arterial injury. A hematoma forms in the site where bleeding occurs into surrounding tissues from a perforated artery. The hematoma usually resolves after several weeks or months, but occasionally an aneurysm develops in the site. Signs of an aneurysm include a pulsating soft tissue mass with a systolic bruit. If there are symptoms, they result from the pressure of the mass on surrounding tissues. The aneurysm can compress a nerve or erode bone.

The possibility of venous communication must be ruled out before excision of the aneurysm. When an artery and a vein are perforated simultaneously, an arteriovenous fistula can form during the healing process. This mass is pulsatile, but the bruit is heard throughout the cardiac cycle. Distended veins are observed in the area. This results from the large increase in venous pressure as arterial blood leaks directly into the venous system, bypassing capillary beds. Digital pressure on the artery proximal to the suspected fistula may cause slowing of the pulse and an increase in blood pressure. The arteriogram and a vascular consult should determine the treatment of this disorder. The operation consists of ligating the artery and vein proximal and distal to the fistula and excision of the fistula.

CONCLUSION

The evaluation and treatment of closed pedal fractures has been presented. A thorough history and physical examination is important. Diagnosis is made by symptoms, signs, and radiographic analysis. Treatment is based on the classification of the fracture, the degree of soft tissue involvement, and the medical status of the patient. Complications can cause serious long-term disability and are best avoided by careful early care.

Ideal care involves gentle, effective reduction as indicated; fixation that immobilizes the fragments but that interferes as little as possible with the function of surrounding tissues; and an early return of the patient to normal function.

REFERENCES

1. Rockwood CA, Green OP: Fractures in Adults. JB Lippincott, Philadelphia, 1984
2. Matsen FA: Compartment syndrome: a unified concept. Clin Orthop 113:8, 1975
3. Mubarak S, Owen CA: Compartment syndromes. Surg Gynecol Obstet 147:943, 1978
4. Matsen FA, Clawson DK: The deep posterior compartmental syndromes of the leg. J Bone Joint Surg 57A:34, 1975
5. Hardcastle PH, Reschauer R, Kutscha-Lissberg E et al: Injuries to the tarsometatarsal joint. J Bone Joint Surg 64B:349, 1982
6. Martorana V, Denick I: Tarsometatarso fracture dislocations: an alternate technique for closed reduction. J Foot Surg 20:17, 1981
7. Anderson L: Injuries of the forefoot. Clin Orthop 122:18, 1977
8. Ryan J: Fractures and dislocations encountered by the general surgeon: general principles. Surg Clin North Am 57:197, 1977
9. Compere EL, Banks S: Pictorial Handbook of Fracture Treatment. Year Book Medical Publishers, Chicago, 1971
10. Simpson A, Schulak D, Spiegel P: Intra-articular fractures of the calcaneus: a review. Contemp Orthop 6:19, 1983
11. Main B, Jowett R: Injuries of the midtarsal joint. J Bone Joint Surg 57B:89, 1975
12. Dewar F, Evans D: Occult fracture-dislocation of the midtarsal joint. J Bone Joint Surg 50B:386, 1968
13. Squire LF: Fundamentals of Radiology. Howard University Press, Cambridge, 1975
14. Weissman SD: Radiology of the Foot. Williams & Wilkins, Baltimore, 1983
15. De Palma A: The Management of Fractures and Dislocations. WB Saunders, Philadelphia, 1953
16. Maxwell J: Open or closed treatment of metatarsal fractures. J Am Podiatry Assoc 73:100, 1983
17. Adams JC: Outline of Fractures. Churchill Livingstone, Edinburgh, 1983
18. Clisham MW, Berlin SJ: The diagnosis and conservative treatment of calcaneal fractures: a review. J Foot Surg 20:28, 1981
19. Pozo JL, Kirwan E, Jackson A: The long term results of conservative management of severely displaced fractures of the calcaneus. J Bone Joint Surg 66B:386, 1984
20. Charnley J: Closed Treatment of Common Fractures. Williams & Wilkins, Baltimore, 1963
21. Tachdjian M: Pediatric Orthopedics. WB Saunders, Philadelphia, 1972
22. Watson F, Whitesides TE: Acute hematogenous osteomyelitis complicating closed fracture. Clin Orthop 117:296, 1976
23. Watson-Jones R: Fractures and Joint Injuries. Williams & Wilkins, Baltimore, 1962

24. Perren SM: Physical and biological aspects of fracture healing with special reference to internal fixation. Clin Orthop 138:175, 1979
25. Desai A, Alavi A, Dalinha M et al: Role of scintigraphy in the evaluation and treatment of nonunited fractures: concise communications. J Nucl Med 21:931, 1980
26. Haymaker W, Woodhall B: Peripheral Nerve Injuries. WB Saunders, Philadelphia, 1953
27. Hawkins L: Fractures of the neck of the talus. J Bone Joint Surg 52A:991, 1970
28. Christensen S, Lorentzen J, Krogsoe O et al: Subtalar dislocation. Acta Orthop Scand 48:707, 1977

3

Management of Open Fractures

Jeffrey M. Karlin, D.P.M.

The management of open fractures tests the skills of the surgeon to deal with injury to skin, soft tissue, muscle, and neurovascular structures in addition to the fracture. An open fracture is defined as a fracture in which the bone ends have penetrated through the skin and there is injury to the underlying soft tissue of varying degree. The surgeon's overall objective is to prevent wound sepsis, obtain fracture healing, and restore function.[1-4] The most important objective is to avoid infection, the most common event leading to nonunion, malunion, loss of function, and increased morbidity.[1,2,5] Factors to consider in preventing infections are the patient's host defense mechanism, antibiotics, surgical debridement and irrigation, wound management, and fracture care. It is the amount of devitalized soft tissue and contamination of the wound rather than the comminution or configuration of the fracture that determines the prognosis of open fractures (Fig. 3-1).[6]

Gustilo recognizes four essential features of open fractures that must be addressed to treat these injuries properly.[3] It is of primary importance to recognize life-threatening situations; open fractures themselves rarely cause mortality. Life-threatening problems must be recognized and the patient stabilized prior to formal treatment of the open fracture in the operating suite. Thirty percent of all trauma patients are polytrauma victims. A patient may have two or more system injuries, involving the head, chest, abdomen, spine, or pelvis, along with the extremities.

Second, the degree of soft tissue and bony damage varies greatly. This is discussed in greater detail below.

Third, all open fractures are considered contaminated wounds. Studies have shown a 60 to 70 percent incidence of bacterial growth in open fractures at initial inspection.[4,7,8]

Fourth, open fractures are a surgical emergency. All open fractures should be treated within 8 hours. An open fracture left open longer than 8 hours has been converted from a contaminated wound to an infected wound.

CLASSIFICATION OF OPEN FRACTURES

As noted by Gustilo[3,4] and Anderson,[9] open fractures are classified into three categories depending on the mechanism of injury, soft tissue damage, and degree of skeletal involvement.

Type I

A type I fracture is an open fracture with a clean wound less than 1 cm long. There is little soft tissue involvement or muscle contusion and no crushing component. The fracture is usually a simple transverse or short oblique fracture with minimal comminution.

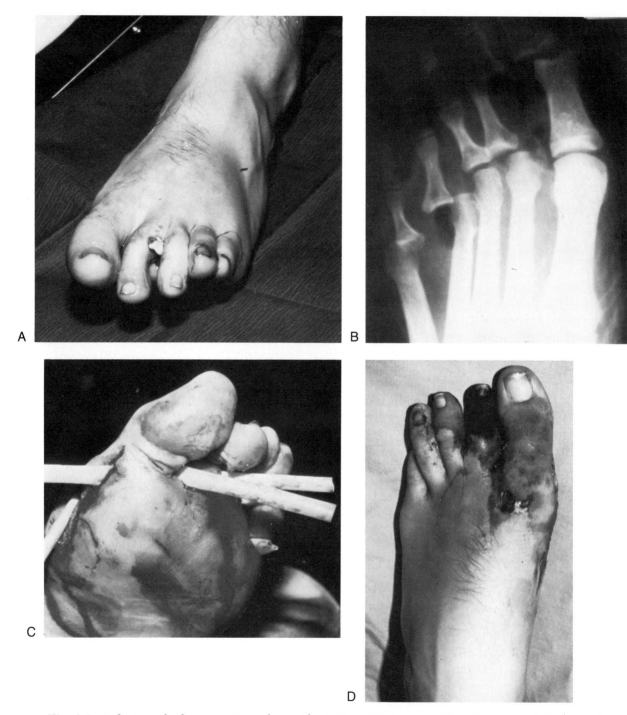

Fig. 3-1. A foot crushed in a motorcycle accident. Type III injury with extensive soft tissue and neurovascular damage. (**A**) Open fracture of second toe with cyanosis of second and third toes. (**B**) Radiograph showing dislocated interphalangeal joint of hallux with open dislocated second toe and dislocated fourth and fifth metatarsal phalangeal joints. (**C**) Postdebridement with Penrose drains protruding through lacerations caused by the severe crush injury. There were lacerations of the medial aspect of the first metatarsal and within each interdigital space. (**D**) Gangrene of second and third toes. (From Karlin,[6] with permission.)

Type II

A type II fracture is an open fracture with a laceration more than 1 cm long without extensive soft tissue damage, skin flaps, or avulsions. Type II wounds have minimal muscle damage and moderate amounts of contamination. The fracture is usually simple transverse or short oblique fracture with minimal comminution.

Type III

A type III fracture has a wound greater than 5 cm long with extensive soft tissue damage to muscle, skin, and neurovascular structures. It is often accompanied by a high-velocity injury or a severe crush component. Type III fractures include farm injuries, gunshot wounds, open fractures with neurovascular injury, traumatic amputations, high-velocity automobile injuries, and open fractures over 8 hours old (Fig. 3-2).[6]

Type III fractures have an increased morbidity associated with sepsis, nonunion, and amputation. Impaired function often results.

Gustilo and Williams further classify type III injuries into three subtypes in order of worsening prognosis.[10]

Type IIIA
Type IIIA fractures have adequate soft tissue coverage of the fracture with limited periosteal stripping, despite extensive soft tissue laceration of flaps, or high-energy trauma irrespective of the size of the wound.

Type IIIB
Type IIIB fractures show extensive soft tissue injury with periosteal stripping and considerable bone exposure, usually with massive contamination.

Type IIIC
Type IIIC fractures are open fractures associated with arterial injury requiring repair.

This classification of open fractures will help in planning the appropriate treatment as well as aid in predicting the eventual outcome of the wound.

PRINCIPLES OF TREATMENT

Gustilo has listed eight principles essential to the treatment of open fractures[3]:

1. All open fractures treated as an emergency.
2. Evaluation of patient for other life-threatening injuries.
3. Appropriate and adequate antibiotic therapy.
4. Adequate debridement and irrigation.
5. Stabilization of the open fracture.
6. Appropriate wound coverage.
7. Early cancellous bone grafting.
8. Rehabilitation.

Antibiotic Therapy

A primary objective in the treatment of open fractures is the prevention of infection. Antibiotic therapy in open fractures is secondary only to adequate debridement, irrigation, and definitive wound care. The patient's local host defense mechanisms may be less able to resist infection owing to the presence of soft tissue damage, edema, ischemia, and necrosis.

The use of antibiotics in prevention of infection in open fractures has been extensively reported.[4,8,9,11,12] Patzakis et al. in a randomized double-blind prospective study of the effectiveness of antibiotic therapy in open fractures demonstrated an infection rate of 13 percent with a placebo, 9 percent with penicillin-streptomycin, and 2.4 percent with a cephalosporin.[11] Gustilo[4,7] and Anderson[9] have shown an infection rate of only 2.4 percent in more than 1,200 fractures when appropriate and adequate doses of antibiotics were given over a short period of time. Antibiotic treatment of open fractures should, therefore, be considered therapeutic rather than prophylactic.

All open fractures should be considered contaminated wounds (Figs. 3-2A and 3-3A). Gram stains and appropriate cultures and sensitivities should be obtained. In the experience of Patzakis et al., the cultures that are most likely to be of value are those taken before any treatment is instituted and immediately after thorough irrigation and debridement are performed.[11] The ini-

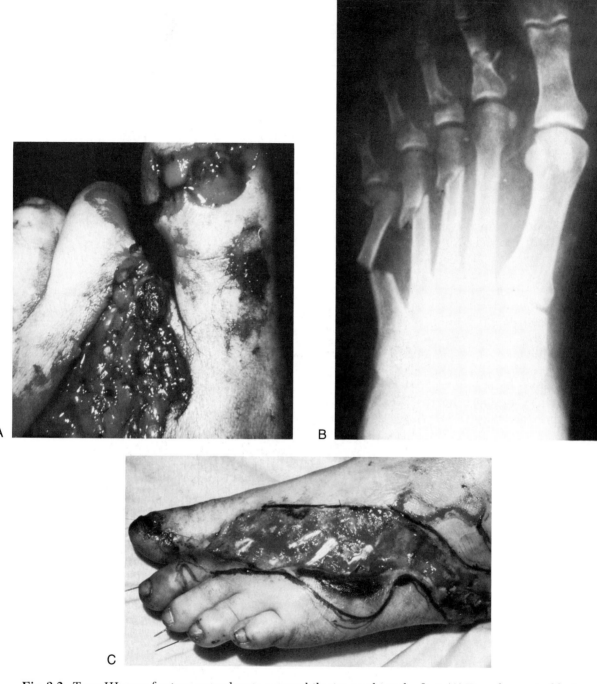

Fig. 3-2. Type III open fracture secondary to automobile tire crushing the foot. (**A**) Dorsal aspect of foot showing extensive devitalized soft tissue and contamination with dirt and gravel embedded in soft tissues and bone. (**B**) Radiograph showing fracture dislocations of toes and of third, fourth, and fifth metatarsal bones. (**C**) Foot prior to second debridement and skin grafting. Fluorescein used to determine nonviable skin. Picture shows extensive degloving injury with pregangrenous second toe requiring amputation. (*Figure continues.*)

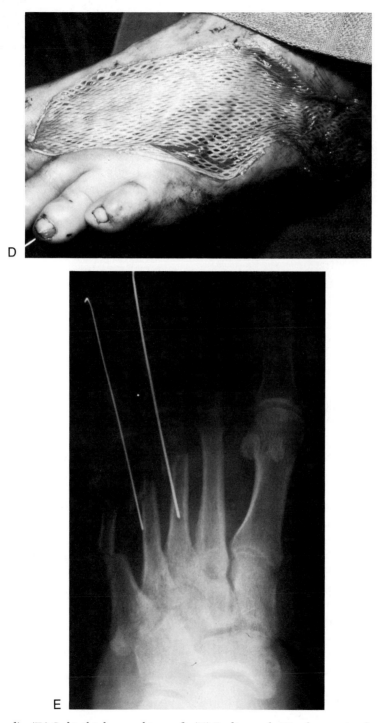

Fig. 3-2 (*Continued*). (**D**) Split-thickness skin graft. (**E**) Radiograph Kirschner-wire fixation and amputation of second toe. (From Karlin,[6] with permission.)

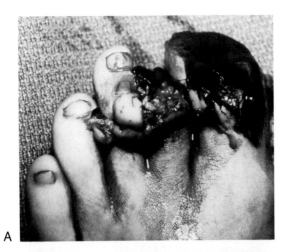

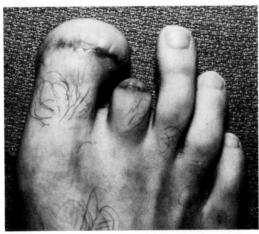

Fig. 3-3. (A) Traumatic amputation following lawn-mower accident with severe soft tissue, osseous, and neurovascular injury. **(B)** Postoperative debridement and delayed primary closure. (From Karlin,[6] with permission.)

tial specimen should be obtained from the deep tissues rather than the skin or superficial tissue. Specimens should be obtained for both aerobic and anerobic cultures. Intraoperative cultures obtained from the depths of the wound aid in assessing the effectiveness of debridement.

The appropriate antibiotic should be given within the first 3 hours of injury. The antibiotic or antibiotics should be effective against both gram-positive and gram-negative organisms. The primary organism encountered in open fractures is penicillinase-producing *Staphylococcus aureus.*

Patzakis has noted a recent increase in gram-negative organisms in infected wounds, predominantly *Pseudomonas* and *Enterobacter* species.[8] The antibiotic of choice for type I and II wounds initially should be a cephalosporin, preferably cefazolin owing to its long half-life. The initial dose of cefazolin is 1 to 2 g intravenously followed by 1 g every 8 hours for 3 days.[13] In type III open fractures, the cefazolin dosage should be doubled. In severely contaminated wounds, and particularly type IIIB and IIIC fractures, anaminoglycoside plus an antistaphylococcal agent or a broad-spectrum cephalosporin should be used. The use of tobramycin-gentamicin beads may be necessary in type III wounds. In open fractures sustained in farming environments where clostridia infections may occur, penicillin G in a dose of 10 to 20 million units intravenously daily should be given. In children, 100,000 units/kg/day intravenously in four to six divided doses is indicated.[8]

Antibiotics are usually administered for a total of 3 days. By this time it will be known whether the wound is infected. Culture reports should then be available, and if infection is present, appropriate antibiotic therapy can then be instituted. If the infection has not been controlled after 3 days, antibiotics alone will not be adequate and further debridement and reevaluation of the antibiotic will be necessary.

Gustilo recommends that antibiotic therapy be instituted for an additional 3 days during delayed primary closure or secondary wound closure, when elective open reduction and internal fixation are performed and when internal or external fixating devices are changed or bone grafting is performed.[3]

The patient must always be appropriately immunized for tetanus prophylaxis (Table 3-1).

Debridement

In the treatment of patients with open fractures, it is important that appropriate irrigation and debridement be performed in the operating room as soon as possible. Adequate debridement is of primary importance in the management of open fractures. In the emergency room, the skin

Table 3-1.   Tetanus Prophylaxis[a]

Immunization Data	Action To Be Taken
Immunization completed previously; last booster within 1 year.	None.
Immunization completed within the previous 10 years; no subsequent booster dose.	0.5 ml of tetanus and diphtheria toxoid, adult type (Td).
Immunization completed more than 10 years previously; last booster within the previous 10 years.	0.5 ml of Td.
Immunization completed more than 10 years previously; no booster with the previous 10 years; wound minor and relatively clean, treated promptly and adequately.	0.5 ml of Td.
Immunization completed more than 10 years previously; no booster within the previous 5 years; wound other than minor and clean or not treated promptly.	0.5 ml of Td and 250 to 500 units of human tetanus immune globulin (TIG[H]): 500 units if wound is clostridia prone, otherwise 250 units. Give Td and TIG(H) by separate syringes and needles at separate sites.
No history or record of immunization; wound minor and clean; wound surgery prompt and adequate.	Begin immunization program with 0.5 ml of Td; schedule further immunization.
No record of immunization; wound other than clean or treated promptly and adequately.	250 units of TIG(H); begin immunization with 0.5 ml of Td. Give 500 units of TIG(H) if wound is clostridia prone; otherwise give 250 units. Give Td and TIG(H) by separate syringes and needles at separate sites.

[a] Tetanus prophylaxis is indicated in all open fractures.
(Data from Gustilo,[7] and Sandusky.[14])

around the wound should be scrubbed and the wound copiously irrigated with a sterile physiologic solution. Foreign debris can be removed with sterile forceps in the emergency room, but sharp debridement may not be indicated at this time.

In the operating suite, the wound is inspected using aseptic technique. At this time, cultures from the depths of the open fracture should be obtained if not already done in the emergency room. The surgical site may then be prepared and draped in the usual sterile manner. A tourniquet may be applied midthigh but is rarely used unless there is severe arterial bleeding. The use of a tourniquet may increase tissue ischemia, increase edema, and further insult the traumatized tissues. It also can interfere with determining tissue viability. A tourniquet may be used for short periods to determine skin viability by observing for the postischemic capillary flush.

Debridement must be systematic, complete, and meticulous to remove all devitalized tissue. If the wound is dirty, a brush is used to remove foreign bodies from soft tissue and bone (Figs. 3-2A and 3-4B and C).[6] It may be necessary at times to extend the wound surgically to remove dead skin, to examine the extent of deep muscle damage, or to remove foreign material.

Skin
All nonviable, macerated, mutilated skin and soft tissue should be sharply excised (Fig. 3-4B and C). Skin debridement should be as conservative as possible, especially on the lower leg and foot. Type I and II open fractures are elliptically enlarged to remove avascular skin. Distally based skin flaps in the foot and lower leg, frequently seen in crush wounds and avulsion injuries, may become frankly necrotic, although they initially appear viable. If the viability of skin

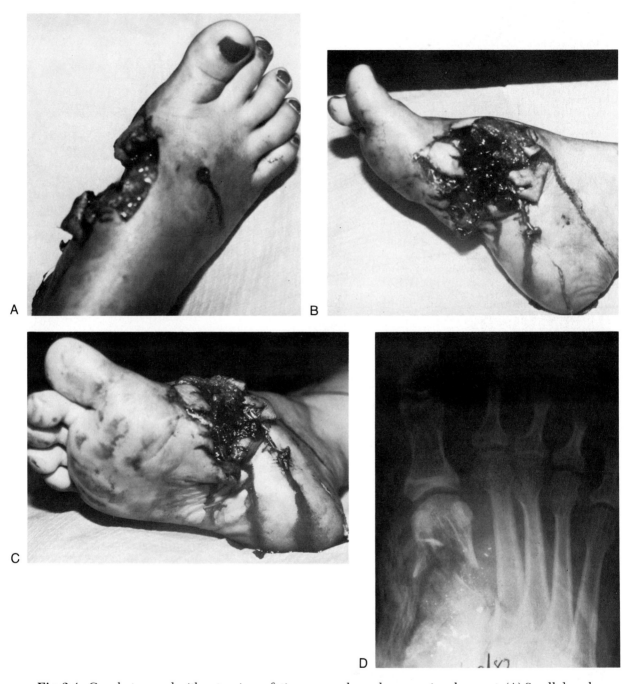

Fig. 3-4. Gunshot wound with extensive soft tissue, muscle, and osseous involvement. **(A)** Small dorsal entrance wound with large exit wound secondary to bullet and bone acting as missiles. **(B & C)** Extensive medial soft tissue necrosis with the distal vascular status intact. **(D)** Radiograph shows first metatarsal fracture with bone loss. (*Figure continues.*)

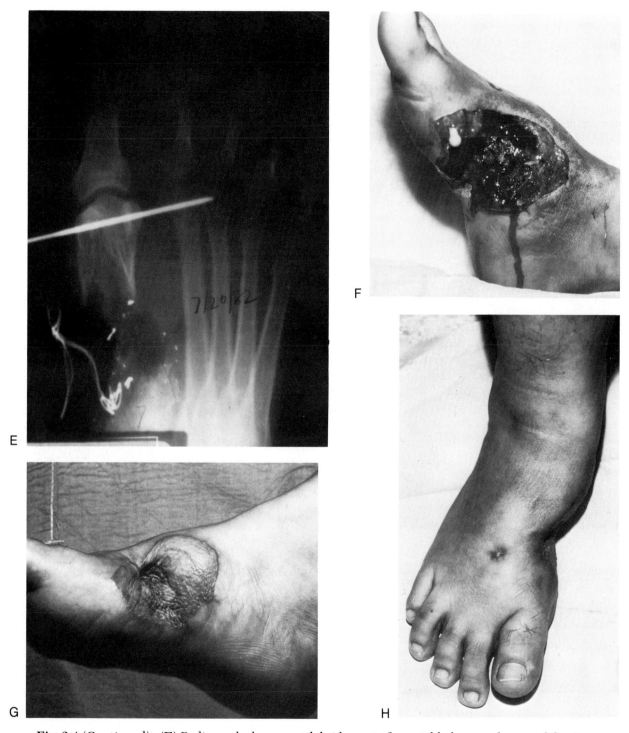

Fig. 3-4 (*Continued*). (**E**) Radiograph shows postdebridement of nonviable bone and external fixation with Kirschner wire for stabilization and distal distraction of bone to prevent shortening. (**F**) Postdebridement of necrotic soft tissue and external fixation. (**G & H**) Appearance of foot with split-thickness skin graft, soft tissue defect, and a functional result. (From Karlin,[6] with permission.)

flaps is difficult to determine, tourniquet technique or the fluorescein dye test may be utilized[15] (Fig. 3-2C). If the tourniquet is released without a flush of initial pink color in the skin, then most likely the skin is nonviable. The margins of viable skin can also be determined by intravenously injecting 10 to 15 mg of fluorescein per kg and observing the skin under a Wood's light. If there is no diffusion of fluorescein dye to the skin, the skin should be considered nonviable. Vomiting, nausea, and urticaria have been observed in 0.6 percent of patients injected intravenously with fluorescein.[16] An antiemetic may be utilized prior to injecting the intravenous fluorescein.

Fascia and Tendon

Fascia is expendable. Fat and deep fascia can be radically excised since they are poorly vascularized and prone to infection. For tendon to remain viable, paratenon must be preserved. Tendon devoid of its paratenon, its primary blood supply, will not survive for long periods. For tendon to remain viable, early coverage must be performed by utilization of skin grafts, skin flaps, primary closure, or muscle coverage (Figs. 3-2D and 3-4G).

Muscle

Scully et al. noted four criteria for muscle viability by both clinical and histological study: consistency, contractility, ability to bleed, and color.[17] The best method to determine muscle viability is local muscular contractility and consistency rebound. Muscle viability may be determined by pinching the muscle with a forceps or stimulating it with low-power coagulation. Bleeding and color are not reliable indicators of muscle viability.

Osseous Structures

The debridement of bone should be conservative. Bony fractures with intact periosteum, soft tissue attachments, and ligamentous or tendinous insertions should be preserved. Small bony fragments that are dirty or contaminated or add no stability may be removed (Fig. 3-4D and E). Most free bone fragments in the foot or lower leg should be preserved since they will provide stability and promote fracture healing. Cancellous bone that is clean should be preserved for use as a possible bone graft. Bone ends of all open fractures must be visualized so that any foreign materials can be removed.

Irrigation

Copious irrigation with warm physiologic saline or lactated Ringer's solution provides mechanical cleansing of debris and aids in reduction of bacterial flora. Gross et al. have demonstrated the use of pulsating water jet lavage in reduction of contamination and removal of foreign material in open and crush wounds.[18] Type I wounds of the foot should be irrigated with 1 to 2 L of solution.[19] Type II and III wounds should be irrigated with a minimum of 2 to 4 L.[7] If the wound is large and heavily contaminated up to 10 L may be needed.[7] Gustilo[3] and Patzakis[8] recommend irrigating the wound with an antibiotic solution. I have found the use of 1 g of cefazolin in 1 L of irrigant to be useful.[19] Patzakis uses 50,000 units of bacitracin and 1 million units of polymycin to 1 L of irrigant.[8] A cephalosporin utilized with an aminoglycoside may be used in highly contaminated wounds when *Pseudomonas* infection is suspected.[19] Sodium bicarbonate increases the pH of the solution, allowing the aminoglycoside to be more active against gram-negative bacteria.[19]

Gustilo recommends that all type III wounds be inspected within 24 to 48 hours after initial surgery and again be debrided and irrigated if necessary.[3] It may be difficult, even for the most experienced surgeon, to recognize nonviable tissue immediately after the first debridement. What may appear to be viable after the initial debridement may become nonviable within 24 to 48 hours if circulation is insufficient. If arterial injury is documented, it may be necessary to reexplore the wound in 12 to 24 hours.[3]

Open fractures that enter a joint or open joint injury without fracture demand an open arthrotomy and cleansing of the joint. An arthrogram may be beneficial in determining whether a joint has been violated. Extravasation of dye from the joint through the entrance wound may be noted.

Stabilization of Open Fractures

Fracture stability is essential to preserve the remaining viable soft tissue, neurovascular, and muscular structures. Immediate stability offers relief of pain, ease of patient care, and early mobility of the extremity, which decreases swelling, muscle atrophy, and stiffness (Fig. 3-4E and F). Realigning and stabilizing the fracture optimizes local wound conditions for soft tissue healing and thereby plays a major role in the prevention of infection.

Plaster splint immobilization along with Kirschner wires or pins is an ideal method for stabilizing open fractures of the foot and lower extremity. Splints enable easy inspection and care of wounds and prevent circular compression of the limb with associated neurovascular compromise. Plaster splints are an excellent method of immobilization of the foot and lower extremity for type I and II open fractures for the first 7 to 10 days for ease of wound inspection.[19] The application of a walker to a circular cast should be initially avoided in the treatment of open fractures.

Kirschner wires are easy to use and provide stability of fractures and viability of soft tissue as well as offering the advantage of a minimal amount of hardware at or near the fracture site. They are easy to insert percutaneously without excessive dissection at the traumatized site. This method of fixation is very useful with multiple phalangeal and metatarsal fractures (Fig. 3-2C–E).

External fixation devices are advantageous in patients with extensive soft tissue involvement because the pins are remote from the fracture site and can still render rigid stability (Fig. 3-5). External fixation devices in the foot have limited use, except in cases of segmental bone loss, where maintenance of length is permitted until the wound and bone are ready for further definitive treatment such as grafting. External fixation may be used to stabilize major open fracture-dislocations, maintain length, prevent soft tissue contractures, and control joint alignment for arthrodesis. Type I and II wounds of the foot in which there are isolated fractures or dislocations are less suitable for external fixators. Other methods are easier to use and usually work well. Ken-

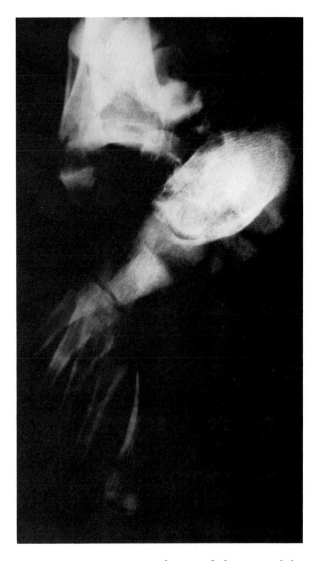

Fig. 3-5. Type IIIB open fracture-dislocation of the foot and ankle following train accident.

zora et al. do not recommend full weight bearing with an external fixator device.[20] Only touchdown gait with crutches or walkers when possible are permitted.

The role of rigid internal fixation in achieving stability of open fractures remains controversial. Rigid fixation by osteosynthesis provides for accurate anatomic alignment, compression, and restoration of functional parameters. Rigid fixation by screws or plates requires more foreign material at the fracture site and may require further extension of the wound, which increases the risk of sepsis, fibrosis, and further soft tissue loss. In view of reported infection rates of 5.2 to 8 percent after initial fixation of type II open fractures and 26 to 41 percent in type III fractures, extensive surgery to achieve complete stability at the time of initial debridement is most probably contraindicated.[1,5,21] Chapman states, regarding internal fixation, that excellent surgical results demand intelligent indications, precise and correct technical execution, and compulsive postoperative care.[1] The room for error is small, and the consequences are usually more severe than the sequelae of less complicated methods of osseous immobilization. Rigid internal fixation for fractures of small bones is technically more difficult than that utilized for fractures of larger bones.

Rigid internal fixation is probably indicated for type III wounds of the rear foot and ankle and in most intra-articular fractures. Open fractures in polytraumatized limbs with arterial injury requiring repair are also suitable for this technique. However, owing to the complexity of type II and type III wounds of the forefoot, internal fixation with screws or plates may not be advisable (Figs. 3-2B and 3-4D).

When immediate internal fixation techniques are used in open fractures, the wounds must *not* be closed primarily, except in selected type I fractures.[1,7,9] Anderson and Gustilo recommend immediate internal fixation in polytraumatized patients and in multiple fractures of one extremity on both sides of the joint, to facilitate care of the soft tissue.[9] Franklin et al. advocate that all open fractures of the ankle should have immediate internal fixation to maximize the ability of the soft tissues to resist infection and to heal, so that optimum functional results can be obtained.[22] They reported a low incidence of infection with a strict protocol of prophylactic antibiotics beginning in the recovery room, copious irrigation and thorough debridement, immediate internal fixation, and delayed primary closure in 5 to 7 days. It is imperative to remember that type III open fractures must be left open, and wound closure performed in 5 to 6 days utilizing delayed primary closure, split-thickness skin grafts, or other reconstructive procedures.

Bone Grafting

Bone grafting may be necessary to achieve osseous stability. Type I open fractures may be grafted at the time of fixation. Gustilo recommends early cancellous bone grafting in type III open fractures with extensive soft tissue injury, large bone exposure or bone loss, or when there is no evidence of early callus formation after 3 months.[3] In most cases, autogenous cancellous bone should be used. This is best utilized at the time of delayed primary closure when there is no evidence of infection.[1,3] In cases in which the graft is important for stabilization, it may be necessary to graft at the time of fixation. Even if infection occurs, the graft may still remain viable. If it is nonviable, the graft can be debrided. Bone grafting should be delayed for 4 to 6 weeks following utilization of local flaps or free muscle microvascular transfer for wound coverage.

Wound Coverage

Primary Closure in Open Fractures

Wound coverage in open fractures has always been the subject of controversy among those who advocate primary closure and those who favor delayed primary closure.[3,5,23,24]

Gustilo has shown that type I and the majority of type II open fractures can be closed primarily if the wound has been adequately debrided and irrigated.[7] Patzakis uses partial closure for type I and type II open fractures.[25] Partial closure is defined as leaving the original wound open and closing the extension of the surgical wound made to facilitate surgical debridement. The fracture is closed, but the wound is left open on one or both sides of the fracture site. Primary closure should only be performed if there is no tension and no evidence of contamination or crushing component and the wound has not been left open for more than 8 hours. After 8 hours, a wound is no longer considered contaminated, but infected. If there is any doubt that debridement and irrigation have not been adequate, the wound should be left open and delayed primary closure performed in approximately 5 to 7 days (see Fig. 3-3A and B).[6]

Delayed Primary Closure

Delayed primary closure is defined as closure of the wound within 3 to 10 days. Wound closure can only be performed if there is no infection. Also, the Gram stain should be negative and the wound clean prior to closure. A clinical decision based on local signs and symptoms as well as culture reports must be made. Quantitative tissue cultures can be performed to determine whether the wound can be closed without the risk of an infection developing.[26] If the quantitative biopsy culture shows less than 10^5 bacteria per gram of tissue, then the wound can be safely closed. If there is adequate skin, direct skin closure can be performed or the wound can be closed with a meshed split-thickness skin graft (Figs. 3-2D and 3-4G). Exposed bone or areas of significant bone loss may require a local muscle flap, myocutaneous flap, or free vascular bone-muscle composite transfer (Fig. 3-6). In wounds without exposed bone or in which only exposed muscle and soft tissue are noted, a meshed split-thickness skin graft may be used.

My experience with major type II and type III open fractures of the foot and ankle has shown that wound coverage can usually be achieved utilizing meshed split-thickness skin grafts or the wound may be allowed to heal by secondary intention. There is rarely indication in the foot and ankle for primary skin grafting of major type II or type III wounds.

Type III open fracture wounds should be closed within 3 to 7 days after injury, if clean. Exposed bone not covered within this period may become desiccated or become secondarily infected. Wounds with good granulation tissue can heal by epithelialization, thus covering the soft tissue defect. This is referred to as healing by secondary intention.

Complications

Complications may occur from the severity of the original injury or the management of the open fracture itself. Major complications include early and late soft tissue infection, delayed union, nonunion, skin loss, osteomyelitis, and gangrene and resulting amputation. Infection remains the major complication to avoid. When infection is prevented, there is less chance of other complications. Morbidity is decreased and overall functional results are increased. It is essential to treat early and late infections with appropriate antibiotics, debridement, and copious irrigation. If infection is not controlled, osteomyelitis, delayed union, skin slough, or gangrene may occur and amputation may become necessary.

Nonunion of fractures in the foot may be ignored if they are asymptomatic.[18] Many times radiographs of fractures of the small bones of the foot will not show union at 6 months, yet

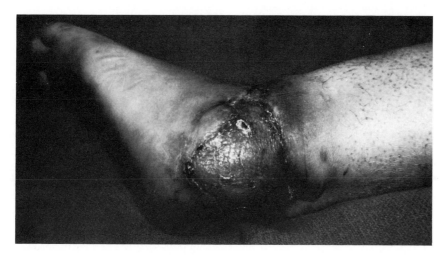

Fig. 3-6. Myocutaneous flap over an open calcaneal fracture with poststatus osteomyelitis.

will show union after 9 to 12 months[18] (see Ch. 32).

Indications for Immediate Amputation

The patient with irreversible blood vessel injury in the foot will require an amputation (see Figs. 3-3A and B).[6] Primary amputation, however, is rarely indicated in the severely injured foot. Elective amputation should be staged to attain the most distal viable level[27] (Figs. 3-1D and 3-2C).

An immediate amputation may be necessary when there is severely crushed or devitalized muscle and skin or loss of the neurovascular supply to the involved part (Fig. 3-7). This is more commonly seen with lawn mower trauma, farming injuries, and military trauma such as landmine explosions. The decision is best made early to prevent agonizing mental and physical periods and expense for both the patient and surgeon (Fig. 3-7A–D).

Rehabilitation

Rehabilitation plays an essential part in reducing morbidity and aiding the patients return to a functional state and gainful employment. Gustilo noted the average hospital stay to be 5 to 7 days for type I injuries, 12 to 14 days for type II injuries, and 67 days for type III tibial fractures.[3] The patient and involved family must be informed of the seriousness of each injury and its socioeconomic implications.

Rehabilitation must be started early to prevent muscle atrophy, disuse, and joint stiffness and to promote improvement of circulation to the injured site. The physical therapist must be involved, providing an exercise program for nonambulatory patients to maintain an optimum of strength in all extremities. If needed, social services and home health care should be made available to the patient.

GUNSHOT WOUNDS

One particular type of injury causing open fractures that should be discussed is shotgun injuries. Gunshot wounds are internal explosions and can fracture bones remote from the missile tract (Figs. 3-4A–H and 3-7A–D). All injured extremities must be examined for arterial and nerve inju-

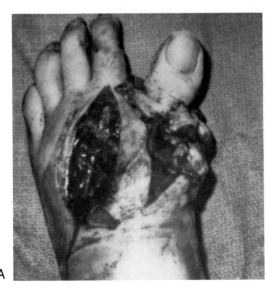
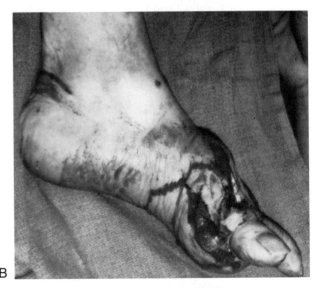

A   B

Fig. 3-7. Accidental gunshot injury at close range. (**A & B**) Extensive soft tissue, muscle, osseous, and neurovascular involvement of the dorsal and medial aspect of the foot requiring transmetatarsal amputation. (*Figure continues.*)

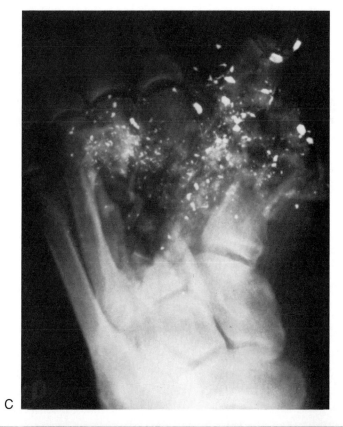

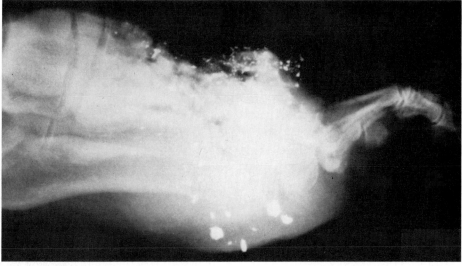

Fig. 3-7 (*Continued*). (**C & D**) Radiographs show severe bone loss and fracture comminution with numerous pellets. (From Karlin,[6] with permission. Courtesy of Gordon Sinclar, D.P.M., Kaiser/Permanente Medical Center, Vallejo, CA.)

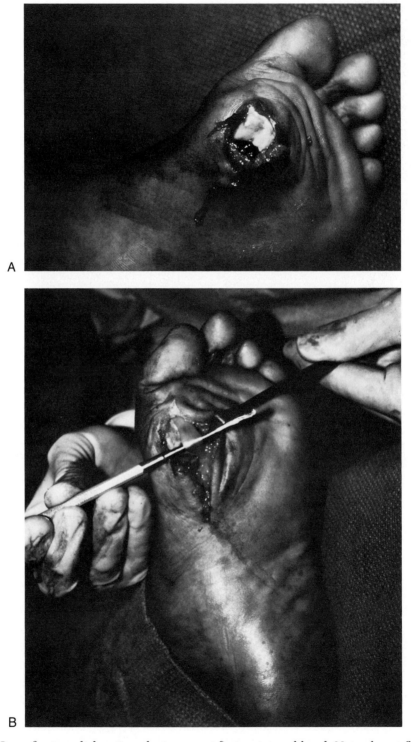

Fig. 3-8. **(A)** Open fracture-dislocation plantar aspect first metatarsal head. Note absent flexor hallucis longus tendon and sesamoids. **(B)** Extension of wound for debridement, inspection of vital structures with repositioning of sesamoids and flexor tendon. (*Figure continues.*)

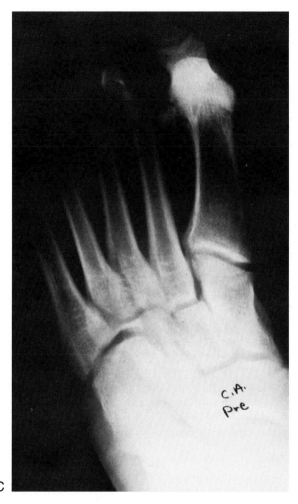

C

Fig. 3-8 (*Continued*). (**C**) Radiograph shows fracture-dislocation of first metatarsal phalangeal joint.

ries. The proper management of open fractures caused by gunshot injuries demands knowledge of the type of firearm and missile and the distance between the firearm and the victim. Therefore, firearm injuries have been classified as low- versus high-velocity missile wounds.

Low-velocity gunshot wounds with fractures need minimal debridement. Wound margins are debrided by ellipsing the entrance and exit wounds and providing copious irrigation. Primary or delayed primary closure and antibiotics for 3 days with tetanus toxoid and immobilization of the fractures are usually indicated.[20] Bretter et al. recommend arthrotomy for penetrating wound

of a joint, repair of ruptured vessels, and removal of subcutaneous bullets when necessary.[28]

High-velocity[29,30] gunshot wounds and close-range gunshot wounds cause substantial soft tissue loss, bone defects with comminution, and damage to nerves and vessels (Figs. 3-4A–H and 3-7A–D). These types of wounds require aggressive treatment with adequate debridement and copious irrigation with jet lavage. They require stabilization of unstable fractures, delayed primary closure, and neurovascular repair when indicated (Fig. 3-4E–G). In close-range gunshot wounds, an attempt must be made to remove the wadding material. It is not necessary to remove every pellet from the wound, since this may cause further damage to soft tissue, bone, or neurovascular structures. Antibiotics should be given for 3 days and longer if needed.

CONCLUSIONS

The open fracture is a surgical emergency (Fig. 3-8A–C). In treating these wounds, there are three primary goals: (1) to prevent infection, (2) to obtain adequate fracture healing, and (3) to restore normal or optimum function of the injured extremity.

The appropriate initial management of these wounds is essential. Basic principles include obtaining a detailed history and physical examination, radiographs, and wound cultures and providing appropriate intravenous antibiotics and tetanus toxoid immunization (Fig. 3-9). In the operating room, meticulous debridement and copious irrigation of the wound must be performed and the fracture fixated with the most appropriate method for that specific wound.

Primary closure is indicated only in clean type I and type II injuries and only after adequate debridement and irrigation. All type III wounds and extensive lacerations should be treated in an open manner and delayed primary closure performed. Bactericidal parenteral antibiotics are usually indicated for the initial 3 days and again for another 3 days at the time of any secondary closure. Proper static and dynamic splinting must

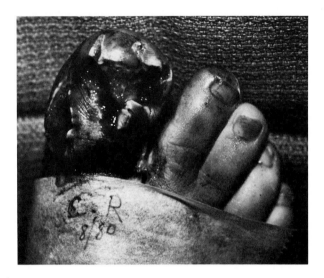

Fig. 3-9. Open fracture of distal phalanx of great toe.

also be provided to achieve optimal and early return to function.

REFERENCES

1. Chapman MW: The use of immediate internal fixation in open fractures. Orthop Clin North Am 11:579, 1980
2. Chapman MW: Role of bone stability in open fractures. p. 75. In Frankel VH (ed): Instructional Course Lectures, American Academy of Orthopaedic Surgeons. Vol. 31. CV Mosby, St. Louis, 1982
3. Gustilo RB: Management of open fractures and complications. p. 64. In Frankel VH (ed): Instructional Course Lectures, American Academy of Orthopaedic Surgeons. Vol. 31. CV Mosby, St. Louis, 1982
4. Gustilo RB: Use of antimicrobials in the management of open fractures. Arch Surg 114:804, 1979
5. Patzakis MJ, Wilkins J, Moore TM: Considerations in reducing the infection rate in open tibial fractures. Clin Orthop 178:36, 1983
6. Karlin JM: Management of open fractures. Clin Podiatry 2:217, 1985
7. Gustilo RB: Management of open fractures and their complications. p. 15. Saunders Monographs in Clinical Orthopaedics. Vol. 4. WB Saunders, Philadelphia, 1982
8. Patzakis MJ: Management of open fractures. p. 62. In Frankel VH (ed): Instructional Course Lectures, American Academy of Orthopaedic Surgeons. Vol. 31. CV Mosby, St. Louis, 1982
9. Anderson JT, Gustilo RB: Immediate internal fixation in open fractures. Orthop Clin North Am 11:569, 1980
10. Gustilo RB, Williams DW: The use of antibiotics in the management of open fractures. Orthopedics 7:1617, 1984
11. Patzakis MJ, Harvey JP, Ivler D: The role of antibiotics in the management of open fractures. J Bone Joint Surg 564:532, 1974
12. Patzakis MJ, Wilkins J, Moore TM: Use of antibiotics in open tibial fractures. Clin Orthop 178:31, 1983
13. Gustilo RB: Current concepts in the management of open fractures. p. 359. In Frankel VH (ed): Instructional Course Lectures, American Academy of Orthopaedic Surgeons. Vol. 36. CV Mosby, St. Louis, 1987
14. Sandusky WR: Prophylaxis of infection in trauma. In Mandell GI, Douglas RG, Bennett JE (eds): Principles and Practice of Infectious Disease. Churchill Livingstone, New York, 1979
15. McCraw JB, Myers B, Shanklin KD: The value of fluorescein in predicting the viability of arterialized flaps. Plast Reconstr Surg 60:710, 1977
16. Marcus NA, Blair WF, Schuk JM et al: Low-velocity gunshot wounds to the extremities. J Trauma 20:1061, 1980
17. Scully RE, Artz C, Sako Y: An evaluation of the surgeons criteria for determining viability of muscle during debridement. Arch Surg 73:1031, 1956
18. Gross A, Cutright DE, Bhaskar SN: Effectiveness of pulsating water jet lavage in treatment of contaminated crushed wounds. Am J Surg 124:393, 1972
19. Karlin JM: Management of open fractures. Clin Podiatr Med Surg 2:217, 1985
20. Kenzora JE, Edwards CC, Browner BD et al: Acute management of major trauma involving the foot and ankle with Hoffmann external fixation. Foot Ankle 1:348, 1981
21. Gustilo RB, Anderson JT: Prevention of infection in the treatment of one thousand and twenty-five open fractures of long bones. J Bone Joint Surg 58A:453, 1963
22. Franklin JL, Johnson KD, Hansen ST: Immediate internal fixation of open ankle fractures. J Bone Joint Surg 66A:1349, 1984
23. Rittmann WW, Perren SM, Matter P et al: Open fractures—long term results in 200 consecutive cases. Clin Orthop 138:132, 1979

24. Wade PA, Campbell RD: Open versus closed methods in treating fractures of the leg. Am J Surg 99:599, 1958

25. Patzakis MJ: Management of open fracture wounds. p. 367. In Frankel VH (ed): Instructional Course Lectures, American Academy of Orthopaedic Surgeons. Vol. 36. CV Mosby, St. Louis, 1987

26. Krizek TJ, Robson MC: Biology of surgical infection. Surg Clin North Am 55:1261, 1975

27. Omer GE, Jr., Pomerantz GM: Initial management of severe open injuries and traumatic amputations of the foot. Arch Surg 105:696, 1972

28. Bretter D, Sealin ED, Mender DG: Conservative treatment of low-velocity gunshot wounds. Clin Orthop 140:26, 1979

29. DeMuth WE: The mechanism of shotgun wounds. J Trauma 11:219, 1971

30. DeMuth WE, Smith JM: High velocity bullet wounds of muscles and bone: the basis of rational early treatment. J Trauma 6:744, 1966

4

Management of Skin Loss

Elliott H. Rose, M.D.

From a historical perspective, the notion of salvage of major foot injuries with extensive soft tissue avulsion is relatively new. Smaller skin defects were covered by traditional plastic surgical methods (skin grafts, local transposition flaps, or cross leg pedicle flaps). Larger avulsion injuries of the sole were treated by below-knee amputations. Over the last decade, however, with improved optics and finer instrument technology, microsurgical techniques have been applied for more successful foot reconstruction.

Selection of flap coverage is predicated on clear-cut anatomic and biomechanical considerations. Clinical rationale for flap usage is based on location and size of the defect, load factors, sensory feedback, and presence of underlying gliding structures.

FUNCTIONAL ANATOMY

The complex structure of the foot is uniquely adapted to the physical demands of weight bearing and ambulation. The skin on the plantar surface is 4 to 5 mm thick, lacking apocrine and sebaceous glands. The sole is tightly bound by fibrous septae to the plantar aponeurosis, and these septae are interspersed by large fat lobules. The thin elastic dorsal skin overlies the synovial sheaths of the extensor tendons.

The dual arch system regulates the transmission of forces during the gait pattern. The mobile *medial longitudinal arch* (calcaneus, talus, navicular, and three medial rays) elevates during the step by "windlass" mechanism. As the toes are brought into extension, the plantar aponeurosis is wrapped around the metatarsal heads, elevating the medial foot and reducing weight bearing.[1] The *lateral longitudinal arch* (cuboid, calcaneous, and two lateral rays) is the more stable weight-bearing portion of the arch.[2] The anatomic *transverse arch* underneath the metatarsal heads is, in fact, obliterated during weight bearing.

During the walk cycle, the line of the center of pressure passes from the heel to the lateral side of the foot and then between the first and second metatarsal head and ends up at the great toe at the time of lift-off.[3] At the time of strike, vertical force exceeds body weight by 10 to 15 percent. Shear forces are greater than 50 lbs (23 kg) at initial floor contact. At the stance phase, vertical toe-off is 15 to 20 percent greater than body weight. The load-bearing function of the forefoot is thought to be three times that of the hindfoot during the walking cycle.[4]

DORSUM OF FOOT

The extensor tendons are enveloped by three separate synovial sheaths extending into the dorsum of the foot from the ankle. With exposure of extensor tendons, the temporalis fascial flap is an ideal cover for exposed tendons.[5] This thin 1-mm vascularized layer convolutes into the intertendonous spaces. If the flap is placed in a reversed fashion, the filmy fascial layer directly apposes the extensor tendons. Gliding is unimpaired. The undersurface of the temporalis fascial flap provides a vascular recipient bed for a split-thickness skin graft. The smooth dorsal contour does not alter footwear sizing.

Case 1

A 28-year-old woman was involved in a motor vehicle accident, sustaining a degloving injury with considerable soft tissue loss to the right foot (Fig. 4-1). On examination, a 12 × 8 cm soft tissue defect over the dorsum of the foot with exposure of the extensor digitorum communis tendons at the depth of the wound was found. The peritenon was denuded. The defect was initially debrided and treated by local wound care. One week after injury, the right foot was reconstructed with a free microvascular temporalis fascial flap plus split-thickness skin graft. The temporalis artery and vein were anastomosed end-to-end to the dorsalis pedis artery and vena comitans. Six months later, the healed graft was flush with the dorsal surface of the foot. Adaptation to footwear was excellent. Full extension of the toes was preserved.

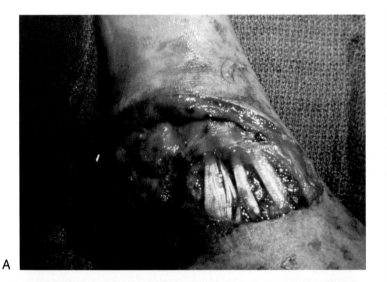

A

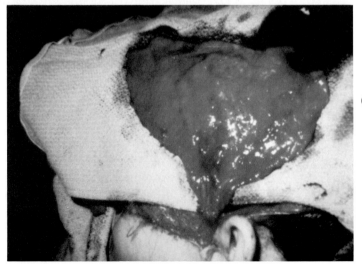

B

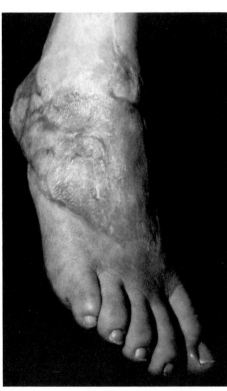

C

Fig. 4-1. (A) Soft tissue avulsion (12 × 8 cm) of dorsum of foot with exposure of extensor tendons. **(B)** Temporoparietal fascial flap from donor scalp. **(C)** Post free flap transfer with split-thickness skin graft.

ANKLE

The thin skin of the ankle is nonessential for weight bearing but must withstand the shear force of footwear and external trauma. I prefer coverage with an ipsilateral arterialized dorsalis pedis flap[6] (Fig. 4-2). This flap contours well over the malleolar prominence. Sensory preservation is not necessary. This method precludes distant pedicle flaps. The nonbulky glabrous skin is satisfactory for high-top shoes and is cosmetically pleasing in women beneath hosiery. Of particular advantage is that the donor skin is confined to the same foot.

Case 2

A 37-year-old woman twisted her left ankle, sustaining a spiral fracture of the distal fibula. This was initially treated by an orthopedic surgeon with open reduction and internal fixation. One day postsurgery, a secondary cellulitis ensued, followed by an open dehiscence of the wound and exposure of the surgical hardware. The metallic hardware was removed and the left ankle was debrided 3 months after injury, resulting in a 7 × 3.5 cm open draining defect. Following intensive topical wound care, the left ankle ulcer was reconstructed with a vascularized dorsalis pedis flap from the dorsum of the foot. The dorsal skin island was brought through a subcutaneous tunnel deep to the tibialis anterior tendon. The donor site was closed with a split-thickness skin graft and bolster dressing. The left ankle defect healed without sequelae.

CALCANEUS

Small defects of the calcaneus of less than 2 cm are easily covered by subfascial axial flaps[7,8] or with adjacent plantar skin preserving the plantar sensory nerve.[9] I prefer the latter procedure.

Case 3

A 66-year-old man sustained a gunshot wound to the left foot in 1947 (Fig. 4-3). Over the last 40 years, a nonhealing ulcer over the distal calcaneus persistently drained. The chronic scar and hypertrophic bony spurs were excised, and the defect was covered with a laterally based arterialized transposition flap. The lateral plantar nerve was preserved by intrafascicular microscopic dissection to allow for mobilization of the sensate flap. The donor defect in the non-weight-bearing area was grafted with split skin.

In larger defects, the dorsalis pedis flap, either as an ipsilateral island[6] or a free microvascular flap,[10] provides durable skin, minimal subcutaneous tissue, and the potential for reinnervation leading to protective sensation (Fig. 4-4). This innervated flap is well suited for the weight-bearing heel.[11] Thin split-thickness skin grafts alone have been used.[12] Patients, however, exhibit the tendency to shift weight from the grafted area to other nongrafted portions of the foot.[13] Flap skin with a thin subcutaneous pad reduces the shear forces and diffuses the weight over the contact surfaces. In my experience, the dorsalis pedis flap adheres to the calcaneus and functionally and cosmetically simulates the normal heel pad.

The ipsilateral island pedicle flap is used in more proximal defects of the heel. Additional length may be achieved by more proximal mobilization of the anterior tibial artery and superficial peroneal nerve to the midcalf. Preoperative assessment by arteriography or by selective Doppler patency of both vessels is essential. If the anterior tibial vessel is disrupted, free flap coverage from the other foot is mandated. Ipsilateral coverage is essential in diabetics, owing to the propensity of donor site graft failure because of small vessel disease.

The recipient nerve is the calcaneal branch of the posterior tibial or the sural nerve. Even in ipsilateral cases the superficial peroneal nerve can be repaired to the more anatomically appropriate nerve. Results have been good protective sensation in all cases. No secondary breakdown after direct weight bearing has been noted.

The donor site graft, which has gained a bad reputation,[14] has not posed a problem in Duncan's five cases[11] and in eight cases in my series with the one exception of loss of split-thickness skin graft in a brittle juvenile diabetic. Careful closure of the epitenon is essential prior to application of the split-thickness graft. In addition, the

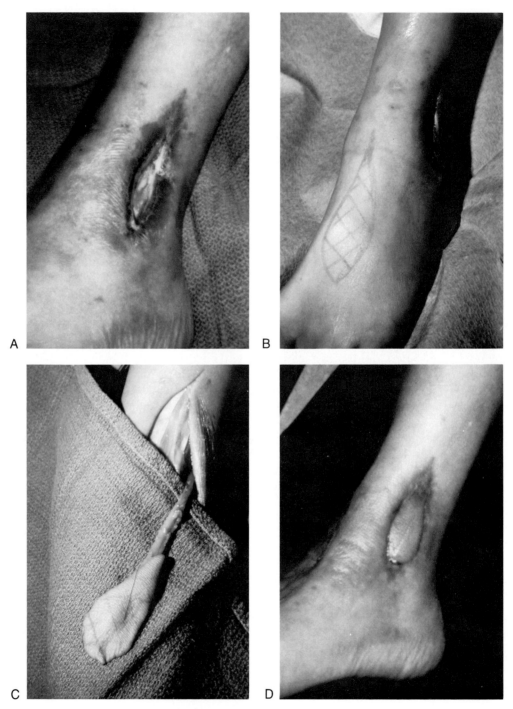

Fig. 4-2. **(A)** Infected ulceration (7 × 3.5 cm) of medial malleolus with exposed hardware. **(B & C)** Ipsilateral dorsalis pedis flap elevated on vascular pedicle. **(D)** Flap healed.

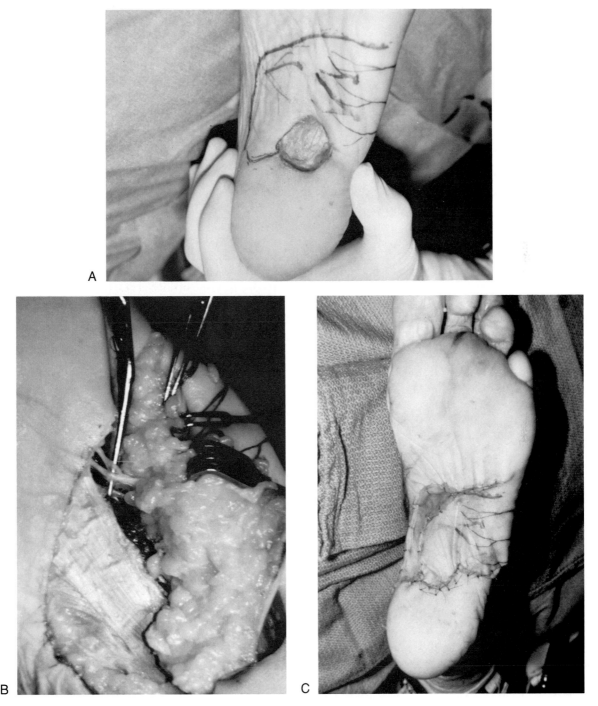

Fig. 4-3. (**A**) Chronic ulcer (3.5 cm) of distal calcaneus. (**B**) Lateral plantar nerve preserved by intrafascicular microscopic dissection. (**C**) Flap rotated onto weight-bearing surface.

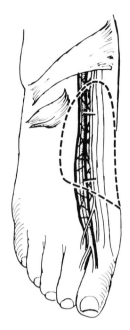

Fig. 4-4. Dorsalis pedis composite flap centered over axial arteriovenous pedicle. Innervation is from superficial peroneal nerve branches.

extensor hallucis longus tendon is displaced beneath the medial foot skin. The foot is immobilized and elevated for 10 days postsurgery prior to partial weight bearing.

Case 4

A 17-year-old boy sustained a severe crush injury to the right foot in a train accident (Fig. 4-5). The right foot was initially debrided and resurfaced with a split-thickness skin graft. The split-thickness skin graft healed satisfactorily, but persistent reulceration occurred with weight bearing. Dorsiflexion contracture of the right ankle with foreshortening of the Achilles tendon occurred secondary to the fracture. The 12 × 15 cm area of split-thickness graft extended over the medial malleous, calcaneus, and lateral aspect of the right foot. Eight months after injury, the right heel was reconstructed with an arterialized neurosensory dorsalis pedis flap from the dorsum of the foot. The superficial peroneal nerve was repaired to the calcaneal branch of the posterior tibial nerve for anatomic accuracy. Postsurgically

the flap healed satisfactorily. No recurrent ulcerations were noted. Secondary lengthening of the Achilles tendon was done 6 months later by an orthopedic surgeon.

Case 5

A 52-year-old man stepped onto a nail, sustaining a puncture wound that developed into a progressive osteomyelitis causing erosion and cystic formation of the calcaneus (Fig. 4-6). Six days preoperatively, the sequestrum of the calcaneus was resected and clindamycin and gentamicin antibiotics were given. Thirteen years after injury, the left heel was reconstructed with a free microvascular transfer of an 8 × 5 cm dorsalis pedis free flap from the other foot. The superficial and deep peroneal nerves were repaired to the recipient sural nerve. Healing was satisfactory. No secondary drainage was encountered at follow-up 2 years later. Full weight bearing was possible.

MEDIAL FOOT

The non-weight-bearing medial foot can accommodate either thick durable skin or muscle for protection against footwear shear. Sensation is not essential. A free muscle flap plus split-thickness skin graft is preferable for exposed or draining bone to reduce infection.[15,16] The dorsalis pedis flap is suitable for replacement of an attenuated skin graft.

Case 6

A 28-year-old woman was involved in a motor vehicle accident sustaining a crush injury of the left foot (same patient as in Case 1) (Fig. 4-7). The exposed first metatarsal and metatarsophalangeal joint were debrided, and chronic drainage was treated by local wound care. One month later, the left foot was reconstructed with a free microvascular gracilis muscle transplant from the left medial thigh and covered with mesh split-thickness skin graft. Postsurgical healing was satisfactory.

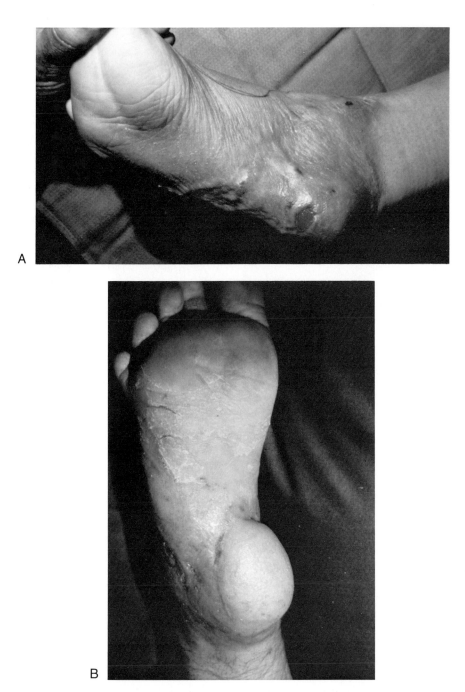

Fig. 4-5. (**A**) Recurrent ulceration on weight-bearing surface. (**B**) Ipsilateral dorsalis pedis flap neurosensory coverage.

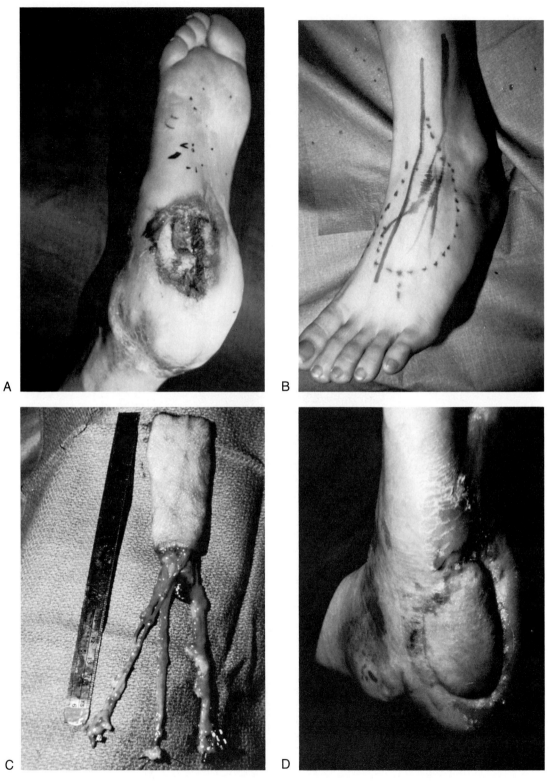

Fig. 4-6. (A) Osteomyelitis of calcaneus. **(B)** Outline of dorsalis pedis flap on contralateral foot. **(C)** Arterial, venous, nerve pedicles. **(D)** Healed flap after microsurgical revascularization and reinnervation.

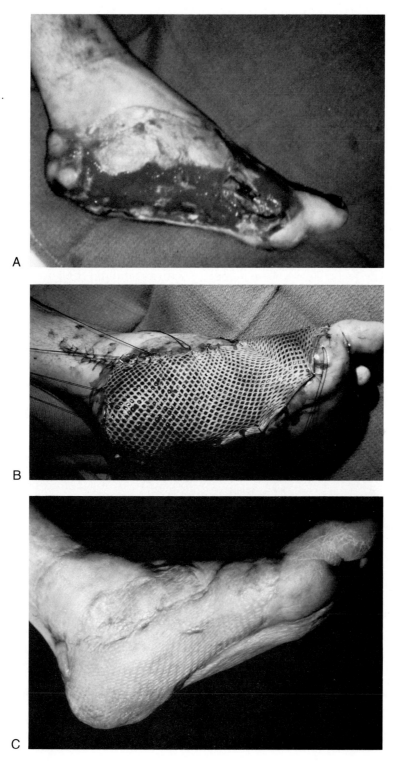

Fig. 4-7. (**A**) Crush avulsion of medial foot with exposed metatarsophalangeal joint. (**B**) Free gracilis muscle flap coverage with mesh skin graft. (**C**) Healed flap coverage.

Special orthotic footwear was designed to redistribute weight to the lateral plantar weight-bearing surface. No recurrent ulcerations were noted. Gait was satisfactory.

Case 7

A 22-year-old laborer caught his left foot in a metal auger, sustaining a severe crush injury. The first metatarsal shaft along with the great toe was resected in the initial debridement. Temporary coverage was with split-thickness skin graft. Recurrent shearing ulcers were encountered with footwear, particularly heavy work boots. Overcompensation caused callus formation on the lateral aspect of the foot. The 8 × 4 cm defect over the medial aspect of the left foot was reconstructed with a free dorsalis pedis flap from the opposite foot. The donor superficial peroneal nerve was repaired to the recipient deep peroneal nerve. Recovery of protective sensation was adequate. No further problems with footwear were encountered.

FOREFOOT

A sensate durable flap is necessary for load bearing across the metatarsal heads during step-off. An innervated muscle flap[17] provides good coverage; however, the bulkiness precludes form-fitting shoes. Durable skin is particularly important if an equinus defect is present as a result of Achilles tendon shortening. I prefer the dorsalis pedis neurosensory free flap.

Case 8

A 22-year-old laborer crushed his right foot with a metal rod (Fig. 4-8). Debridement entailed removal of the toes at the transmetatarsal level. The forefoot was shortened by approximately 3 cm. Ulcers persisted over the bony prominences of the first and fifth metatarsal heads. The right foot was reconstructed with a free microsurgical transfer of neurovascular dorsalis pedis flap from the dorsum of the left foot. The fascicles of both

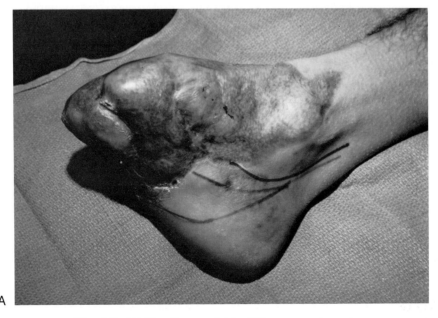

A

Fig. 4-8. (A) Forefoot avulsion. (*Figure continues.*)

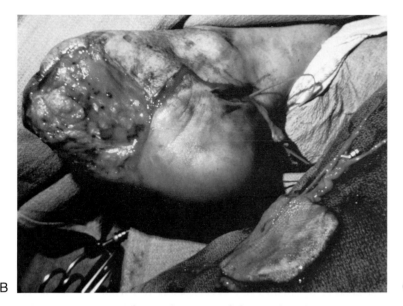

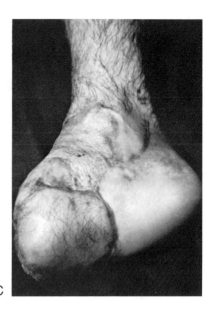

B   C

Fig. 4-8 (*Continued*). (**B**) Excision of skin graft and preparation of free flap. (**C**) Sensate skin coverage.

the superficial and deep peroneal nerves were grouped together and repaired to the medial and lateral plantar sensory nerves. Return protective sensation was satisfactory. Over-the-counter footwear with toe padding was tolerated.

PLANTAR SOLE

The entire plantar foot can be resurfaced with a large free neurosensory flap from the dorsum of the contralateral foot. The flap design combines the anatomic vascular territories of the dorsalis pedis flap[6] and the first webspace flap.[18,19] The dorsalis pedis flap extending from the extensor retinaculum proximally to near the webspace distally can supply as much as 14 × 12 cm of skin if the "random" areas are properly deployed.[6] The maximum size of the first webspace flap with dorsal and plantar extensions is 12 × 8 cm.[20] Both flaps are axial flaps nourished by the dorsalis pedis artery and its terminal branches. Anatomic territories of the two overlap the distal metatarsals, although Mann and Acland have found the

first dorsal metatarsal artery to be absent in 14 percent of 23 dissections. Donor two-point discrimination averages 32 mm on the dorsum of the foot, 11.3 mm on the lateral surface of the great toe, and 16.4 mm on the medial surface of the second toe.[18] Return of pressure sensation reduces neurotrophic ulceration thought to be due to the inability to perceive friction during walking.[21]

Case 9

A 24-year-old woman sustained a degloving injury of the entire left foot when she caught her left foot beneath a train (Fig. 4-9). She initially underwent debridement and wound closure with multiple split-thickness skin grafts. The avulsed plantar surface of the foot was anesthetic. The graft was ulcerated over the exposed first metatarsal head. The plantar foot was resurfaced with a 19 × 12 cm combined dorsalis pedis and first webspace flap. The superficial and deep peroneal nerves were repaired en bloc to the posterior tibial nerve. The bulk of the flap was used to

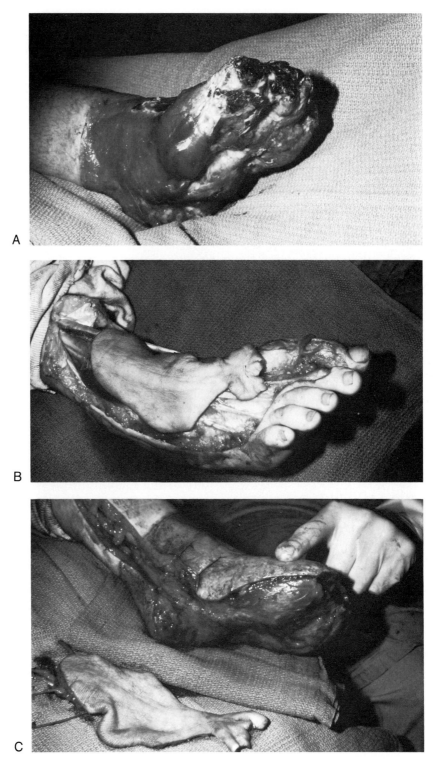

Fig. 4-9. (**A**) Degloving injury of foot. (**B**) Design of 19 × 12 cm flaps from opposite foot. (**C**) Flap ready for inset. (*Figure continues.*)

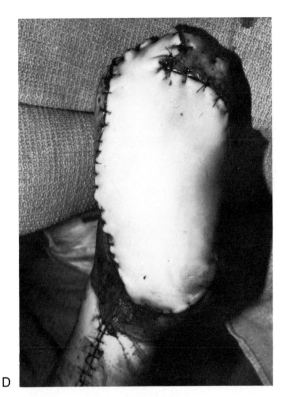

D

Fig. 4-9 (*Continued*). **(D)** Flap inset.

provide durable coverage over the planatar surface of the foot. The first webspace extension was
draped over the exposed first, second, and third
metatarsal heads. Approximately 20 percent of
the distal lateral portion of the flap was lost secondarily to necrosis. Long term, the successful
flap transfer provided thick soft tissue coverage
and protective sensation for weight bearing. A
minor breakdown was noted over the metatarsal
heads because of Achilles tendon shortening (the
patient refused Achilles tendon-lengthening procedure).

Alternative to this approach is the application
of the innervated radial forearm flap (Fig. 4-10).
This flap, originally described by Song et al.,[22]
has been applied to plantar foot defects as large
as 25 × 13 cm.[23]

Case 10

A 44-year-old man crushed his left foot beneath
a forklift, avulsing the sole and fracturing the second through fourth metatarsals (Fig. 4-11). The
wound was initially treated by debridement and
delayed skin grafts. On clinical examination, a 16
× 16 cm plantar defect extended over the calcaneus, medial arch, and midsole. A 3 × 2 cm crater of infected draining bone (*Pseudomonas
maltophilia, Staphylococcus epidermidis, Fusar-
ium*) was present over the fourth metatarsus. The
skin of the forefoot and great, second, and third
toes was insensate. Four months after injury, the
plantar sole was resurfaced with a "custom-fit"
Chinese neurosensory flap from the forearm innervated from the posterior tibial nerve. The superficial sensory branch of the radial nerve was
used to bridge the avulsion gap for interfascicular
repair to the common digital nerves of the great,
second, and third toes. Six months later, protective sensation was restored to the flaps. Advancing Tinel's sign was detected in the forefoot and
toes.

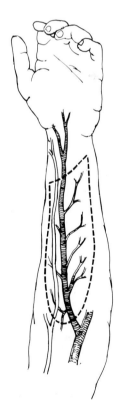

Fig. 4-10. Design of Chinese flap centered over radial
artery and superficial radial nerve of forearm.

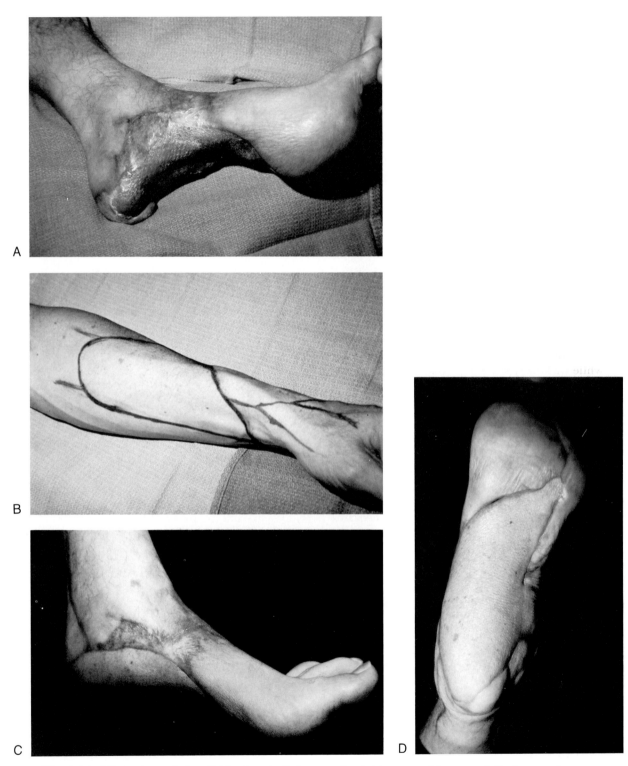

Fig. 4-11. (**A**) Avulsion defect (16 by 6 cm) of plantar sole. (**B**) Design of "custom fit" Chinese flaps on forearm. (**C & D**) Flaps inset.

SUMMARY

I have attempted to present a rational approach to soft tissue coverage of the foot employing microsurgical techniques. Ideal selection of the donor site is determined by optimal thickness, durability, sensibility, and surgeon facility for execution of the flap. Each flap design should be specifically tailored to the recipient's needs.

REFERENCES

1. Hick JH: Mechanics of the foot. II: The plantar aponeurosis and the arch. J Anat 88:25, 1954
2. Jones FW: Structure and Function as Seen in the Foot. p. 252. Williams & Wilkins, Baltimore, 1944
3. Mann RA: Biomechanics. In Jahss RH (ed): Disorders of the Foot. WB Saunders, Philadelphia, 1982
4. Grundy M, Tosh B, McLeish RD et al: An investigation of the centers of pressure under the foot while walking. J Bone Joint Surg 57B:98, 1975
5. Brent B, Upton J, Acland RD et al: Experience with the temporoparietal fascial free flap. Plast Reconstr Surg 76:177, 1985
6. McGraw JB, Furlow CT, Jr: The dorsalis pedis arterialized flap. Plast Recontr Surg 55:177, 1975
7. Reiffel RS, McCarthy JG: Coverage of heel and sole defects: a new subfascial arterialized flap. Plast Reconstr Surg 66:250, 1980
8. Shanahan RE, Gingrass RP: Medial plantar sensory flap coverage of heel defects. Plast Reconstr Surg 64:295, 1979
9. Shaw WW, Hidalgo DH: Anatomic basis of plantar flap design: clinical applications. Plast Reconstr Surg 78:415, 1986
10. Robinson DW: Microsurgical transfer of the dorsalis pedis neurovascular island flap. Br J Plast Surg 29:209, 1976
11. Duncan MJ, Zuker RM, Manktelow RT: Resurfacing weight bearing areas of the heel: the role of the dorsalis pedis innervated free tissue transfer. J Reconstr Microsurg 1:201, 1985
12. Woltering EA, Thorpe WP, Reed JK, Rosenberg SA: Split thickness skin grafting of the plantar surface of the foot after wide excision of neoplasms of the skin. Surg Gynecol Obstet 149:229, 1979
13. Sommerland BC, McGrouther DA: Resurfacing of the sole: long term follow up and comparison of techniques. Br J Plast Surg 35:107, 1978
14. Serafin D, Voci VE: Reconstruction of the lower extremity: microsurgical composite tissue transplantation. Clin Plast Surg 10:55, 1983
15. Mathes SJ, Alpert BS, Chang N: Use of the muscle flap in chronic osteomyelitis; experimental and clinical correlation. Plast Reconstr Surg 69:815, 1982
16. Stevenson TE, Mathes SW: Management of foot injuries with free muscle flaps. Plast Reconstr Surg 78:665, 1986
17. Dabb RW, Conklin WT: A sensory innervated latissimus dorsi musculocutaneous free flap: case report. J Microsurg 2:289, 1981
18. May JW, Chait LA, Cohen BE, O'Brien BMC: Free neurovascular flap from the first web space of the foot in hand reconstruction. J Hand Surg 2:387, 1977
19. Strauch B, Tsur H: Restoration of sensation to the hand by a free neurovascular island flap from the first web space of the foot. Plast Reconstr Surg 52:361, 1978
20. Morrison WA, O'Brien BMC, MacLeod AM, Gilbert A: Neurovascular free flaps from the foot for innervation of the hand. J Hand Surg 3:235, 1978
21. Snyder GB, Edgerton MT: The principle of the island neurovascular flap with management of ulcerated anesthetic weight areas of the lower extremity. Plast Reconstr Surg 36:518, 1965
22. Song R, Gao Y, Song Y et al: The forearm flap. Clin Plast Surg 9:21, 1982
23. Chicarilli ZN, Price GJ: Complete plantar foot coverage with the free neurosensory radial forearm flap. Plast Reconstr Surg 78:94, 1986

5

Fixation Techniques for Fractures

Stephen V. Corey, D.P.M.
Bradley D. Castellano, D.P.M.
John A. Ruch, D.P.M.

Open reduction and internal fixation of fractures has traditionally implied that closed reduction methods failed to provide satisfactory alignment. There are, however, many reasons for choosing operative treatment of a fracture, only one of which is poor alignment.

The goal of all fracture treatment is to obtain union of the fractured bones. Some fractures have a greater propensity to heal without the benefit of assistance. The prognosis innate to a specific fracture can be helpful in the decision-making process when open reduction is contemplated.[1]

The rate of healing of fractures is directly proportional to the gap distance.[2–4] Therefore, efforts to reduce the gap between fracture ends are well founded. Often a satisfactory reduction can be obtained with closed manipulation and external splintage. The decision to perform open reduction and internal fixation should then be based on sound understanding of the functional and structural requirements of the injured part. Fractures that poorly tolerate even minimal displacement such as intra-articular fractures are often best treated operatively.

Internal fixation can be achieved by two methods: splintage or interfragmental compression. This chapter attempts to place in perspective the role of open reduction and internal fixation. We describe the materials and techniques available to the modern surgeon as well as discuss their application in foot and ankle surgery.

FACTORS AFFECTING THE METHOD OF FIXATION

There are many factors that will influence the type and method of fixation. The most elementary and important of these is the inherent stability of the fracture itself.[5] This is determined by intrinsic and extrinsic factors.

Intrinsic Factors

Intrinsic factors include fracture configuration, bone composition, and bone quality. Transverse fracture configurations are inherently more stable than obliquely oriented fractures. Oblique or spiral fractures tend to be displaced with axial loads, resulting in shortening of the segment. Fractures with intact cortical walls such as greenstick or torus fractures are less likely to displace. Finally, comminution has a deleterious effect on fracture stability (Fig. 5-1).

Bone composition refers to cancellous and cortical makeup. Fractures in cancellous bone usually have a greater degree of friction between fragments owing to bone to bone contact. Fractures that occur in areas that are primarily cortical will have less stabilizing effect because of friction. Surface contact, however, could be a resistant force in achieving closed reduction. Finally methods of internal fixation often will be influ-

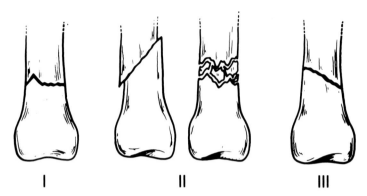

Fig. 5-1. Charnley's classification of fractures is based on intrinsic stability of fracture to withstand forces that tend to telescope the fragments. (I) Stable. (II) Unstable. (III) Potentially stable. (From McGlamry,[24] with permission.)

enced by bone composition since some devices work well in cancellous areas while others are better adapted to cortical bone.

Bone quality is the last intrinsic factor affecting the stability of the fracture. Pathologic fractures and fractures occurring in osteopenic bone may require the added support afforded by internal fixation. Poor bone quality will also affect the choice of fixation since purchase is compromised in these regions.

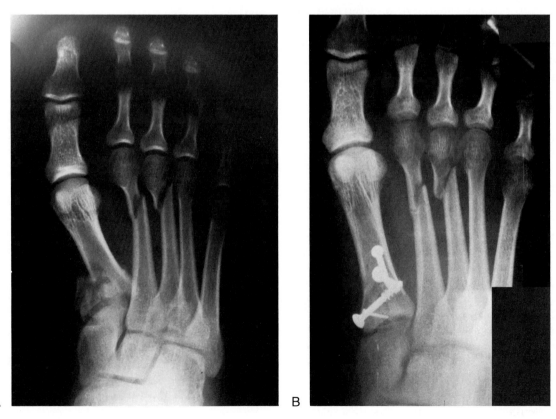

Fig. 5-2. (A & B) Vassal's principle is depicted by the fracture reduction shown. Reduction and fixation of the first metatarsal fracture resulted in spontaneous reduction of the lesser metatarsal fractures.

Extrinsic Factors

Soft tissue attachments play a major role in the stability of a fracture, and their influences are important in reduction. Tendons, ligaments, and periosteum can either aid in manipulation of a fracture or prevent successful reduction. Some operative methods utilize the tensile forces applied by tendons and ligaments to add compression and stabilization, i.e., tension banding.[6]

When multiple fractures exist, soft tissue attachments between larger fragments can be instrumental in providing satisfactory realignment and stabilization. This principle is known as the vassal rule and states that fixation of the dominant fracture will afford stabilization to the subordinate fracture (Fig. 5-2).

Forces that tend to cause a bone to fracture will also affect the stability of the fracture. These forces must be controlled by the fixation device employed if lasting immobilization is to be achieved. The mechanical forces that affect fracture stability include bending, torsion, and shear. Compression tends to cause fracture of bones; however, once the fracture occurs it will usually be a stabilizing force. Control of extrinsic forces is based on the two mechanical principles of rigid internal fixation and splintage.

GOALS OF FIXATION

There are numerous methods and materials available for operative management of fractures. There are many good choices for a specific fracture situation, and there are also some poor choices.

The goals of internal fixation techniques were clearly designated by the Swiss Arbeitgemeinshaft für Osteosynthesisfragen (AO) group (Association for the Study of Internal Fixation) (ASIF). They described four conditions that were prerequisite for "perfect internal fixation."[7] The first of these is anatomic reduction of the fracture. As stated earlier, this is especially critical in the intra-articular fracture. Stable internal fixation is the second principle and is fundamental to all fracture healing.[8] The fixation methods should

comply with the biomechanical demands of the lower extremity. The surgical technique should maintain the vascular supply to the injured tissue. Atraumatic surgery, therefore, is the third important concept. The final goal is early active mobilization of the injured limb to prevent the stiffness and atrophy caused by cast disease.

Some of the methods presented here comply with these principles. All of these goals may not be achievable or implemented in some fracture situations. However, these criteria should always remain the standard by which any fixation technique is measured.

SPLINTAGE TECHNIQUES

Reapproximation and fixation of fracture fragments utilizing the most basic techniques often provides adequate stabilization. Combining basic internal fixation devices with casting is a frequently used treatment regimen. Non-weight bearing will also sometimes be a necessary adjunct. Proper application of these splintage techniques will usually give a quite satisfactory result for many fracture situations.

Kirschner Wires and Steinmann Pins

Pin fixation is one of the simplest forms of fixation; however, since it is an easily applied technique it is also often misused. Most surgeons agree that pin fixation can be useful in maintaining fragment alignment. For this reason they are frequently used as temporary fixation while more permanent methods are applied. Pin fixation does have several applications as a singular or combination technique.

Kirschner wires are supplied in various sizes. The most frequently used sizes are 0.035, 0.045, and 0.062 inches in diameter. Both smooth and threaded versions are available. The tips are usually pointed to allow ease in bone penetration.

Steinmann pins are larger than Kirschner wires. The most frequently used size in foot surgery is 5/64 inches in diameter. These pins also are pointed at each end. They are used in a similar manner as Kirschner wires when a more substantial device is desirable.

Single pin fixation has few advantages over other techniques. Stabilization of small fragments that have only minor propensity for disruption may be an indication for this method. Another application of this technique is intramedullary fixation of displaced transverse metatarsal fractures. Smooth Kirschner wire fixation is the method of choice when a physeal plate must be traversed. (Fig. 5-3).

The disadvantages of single pin fixation include poor resistance to distraction and rotatory forces. Resistance to bending forces will depend on the diameter of the pin being utilized. Failure of pin fixation caused by any of the above forces can be diminished by adding additional pins in divergent directions. Numerous investigators have demonstrated that crossed Kirschner wire fixation is far superior to single pin fixation.[9]

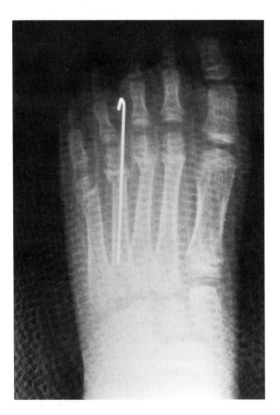

Fig. 5-3. Pinning across an open physis should always be performed with a smooth wire to help prevent destruction and early closure of the physis.

Threaded Kirschner wires offer the advantage of resistance to distraction or pull-out. However, care should be taken to prevent separation of the fracture fragments as the far fragment is penetrated. This is accomplished by holding the fragments compressed as the wire is inserted. When bending and torsional forces are also present, these devices become less reliable. Fatigue and failure are more likely to occur since threaded Kirschner wires have a decreased core diameter and grooved stress risers.[10]

Pins can be buried within the surgical wound or left transcutaneous if ease in removal is preferred. Pins exiting the skin are more likely to cause skin irritation, and infection of the pin tract site is always possible. These complications can be minimized by taking measures to reduce motion at the skin–pin interface. Disruption of the seal at the exit site is the major cause of opportunistic pin tract infection.

Smooth pins have a tendency to migrate. Accidental dislodgement or loss of the pin into the deeper tissues can easily complicate even the best fixation method. Bending of the wire is an easy remedy to prevent pin migration into the wound. Proper bandaging over the pin is the best prevention of accidental extraction.

Another method of utilizing Kirschner wires and Steinmann pins is through percutaneous fixation. While using pins in this manner may seem attractive, experience has shown that it is difficult to maintain the reduction and to place the fixation accurately. Fluoroscopy guidance can be beneficial; however, intraoperative triplanar radiographic evaluation is necessary to confirm accurate reduction and pin position. Additionally, the wire will be external and carry with it the disadvantage of possible pin tract infection. Therefore, this method should be reserved for situations in which the above disadvantages are outweighed by this less invasive technique.[11]

Surgical Stainless Steel Wire

There are two basic techniques that utilize surgical stainless steel wire: intraosseous wire loop and cerclage wire. These techniques have been described and used for many years with varying degrees of success. Proper application and insight into reasons for failure are presented.

Surgical stainless steel wire is supplied in numerous sizes. Sizes are measured in gauges. The larger the gauge, the smaller the diameter of the wire. Commonly used gauges occur in the range of 30 to 18. Thinner gauge wire has less tensile strength but is more flexible and easier to manipulate. Thicker gauge wire offers the advantage of greater tensile strength; however, it is more likely to kink when bent at acute angles. Thicker gauge wire is generally used for bone fixation, while thinner gauge wire is usually reserved for suturing of soft tissues such as skin and tendon.

Fatigue and failure of wire has been a common complication of its use in internal fixation. In most cases, the failure is caused by back-and-forth intermittent bending forces. Unidirectional bending is well tolerated by stainless steel and is one of the reasons it is chosen over carbon steel.[12] For this reason, care should be taken to manipulate the wire as little as possible during insertion of the fixation to prevent fatigue and failure.

Cerclage wire techniques have been condemned by numerous researchers, who state that a high propensity for nonunion exists. The failure was thought to be the result of avascular necrosis caused by strangulation of the bone ends by the encircling wire.[5] However, Boehler thought that excessive periosteal stripping and traumatic surgical technique was a more likely cause for the nonunion phenomenon.[13] Motion across the fracture secondary to insufficient stability is more likely cause for the failure seen following use of this type of fixation.[14]

Cerclage or circumferential wiring can be used in two ways. The first application is to prevent telescoping of an oblique fracture (Fig. 5-4). Single or multiple loops can be used to achieve stabilization. The second method is as a gathering influence to control small fragments in combination with other forms of fixation.

Intraosseous wire loops are generally used to stabilize small fracture fragments. Bones with thick cortical walls are best suited for this type of fixation since pull-through is a common complication. This form of fixation has proved to be effective in many fracture situations that occur in the foot and ankle. The degree of stability has

been shown to be directly related to the number of cortices purchased by the wire loop. Purchase of only two cortices is far inferior to purchase of four or more cortices. Wire loops should be placed perpendicular to the fracture in either a horizontal or vertical mattress fashion. When two loops are used, they should be oriented 90 degrees to each other to obtain maximum stabilizing affect.[15] Outer metatarsal fractures (first and fifth metatarsals) are somewhat more amenable to this method since access to three cortical walls is readily available. Oblique loops will often be necessary for fixation of inner metatarsals.

Staple Fixation

Staples have traditionally been used for the fixation of elective osteotomies and anchoring of detached ligaments and tendons. Their use in the treatment of fractures is somewhat limited since other forms of fixation generally have advantages over staples. However, some fracture situations may be effectively managed by this technique.

Staples are supplied in various forms but are generally made up of two or more prongs and an intervening bar or plate. The simplest form of staple is the Blount staple. Richards and Stone staples are other forms that will be discussed. A pneumatically driven staple gun is currently being marketed by 3-M (3-M Orthopedic Division, St. Paul, MN). This power stapler has several advantages over manually driven staples.

Staples are almost exclusively designed for use in cancellous bone. The force of impact as a staple is driven is generally quite substantial. Insertion of staples into thick cortical bone carries a significant risk of secondary fracture. Predrilling of the insertion sites may be helpful in preventing secondary fracture lines. Most manufactures suggest that staple use be restricted to cancellous regions. Therefore, staples have been applied to fractures of the malleoli and tarsal bones.[16]

The limitations of staple fixation in trauma surgery lie in their lack of precision and finesse. Instrumentation is somewhat crude and exact placement can be difficult. Reduction of the fracture by a second person while the surgeon places the staple will often be necessary. Even when

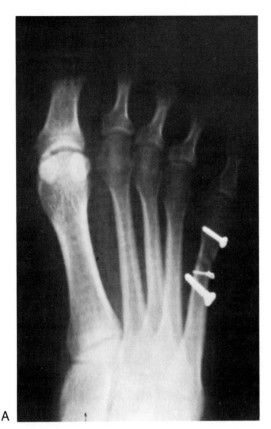
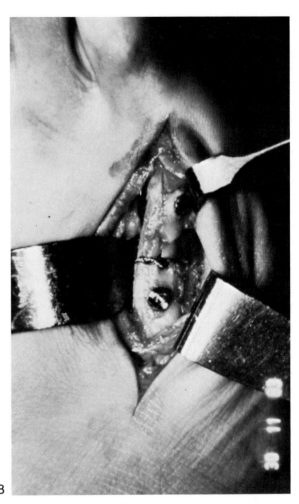

A   B

Fig. 5-4. (A & B) This oblique fracture of the fifth metatarsal is shown fixated with a combination of screw and cerclage wiring. The wire helps prevent telescoping of the oblique fracture and gathers the comminuted portions of the fracture.

extra help is available, dislodgement of the fragments during impaction of the staple is possible.

Fracture configuration and stability is rarely ideal for staple fixation. Transverse fractures within cancellous bone that also will resist the force of impaction of the staple are not common situations. Staples resist distraction forces across the fracture site but generally do not withstand shear and bending forces. Shear and bending forces dislodge the staple and the device backs out. This has been compensated to some degree by placing barbs on each of the prongs of the staple. Square rather than rounded prongs give

additional resistance to torsional forces. As with most fracture situations, two or more points of fixation provide better resistance to rotational forces. A 90-degree angle between staples affords the most secure fixation.

One fracture situation in which staple fixation has traditionally been utilized is the joint depression calcaneal fracture. However, staple prongs are usually not long enough to perform the vital task of fixating the lateral portion of the posterior facet to the medial sustentacular fragment.[17] Finally this intra-articular fracture probably warrants a greater degree of precision in operative technique than is afforded by this somewhat crude method of fixation.

Staples are usually inserted with a specialized driver that grips the staple while it is being impacted with a mallet. Proper technique and careful placement of the staple are very important since removal of a misdirected staple and repeated insertion significantly compromises the bones being fixated. The fracture should be held reduced and the limb supported while the staple is impacted. The staple should be driven with as few strokes of the mallet as possible. Rocking occurs when the staple is driven in slightly different directions with each stroke of the mallet. This results in loss of contact between the staple and the bone and compromised fixation.[18]

Many of the problems associated with staple fixation are directly related to the method of insertion. A recent advance in staple fixation technique has employed a pneumatic-powered staple driver system. The manufacturer emphasizes that the 3-M stapler is intended for metaphyseal regions with cortical thickness less than 2 mm. Therefore, its use is contraindicated in diaphyseal regions. Other contraindications include areas where the staple bridge is exposed to significant compression, pure shear, or torsion. Ostgaard and Herberts warn that osteopenic bone is another relative contraindication.[16]

RIGID INTERNAL FIXATION

Methods of fixation can be categorized based on the degree of stability between the fracture fragments. Relative motion across a fracture site will almost certainly occur if simple splintage is used to stabilize the fragments. Motion between healing bone ends is the primary cause for unpredictable healing and lack of differentiation of callus to bone tissue.[3] It is possible for fractures to heal without callus formation, and this form of healing is the result of fractures that heal while rigidly fixated.

Advances in the technology of internal fixation have been led by the Swiss ASIF group. The complications of delayed union and nonunion associated with fractures treated by simple splint-

age prompted the development of more sophisticated materials and methods of fixation. The ASIF instrumentation has been copied by many surgical instrument manufacturers. However, the original ASIF implants that are distributed by Synthes (Synthesis Ltd. (USA), Wayne, PA) have been the most thoroughly tested by the technical commissions of the ASIF.

One difference between splintage and rigid internal fixation lies in the type of bone union that occurs. Typically, splinted fractures heal by means of callus formation. The amount of bone callus that forms is directly related to the gap and motion across the fracture site. The function of the callus is to reduce the motion and bridge the gap between bone fragments. This callus must undergo differentiation from fibrous to cartilaginous tissue and finally to bone. It is during this stage of differentiation that delay and arrest of bony union can occur. Shenk and Willenegger were the first to demonstrate that fractures of the extremities can occur without callus formation when fragments are rigidly fixated.[19] This is known as primary vascular bone healing. Rigid internal fixation implies that minimal gap exists between fracture fragments and that no motion occurs across the fracture site.

The advantages of rigid internal fixation over simple splintage are well documented.[4,20] The most significant advantages include more predictable bone healing and decreased convalescence.

Interfragmental Compression

Rigid internal fixation implies that compression exists between the fracture fragments. Interfragmental compression requires that the implants be placed under tension and that the bone fragments be relatively large. Interfragmental compression can be either static or dynamic.

Static interfragmental compression is the result of the tension exerted by the prestressed implant at the fracture interface. The lag effect exerted by properly inserted screws is the typical example of this form of interfragmental compression. Dynamic compression utilizes a combination of static force in conjunction with physiologic loads that naturally occur about the extremity. The classic example of dynamic compression is the tension-band technique.[6]

Lag Screw Technique

The most significant and versatile method of achieving static interfragmental compression is with the use of screws. Compression between fracture fragments requires that a screw be placed under tension by the lag technique. A lagged screw is one that engages only the far fragment with its threads. Compression occurs as the head of the screw contacts the near cortex and the threads purchasing the far fragment pull the fragments together. (Fig. 5-5).

Two basic screw designs exist—cortical and cancellous. Cortical screws have a fully threaded shaft, whereas cancellous screws are only threaded at the distal end. Both types of screws can be used to create interfragmental compression when properly inserted (Fig. 5-6).

Cortical Screws. Fully threaded screws are known as cortical screws. Since the degree of purchase is directly related to the number of threads in contact with the bone, the thread pattern for cortical screws is narrow. This allows the maximum number of threads to purchase the relatively thin cortical wall.

Cortical screws are supplied in various sizes that are based on the diameter of the threads (Fig. 5-7). The screw size should match the size of the fragments being fixated. Thinner cortical

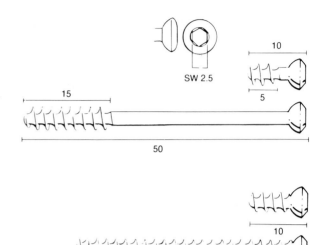

Fig. 5-6. Cancellous screws have a smooth shaft and contain threads at the distal aspect. Cortical screws are fully threaded. Each screw has advantages depending on the fracture situation. (From McGlamry,[24] with permission.)

walls are best purchased by the smaller screws with narrow thread patterns.

The techniques developed by the ASIF group for the insertion of cortical lag screws is well outlined in the *Manual of Internal Fixation*[7] and in *Internal Fixation of Small Fractures*.[21] As previously stated, to enable a screw to produce interfragmental compression the threads must purchase only the far fragment. Therefore, to achieve interfragmental compression with the fully threaded screw, the near fragment must be over-drilled to prevent purchase of the threads. Creating a hole slightly larger than the thread diameter allows the screw to glide through the near cortex.

Cancellous Screws. The cancellous screw is partially threaded, that is, the neck of the screw consists of a smooth shaft. Therefore, in most fracture situations over-drilling of the near fragment will not be necessary to produce interfragmental compression. However, care should be taken to ensure that no threads cross the fracture line, especially when the near fragment is significantly larger than the far fragment. (Fig. 5-8).

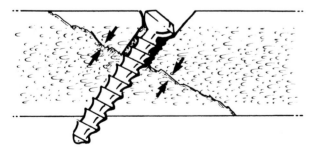

Fig. 5-5. Proper insertion of a cortical screw is shown. Note that the near fragment is over-drilled to allow gliding of the threads. As the screw head contacts the near cortex compression occurs across the fracture interface. (Adapted from McGlamry,[24] with permission.)

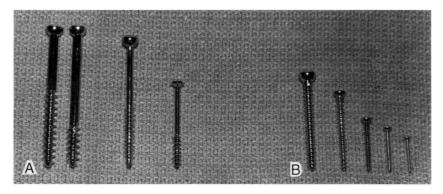

Fig. 5-7. The types of ASIF screws available. (**A**) Cancellous screws: 6.5 mm, long and short thread; 4.5 mm malleolar; 4.0 mm. (**B**) Cortical screws: 4.5 mm; 3.5 mm; 2.7 mm; 2.0 mm; and 1.5 mm.

Cancellous screws have a wider thread pattern and a thinner core diameter (Fig. 5-6). This allows a greater degree of bone-to-screw contact in the more porous trabecular bone found in metaphyseal regions. Variations of the cancellous screw consist of a fully threaded version, different thread lengths, and a self-tapping malleolar screw (Fig. 5-7).

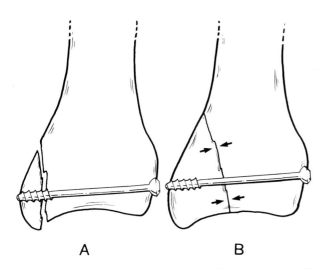

Fig. 5-8. Even when using cancellous screws, all threads must be distal to the fracture line. (**A**) When screw threads span the fracture line, distraction occurs. (**B**) Fracture line is spanned by smooth shaft, and interfragmental compression is produced. (From McGlamry,[24] with permission.)

Techniques of Screw Fixation

Fixation of fractures with screws demands that proper technique and screw orientation be used to ensure that the fracture remains anatomically reduced. Compression at the fracture interface should be directed as perpendicular to the fracture line as possible. Therefore, the ideal fracture situation is one in which the fracture line and the near cortex are parallel and the screw is oriented 90 degrees to both. Unfortunately, the ideal situation rarely exists and compromise is a frequent necessity.

Oblique fractures will often require that a lag screw be oriented at an acute angle to the cortex to achieve interfragmental compression. Although the maximum amount of compression is gained if the screw is oriented 90 degrees to the fracture line, poor stability results under axial loads.[21] Axial loading of the oblique fracture results in telescoping of the fragments and loss of stability (Fig. 5-9). When a single screw is used to produce compression at the fracture interface, it must be oriented at an angle halfway between perpendicular to the cortex and perpendicular to the fracture line.

Long oblique or spiral fractures are often amenable to multiple screw fixation. In this situation, the first screw inserted should maintain the reduction by its orientation perpendicular to the cortex (Fig. 5-10). Subsequent screws can then be placed at right angles to the fracture line to distribute interfragmental compression evenly

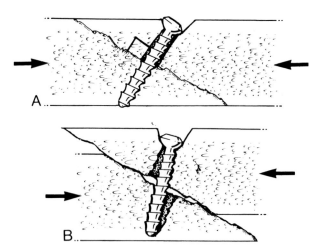

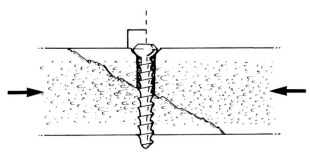

Fig. 5-10. In oblique fractures, the first screw should be inserted perpendicular to the cortex to maintain alignment. (Adapted from McGlamry,[24] with permission.)

Fig. 5-9. (A & B) When screw is placed perpendicular to fracture line and oblique to cortex, loading forces can cause loosening of the screw and telescoping of the fragments. (From McGlamry,[24] with permission.)

along the length of the fracture. Two screws are almost always preferable to one since resistance to bending and shear forces is greatly enhanced by the addition of fixation points.[21,22]

Screw Insertion Sequence

The technique of screw insertion is quite standardized and varies only slightly depending on the type of screw being inserted and to some degree on the fracture situation itself (Tables 5-1 and 5-2). When properly used the instrumentation supplied by the ASIF will result in predictable and secure stabilization of all fractures. It is assumed that preparation of the fracture site has been performed prior to the insertion of the fixation devices. Careful dissection of the soft tissues and reflection of the periosteum allows proper

visualization of the fracture line to ensure anatomic alignment. The fracture should be held opposed by temporary fixation with either bone clamps or smooth Kirschner wires.

Guide Hole. The initial or guide hole penetrates through both fragments. It can be made with a power drill or wire driver. The guide hole should be slightly smaller than the thread hole. ASIF guidelines omit this step in the fixation sequence; however, experience has shown this step to be important for several reasons.[22] Power instrumentation reduces the force necessary to penetrate the bone and provides more precise placement with less torque applied across the fracture. Power-driven drills are especially useful when placing screws oblique to the bone. When manually drilling in an oblique fashion, the bit has a greater tendency to glance off the inner side of the opposite cortex and cause fracture of the drill bit or unwanted increase in the angle of insertion (Fig. 5-11).

Glide Hole (Over-drill). Next, the initial guide hole of the near fragment is increased in diame-

Table 5-1. Proper Instrumentation for Each Cortical Screw

Thread Diameter	Spherical Head Diameter	Core Diameter	Drill Bit Thread Hole	Drill Bit Gliding Hole	Tap Diameter
1.5	3.0	1.0	1.1	1.5	1.5
2.0	4.0	1.3	1.5	2.0	2.0
2.7	5.0	1.9	2.0	2.7	2.7
3.5	6.0	1.9	2.5	3.5	3.5
4.5	8.0	3.0	3.2	4.5	4.5

Table 5-2. Related Instrumentation for Each Cancellous Screw Provided by Synthes

Thread Diameter	Spherical Head Diameter	Shaft Diameter	Core Diameter	Drill Bit Thread Hole	Tap Diameter
4.0	6.0	2.3	1.9	2.5	3.5
4.5	8.0	3.0	3.0	3.2	4.5
6.5	8.0	4.5	3.0	3.2	6.5

ter by over-drilling. This enables the threads of the screw to pass through the near fragment without purchase. Therefore, over-drilling is necessary only when using a fully threaded (cortical) screw. This glide hole is made by manually drilling with a drill bit that equals the thread diameter of the screw being inserted. Care must be taken to avoid inadvertent over-drilling of the far fragment since this would result in total loss of thread purchase (Fig. 5-12A).

Thread Hole. The guide hole is next enlarged in the far fragment by the use of a hand-driven

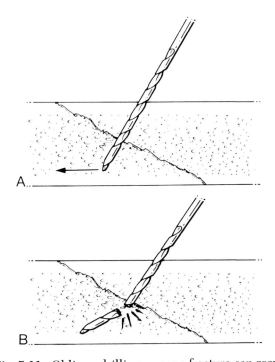

Fig. 5-11. Oblique drilling across a fracture can result in glancing of the drill bit on the far cortex (**A**) and may result in fracture of the drill bit (**B**). (Adapted from McGlamry,[24] with permission.)

drill bit. This creates the thread hole that allows the core of the screw to pass through the entire bone without impingement. To ensure that concentric drilling of the far fragment occurs, a drill guide is first inserted in the glide hole of the near fragment. The outer diameter of the drill guide equals that of the glide hole, while the inner diameter allows the passage of the thread hole drill bit. The drill guide accurately centers the thread hole in line with the proximal glide hole (Fig. 5-12B).

Countersink. Countersinking serves two functions in the insertion sequence. First, it recesses the screw within the near cortex and reduces the prominence of the screw head. The more important function is to distribute the forces evenly at the screw-bone interface. This is accomplished by shaping the near cortex to fit the undersurface of the screw head. Uneven distribution of force results in increased incidence of stress fracture of the near cortex. Therefore, it is also important that countersinking be performed in the same direction as the screw path (Fig. 5-12C).

Depth Gauge. The distance between the near and far outer cortices is measured with a depth gauge. The appropriate screw length is obtained by inserting the tip of the depth gauge through the thread hole and hooking the far cortex. When traversing bone at an oblique angle, the hook should be faced so that the longest measurement is obtained. The barrel of the depth gauge, which is the same shape as the undersurface of the screw head, is advanced until it is seated within the countersunk near cortex. Uneven seating of the barrel tip on the near cortex provides the first hint that additional countersinking will be necessary for proper screw contact. The screw length chosen should measure 1 to 2 mm longer than the actual measured distance to ensure purchase of the full thickness of the far cortex (Fig. 5-12D).

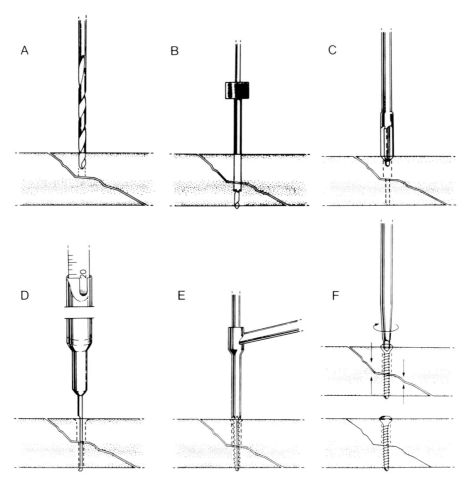

Fig. 5-12. The technique for inserting a cortical screw. (**A**) Gliding hole is drilled in the near fragment. (**B**) Drill sleeve is inserted in the glide hole and the thread hole is drilled in the far fragment. (**C**) Countersinking is performed in the direction of the screw path. (**D**) Measurement of the screw path is performed with a depth gauge. (**E**) The threads are tapped into the far fragment through the thread hole. Note: a tap sleeve is used to protect soft tissue. (**F**) Insertion of the screw. (Adapted from McGlamry,[24] with permission.)

Tapping. Tapping cuts the thread pattern through the thread hole. This step allows the screw to engage the bone and function correctly. Without precut threads, additional force will be necessary to insert the screw, increasing the risk of fixation failure. Self-tapping screws while attractive are not highly recommended by the ASIF. A tap sleeve should always be employed to prevent the soft tissue from winding about the tap.

The tap size is the same diameter as the screw thread except in the 4.0-mm cancellous screw (Table 5-1). When the screw is being inserted into only the cancellous bone of the far fragment, partial tapping is recommended to increase purchase of the screw. However, if the screw is to traverse the cortex of the far fragment, complete tapping is essential (Fig. 5-12E).

Screw Insertion. The screw is finally inserted into the hole of the near cortex. The screw is advanced by turning the driver in a clockwise direction. The cortical screw should glide until the far fragment is encountered. It is important to maintain the reduction of the fracture while the screw is being inserted. Notably, the cancellous screw will cause distraction of the fragments until all of the threads have crossed the fracture line.

Prior to the final tightening of the screw, all temporary fixation should be removed. Two-finger technique is used to ensure adequate compression without risk of stripping the screw threads through the opposite fragment. If compression does not occur between the fractures, one of two situations exists. First, all of the threads may not be across the fracture line. Second, spinning of the screw despite screw head contact with the near cortex indicates that the far fragment has been stripped or that the screw is too short and is not reaching the far cortex (Fig. 5-12F).

Generally, innovation in screw fixation is not recommended. However, in some circumstances variation in sequence of screw fixation may be instituted without significant compromise in the final result.

Plate Fixation

Another method of obtaining rigid internal fixation is with the use of plates. Plates can be used in some fracture situations to create interfragmental compression. However, in many instances plates are used as splintage to provide protection of the interfragmental compression provided by lag screws. There are many types of plates, and all can be used to provide either of the forms of fixation described above.[21,22]

The types of plates most commonly used in fractures of the lower extremity include straight and shaped plates. The type of plate chosen will depend on the biomechanical function required and on the actual configuration of the fracture and bone fragments. In general, straight plates are used to fixate diaphyseal fractures. Straight plates include tubular, round hole, and dynamic compression plates. Shaped plates are meant for metaphyseal and epiphyseal regions and in irregularly shaped bones. These include clover leaf, T-, and L-plates (Fig. 5-13).

Functions of Plates

There are three categories of plate fixation based on function-axial interfragmental compression, neutralization, and buttress.[17,18]

Axial Interfragmental Compression. Axial compression applied to fracture can be achieved with a prestressed plate. A relatively transverse fracture configuration is required to obtain this form of fixation since oblique fractures under axial compression are displaced. Axial compression is obtained by the eccentric drilling of either a tubular or dynamic compression plate (DCP) or a tension device. The thicker DCP allows for more stable fixation across the fracture interface. How-

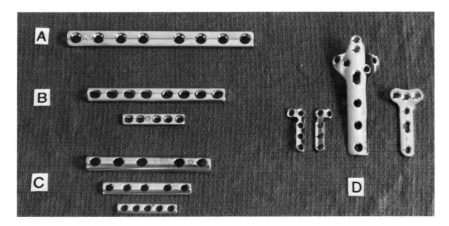

Fig. 5-13. Straight plates. **(A)** Round hole plate; **(B)** DCP; **(C)** semi-tubular, one-third tubular, and one-quarter tubular plates. **(D)** Shaped plates: L-, cloverleaf, and T-plates.

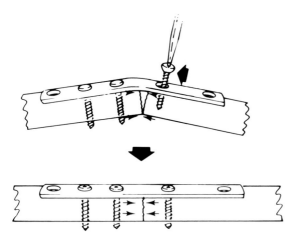

Fig. 5-14. Uniform compression is encouraged with prebending of the plate prior to screw tightening. (Adapted from McGlamry,[24] with permission.)

ever, prebending of tubular plates compensates for the loss of thickness and thereby allows more uniform compression (Fig. 5-14). Short oblique fractures should be compressed by the lag screw technique prior to the addition of axial compression. Oval holes are provided in the long arm of shaped plates so that axial compression can be achieved. A tension device temporarily applies tension to the plate until it is affixed to the fragments in the prestressed attitude (Fig. 5-15).

In some situations the placement of the plate will be dictated by the fracture configuration. However, when possible, the plate should take advantage of the tension-band principle. Therefore, the plate should be applied on the side of

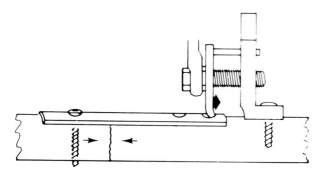

Fig. 5-15. A tension device can be utilized to prestress a plate prior to screw fastening. (Adapted from McGlamry,[24] with permission.)

the bone that would normally be under tension. Bones that are eccentrically loaded with weight bearing or have tension placed on them owing to the pull of soft tissue attachment are ideal for this type of dynamic compression (Fig. 5-16).

Neutralization. Some fracture situations are not amenable to axial compression. These include spiral oblique and comminuted fractures (Fig. 5-17). In these situations, interfragmental compression can usually be obtained with the use of lag screws. However, protection of the stabilization will often be required to neutralize the shear, bending, and torsional forces about the fracture site. Plates applied for this purpose are called neutralization plates. Virtually any ASIF plate can be used in this manner. The only condition is that the plate be well molded to fit the bone to which it is being applied. Therefore, malleable plates such as the tubular type are well suited for this function.

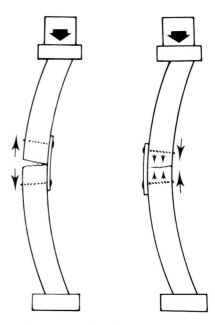

Fig. 5-16. The tension-band principle is illustrated by the curved bone placed under an axial load. Loading results in eccentric dispersement of the force with the concave portion of the bone under tension and the convex side under compression. The plate is placed to absorb the tension force and the bone resists the resulting compression. (Adapted from McGlamry,[24] with permission.)

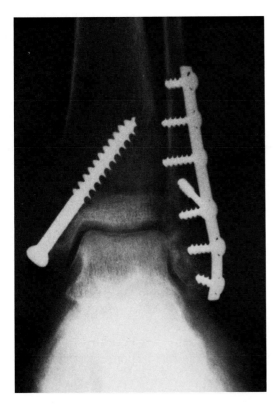

Fig. 5-17. An example of a neutralization plate is shown in this anteroposterior radiograph of an ankle. Note that an interfragmental screw is providing compression across the fracture and that the well-contoured plate has centrally placed screws.

Buttressing. Buttressing is the final manner in which plates can be utilized in the fixation of fractures. They are used in very unstable fractures to maintain alignment of the fracture fragments. However, no interfragmental compression is achieved with this method of fixation. Instead, the plate serves as a bridge between larger fragments with intervening small fragments. Devitalized bone fragments that are removed can be replaced with cancellous bone graft under the protection of a buttress plate.

Techniques of Plate Fixation

The method of securing a plate to a fractured bone will vary depending on the type of fixation being attempted. Cortical screws are generally used to affix the plate. However, in some situa-tions a lagged screw can be used through a hole in the plate. The number of screws and the amount of thread purchase used to press the plate against the bone are important. In general, the more peripheral the fracture, the less screw threads will be necessary to provide stable fixation. The ASIF recommends that four cortices be purchased per main fragment in metatarsal fractures. In the more proximal skeleton, purchase of five cortices is recommended. However, in transverse fractures stabilized by axial compression, six cortices should be purchased to withstand the shearing forces across the fracture.[22]

Axial Compression with Tubular Plates. Once the fracture has been reduced and temporarily fixated, a plate of the proper size and shape is chosen. The plate is contoured and prebent as necessary to fit the surface of the bone to which it is being applied. The plate is initially secured to the smaller fragment in most circumstances. The holes in the plate adjacent to the fracture are utilized first. Eccentrically drilled holes (away from the fracture line) are made with a power drill. In most cases, the screws are inserted without overdrilling since purchase of the near cortex is desired. As the head of the screw contacts the far rim of the plate, the screw along with the bone to which it is purchasing must slide centrally, resulting in compression at the fracture interface (Fig. 5-18). Finally, the remainder of the screws are placed in holes drilled centrally within the plate holes.

Another method of achieving axial compression with a tubular plate is with a tension device. This requires additional soft tissue exposure, which tends to limit its usefulness in fractures of the foot and ankle.

Axial Compression with Dynamic Compression Plates. DCPs are specially designed to provide axial compression without a tension device.[17] This decreases the amount of exposure necessary for plate fixation. These plates are thicker and sturdier than tubular plates. The holes in the plate are grooved to produce gliding of the eccentrically drilled screw. The grooved holes also allow for angulation of the screws.

The DCP is applied in the same manner as described above for tubular plates. However, the eccentric and centrally drilled screw holes are

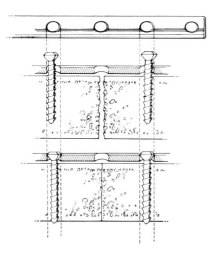

Fig. 5-18. Axial interfragmental compression achieved by eccentric drilling of a tubular plate. As the head contacts the plate, the screw and the bone to which it is attached is forced centrally, resulting in compression at the fracture interface.

guided by a special color coded DCP drill guide. The first screw is inserted in the hole adjacent to the fracture line utilizing the central (green-tipped) drill guide. The second screw is inserted in the hole opposite the fracture line with the eccentric (yellow-tipped) drill guide. A second eccentrically drilled screw can be placed adjacent to the first eccentric screw to increase the amount of compression between the fracture fragments. The first eccentric screw must be loosened before tightening of the second eccentric screw. The remainder of the screws are placed centrally.

Neutralization Plates. Careful planning is necessary when applying plates to protect interfragmental compression achieved by screw fixation. The orientation of the fracture and the shape of the fragments will often dictate whether the interfragmental screw is placed separately or through the neutralization plate. All screws placed through the plate are centrally drilled. The interfragmental screw is of primary importance in either situation, and the plate application should not disrupt the compressed fragments (Fig. 5-19).

Buttress Plates. Bridging of defects between fracture fragments and prevention of displace-

ment is the goal of the buttress plate. Since axial compression is not a desired effect of this type of plate fixation, all screws are centrally drilled. The large fracture fragments are aligned by the plate, and defects are filled as necessary with cancellous bone graft material. All forces crossing the fracture will be transmitted to the plate since there is no inherent stability of the fracture itself. Therefore, the plate should be of sufficient strength to resist all forces that will be conveyed across the fracture (Fig. 5-20).

Tension-Band Principle

As previously described, rigid internal fixation can be divided into static and dynamic methods. For dynamic compression to occur, a physiologic load must be present in combination with static compression.

When bone is loaded eccentrically, it is subjected to bending forces. This creates tension on the concave side and compression on the convex side of the bone. Failure of the bone results in dissipation of these forces. Fixation of the fragments replaces the loads about the bone. However, the tensile forces must be resisted by the fixation device itself if dynamic compression is to occur. Therefore, to achieve tension banding, the bone must be able to withstand compression and the plate or wire must be able to absorb the ten-

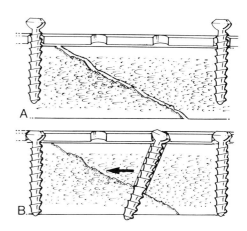

Fig. 5-19. (A & B) Interfragmental compression with a lag screw used through a neutralization plate. (Adapted from McGlamry,[24] with permission.)

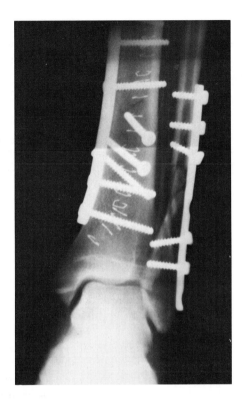

Fig. 5-20. A buttress plate on the fibula of this distal leg fracture is shown. Note the comminution of the intervening bone being bridged by the plate.

sile forces. Fixation devices placed on the compression side of the bone will often result in gapping of the tensile side cortex and loss of stable fixation (Fig. 5-21).

Tension-Band Technique
The two components of the tension-band technique include the osseous beam and the fixation

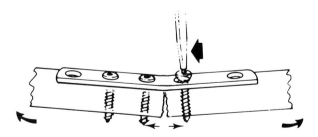

Fig. 5-21. When compression plates are placed on the compression side of a fracture, the tension side will have a tendency to gap. (Adapted from McGlamry,[24] with permission.)

device. Separation of the fragments on the tension side is resisted by the tension-band device. The tension-band device can be either stainless steel wire or a plate. Avulsion fractures are the most amenable to dynamic compression with the tension-band technique. Fractures of the ankle malleoli and the base of the fifth metatarsal are commonly fixated by this method (Fig. 5-22).

Kirschner wires are frequently added to tension-band wiring to enhance rotational stability and provide a anchoring post for the wire loop.[22] The Kirschner wires are placed parallel in the initial step of this technique, aiding in the reduction of the fracture (Fig. 5-23). The wire is placed through an osseous tunnel or a tendinous structure. The wire loop is then crossed and directed around the Kirschner wires and twisted tight. Crossing the wire over the fracture line centers the compressive force. Pulling tension should be placed on the wire as it is twisted to ensure that a tight coil occurs (Fig. 5-24).

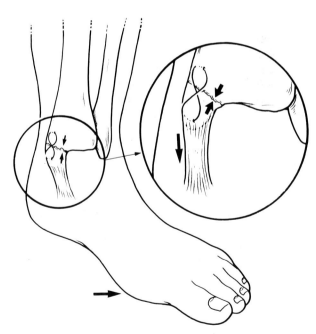

Fig. 5-22. This example of the tension-band concept shows how movement of the foot and an intact deltoid ligament can produce dynamic interfragmental compression. The wire loop is placed to resist the tension at the outer malleolus. (Adapted from McGlamry,[24] with permission.)

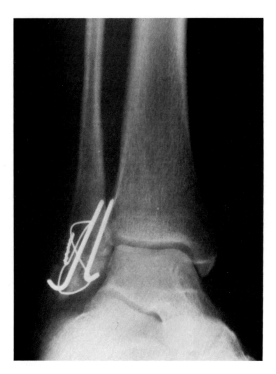

Fig. 5-23. Kirschner wires added to the tension-band loop result in greater stability of this avulsion fracture of the fibular malleolus.

EXTERNAL FIXATION

The primary application for external fixation is for fractures that are associated with soft tissue defects, comminuted or osteoporotic bone, and infection. External fixators can create rigid fixation or function as a splint. However, since transverse fracture configuration is necessary to obtain axial compression, their use is limited for this type of fixation. When a relatively transverse fracture is present, pins can be placed percutaneously through the proximal and distal fragments parallel to the fracture line. The pins can then be secured to the frame and simultaneously tightened to create axial compression.[23]

The external fixator can be utilized as a splint to neutralize disruptive forces or to maintain distraction of fracture fragments. Distraction maintenance is especially useful in open comminuted fractures. The technique is the same as previously described; however, the fragments are distracted instead of compressed.

The disadvantages of external fixation are directly related to the percutaneous pinning. Not

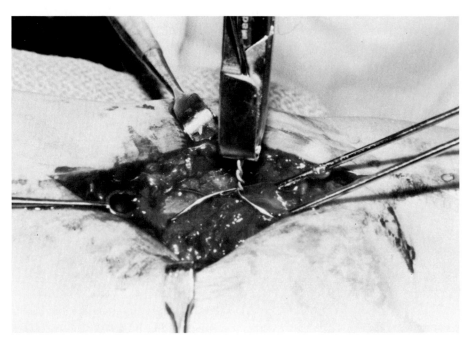

Fig. 5-24. Tightening of the wire loop with the ASIF wire twister is shown. The tension placed on the wire during tightening creates tight coiling and equal dispersion of the compression.

only are these pins somewhat difficult to place, they require special aftercare. The incidence of pin tract infections is well documented. If the bone itself become secondarily infected, disastrous results can occur.[23] A major disadvantage is that the external frames are usually quite bulky and inconvenient.

REFERENCES

1. Hughes JL, Weber H, Willenegger H, Kuner EH: Evaluation of ankle fractures: non-operative and operative treatment. Clin Orthop 138:111, 1979
2. Peacock E: Healing and repair of bone. p. 398. In Peacock E (ed): Wound Repair. WB Saunders, Philadelphia, 1984
3. Shenk R: Histology of Fracture Repair and Non-Union. p. 14. Buchdruck-Offset, Bern, Switzerland, 1978
4. Rhinelander F, Phillips R: Microangiography in bone healing. II: Displaced closed fractures. J Bone Joint Surg 50A:643, 1968
5. Charnley J: Conservative versus operative methods. p. 3. In Charnley J (ed): The Closed Treatment of Common Fractures. Churchill Livingstone, London, 1974
6. Pauwels, F: Der Schenkelhalsbruch ein mechanishes Problem. Enke, Stuttgart, 1935
7. Muller ME, Allgower M, Willenegger H: Manual of Internal Fixation. Springer-Verlag, Berlin, 1979
8. Heppenstal RB: Fracture Treatment and Healing. WB Saunders, Philadelphia, 1980
9. Vanik R, Weber R, Matloub M et al: The comparative strengths of internal fixation techniques. J Hand Surg 9A:216, 1984
10. DiGiovanni J, Martin R: Pins, wires, and staples in foot surgery. Clin Podiatry 1:211, 1984
11. Mears D: Materials in Orthopaedic Surgery. p. 412. Williams & Wilkins, Baltimore, 1979
12. Frost H: Orthopaedic Biomechanics. p. 58. Charles C Thomas, Springfield, IL, 1973
13. Boehler J: Percutaneous cerclage of tibial fractures. Clin Orthop 105:276, 1974
14. Mears D: Materials and Orthopaedic Surgery. p. 6. Williams & Wilkins, Baltimore, 1979
15. Cavaliere RG, Ruch JR: Fixation of first metatarsal osteotomies. p. 136. In McGlamry ED, McGlamry R (eds): Doctors Hospital Podiatry Institute Seminar Manual. Atlanta, GA, 1985
16. Ostgaard HC, Herberts P: Evaluation of the 3-M Stapilizer: a new internal fixation system. Injury 19:28, 1988
17. Palmer I: The mechanism and treatment of fractures of the calcaneus. J Bone Joint Surg 30A:2, 1948
18. Alldridge RH, Riordan DC: The use of staples and bone-chip grafts for internal fixation in foot stabilization operations. J Bone Joint Surg 35A:951, 1953
19. Shenk R, Willenegger H: Zur histologie der primaren knochen neileng. Lagenbecks Arch Chir 308:440, 1964
20. Perren S, Matter P, Ruedi T, Allgower M: Biomechanics of fracture healing after internal fixation. p. 361. In Nyhus LM (ed): Surgery Annals. Appleton-Century-Crofts, East Norwalk, CT, 1975
21. Heim U, Pheiffer KM: Internal Fixation of Small Fractures. Springer-Verlag, New York, 1988
22. Ruch JR, Merrill T: Principles of rigid internal compression fixation and its application in podiatric surgery. p. 246. In McGlamry ED (ed): Fundamentals of Foot Surgery. Williams & Wilkins, Baltimore, 1987
23. Mears D: External Skeletal Fixation. Williams & Wilkins, Baltimore, 1983
24. McGlamry ED: Fundamentals of Foot Surgery. Williams & Wilkins, Baltimore, 1987

6

Soft Tissue Trauma: An Overview

Claudia Sands, D.P.M.
Thomas H. Walter, D.P.M.
Barry L. Scurran, D.P.M.

The physician's role in the management of all trauma is to reestablish tissue homeostasis and to aid the rapid return to normal function. This is achieved through accurate assessment and appropriate treatment. Soft tissue trauma consists of injuries that disrupt a complex system of closely integrated metabolic and physiologic components. Wound management therefore must begin with the emergent care of the entire patient. Life-threatening injuries are addressed initially. Once the patient is medically stable, evaluation of soft tissue trauma can begin.

Trauma to the foot may certainly involve more than soft tissues, so each tissue system must be specifically evaluated and addressed. Principles of treatment include maintenance of adequate blood supply, realignment of osseous structures, expedition of wound healing through appropriate debridement, prevention of infection, and restoration of skin coverage. The clinician should strive to restore or preserve anatomic structure and function while attempting to achieve cosmetically acceptable results.

Careful evaluation of the injury with subsequent exploration, irrigation, and debridement are often necessary in the initial management of the traumatic wound. Osseous injury must be stabilized when appropriate to provide a structural framework to prevent further injury or neurovascular compromise (Fig. 6-1). Vascular and neuro-logic status should be documented. Wounds must be assessed for potential primary closure, for delayed closure, or for future, more extensive plastic or reconstructive procedures when necessary. Tetanus prophylaxis[1] and antibiotic therapy may be indicated.

The potential for local pedal vascular insufficiency secondary to gross ischemia or hemorrhage must be evaluated. Unstable fractures are splinted to prevent further damage to surrounding soft tissues. Comprehensive history and physical examinations may then ensue.

HISTORY

A thorough history should include a detailed description of the injury with specific regard to the nature and time of the offending trauma. The examiner should determine whether foreign material penetrated the skin and whether debris, including parts of shoes or socks, could potentially remain in the wound. The environment of the injury should be noted. Was the offending object a clean kitchen knife or a lawn mower blade? The gross appearance of the wound after injury should be elicited. A description of the amount of blood loss and initial treatment, if any, can give useful clues to the extent of the wound and possi-

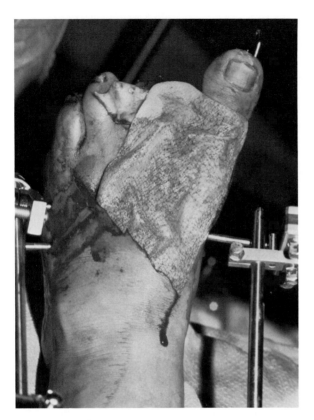

Fig. 6-1. Stabilization and realignment of osseous structures in the presence of soft tissue trauma. An external fixator was utilized to stabilize soft tissues as well as osseous structures in this motorcyclist who suffered a skin avulsion injury to the foot with multiple fractures and traumatic amputations of the second and third toes. A porcine xenograft is the initial wound dressing.

ble underlying damage. Queries should be made as to potential industrial injury, alcohol use, previous injuries, disabilities, and neurologic or functional deficits of the foot or legs. In the event that general anesthesia for surgery is indicated, an estimate of the time food or drink was last ingested becomes necessary.

Information regarding current medications, drug allergies, illnesses, or disabilities is obtained, noting any condition that may compromise the patient's healing or immune response (e.g., current steroid therapy, sickle cell anemia, arterial or venous insufficiency, or diabetes mellitus). Determination of current tetanus immuni-

zation status is mandatory. A review of systems and family and social history including occupation and activity level is routinely sought.

PHYSICAL EXAMINATION

Although complete physical examinations are generally performed, emphasis in this discussion is directed toward the lower extremity. Initial examination of the injury should include assessment of vascular and neurologic status as well as dermatologic and musculoskeletal evaluation. Hemostasis can be achieved by elevation, proximal or direct pressure, or short-term tourniquet use. The presence of a retained foreign body may contraindicate direct pressure. A proximal tourniquet used judiciously allows better visualization, yet one must consider the risk of further ischemic damage to already compromised tissue. Blind clamping of blood vessels is contraindicated, as adjacent structures might be damaged.

Vascular and neurologic status should be assessed prior to administrating a local anesthesia. Patency of the dorsalis pedis and posterior tibial pulses is noted. If pulses are absent or the presence of edema precludes palpation, Doppler evaluation may prove useful in assessing blood supply. Clinical signs of decreased or absent pulses, pallor, pain, paresthesias, paralysis, and decreased temperature should be considered indications of arterial compromise.[2] If the injury is unilateral, the contralateral foot must be logically used for comparison. The neurologic examination should clearly document any sensory or motor deficit.

The practitioner should observe the degree of integumentary damage or loss and inspect for possible osseous and tendinous damage, testing for strength, range of motion, and stability of the joint or joints involved. If the presence of a fracture or foreign body is suspected, radiographs should be taken and reviewed prior to any manipulation required for accurate examination.

If further exploration is indicated, appropriate anesthesia should be used to permit adequate assessment without undue discomfort to the patient. Sedation may be especially helpful for young children or uncooperative patients. If extensive exploration or debridement is anticipated, general or spinal anesthesia should be considered.

When local anesthesia is used, a peripheral nerve block or infiltration proximal to the site of injury is indicated. The smallest effective amount of local anesthetic without epinephrine is used to avoid increasing local tissue pressures or vasoconstriction that might contribute to further vascular compromise.

Gentle cleansing of the surrounding skin using mild antiseptics is undertaken prior to deeper exploration. Using aseptic technique, the depth and extent of the wound is established, and all tissue planes and structures involved are documented.

Unless there is little doubt that one is dealing with a clean, fresh wound, deep wound cultures and Gram stains should be obtained. Laboratory evaluation should include complete blood count, urinalysis, electrolytes, and other specific tests (e.g., blood alcohol), when indicated. Radiographs of the foot in three body planes should be obtained when appropriate. Comparison views and special studies are utilized when specific indications are noted.

CLASSIFICATION

Categorization of soft tissue injuries facilitates decisions regarding treatment options including planning for wound closure. With any attempt at classification there exists possible overlap or ambiguity. It is recommended that each examiner formulate a methodology that provides a framework for evaluation allowing all injuries to be approached in a systematic fashion.

Many attempts to formulate wound classification systems have been suggested.[3–5] Rank[6] and Thompson[7] proposed four categories for wound classification: tidy, untidy, wounds with tissue loss, and infected wounds. Utilizing this general format, injuries discussed in this chapter are loosely described as clean (tidy), contaminated

(untidy or those with extensive tissue loss or damage), or infected wounds. Injuries are also described by the specific tissue damage involved.

It may be helpful to divide wounds into those that can be closed primarily and those that cannot. Clean, recent wounds are closed primarily when feasible (Fig. 6-2). Contaminated wounds cannot be closed primarily unless, by appropriate local treatment (i.e., debridement and copious lavage), they can be converted to clean wounds (Fig. 6-3). Infected wounds are not closed until clear transformation into clean wounds is obtained (Fig. 6-4). Use of systemic antibiotics after identification of the offending organism is clearly indicated. Debridement of infected necrotic tissue and intensive local wound care must be used. Generally, serial negative cultures and clinical resolution of the infection are mandatory before consideration for wound closure.

Clean wounds usually involve minimal soft tissue damage or contamination and do not require extensive debridement prior to closure. These wounds are not likely to become infected. Included in this category are those injuries converted to clean wounds. Incisions and lacerations—without undue contamination—are exam-

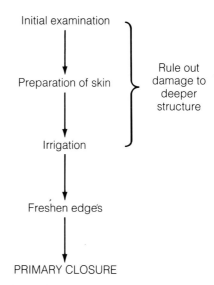

Fig. 6-2. Schema for treatment of clean wounds. (Modified from Noe and Kalish,[17] with permission.)

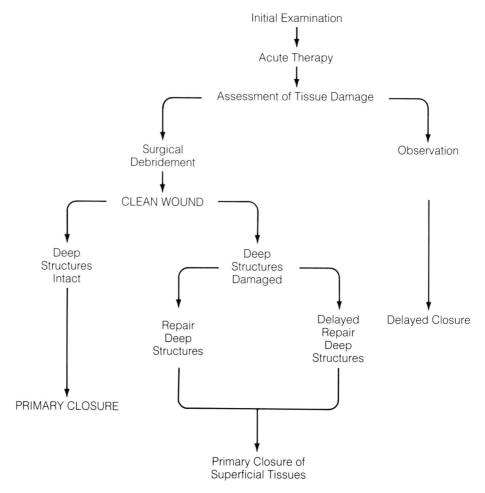

Fig. 6-3. Schema for treatment of contaminated wounds. (Modified from Noe and Kalish,[17] with permission.)

ples of injuries that are generally considered clean wounds (Fig. 6-5).

Contaminated wounds or those that exhibit a high degree of soft tissue damage are considerably more predisposed to infection (Fig. 6-6). Factors that increase the potential for wound infection include a significant amount of contamination or retained necrotic material, vascular compromise, extensive tissue loss, and excessive desiccation of tissues. A clean wound may progress to contaminated wound status if it is left exposed and untreated for more than 6 hours after the initial trauma owing to the amount of tissue desiccation and bacterial colonization present.

A wound should be considered infected if any clinical sign of infection or gross contamination exists. Treatment includes appropriate local wound care, debridement, and broad-spectrum antibiotic coverage against the most likely pathogen until Gram stain and culture results are available. Delayed primary closure or skin grafts may be performed if indicated once the infection has been resolved. A more complete discussion of infections in traumatic wounds is presented in Chapter 30.

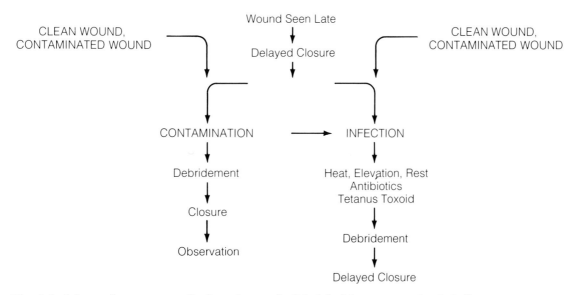

Fig. 6-4. Schema for treatment of infected wounds. (Modified from Noe and Kalish,[17] with permission.)

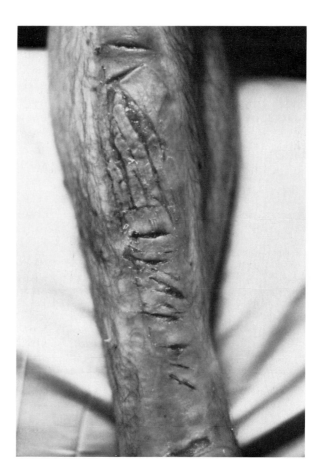

Fig. 6-5. Lacerations. This psychiatric patient created these factitious wounds on the desensitized site of a previous skin graft.

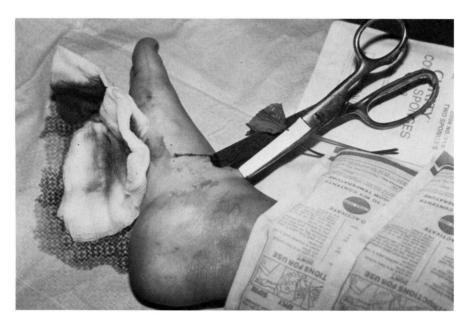

Fig. 6-6. Contaminated wound. An 8-year-old girl dropped scissors on her foot while cutting flowers in the garden.

CLOSED WOUNDS

Wounds may also be described by their effect or action upon the skin and surrounding tissues. Closed trauma, when no interruption of the integument is evident, may be simple or complex (Fig. 6-7). The injury is usually the result of blunt

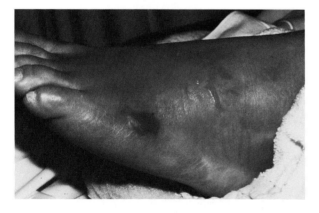

Fig. 6-7. A closed, crush injury with multiple foot fractures, contusions, and fracture blisters after a horse rolled over the foot and leg.

trauma causing a contusion, compression, or crush injury. There is no external bleeding, and variable amounts of ecchymosis and edema may be present. The effects of this type of injury may be subtle and the extent not immediately discernable. These wounds should be observed since extensive vascular, neurologic, or soft tissue damage may become evident hours or days after the injury. The objective of initial treatment is to reduce pain and swelling and to alleviate or control future swelling. Compression, elevation, the intermittent application of ice, and rest may be sufficient.[4] Physical therapy may also be a useful aid to rapid functional return.

Complications of closed soft tissue injury include compartment syndrome and hematoma formation. Compartment syndrome can result from excessive edema of the foot or leg secondary to a crush injury, contusion, burn, or infection. Muscle compartments are bordered by bone and relatively inelastic fascia that can become constricting forces with increasing volume within the closed compartment. This expansion of tissues causes the fascial compartments to become very tense, intracompartmental pressures increase, and neurovascular bundles may be compressed.

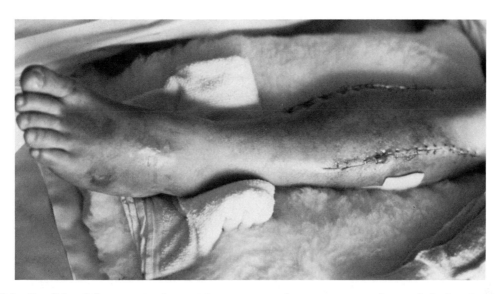

Fig. 6-8. Careful and frequent evaluation for neurovascular compromise ultimately led to decompression compartmental fasciotomies of the leg. The cutaneous layer is closed only if this can be accomplished without tension. The fascial layer beneath is not closed.

Treatment consists of compartmental fasciotomies when this entity is suspected (Fig. 6-8). Compartment pressures can be measured to substantiate clinical impressions, but it is the clinical picture of decreased or absent pulses, increased ischemic pain, and rapidly advancing trophic changes that must be addressed. Treatment should be immediate, as permanent sequelae secondary to neurovascular compression can result (see Ch. 15 on vascular trauma).

Hematoma formation in a closed wound can delay healing and also serve as a culture medium for bacterial infection secondary to hematogenous dissemination of blood-borne flora into an enclosed dead space. A large-bore needle can be used for hematoma aspiration until the hematoma begins to consolidate. After this, removal may require open surgical debridement.

OPEN WOUNDS

Open injuries range from very superficial soft tissue injuries, such as abrasions, to more extensive trauma including lacerations, avulsions, degloving, burns, gunshot wounds, and puncture wounds. Abrasions are superficial wounds with only partial-thickness skin loss. Lacerations or incisions should be considered full-thickness injuries. Avulsions and deglovings involve the undermining and removal of tissue with variable amounts of tissue loss (Fig. 6-9). Detailed discussions of other types of soft tissue trauma, such as gunshot or puncture wounds, foreign bodies, and burns, are found elsewhere in this text.

CLINICAL ASPECTS OF WOUND HEALING

The healing process, described in detail in Chapter 1, begins immediately after injury. Healing implies a return to "normal" tissue. Skin and other superficial tissues do not, however, regenerate to normal but are repaired through granulation, fibrosis, and scarring.

The first phase of healing is the exudative phase. Capillary permeability is increased, resulting in increased tissue perfusion in the first 3 to 5 hours after injury. Theoretically, during this time delivery of fluids to tissue is enhanced and the early antibacterial response of the host may

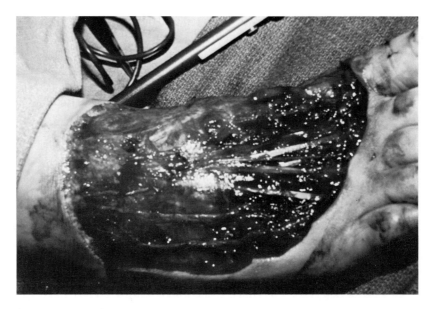

Fig. 6-9. Degloving injury suffered in motorcycle accident. Note the full-thickness tissue loss that will necessitate coverage with a skin graft.

be supplemented by the use of antibiotics.[8] A leukotactic substance is released from traumatized tissue, summoning polymorphonuclear leukocytes to aid in phagocytosis of nonviable tissue. The host immunologic response "lags" by 4 to 5 days. During this time, nonviable tissue is separated by phagocytosis or enzymatic digestion. This is the body's attempt to create a clean wound. Surgical or mechanical debridement of the wound will expedite this phase of healing.[9] Conversely, this phase can be prolonged through tissue desiccation, poor tissue handling, hematoma formation, or incomplete debridement.

The proliferative or exudative phase begins approximately 5 days after the injury and produces granulation tissue to cover and protect the wound. The development of granulation tissue is the wound's response to bacterial contamination.[10] This tissue is not true regenerative tissue but is indicative of a revascularization process occurring beneath the wound surface. Granulation tissue is debrided prior to delayed primary closure or grafting but should remain intact in wounds left to heal by secondary intention. This tissue will later become dense, fibrous tissue that will contract, allowing epithelialization of the wound. Contracture, the final phase, in which wound margins are brought closer together, can create unsatisfactory scars that potentially limit motion.

WOUND TREATMENT

Surgical debridement is performed to remove all foreign or devitalized tissue.[11] For effective debridement, hemostasis must be optimal. Bleeding vessels, once visualized and isolated, can be clamped and ligated or cauterized. Atraumatic tissue handling is essential to avoid further damage to already tenuous tissues.[12] Skin edges are gently retracted with sharp instruments rather than with blunt forceps or clamps, which may crush already traumatized soft tissue.

Only tissue that is clearly nonviable, avascular, or necrotic should be removed. Secondary debridement may be indicated after demarcation into viable and nonviable tissue is evident. Remove foreign debris and only very small bone fragments. Hematomas are avascular and must be evacuated. Use drains placed in dependent corners of the wound, wound packing, and pressure dressings to prevent further hematoma formation. Fresh bleeding may indicate an adequate blood supply; however, further debridement may be necessary.

Irrigation with copious amounts of physiologic saline or lactated Ringer's solution aids in debridement, decreases local wound flora, and may prevent desiccation. Topical irrigation, however, usually only decreases surface contamination or inoculation. Jet lavage has been shown to decrease bacteria in deeper tissue once this tissue has been properly exposed.[13] The use of strong antiseptic solutions is discouraged since these solutions may be locally toxic.[9]

After cleansing and irrigation, most wounds remain essentially contaminated, but not all become clinically infected. Factors that might predispose to wound infection include virulence of the bacteria, size of the inoculum, presence of necrotic or foreign material, as well as host resistance and immune response. Quantitative bacteriology has shown that approximately 10^5 to 10^6 organisms per gram of tissue in a surgical wound will cause a clinical infection.[10,14] The presence of a single suture decreases the number of bacteria needed to 10^4 organisms per gram of tissue.[14]

Wound care necessary to prevent infection includes appropriate irrigation to reduce the quantity of bacteria, debridement to remove compromised, nonviable tissue and debris, and appropriate systemic antibiotics to assist the host immune response. Antibiotics against the most likely organism are used if the past medical history reveals no allergy or sensitivity. Serial Gram stains and wound cultures can be effective in evaluating progress of wound therapy. Wounds suspected of contamination include wounds in which there has been an excessive time lapse before treatment, and wounds in which excessive amounts of soft tissue damage exist. In either case primary closure is not recommended.

SEQUENCE

A logical approach to wound debridement includes attention to those aspects of debridement mentioned above. Skin edges, unless nonviable, require only a thin debridement of wound margins, if any at all. Care is taken to preserve subcutaneous layers unless already exposed or contaminated to avoid further integumentary compromise. Muscle tissue is perhaps the most difficult tissue in which to assess viability early in wound management. Generally, muscle may be debrided until fresh bleeding is noted. Nonviable muscle may appear beefy red early after injury but can progress to a dusky, red-brown appearance in 48 to 72 hours. Serial debridement may be necessary. Low-grade electrical stimulation (e.g., Bovie) may be useful to assess contractility in an attempt to ascertain muscle viability.

Tendons should be identified, and if they are traumatized or lacerated, either primary or delayed primary closure may ensue, as discussed in Chapter 12. Certain tendons may not require repair (e.g., lesser digital extensor tendons), as these are often sacrificed in elective surgical procedures.

Trauma to vascular and neurologic structures is also discussed in detail in subsequent chapters; however, the presence, absence, and degree of damage should be clearly documented and addressed when appropriate.

"Leave alone the bone except bits quite alone" states the adage addressing early traumatic wound debridement. Excessive removal of even small pieces of bone may delay osseous healing, create instability, or eliminate the foundation for future osseous repair. Specific osseous repairs are also discussed in great detail in subsequent chapters.

WOUND CLOSURE

Primary closure of a clean wound may be performed after a gentle scrub with mild soap and water. The wound margins are freshened 1 to 2 mm and irrigated with physiologic solution or lactated Ringer's solution. Deeper structures are inspected and repaired as indicated. Specific techniques for repair of neurovascular, tendinous, and osseous structures are discussed elsewhere in this text. Skin edges must be reapproximated without tension. Non-weight bearing or immobilization, especially for plantar incisions or tenuous closures, is considered to specific injuries.

Absorbable sutures should be used sparingly as the materials tend to lower local tissues' resistance to infection. Material selected for repair of deeper structures should have low tissue reactivity and resist degradation in the presence of infection. According to Yu et al., polyglycolic acid and polyglactin 910 are the absorbable sutures best meeting the previous criteria.[15] Nonabsorbable polypropylene sutures are the least reactive, exhibit good handling properties, and are the sutures of choice in compromised tissue.[15]

Sutures remain in place approximately 14 days in the foot and leg and up to 21 days in the thicker plantar skin. Adhesive closure strips can be used for small incisions or in addition to sutures to further reinforce closures. They may also be utilized to maintain or even draw skin margins closer together in open wounds in which primary closure is not yet feasible or indicated.

Alternatives to primary closure include delayed primary closure, healing by secondary intention, coverage with skin grafts, or utilization of local or distant neurovascular flaps. Delayed primary closure usually is undertaken 4 to 6 days after the initial injury, which corresponds to the end of the lag phase of the host immunologic response. Delayed primary closure is considered once viability of surrounding tissues is reasonably ensured and the wound can be considered clean. The surgical technique is similar to that of primary closure. If the possibility of contamination exists, closure may be undertaken loosely over a drain placed in a dependent portion of the wound. Drains should be removed or changed every 24 to 48 hours until one is certain that wound healing has progressed satisfactorily without infection or complication. Prophylactic antibiotic therapy may be discontinued; however, the wound should be observed closely for developing signs of infection.

An open wound that may be in jeopardy of infection, increased metabolism, protein loss, and functional impairment may benefit from biologic dressings, such as allografts, porcine xenografts, and amniotic membranes.[16] These dressings may establish an environment that lessens desiccation and decreases bacterial flora. Dressings may also be utilized to create low-grade compression that will decrease edema and potential dead space for hematoma or seroma formation.

For minor soft tissue trauma, ice, elevation, compression, and cleansing of superficial abrasions remains the treatment of choice. More complex injuries may require further procedures and reconstruction, as described in subsequent chapters of this text.

REFERENCES

1. Rakel RE: Family Practice. p. 532. WB Saunders, Philadelphia, 1978
2. Abramson DI, Miller DS: Vascular Problems in Musculoskeletal Disorders of the Limbs. p. 79. Springer-Verlag, New York, 1981
3. Grossman JA: The repair of surface trauma. Emerg Med 12:220, 1982
4. Hirata I: Soft tissue injuries. Coll Health 23:215, 1975
5. Mills J et al: Current Emergency Diagnosis and Treatment. Lange Medical Publications, Los Altos, CA, 1985
6. Rank BK: Surgery of Repair as Applied to Hand Injuries. p. 88. 3rd Ed. Williams & Wilkins, Baltimore, 1968
7. Thompson RVS: Primary Repair of Soft Tissue Injuries. Melbourne University Press, Melbourne, Australia, 1969
8. Burke JF: Elements affecting susceptibility to infection. Contemp Surg 10(4):38, 1977
9. Hoover NW, Ivins JC: Wound debridement. AMA Arch Surg 79:701, 1959
10. Krizek TJ, Robson MC: Biology of surgical infection. Surg Clin North Am 55:1261, 1975
11. Bulletin of the American College of Surgeons, Committee on Trauma: A Guide to Initial Therapy of Soft Tissue Wounds. June, 1974
12. Converse JM: Plastic and Reconstructive Surgery. Vol. 1. p. 9. WB Saunders, Philadelphia, 1964
13. Krizek TJ: Local factors influencing incidence of wound sepsis. Contemp Surg 10(4):45, 1977
14. Elek SD: Experimental staphylococcal infections in the skin of man. Ann NY Acad Sci 65:85, 1956
15. Yu VG, Cavaliere R: Suture materials. Am Podiatry Assoc 73:57, 1983

16. Robson ML et al: Amniotic membranes as a temporary wound dressing. Surg Gynecol Obstet 136:904, 1973
17. Noe JM, Kalish S: Wound Care. Cheesebrough-Ponds, Greenwich, CT, 1975

SUGGESTED READINGS

Bolognini N, Goldman F: Management of forefoot trauma. J Foot Surg 24:88, 1985

Blair VP: The influence of mechanical pressure on wound healing. IMJ 46:229, 1924

Branemark PI et al: Local tissue effect of wound disinfectants. Acta Chir Scand 357(Suppl):166, 1966

Brown PW: The prevention of infection in open wounds. Clin Orthop 96:42, 1973

Burke JF: The effective period of preventive antibiotic action in experimental incisions and dermal lesions. Surgery 50(1):161, 1961

Burke JF, Morris PJ: Recent trends in surgical bacteriology. J Surg Res 7(2):95, 1967

Campbell E, Colton JB: Theodoric: master surgeon of the 13th century. NY State J Med 54:191, 1954

Clancey GJ et al: Open fractures of the tibia. J Bone Joint Surg 60(A):118, 1978

Graziano TA et al: Crush and avulsion injuries of the foot: their evaluation and management. J Foot Surg 23(6):445, 1984

Milholland AV, Cowley RA: Anatomical injury code. Am Surg 45:93, 1979

Shaftan GW, Gardner B: Surgical Emergencies. JB Lippincott, Philadelphia, 1974

Weeks PM, Wray RC: Management of Acute Hand Injuries. CV Mosby, St Louis, 1973, p. 109

7

Injuries to the Nail Bed and Associated Structures

D. Scot Malay, D.P.M.

Digital trauma with resultant nail bed and associated soft tissue and osseous injury is frequently encountered by the podiatric physician. For this reason, the podiatrist must be familiar with the anatomic structures that form the tip of the toe. An understanding of the function of these intimately related components will make clear the necessity for appropriate initial treatment of a wide variety of digital injuries. Anatomic structures of concern include the nail bed and its overlying nail plate; the nail matrix proximally; the medial, lateral, and proximal nail folds that aid in anchoring the nail plate to the nail bed; the subungual neurovascular plexus that courses between the nail bed and distal phalanx; the distal phalanx that, along with the overlying nail plate, supports the sensate digital pulp against the substrate during stance; and the digital pulp itself with its neurosensory end-organs that aid in proprioception and fine tactile sensation (Fig. 7-1). The overriding goal in the treatment of injuries to the nail bed and associated structures is to maintain the functional unity of these intimately related component parts.

The mechanisms of acute injury to the nail bed and its associated structures include primarily crushing or stubbing forces and, to a lesser degree, lacerations and puncture wounds. Such injuries require appropriate initial therapy to prevent the development of undesirable functional and cosmetic sequelae. The sequelae include malalignment of the nail plate with resultant cryptosis, onycholysis with predisposition to fun-

gal as well as bacterial infection, and discoloration with loss of nail plate sheen. Trauma may result in the regeneration of a deformed nail plate that may be thickened, split, or transversely grooved in the form of a Beau's line (Fig. 7-2). Injuries that disrupt the proximal nail fold with concomitant nail plate avulsion may result in the development of a split-nail (canaliformis) deformity, should the dermis of the proximal nail fold adhere to the damaged nail bed proximally. Post-traumatic sequelae may create symptomatology that ranges from the severe pain associated with onychocryptosis to the aggravation and pain associated with a deformed nail plate that continually snags stockings or causes excessive pressure in snug-fitting footwear. One should be aware that toenail plate regeneration will progress over 7 to 9 months in the typical adult following complete, traumatic avulsion. The degree of tissue disruption affecting the proximal nail fold, nail matrix, and proximal segment of the nail bed greatly influences the final regeneration product. Injuries that severely disrupt proximal structures dictate a poor prognosis for satisfactory nail plate regeneration.

Injuries to the nail bed and associated structures can be categorized as follows:

1. Primary onycholysis.
2. Subungual hematoma.
3. Simple nail bed laceration.
4. Complex (stellate) nail bed laceration.
5. Nail bed laceration with phalangeal fracture.

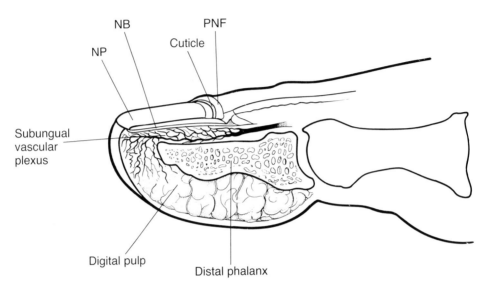

Fig. 7-1. Perionychial anatomy: NP, nail plate; NB, nail bed, PNF, proximal nail fold.

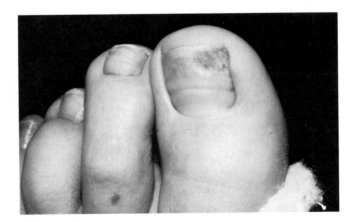

Fig. 7-2. Post-traumatic Beau's line 4.5 months following stubbing injury that caused subungual hematoma formation. Note distomedial dystrophic nail plate and the normal appearance of the nail plate proximal to the transverse defect. (From McGlamry,[10] with permission.)

6. Nail bed and toe tip tissue loss including nail bed avulsion, partial digital amputation, and digital degloving.

With the exception of primary onycholysis, these acute injuries require prompt initial treatment in an effort to prevent significant post-traumatic sequelae.

PRIMARY ONYCHOLYSIS

Minor separation of the overlying nail plate from the nail bed can occur secondary to mechanical disruption of the nail plate. This commonly occurs in the toenails secondary to recurrent microtrauma associated with chronic digital deformities and tight-fitting shoegear. The clinical result of minor nail plate separation from the underlying nail bed is the appearance of small, irregular white spots visible in the nail plate. The whitish coloration occurs owing to a change in the refractile index of the nail-plate–nail-bed complex following separation. This disorder is by no means an acute injury that requires emergency treatment. It is, however, a common finding, and one about which patients frequently question their podiatrists. The significance of accurately diagnosing this mechanically induced minor onycholysis lies in its distinction from dermatophyte or yeast infection.[1] Indeed, the mechanical onycholysis itself may predispose to a secondary dermatophyte infection. The goal of treatment for this minor disorder is the alleviation of the causative mechanical forces, typically involving routine nail care and properly fitting shoegear.

SUBUNGUAL HEMATOMA

Crushing and stubbing injuries affecting the toes frequently result in the formation of a subungual hematoma. The presence of hemorrhage beneath the nail plate indicates nail bed and subungual vascular disruption. Disruption of the nail bed allows the hemorrhage to fill the potential space existing between the nail plate and nail bed (Fig. 7-3). Hemorrhage confined deep to the nail plate creates pressure that the patient characteristically describes as throbbing pain of a deep, aching nature. Clinically, the subungual hematoma appears as a bluish-red discoloration in the initial phase, and a brown to black coloration after approximately 1 week when visualized through the nail plate. The presence of subungual hematoma indicates the need for radiographic evaluation of the distal phalanx, as approximately 20 percent of subungual hematomas present with an associated distal phalangeal fracture.[2]

A subungual hematoma is treated by drainage of trapped blood beneath the nail plate and inspection and repair of the nail bed. Following appropriate cleansing of the traumatized digit and forefoot, drainage can be obtained by penetrating the intact nail plate utilizing one of a variety of techniques. Useful techniques include penetrating the nail plate with a hand cautery unit (Fig. 7-4) or a heated paper clip, or twisting a #11 scalpel blade or an 18-gauge needle under gentle pressure, or applying a high-speed rotary ball burr. Upon penetration of the nail plate, the hemorrhage is expressed through the opening and subungual pressure is relieved. A dry sterile dressing is then applied, and the wound is inspected in 3 to 5 days. These simple techniques are useful when the subungual hematoma involves up to 25 percent of the visible nail plate. Should the hematoma involve greater than 25 percent of the visible nail plate, with or without significant disruption of the surrounding nail folds, the underlying nail bed should be inspected for major laceration[3] (Fig. 7-5). Obviously, the presence of a large subungual hematoma and nail fold disruption with loosening of the nail plate (partial nail plate avulsion) strongly suggests significant nail bed injury.

SIMPLE NAIL BED LACERATION

Appropriate local anesthesia must be achieved for all nail bed injuries requiring nail plate avulsion and nail bed repair. Local anesthesia is obtained with a digital block, or in the presence of

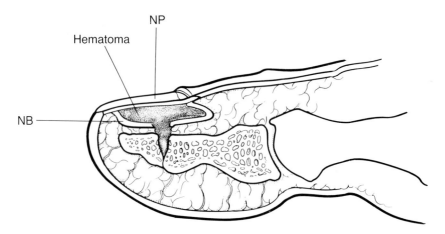

Fig. 7-3. Nail bed disruption with subungual hematoma and distal phalangeal fracture.

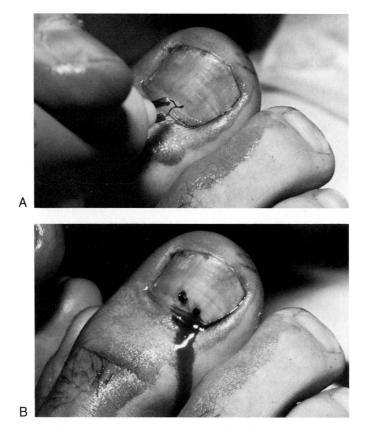

Fig. 7-4. (**A**) Drainage of subungual hematoma by using the hand cautery unit for nail plate penetration. (**B**) Hemorrhagic drainage associated with decompression and pain relief. (From McGlamry,[10] with permission.)

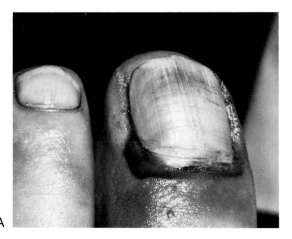
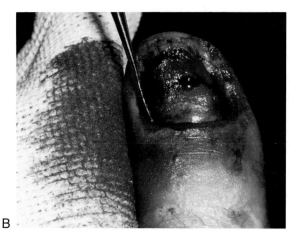

Fig. 7-5. (A) Subungual hematoma involving the entire nail plate. Note the disruption of the proximal nail fold, indicative of partial nail plate avulsion. (B) Simple nail bed laceration visualized after nail plate removal. (From McGlamry,[10] with permission.)

significant proximal digital soft tissue injury, a more proximal block is performed at the metatarsal level. Epinephrine should not be used in traumatized tissues. Hemostasis can be achieved with either a digital Penrose tourniquet at the base of the toe or a pneumatic tourniquet (such as a blood pressure cuff) at the ankle level. In general, tourniquets are not utilized unless enhanced visualization is necessary during the brief period in which the nail bed is accurately reapproximated. It is also important to realize that the presence of a nail bed laceration represents a violation of the cutaneous barrier to bacterial contamination of underlying tissues, notably, the distal phalanx. Appropriate surgical scrub and preparation are necessary prior to nail plate avulsion, and tetanus prophylaxis as well as systemic antibiotic therapy must be administered as necessary.

Following avulsion of the nail plate, the nail bed is lavaged and inspected. The simple nail bed laceration typically appears as a short, transverse defect without significant disparity between the wound margins (Fig. 7-5B). The surgeon must keep in mind that the nail bed is composed of a rather friable tissue in comparison with the skin of the surrounding nail folds. For this reason, debridement should be kept to a minimum in an effort to avoid loss of large segments of nail bed and exposure of the underlying

phalanx. Simple nail bed lacerations usually require debridement in the form of high-pressure lavage using a 10-to-20-ml syringe and an 18-gauge needle with either normal saline or a dilute povidone-iodine solution.

Primary suture repair of simple nail bed lacerations is performed utilizing 4-0 or 5-0 synthetic absorbable suture material on a taper-tip needle in a simple interrupted fashion. Ideally, primary suture closure should be performed within 1 week of the nail bed injury in an effort to avoid excessive granulation tissue and resultant undesirable scar formation.[3] Care must be taken when suturing the nail bed to avoid the underlying distal phalanx. Absorbable suture material is preferred for nail bed repair because suture removal is unnecessary. When nonabsorbable sutures are used, their removal can be difficult for the surgeon and uncomfortable for the patient owing to covering of the suture material with organized wound exudate. Should the wound be heavily contaminated with bacteria, consideration should be given to using nonabsorbable sutures if primary nail bed repair is to be performed.

Simple nail bed lacerations that propagate into the adjacent nail folds are not very common. When the nail fold is lacerated, it should be repaired utilizing 4-0 or 5-0 nonabsorbable sutures on a reverse cutting needle in a simple interrupted fashion. Care must also be taken to preserve the cul-de-sac nature of the proximal nail groove and the overlying proximal nail fold. It is crucial to prevent contact between the dermis of the proximal nail fold and the damaged nail bed during healing. Should this occur, there is risk of developing permanent adherence of the proximal nail fold to the nail bed and resultant disruption of the nail plate as it grows out of the proximal nail groove and over the scarred nail bed. Following suture of the nail bed laceration, it is recommended that a smooth, appropriately contoured splint or template be applied to the nail bed. The goal behind this is to prevent surface irregularities in the healing nail bed and thereby minimize the post-traumatic sequelae associated with onycholysis. To this end, a number of techniques have been described for maintaining the contour of the nail bed as well as the cul-de-sac configuration of the proximal nail groove. Schiller described utilizing the cleansed and trimmed old nail plate, sutured to the medial and lateral nail folds, as the template for guiding the regeneration of the nail bed and proximal nail fold as the new nail plate grows outward.[4] Another common technique is the use of a 0.02-inch (0.5-mm) silicone elastomer sheet as a template, fashioned to fit the nail bed and proximal nail groove. This is a convenient technique as the silicone elastomer can be maintained in a sterile container and readily fashioned at the time of nail bed repair. I have found the use of a nonadherent sterile gauze (Xeroform, Adaptic) to be useful as an adequate template for the maintenance of the contour of the nail bed and the proximal nail groove. This material is also sterile, and is convenient to use. Studies comparing long-term follow-up of nail bed injuries treated with the use of the old nail plate, the silicone elastomer template, and the nonadherent gauze revealed no significant clinical variation among the three techniques with respect to final regeneration product.[5] Following application of the nonadherent gauze, a moistened saline dressing sponge is applied followed by the application of a dry sterile dressing and the use of a Darby shoe. Consideration should be given to the use of a forefoot splint or a below-the-knee cast and non-weight bearing as necessary. The wound is redressed at 3 to 5 days following primary suture repair. Sutures are typically removed at 10 to 14 days.

COMPLEX NAIL BED LACERATIONS

Complex, or stellate, nail bed lacerations result from the application of a violent crushing force to the digit. This type of crushing laceration presents with an irregular defect that often propagates outward through the surrounding nail folds and even plantarly into the digital pulp (Fig. 7-6).

The principles of management for a stellate nail bed laceration are identical to those for the treatment of simple nail bed lacerations. Because of the significant increase in tissue disruption, repair of the complex laceration can be more difficult. There is almost always an associated distal phalangeal fracture. Moreover, these injuries are often highly contaminated, and initial surgical debridement followed by delayed definitive reconstruction may be necessary.

NAIL BED LACERATION WITH PHALANGEAL FRACTURE

Simple and comminuted distal phalangeal tuft fractures often result from digital crush injuries (Fig. 7-7). Such injuries must be considered open fractures, and initial management involves ap-

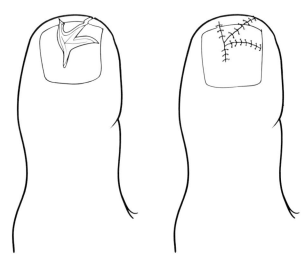

Fig. 7-6. Irregular stellate nail bed laceration.

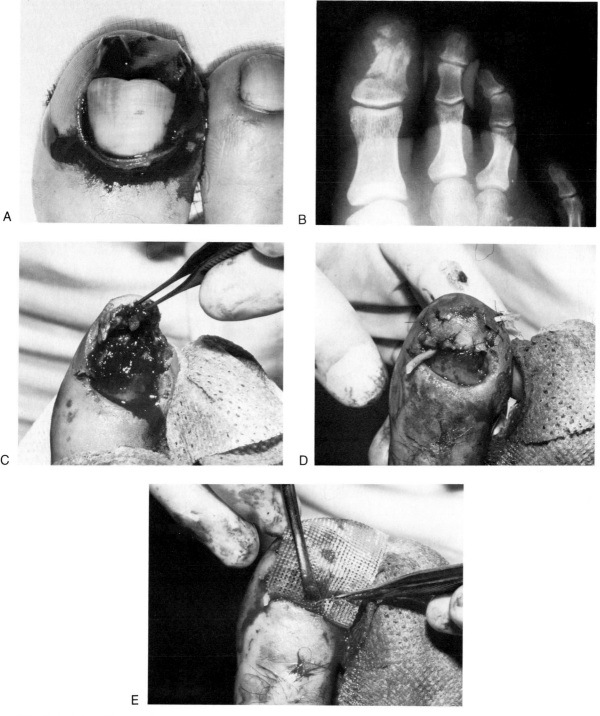

Fig. 7-7. **(A)** Stellate nail bed laceration caused by crush injury of the hallux. Note the plantar propagation of the laceration into the digital pulp. The nail plate is almost completely avulsed, and the cuticle has been separated from the proximal nail fold. **(B)** Comminuted fracture of the distal phalanx. **(C)** Complex nail bed laceration observed following nail plate removal. **(D)** Primary suture repair of the nail bed and adjacent folds, as well as the digital pulp. Because of the high risk of infection associated with this type of injury, closure is made over a sterile rubber band drain. **(E)** Nonadherent gauze being evenly applied over the nail bed and into the proximal nail groove. (From McGlamry,[10] with permission.)

propriate debridement and local wound care, as well as the use of systemic antibiotics. Markedly displaced, small, unstable distal phalangeal fracture fragments are usually excised. Minimally displaced fragments usually realign satisfactorily upon repair of the nail bed. Rarely, an axial Kirschner wire is required to stabilize large distal phalangeal fragments. Placement of a drain, such as a sterile rubber band, is recommended prior to closure of the nail bed and surrounding nail folds. In the presence of heavy contamination or infection, open packing and subsequent surgical debridement with delayed wound closure are indicated.

NAIL BED AND TOE TIP TISSUE LOSS INJURIES INCLUDING NAIL BED AVULSIONS, PARTIAL DIGITAL AMPUTATIONS, AND DIGITAL DEGLOVING

Injuries involving nail bed tissue loss markedly increase the likelihood of a cosmetically as well as functionally poor outcome. Such injuries are categorized according to both the level and direction of tissue loss, as described by Rosenthal[6] (Figs. 7-8 and 7-9).

The initial treatment of fresh zone 1 nail bed tissue loss injuries focuses on adequate cleansing debridement followed by appropriate wound closure. The majority of these injuries are allowed to granulate closed by secondary intention. Occasionally, skin grafting will be useful for coverage of hallucial defects larger than 1 cm². Newmeyer and Kilgore described a very useful and simple technique for procuring and transplanting a small split-thickness skin graft for coverage of large zone 1 injuries in the hand.[7] This technique has also proved useful in cases of toenail bed injuries associated with significant digital pulp skin loss. One must keep in mind that a split-thickness skin graft is generally not very durable and that significant graft contraction should be anticipated. For these reasons, full-thickness skin grafts have been advocated for resurfacing weightbearing and contact areas. Full-thickness skin grafts may be harvested from the volar surface of the antebrachium or from the groin, buttock, thigh, calf, and the skin over the sinus tarsi. Full-thickness skin grafts display less tendency for complete "take"; however, graft contraction is minimal in comparison with that of a split-thickness skin graft, and this form of wound coverage is very durable.

Zone 2 nail bed tissue loss injuries result in the exposure of the distal aspect of the terminal phalanx. Debridement of these injuries requires reduction of the prominent bone and removal of any grossly infected and necrotic soft tissue and bone. Coverage of the tip of the digit and distal augmentation of the nail bed are usually achieved with a local adjacent neurovascular V-Y advancement flap. These techniques provide sensate skin for coverage of the tip of the toe and robust coverage of the remnant bony phalanx. The orientation of the flap of the V-Y skin plasty is determined by the direction of tissue loss. The plantar V-Y advancement flap (Fig. 7-10), as described for the finger by Atasoy et al.,[8] and the mediolateral biaxial V-Y advancement skin plasty (Fig. 7-11), as described for the finger by Kutler,[9] are frequently used for pedal nail bed and distal digital reconstruction. These techniques are readily used in the emergency room or office setting. Obviously, grossly contaminated or "old" wounds (untreated for longer than 4 to 6 hours) should undergo initial debridement followed by definitive reconstruction on a delayed basis.

Zone 3 tissue loss injuries (Fig. 7-12) are generally not amenable to initial definitive treatment in the emergency room or office setting. The prognosis for nail bed survival is extremely guarded in this type of digital trauma. Surgical debridement in the operating room is followed, either immediately or on a delayed basis, by revision of the distal aspect of the digit. The entire nail matrix is typically excised to prevent aberrant nail plate regeneration, and every attempt is made to preserve the distal interphalangeal joint and digital tendon function. Distal digital ablation, often in the form of a terminal Symes-type revisional amputation, may be necessary.

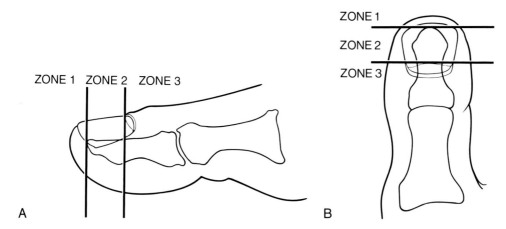

Fig. 7-8. The level of nail bed tissue loss. Zone 1, distal to the bony phalanx; zone 2, distal to the lunula; zone 3, proximal to the distal end of the lunula. (**A**) Sagittal plane view. (**B**) Transverse plane view.

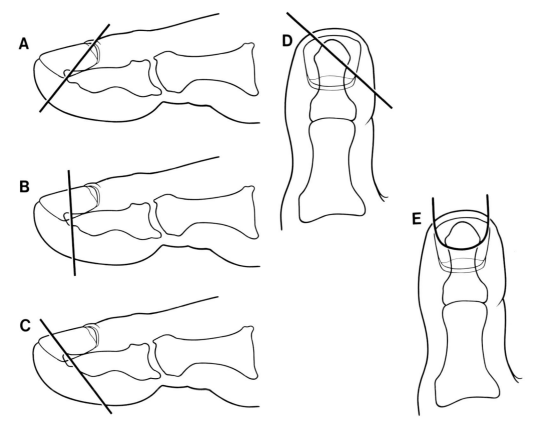

Fig. 7-9. Direction of nail bed tissue loss. (**A**) Dorsal oblique. (**B**) Transverse or guillotine. (**C**) Plantar oblique. (**D**) Tibial (or fibular) axial. (**E**) Central or gouging.

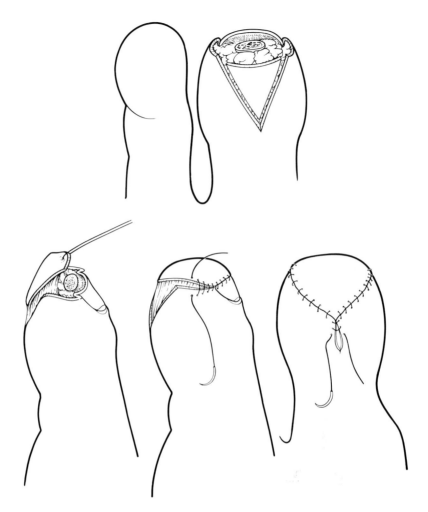

Fig. 7-10. Plantar V-Y local neurovascular advancement flap.

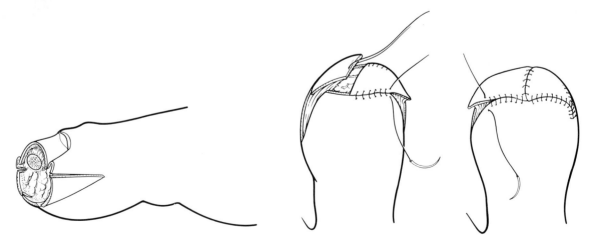

Fig. 7-11. Mediolateral V-Y local neurovascular advancement flaps.

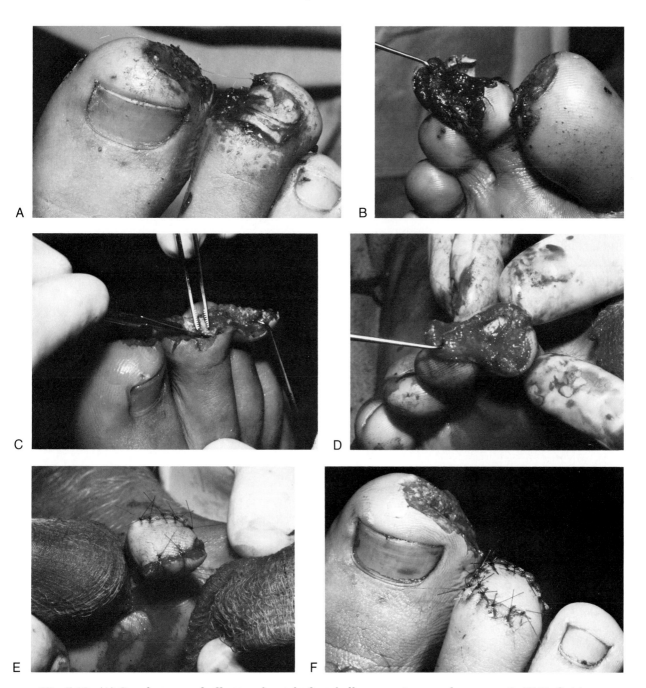

Fig. 7-12. (**A**) Gunshot wound affecting the right foot: hallux, zone 1; second toe, zone 3. (**B**) Definitive surgical debridement performed in the operating room approximately 36 hours after initial debridement in the emergency room. All necrotic soft tissue and bone are removed. (**C**) Total excision of the nail matrix of the second toe in preparation for ablative revision of the digit. (**D**) Large, robust lateral flap designed to cover the tip of the second toe. The largely necrotic distal phalanx has been excised, and the middle phalanx has been remodeled distally. (**E**) Initial closure of the laterally based pedicle flap. (**F**) Immediate postoperative appearance. The hallux was allowed to close by secondary intention. (Courtesy of WD Secrest, DO, Tucker, GA.)

CONCLUSION

Nail bed injuries are frequently encountered by the podiatric physician. In the foot, the most common mechanisms of injury are crushing and stubbing. Lesions requiring immediate care include subungual hematomas and nail bed lacerations with associated phalangeal fracture, as well as digital tissue loss injuries. In the acute setting, every effort should be made to restore the functional unity of the intimately related anatomic structures of the distal aspect of the toe. Appropriate emergency treatment ranges from the drainage of subungual hematoma to the accurate anatomic reconstruction of the nail bed and its associated structures.

REFERENCES

1. Baran R, Badillet G: Primary onycholysis of the big toenails: a review of 113 cases. Br J Dermatol 106:529, 1982
2. Farrington GH: Subungual hematoma: an evaluation of treatment. Br Med J 21:742, 1964
3. Zook EG: The perionychium: anatomy, physiology, and care of injuries. Clin Plast Surg 8:21, 1981
4. Schiller C: Nail replacement in fingertip injuries. Plast Reconstr Surg 19:521, 1957
5. Zook EG, Guy RJ, Russell RC: A study of nail bed injuries: causes, treatment, and prognosis. J Hand Surg 9A:247, 1984
6. Rosenthal EA: Treatment of fingertip and nail bed injuries. Orthop Clin North Am 14:675, 1983
7. Newmeyer WL, Kilgore ES: Fingertip injuries: a simple, effective method of treatment. J Trauma 14:58, 1974
8. Atasoy E, Iokimidis E, Kasdan ML et al: Reconstruction of the amputated fingertip with a triangular volar flap. J Bone Joint Surg 52A:921, 1970
9. Kutler W: A new method for fingertip amputation. JAMA 133:29, 1947
10. Malay DS: Trauma to the nail and associated structures. pp. 997, 998, 999. In McGlamry ED (ed): Comprehensive Textbook of Foot Surgery. Vol. 2. Williams & Wilkins, Baltimore, 1987

8

Foreign Bodies

Robert A. Cooke, D.P.M.

Foreign body injuries of the foot and ankle often present the physician with the dilemma of formulating an effective treatment plan. This becomes particularly perplexing when there is no history of recent penetrating injury or when radiographic findings are negative. Fortunately, the majority of these types of injuries have a clear history. However, the initial clinical signs and symptoms often do not correspond with the extent or severity of the injury. The presence of localized tenderness, erythema, and edema should always raise a degree of suspicion that a retained foreign body is the source of the problem. It should additionally be recognized that the sequelae of a foreign body injury may range from a simple foreign body reaction to a functional deficit of the involved part to a potentially limb-threatening infection.[1] Thus, complete, thorough evaluation and treatment are imperative.

METALLIC FOREIGN BODIES

Needles

The most commonly encountered foreign body in the foot is a pin or needle.[2] This generally results from a puncture wound in which the needle tip has broken off after penetrating the skin (Fig. 8-1). They are usually superficial; however, given the forces of weight bearing and delayed detection, the needle may migrate to deeper layers[3] (Fig. 8-2).

Removal of the needle is often not necessary. These injuries usually heal without sequelae providing there is no involvement of the bone, joint spaces, or neurovascular structures. This is particularly true if the needle is lying parallel to the weight-bearing surface or is present in a non-weight-bearing area. If the needle lies vertical to the weight-bearing surface, its presence is more likely to become symptomatic as a result of movement of the object with the compression and expansion of the foot during ambulation.

Indications for removal include persistent discomfort with or without weight bearing, intra-articular involvement, or the presence of a chronically draining wound.[3]

The initial identification and diagnosis of metallic foreign bodies is easily made by standard radiographic techniques. Intraoperative localization, on the other hand, can be extremely difficult. Needles can be particularly elusive by the nature of their size and shape. Additionally, they can lie along tissue planes, aiding detection, or they may be embedded within the substance of a muscle or tendon, making detection more difficult (Fig. 8-3). Because needles can remain as inert objects for long periods, the tissue reactions seen with other foreign objects such as local inflammation, abscess, or foreign body reaction may not be present. These reactions are often helpful in locating the foreign body during surgical exploration.

Multiple instruments and methods have been devised over the years to facilitate localization of

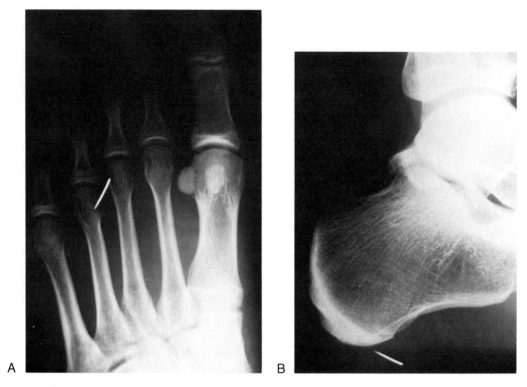

Fig. 8-1. (**A**) Needles embedded in the soft tissue of the forefoot. (**B**) Needle embedded in the subcalcaneal fat pad.

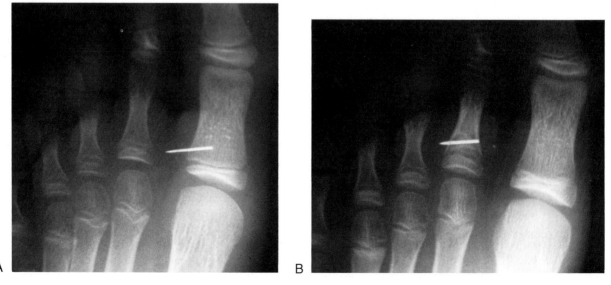

Fig. 8-2. (**A**) Initial radiograph of a child's foot with a sewing needle embedded in the proximal soft tissue of the great toe. (**B**) Demonstrates migration of the needle to the level of the proximal phalanx of the second toe, which was found to be penetrated at the time of surgery.

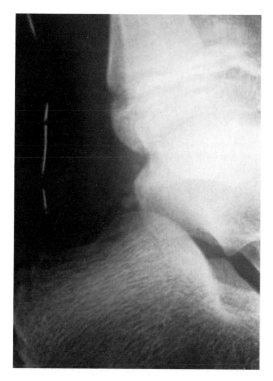

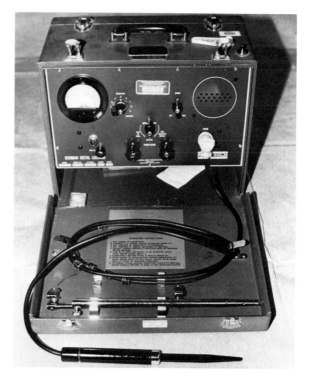

Fig. 8-3. Multiply fragmented needle extending through the substance of the Achilles tendon in a young child. (Courtesy of Barry L. Scurran, D.P.M.)

Fig. 8-4. Berman Metal Locator, one of the early instruments devised to detect and localize metallic foreign bodies.

metallic foreign bodies at the time of surgery. Electromagnetic metal locators have been used for many years (Fig. 8-4). These instruments have a hand-held probe connected to a speaker that emits a rising pitch and to a meter that numerically rises as the probe nears the foreign object while the skin surface is scanned. It is more effective at detecting magnetic metals (iron and steel) than nonmagnetic metals (brass, copper, and aluminum). Localization with hypodermic needles inserted into the area of the foreign body has been a popular technique.[4] There are many variations using different gauge needles inserted at various angles.[5] One of the more common methods is triangulation.[6] Triangulation involves placing needles at 90 degree angles to pinpoint the depth and location, making dissection more accurate (Fig. 8-5). This is a good intraoperative technique; however, it involves delays for radiographs to be taken and processed.

C-arm fluoroscopy[1,7] is now the technique of choice for localization of radiopaque foreign bodies (Fig. 8-6). It is an imaging technique that produces instantaneous projections of intraoperative radiographs on a television screen. The resultant image can be cleared from the C-arm fluoroscope, stored in its memory for later reference, or converted to a hard x-ray copy. It is easily utilized and eliminates surgical delays resulting from x-ray-processing time. In using the C-arm fluoroscope, multiple exposures are made while advancing a metallic surgical instrument closer to the foreign body. Once the incision is made, dissection to the foreign body can then be directed by producing periodic images.

Gunshot Wounds

Gunshot wounds to the lower extremity frequently result in retained foreign bodies. Debridement of these wounds and removal of mis-

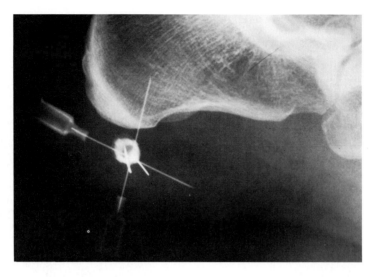

Fig. 8-5. Triangulation of hypodermic needles to facilitate intraoperative localization of foreign bodies.

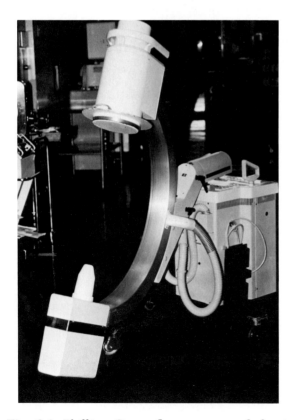

Fig. 8-6. Phillips C-arm fluoroscope used for intraoperative localization of radiopaque foreign bodies.

sile or pellet fragments depend, in a large part, on the distance between the firearm and the victim as well as the missile type and velocity.[8] Missiles are classified into low and high velocity. In general, low-velocity injuries such as shotgun wounds from a large distance require superficial initial debridement. The entrance and exit sites are irrigated and debrided. Retained pellets or missiles are not removed (Fig. 8-7), unless they are superficial or involve a joint space.[9] Fragments that become superficial and symptomatic as the body attempts to extrude them should be removed. Secondary wound infection resulting from the foreign body may additionally require removal in conjunction with antibiotic therapy.

High-velocity gunshot or close range shotgun wounds[10,11] create extensive internal soft tissue and bone damage (Fig. 8-8) as well as cause large superficial tissue deficits. As the missile passes through the body part, it may leave a path of metallic fragments that are quite apparent on standard radiographs (Fig. 8-9). Aggressive superficial and deep wound debridement is indicated, including removal of all visible missile fragments. Attempts should not be made to remove deeply imbedded fragments or pellets since further neurovascular and tissue damage may result.[12]

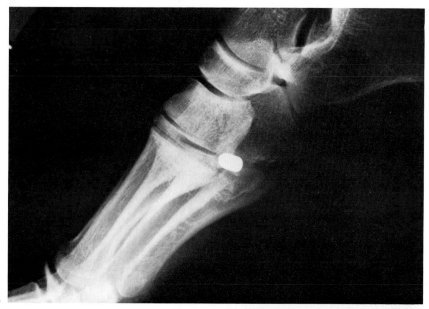

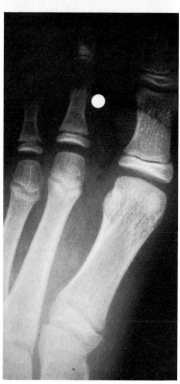

Fig. 8-7. (**A**) Low-velocity pellet lodged in the midfoot. (**B**) Self-inflicted gunshot wound with a BB embedded in a child's second toe.

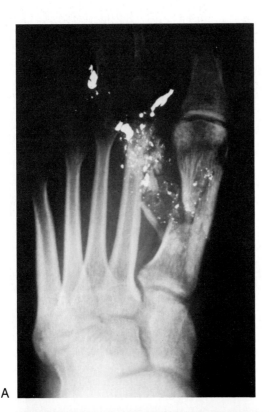

A

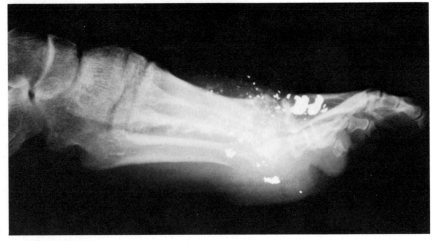

B

Fig. 8-8. (A & B) High-velocity gunshot wound to the forefoot resulting in massive destruction of the first metatarsal.

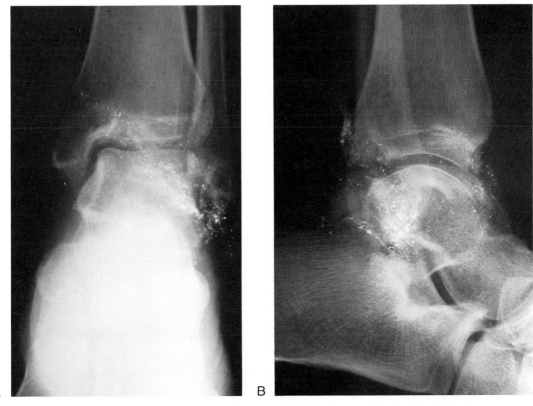

Fig. 8-9. **(A & B)** High-velocity gunshot wound to the posterior ankle showing a track of metallic debris passing from medial to lateral.

NONMETALLIC FOREIGN BODIES

Wood

Wood splinters, toothpicks, and thorns are among the most frequently encountered nonmetallic foreign bodies in the foot. They are the most difficult to diagnose and treat. Wood is one material that is consistently missed by standard radiographic techniques.[13] In the past, this had led to attempts to utilize alternate diagnostic techniques such as xeroradiography. Xeroradiography is a radiographic technique used for soft tissue enhancement. Unfortunately, it has been used with less than successful results in localizing wood foreign bodies. This technique has been shown to be no more superior than standard radiographs in terms of visualization of wood.[14]

Recently, computed tomography (CT) has proved to be the most reliable method of localizing retained wooden objects[15] (Fig. 8-10). Bernardino et al. compared ultrasound, xeroradiography, and CT, demonstrating the superiority of CT to the other techniques in both consistency of identification and size approximation.[16] CT has been shown to be one hundred times more sensitive in detection of wood than radiography as well as giving the added advantage of three-dimensional localization.[17] Until CT became more readily available, physicians had to rely on the history of injury and the clinical signs and symptoms. This particular injury remains one in which a thorough history is especially important and may aid in the formulation of a treatment plan. Early clinical signs and symptoms usually include localized pain, edema, and inflammation with the presence of a puncture wound. If the injury is

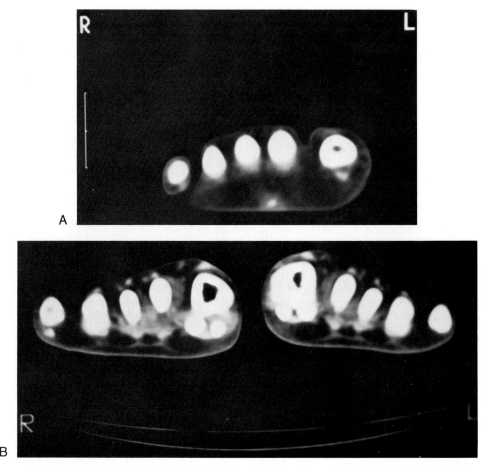

Fig. 8-10. (**A**) CT scan of the forefoot demonstrating a wood foreign body inferior to the second inter-space. Standard radiographs were negative. (**B**) CT scan of the forefoot confirming the presence of a wood foreign body inferior to the fifth metatarsal, unable to be visualized on initial radiographs.

superficial, local debridement with removal of the foreign body may be all that is necessary. Deep wood foreign bodies, if undetected, may become asymptomatic. However, symptoms may eventually return, producing differing reactions depending on the tissue involved. Intra-articular lesions can produce synovitis.[18] Where bone such as a metatarsal has been involved, a perios-teal reaction with cortical thickening may occur as well as osteolysis where the bone has been penetrated.[14,18–20] Pathologically, in areas where joint destruction, osteolysis, and periostitis have occurred as a late result of a retained piece of

wood or thorn, a foreign body granuloma is commonly demonstrated. Standard radiographic evaluation will detect these late osseous changes. It is important to note that these changes can simulate a Ewing's sarcoma, which should be part of the differential diagnosis, espe-cially when there is a vague history of injury. Foreign body granulomas commonly form chronic draining wounds. Generally these are sterile, but they can become secondarily in-fected.[3] This is in contrast to infection of metal foreign bodies, in which *Pseudomonas aeru-ginosa* is a strongly suspected pathogen.[21]

Glass

Glass foreign bodies in conjunction with wood make up the most frequently encountered non-metallic foreign bodies in the foot. They are most often a direct result of a plantar puncture wound in which the glass fragment becomes subcutaneously embedded. These fragments are usually visible on standard radiographs depending on their size and density (Fig. 8-11). Pigmented or lead-containing glass is easily visualized. Most other commonly occurring glass fragments measuring greater than 0.5 mm can be readily demonstrated by standard radiographs providing there is no overlying bone.[12,22] Radiographs taken at oblique angles alleviate the impairment in visualization caused by overlying bone. Glass fragments measuring greater than 2 mm can be easily seen even where overlapping bone is present. Anderson et al. found in a retrospective study of foreign bodies occurring in the hand that 96 percent of all glass fragments were visible on standard radiographs.[13]

Glass foreign bodies do not usually result in severe infections and thus do not always require removal. Removal is indicated if the foreign body is intra-articular, involves bone, threatens neurovascular structures, or becomes symptomatic. As with metallic foreign bodies, they may migrate; however, migration of foreign bodies in the foot is almost always restricted to a very small area. The more likely sequela is for the body to encapsulate the glass fragment and gradually attempt to extrude it over an extended period of time. During this process, the area of extrusion is likely to become erythematous and tender, necessitating removal of the foreign body.

MISCELLANEOUS FOREIGN BODIES

Plastic

Plastic may or may not be seen by standard radiography depending on the size, configuration, and orientation of the fragment within the soft tissue.[14] Plastic foreign bodies should be treated in the same manner as glass.

Hair

Segments of hair may occur as a foreign body. Heavy coarse hair such as that from a beard or from the terrier dog breeds is the most common foreign body. When stepped on, these stiff hairs can cause a puncture wound. This can go undetected until an eventual abscess develops. Upon debridement of the lesion, the hair is frequently detected as an incidental finding. Removal of the hair is usually the only treatment needed. Antibiotics are seldom required, depending on the clinical signs and symptoms.

Longer, finer texture hairs occasionally occur as external foreign bodies circumferentially wrapped around the toe of an infant (Fig. 8-12). This can be a potential threat to the viability of the involved toe if undetected for a long period. The hair will stretch minimally as the toe grows, which may result in vascular compromise. The physician may be the first to detect the hair when the parent complains of a dusky appearance to the digit. Removal of the hair should be immediate and done with great care. If the end of the strand can be detected, it may simply be unwound. More frequently, the end of the hair cannot be found and the circumferential ring must be sharply incised in a longitudinal direction so as not to traverse the digital arteries. After the ring is broken, each strand can be meticulously removed.

OTHER FOREIGN BODIES

Gravel, dirt, grass, or portions of shoe and sock are most often the result of a plantar puncture. These wounds should be treated as dirty wounds. Treatment should consist of aggressive initial wound debridement and irrigation, tetanus prophylaxis, and appropriate antibiotic therapy. Initial laboratory tests and radiographs should be obtained. The wound is kept open when possible with packing material that is changed every 24 to 48 hours.

Subsequent treatment depends on the clinical signs and symptoms. A progressively improving

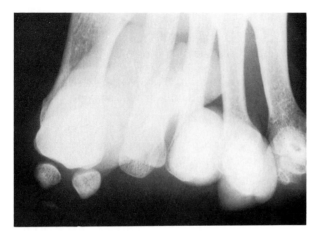

Fig. 8-11. Glass fragment embedded in the soft tissue inferior to the sesamoids.

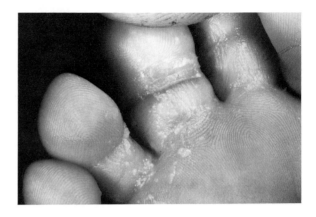

Fig. 8-12. Hair wrapped circumferentially around an infant's third toe. (Courtesy of Barry L. Scurran, D.P.M.)

wound generally requires only local wound care with eventual discontinuation of antibiotic therapy based on clinical, laboratory, and radiographic findings. Delayed primary wound closure is done after 3 to 4 days as improvement continues. On the other hand, when a wound is clinically deteriorating, more aggressive management may be necessary. This may include incision and drainage of the lesion when an abscess or osteomyelitis is suspected. Adjusting the antibiotic regimen based on both clinical response and culture and sensitivity results may be necessary. Wound closure and discontinuation of antibiotic therapy is done as previously noted.

REFERENCES

1. Puhl RW, Altman MI, Seto JE, Nelson GA: The use of fluoroscopy in the detection and excision of foreign bodies in the foot. J Am Podiatry Assoc 73:514, 1983
2. Mann R: Surgery of the Foot. 5th Ed. CV Mosby, St. Louis, 1986
3. Jahss MH: Pseudotumors of the foot. Orthop Clin North Am 5: 67, 1974
4. Jeffery JI: Surgical excision of foreign bodies. J Am Podiatr Med Assoc 74:229, 1984
5. Rickoff SE, Bauder T, Kerman BL: Foreign body and localization and retrieval in the foot. J Foot Surg 20:33, 1981
6. Hunt GB: Triangulation for removal of foreign bodies: two illustrative cases. Texas Med 71:84, 1975
7. Wilner JM, Lepon GM: The use of C-arm fluoroscopy and its application to podiatric surgery. J Foot Surg 22:283, 1985
8. Karlin JM: Management of open fractures. Clin Podiatry 2:217, 1985
9. Bretter D, Sealin ED, Mender DG: Conservative treatment of low velocity gunshot wounds. Clin Orthop 140:26, 1979
10. DeMuth WE, Smith JM: High velocity bullet wounds of muscles and bone: the basis of rational early treatment. J Trauma 6:744, 1966
11. DeMuth WE: The mechanism of shotgun wounds. J Trauma 11:219, 1971
12. Alfred RH, Jacobs R: Occult foreign bodies of the foot. Foot Ankle 4:209, 1984
13. Anderson MA, Newmeyer WL, Kilgore ES: Diagnosis and treatment of retained foreign bodies in the hand. Am J Surg 144:63, 1982
14. Charney DB, Manzi JA, Turlik M, Young M: Nonmetallic foreign bodies in the foot: radiography versus xeroradiography. J Foot Surg 25:44, 1986
15. Kuhns LR, Borlaza GS, Seigel RS et al: Technical notes: an in vitro comparison of computed tomography, xeroradiography, and radiography in detection of soft tissue foreign bodies. Radiology 132:218, 1979
16. Bernardino ME, Jing BS, Thomas J et al: The extremity soft tissue lesion: a comparative study of ultrasound, computer tomography, and xerography. Radiology 139:53, 1981

17. Nyska M, Pomeranz S, Porat S: The advantage of computed tomography in locating a foreign body in the foot. J Trauma 26:93, 1986

18. Cracchiolo A: Wooden foreign bodies in the foot. Am J Surg 140:585, 1980

19. Swischuk LE, Jorgensen F, Jorgenson A, Capen D: Wooden splinter induced "pseudotumor" and osteomyelitis-like lesions of bone and soft tissue. Am J Roentgenol Radium Ther Nucl Med 122:176, 1974

20. Simmons BP, Southmayd WW, Schwartz HS, Hall JE: Wood: an organic foreign body of bone. Clin Orthop 106:276, 1975

21. Johanson RH: Pseudomonas infections of the foot following puncture wounds. JAMA 204:170, 1968

22. Tandberg D: Glass in the hand and foot. JAMA 248:1872, 1982

SUGGESTED READINGS

Dowling GL: Foreign body: a review of two cases. J Foot Surg 21:70, 1982

Gelfer SD: Foreign body removal with the aid of a metal locator. J Am Podiatr Med Assoc 51:502, 1961

Gilsdorf JR: A needle in the sole of the foot. Surg Gynecol Obstet 163:573, 1986

Parisien JS, Esformes I: The role of arthroscopy in the management of low-velocity gunshot wounds of the knee. Clin Orthop Rel Res 185:207, 1984

Rhoades CE, Saye I, Levine E et al: Detection of a wooden foreign body in the hand using computed tomography. Case report. J Hand Surg 3:306, 1982

Sanford CC: Puncture wounds of the foot. Am Fam Physician 24:119, 1981

Weinstock RE: Noninvasive technique for the localization of radiopaque foreign bodies. J Foot Surg 20:73, 1981

Yu JC, Chang KK: Migration of broken sewing needle from the left forearm to the heart. Chest 67:626, 1975

9

Animal Bites

Stephen H. Silvani, D.P.M.

Animal, insect, and reptile bites of the lower extremities occur with a surprisingly high frequency. The unrelenting push of civilization into the wilderness encourages increasing numbers of human-animal encounters. New construction that alters ecosystems; outdoor jobs and recreation; and increasing pet and reptile ownership adds to the potential chance for injury to human feet. Despite the high incidence of these pedal injuries, considerable controversy exists about their management. This is due to the lack of well-designed, prospective studies that examine efficacy of various treatment regimens for bite wounds.[1] Several risk factors that affect bite therapy outcome would have to be controlled and analyzed.[2] These include prehospital management, type of injury (shearing, crushing, puncture, etc.), depth and extent of wounds, anatomic location, type of wound-cleansing agent, extent of debridement, and patient health. One can see that a valid treatment investigation would be very difficult.

The basic principle of trauma management of the total patient takes precedent over local wound care. Airway management, breathing control, and maintenance of adequate circulation are of primary importance. Tetanus immunization status should be ascertained and reinforced if necessary (Table 9-1). In this chapter, it will be assumed that basic emergency care has been rendered and that the patient is stable. The discussion therefore will be limited to local wound management. Consultation with a plastic surgeon, a vascular surgeon, an infectious disease expert, and others should be sought as appropri-

ate. Guidelines for wound management, debridement, antibiotic therapy, and aftercare are presented.

MAMMALIAN BITES

Mammalian bites to the lower extremity, usually from dogs, cats, and human beings, rarely are seen in emergency departments and physicians' offices.[3] While the potential for serious injury is present, the majority of these bites inflict only minor damage. Animal bites accounted for 0.7 percent of all emergency department visits in one study.[4] Pinckney and Kennedy reviewed extensive data, including newspaper articles, and reported 74 deaths from dog bites in the United States.[5] Children represent a majority of fatal and nonfatal bite incidents owing to their proximity and innocence in dealing with animals. Nondomestic mammalian (monkey, rodent, horse, bat, coyote, fox, lion, bear, boar, raccoon, and anteater) bites are even more infrequent.[4,6,7] The constant encroachment of humans on animal habitats increases these occurrences. The true extent of this problem is not known because there is no national reporting system for nondomestic animal bites.

Human bites occur at an estimated rate of 60 bite incidents per 100,000 persons.[8] Statistically, these patients are most often young males, inebriated and not very compliant. The peak incidence is during warm weather months. Pedal injuries occur during karate-type kicks, brawls, and

Table 9-1. Tetanus Prophylaxis in Wound Management[a]

History of Tetanus Immunization Doses	Clean Minor Wounds		Other Wounds	
	Td	TIG	Td	TIG
Uncertain	Yes	No	Yes	Yes
0–1	Yes	No	Yes	Yes
2	Yes	No	Yes	No[b]
3 or more	No[c]	No	No[d]	No

[a] Td, Both tetanus and diphtheria toxoids; TIG, tetanus immune globulin.
[b] Yes, if wound is more than 24 hours old.
[c] Yes, if more than 10 years since last booster.
[d] Yes, if more than 5 years since last booster.
(Data from Centers for Disease Control: Adult immunization: recommendations of the Immunization Practices Advisory Committee (ACIP). MMWR, 33:suppl. 1, 1s–68s, 1984.

altercations involving kick-boxing. Occasionally they occur in cases of child abuse. Biting injuries to the foot may be self-inflicted, as with the infant who becomes startled while sucking toes.

Microbiology and Clinical Manifestations

The flora of mammalian oral cavities, as well as the infection of the inflicted wounds, are well documented. A variety of infections can occur, with cellulitis, lymphangitis, abscesses, and osteomyelitis being relatively common. Subcutaneous gas collection,[9] meningitis,[10] endocarditis,[11] tularemia,[12] and syphillis[13] have all been reported in the literature following various animal bites. In immunosuppressed or compromised patients, a fulminate gram-negative septicemia has been reported[14,15] after dog bites.

Pasteurella multocida is the most common pathogen in dog and cat bites.[4,9] This gram-negative facultatively anaerobic rod is very susceptible to penicillin. Within 48 hours of the bite inoculation, erythema and drainage occur from the bite site. Usually regional lymphadenopathy and a low-grade fever accompany this infection. Even though the organism readily responds to antibiotics, suppurative tenosynovitis, septicemia, and osteomyelitis can occur.

Esoteric unnamed gram-negative rods are also pathogens found in dog bites. These are classified under the alphanumeric Centers for Disease Control system and have been implicated in meningitis,[10] endocarditis,[11] and overwhelming septicemia.[15] More common organisms such as *Streptococcus viridans*, *Staphylococcus aureus*, *Bacterioides* species, and *Fusobacterium* species have also been cultured from animal bite infections.

Human bites are especially contaminated, with multiple anaerobes being found in over 50 percent of these wounds.[16] *Staphylococcus* and *Streptococcus* species may not be as common pathogens as previously believed. With better culture techniques, *Eikenella corrodens*, a gram-negative rod present in dental plaque, is seen in 20 percent of infected human bites.[16] Its resistance to penicillinase-resistant penicillins, aminoglycosides, and clindamycin is worrisome, but it is usually sensitive to cefoxitin and other cephalosporins. *Treponema pallidum* has been cultured from human bites.[13] Human bites, owing to the high incidence of occurrence in the hand and foot, have a long-term unfavorable morbidity. Infections in these anatomic structures can result in decreased function or even amputation.

Cat-scratch disease, probably caused by a chlamydia-like organism, occurs in certain animal bites. No specific antibiotics are indicated because this is a benign, self-limiting condition. Rat bites are associated with two specific infections. Fever and chills, followed by pharyngitis, headache, myalgias, and a diffuse morbilliform rash on the palms and soles are characteristic of streptobacillary rat-bite fever. The causative organism is *Streptobacillus moniliformis*,[17] which usually responds to high-dose penicillins. Sodoku, or spirillary rat-bite fever, is caused by the spirochete *Spirillum minus*. These lesions develop erythema, induration, and eschar formation, with the patient experiencing fever, chills, and a macular rash at the lesion site. This organism is very sensitive to high-dose penicillin.

The tetanus immunization status of the patient should be ascertained and treated appropriately (Table 9-1). Tetanus immune globulin (TIG) of human origin avoids some of the serious allergic

Table 9-2. Rabies Postexposure Prophylaxis

Animal Species	Animal Condition	Treatment
Dog or cat	Healthy and available for 10 days observation	None, unless animal develops rabies[a]
	Rabid or suspected	RIG and HDCV[b]
	Unknown (escaped)	Consult public health department RIG and HDCV
Skunk, bat, fox, coyote, raccoon, bobcat, other carnivores	Regard as rabid unless laboratory test proves negative[c]	RIG and HDCV
Livestock, rodent, rabbits	Consult public health officials	

[a] During the usual 10-day holding period, begin treatment at the first sign of rabies.
[b] RIG, Rabies immune globulin; HDCV, human diploid cell vaccine. Give as soon as possible. Local reactions are common. Discontinue if animal tests are negative.
[c] The animal should be killed and tested as soon as possible. Holding for observation is not recommended.
(Data from Centers for Disease Control: Rabies prevention, United States. 1984 Recommendation of the Immunization Practices Committee. [ACIP]. MMWR 33:393, 1984.

reactions previously seen with horse serum preparations. Rabies is another infection that must be considered with mammalian bites. Most domestic animals can be captured and observed with the cooperation of the local animal control service. However, the rabies status of nondomesticated mammals is seldom known as the animals are rarely captured postinjury. The prophylactic rabies regimen is presented in Table 9-2. Consultation with an infectious disease expert is recommended if rabies is suspected.

Management

Most mammalian pedal bites can be managed on an out-patient basis. Treatment with antibiotics cannot overshadow the importance of meticulous wound cleansing, thorough debridement, and high-pressure irrigation. Unless an iodine allergy is reported, diluted povidone-iodine solution cleansing is initially used with fine-mesh sponges. This initial mechanical scrub, after appropriate local or regional analgesia, cleanses some of the gross contaminating foreign material. This solution has antibacterial and antiviral properties. High-pressure irrigation with normal saline employing a surgical lavage mechanism or a large syringe (50 ml) with an 18-gauge needle is utilized to further cleanse the wounds. This size needle is especially useful for irrigating deep puncture wounds. Meticulous debridement of all

visible devitalized subcutaneous tissue and dermis is extremely important, especially in small puncture wounds. Many animal bites are essentially crush wounds with much deep tissue destruction that may not be obvious for several days (Fig. 9-1). Secondary debridement will optimize the wound for delayed primary closure or perhaps skin grafting.

At this time, the wound is explored for injuries to tendons, nerves, joint capsule, cartilage, or bone. Radiographs are recommended to rule out foreign bodies, retained animal teeth, and fractures or crushed bones.

Most clinicians and investigators agree that wounds on the feet and hands should not be closed initially owing to the proximity of tendons, bones, and joint spaces. Close wound observation and delayed primary closure or healing by granulation are preferred. This will produce greater function and less morbidity than a wound that was closed initially and subsequently became infected.

Organisms recovered from infected wounds often correlate poorly with those cultured from the same site, once it became infected.[1] Therefore, the value of routine prophylactic antibiotics started empirically in nonacral wounds is questionable. Thorough cleansing and extensive debridement will prevent most infections. Once an infection is established, appropriate antibiotics can be used as determined by the culture and sensitivities of the organisms. However, owing to

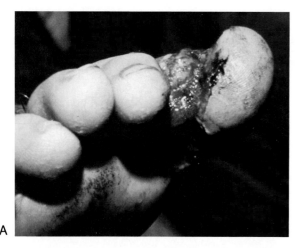

A

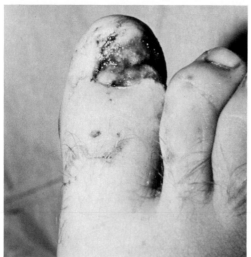

B

Fig. 9-1. (**A & B**) A dog bite to the hallux and treated locally and granulated to heal without sequelae. The nail plate was removed to clean the wound adequately.

the superficial and important structures found in the hand and foot, infections can occur quickly and spread proximally or deeply with great rapidity. Therefore, antibiotic prophylaxis is recommended. With the previous microbiologic discussions in mind, hand and foot wounds, deep or grossly contaminated wounds, or those present in an immunocompromised patient necessitate the use of a semisynthetic penicillin or a cephalosporin (500 mg every 6 hours by mouth). Hospitalization and parenteral antibiotics are encour-

aged in human bites with deep penetration and those wounds that fail to respond to the above therapy. These wounds are rechecked at 48 hours for signs of infections and again at 5 to 7 days. Steri-strips can be used or delayed primary closure with sutures can be achieved at this time. In some cases with extensive necrotic areas secondary to crushing or shearing, skin grafting is appropriate. Physical therapy and occupational therapy may be necessary to resume full function of the involved foot.

SPIDER BITES

Almost all of the 100,000 species of spiders can bite, but only a few have chelicerae strong enough to penetrate human skin. Tarantulas (actually the American mygalomorph)[18] have urticaria-producing hairs on the dorsal surface of the abdomen. Contact with these causes severe local edema and pruritus. Treatment is usually topical corticosteroids or oral antihistamines. If severe, a decreasing, short term course of oral prednisone is recommended.

The brown recluse spider, which belongs to the genus *Loxosceles*, is dull yellow to light brown in color. On the dorsum of the cephalothorax is a dark brown violin-shaped marking. The bite of this spider causes severe necrotic tissue destruction, called necrotic arachnidism (Fig. 9-2). This spider is usually encountered indoors in webs, but because it also spins its webs in low-lying grass and debris, walking barefoot outdoors is the most common method of receiving these injuries to the foot. The most severe reactions, however, occur in fatty areas such as the thigh or buttocks.[19] Local stinging, pain, or pruritus are the initial symptoms experienced. A blue-gray halo appears around the puncture wound in true necrotic arachnidism, indicating that local cyanosis is present. This usually progresses to necrosis, eschar formation, and a large ulceration, which may take 6 to 8 months to heal. Systemic signs may occur as the lesion enlarges. These may include restlessness, generalized urticaria, arthralgias, myalgias, hemolysis, disseminated intravascular coagulation, fever, diarrhea,

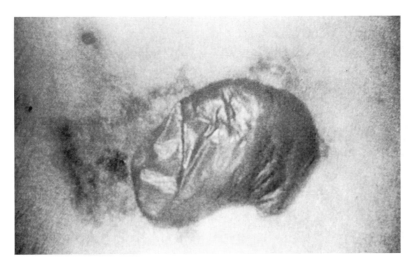

Fig. 9-2. A brown recluse spider bite (3 days old).

proteinuria, hematuria, shock, and coma.[20] Death can result in the true severe viscerocutaneous loxoscelism.[21] Patients with a necrotic bite larger than 1 cm in diameter should be tested for a progressive hemolytic anemia or thrombocytopenia. If this has not occurred by 10 to 12 hours postenvenomation, the likelihood of a severe systemic reaction is low.[21]

The venom of the brown recluse is more potent than that of a rattlesnake, and many enzymes that cause the dermatonecrosis and hemolysis have been isolated. The treatment of the bite is controversial in the literature. Intralesional and oral steroids, surgical debridement, and the use of dapsone have been recommended.[18–23] Cleansing of the wound, protection with sterile, nonadherent dressings, having the patient avoid unnecessary activity, analgesics, and avoiding early surgery are generally agreed upon courses of action. If secondary bacterial infection becomes evident, use of antibiotics is guided by cultures obtained from the wound. Dapsone has been effective in reducing the cutaneous ulceration, as are early cold compresses.[19–21,23,24] Systemic steroids may be necessary if the necrotic area becomes larger than 3 to 4 cm in diameter or if renal problems or coagulopathies develop. Fortunately, most patients respond with just local care and the necrotic ulcer fully epithelizes in several months.

The venom of the black widow spider, which belongs to the genus *Latrodectus*, produces significant neurotoxic symptoms after envenomation. The spider is easily distinguished by its markings, being jet black with a red hourglass marking on its abdomen. The venom of the black widow spider causes a block in neuromuscular transmission by initial release of the acetylcholine or catecholamines, followed by their depletion. This effect can be blocked by *Latrodectus* antivenin.[25] The initial bite may present with two fang puncture marks with slight surrounding erythema. Shortly, within 1 hour, a dull ache to severe pain with some numbness spread proximally to involve the entire torso. It is most severe in the legs and the abdomen where it may mimic an acute abdomen. This peak is several hours postbite, but may last for several days. Anxiety, dizziness, weakness, fever, headaches, nausea, vomiting, chest tightness, respiratory distress, urinary retention, muscle fasciculations, and paresthesias may also be present. The limbs may be contracted with flexor muscle spasms, and there may be burning paresthesias of the plantar pedal surfaces. Renal damage, shock, cardiac and respiratory failure, cerebral hemorrhage, and local bacterial infections may also occur. The young, the old, or those with underlying cardiac dysfunction are most susceptible to death.

There is controversy about the use of the horse

serum antivenin for black widow spider bites. Traditionally, if the patient has severe signs and symptoms of latrodectism, hospitalization is recommended, as well as usage of one ampule of *Latrodectus mactans* antivenin (Lyovac, 2.5 ml). This should be administered with caution owing to the possibility of a severe allergic reaction that can occur even in patients with negative skin testing for horse serum. Serum sickness is also a possibility. An alternative medication is calcium gluconate (20 ml of 10 percent solution intravenously), muscle relaxants (diazepam), methocarbamol, or steroids. It has been stated that there is a higher incidence of severe reactions to the horse serum antivenin than there is to the envenomation.[26] The majority of envenomations are self-limited, peak in severity at 3 to 4 hours, and require only symptomatic treatment. Therefore, hospitalization and close observation are utilized in children, elderly persons, cardiac patients, and pregnant women. The spider bite wound itself requires only local symptomatic treatment.

POISONOUS SNAKE BITES OF THE EXTREMITIES

The treatment of poisonous snake bites is a complex and also controversial issue. No single mode of treatment is accepted by all authorities. Several deaths occur annually in the United States as the result of snake bites. Permanent deformities and amputations of the extremity are a common and serious complication. The hands and feet are commonly involved, and the resultant incapacities contribute to the severe morbidity.[27] The clinician who has the occasion to treat venomous snake bites should have a thorough understanding of the systemic and local effects of the toxins.

The poisonous varieties of snakes in the United States, with the exception of the coral snake, are members of the family Crotalidae. These pit vipers include the rattlesnake, the water moccasin, and the copperhead. The fangs of the coral snake are sharp and permanently erect. Their highly toxic venom is injected into multiple puncture wounds by a series of chewing mo-

tions. In contrast, the fangs of the pit vipers are long and hinged. They are erected during the strike, and as soon as they contact with the victim, the venom is expressed by sudden muscular contractions of the poison glands. Various toxins in the snake venom immobilize its prey. Proteolytic enzymes digest the prey if the snake should swallow an animal whole.

Snake venoms contain various amounts of neurotoxin, hemolysin, cardiotoxin, cholinesterase, phosphatase, nucleotidase, cytochrome oxidase inhibitor, hyaluronidase, and proteolytic enzyme. Thus, all body tissues are subject to attack. Venom causes toxic systemic side effects, local cellular destruction, and necrosis at the puncture site. The venom is activated by body temperature and pH when it is injected into the subcutaneous tissue. The immediate cellular destruction, as well as destruction of lymphatics and blood vessels, occurs by hydrolysis. Swelling rapidly follows because of a rise in tissue osmotic pressure that is secondary to local cellular destruction and the presence of cellular degradation products. Severe pain accompanies the swelling. Ecchymosis and bulla formation also occur.

Some toxins and digested cellular substances may enter intact vessels and thus spread throughout the body to cause systemic effects. Local gangrene of the skin and underlying structures is seen secondary to profound local ischemia. When envenomation occurs in muscle tissue, the hemorrhage is rapid and severe because of the high susceptibility of muscle fibers to enzymatic degradation. Hemorrhage and increased osmotic pressure within an enclosed fascial compartment impair circulation and enhance necrosis.

Glass has stated that circulation to the anterior compartment of the leg can be obstructed as early as 1 hour after the bite.[28] The circulation to the posterior compartment also may be severely impeded within 3 hours. Systemic effects occur when venom and cellular degradation products reach susceptible organs, that is, heart, kidney, liver, and formed blood elements. These effects may include fever, nausea, vomiting, circulatory collapse, anuria, hemorrhage, jaundice, neuropathic muscle cramping, pupillary constriction, disorientation, delirium, coma, and death.

Laboratory abnormalities may be equally varied and can include progressive anemia, poly-morphonuclear leukocyte count of greater than 20,000 mm³, thrombocytopenia, hypofibrino-genemia, and altered coagulation time. Renal failure and other organ involvements are repre-sented by an altered electrolyte balance. Thus, envenomation causes complex local and systemic problems that require complex solutions. These problems are compounded by the fact that the authorities cannot agree on a single mode of treatment.

Treatment of Pedal Snake Bites

Envenomation of the victim can result in defi-brination of plasma, exsanguination, cerebral hemorrhage, coma, and death. The effects of snake bites to the extremities can be physiologi-cally, psychologically, and biomechanically crip-pling (Fig. 9-3). A review of the literature indi-cates that authorities do not agree on first aid techniques. The main objective is to calm the victim and provide transport as quickly as possi-

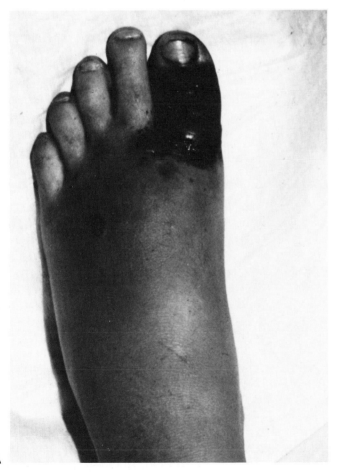

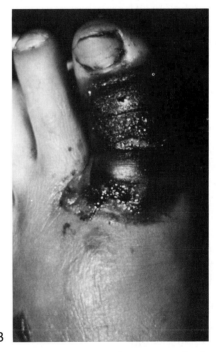

A

B

Fig. 9-3. A rattlesnake envenomation of the left foot. **(A)** Left foot 3 days postbite showing marked edema (to the thigh), bleb formation, and necrosis surrounding the bite. The patient had received nine vials of Crotalidae antivenin initially. **(B)** Extreme gangrene (well demarcated) is present 9 days post-bite. This extended deep, including the extensor tensons, joint capsule, and cortex of the phalanx. (*Figure continues.*)

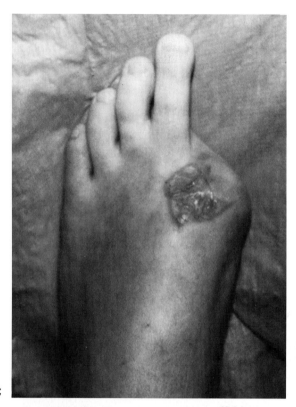

C

Fig. 9-3 (*Continued*). **(C)** Twenty days postbite, the hallux was amputated (after three debridements) and wound closure was achieved by a plantar flap and split-thickness skin graft. (From Silvani, et al.,[27] with permission.)

ble to a physician. Pitts has stated that the best first aid item is a set of car keys.[29]

A snug constriction band should be applied proximal to the bite area and made loose enough to slip a finger underneath. This band should not be applied tightly, and the distal pulse should be palpable. This tourniquet should not be released unless the edema becomes severe or if it has been in place for more than 1.5 hours. Watt and Gennaro described a patient who went into shock upon tourniquet release owing to the sudden injection of venom in the systemic circulation.[30] A splint must be improvised to keep the limb horizontal. Most authorities discourage the use of ice packs, and if they are used at all, it should be for only a very limited time period. Crushed ice applied to the extremity of a conscious victim may decrease the activity of the

venom, but does not neutralize, destroy, or remove it.[28] Extreme cooling can cause frostbite and compound the ischemia already produced by the venom. Ischemia may occur during the reactive hyperemic vascular phase that occurs after removal of ice, when metabolic oxygen demands exceed oxygen delivered by the already compromised arterial circulation. Therefore, ice should be avoided. Incision and suction should be performed only if it can be done within seconds of the bite if medical attention is not immediately available (within 1 hour). These cuts are ineffective in severe bites and may cause damage in minor ones. Glass reported two peroneal and one median nerve transsection in a 1-year period in Texas.[28] When a physician is not nearby, a linear incision to subcutaneous tissue is acceptable. This incision should not go more than 0.3 cm deep, and suction should not be applied for more than 30 minutes. According to McCollough and Gennaro, 22 to 50 percent of the venom can be removed this way in the first 3 minutes after the bite.[31]

When feasible, the snake should be killed and brought safely to the hospital for identification. Many patients have been bitten more than once by the same snake, so extreme care must be exercised in doing so. Most authorities concur on the following early hospital treatment plan. Because some bites do not produce symptoms immediately, the patient must be observed for several hours for pain, edema, ecchymosis, or blebs. Weakness, dizziness, numbness, clammy skin, tachycardia, nausea, vomiting, and diarrhea may be present. The tourniquet is not released until an intravenous line (18 gauge) is secured and patent. A slow infusion of 5 percent glucose and lactated Ringer's solution is started. Antivenin is properly used in cases in which envenomation is suspected on the basis of serious systemic symptoms.

The patient should be questioned for a history of allergy to horse serum, and 1 : 1,000 epinephrine solution should be readily available. A skin or eye test for hypersensitivity is performed before administering one vial of intravenous antivenin with careful monitoring for allergic reaction. Desensitization according to the manufacturer's instructions may be necessary prior to therapy. In the literature there are stories of miraculous survivals of snake bite victims, despite severe anaphalaxis to antivenin, shock, and stormy hospital courses.[32]

There is some controversy about what constitutes the correct dose of antivenin. Insufficient neutralization has been more common than overneutralization.[33] As neutrality approaches, the patient "feels better," the rate of swelling decreases, and vital signs improve. Pitts has provided estimates of venom neutralization potency for various snakes by which the appropriate amount of antivenin can be judged.[29] Severe envenomation may require 20 to 30 vials, and Mojave rattlesnake bites may require 30 to 40 vials. In general, bites of the extremities and bites in children require greater amounts of antivenin. Patients may require decreasing doses of steroids to combat the increasing serum sickness. Immobilization of the extremity, tetanus toxoid, and prophylactic antibiotics are generally recommended.

Many authorities agree that early debridement of the bite area provides the least systemic and local morbidity, although debridement is reserved for those patients who exhibit signs of significant envenomation (moderate to severe toxic systemic side effects and local tissue damage). Early dermotomy on the digits is especially helpful.[24] This is a medial or lateral subcutaneous incision, made in between the neurovascular bundles, that releases the deep fascial compartments. The wound is packed open for 24 hours only and may be closed primarily after several days. If this procedure is done early, functional and cosmetic results are usually satisfactory. Otherwise, the skin and subcutaneous tissue are excised en bloc with a 1-cm margin around each fang mark. Pressure dressings are used for hemostasis. Early wound excision or dermotomy removes most of the local toxins and enzymes and limits tissue necrosis by compression. Adequate early antivenin treatment usually prevents persistent bleeding. Watt described good results and a decrease in systemic manifestations with this method.[33]

It can be seen the treatment of bites to the extremities is an extremely complex matter requiring the coordinated skills of a surgeon and an internist. A hematologist, a plastic surgeon, an infectious disease specialist, or a medical herpetologist may also be necessary. Consultations with local public health departments or poison control centers may be necessary. Following these guidelines and the principles of proper wound management, most patients inflicted with bites upon the extremities should heal successfully with function preserved for the future.

REFERENCES

1. Feder HM, Shanley JD, Barbera JA: A review of 59 patients hospitalized with animal bites. Pediatr Infect Dis 6:24, 1987
2. Trott AT: Principles and Techniques of Minor Wound Care. Medical Examination Publishing, New York, 1985
3. Jaffe AC: Animal bites. Pediatr Clin North Am 30:405, 1983
4. Aghababian RV, Conte JE: Mammalian bite wounds. Am Emerg Med 9:79, 1980
5. Pinckney LE, Kennedy LA: Traumatic deaths from dog attacks in the United States. Pediatrics 69:193, 1982
6. Dibb WL, Digranes A, Tonjum S: *Actinobacillus lignieresii* infection after a horse bite. Br Med J 283:583, 1981
7. Kizer KW: Epidemiologic and clinical aspects of animal bite injuries. JACEP 8:134, 1979
8. Marr JS, Beck AM, Lugo JA: An epidemiologic study of the human bite. Public Health Rep 94:514, 1979
9. Callahan ML: Treatment of common dog bites: infection risk factors. JACEP 7:83, 1978
10. Bracis R, Seibers K, Julien RM: Meningitis caused by group II-J following a dog bite. West J Med 131:438, 1979
11. Shankar PS, Scott JH, Anderson CL: Atypical endocarditis due to gram-negative bacillus transmitted by dog bite. Southern Med J 73:1640, 1980
12. Quenzer RW, Mostow SR, Emerson JK: Cat-bite tularemia. JAMA 238:1845, 1977
13. Fiumara NJ, Exner JM: Primary syphilis following a human ite. Sex Transm Dis 8:21, 1981
14. Fiala M, Bauer H, Khaleeli M: Dog bite, *Bacteroides* infection, coagulopathy and renal microangiopathy. Ann Intern Med 87:248, 1977
15. Findling IW, Pahlmann CP, Rose HD: Fulminant

gram-negative bacillemia (DF-2) following a dog bite in an asplenic woman. Am J Med 68:154, 1980

16. Martin LT: Human bites—guidelines for prompt evaluation and treatment. Postgrad Med J 81:221, 1987

17. Speck WT: Rat bite fever. p. 649. In Behrman R, Vaughn V (eds): Textbook of Pediatrics. WB Saunders, Philadelphia, 1983

18. Hunt GR: Bites and stings of uncommon arthropods. I: Spiders. Postgrad Med J 70:91, 1981

19. King LE, Rees RS: Management of brown recluse spider bites. JAMA 251:889, 1984

20. Pitts NC: Necrotic arachnidism. N Engl J Med 267:400, 1962

21. Dillaha CS, Jansen GT, Honeycutt WM: North American loxoscelism. JAMA 188:33, 1964

22. Russell FE, Gertsch WJ: Letter to the editor. Toxicology 21:337, 1983

23. Berger RS: A critical look at therapy for the brown recluse spider bite. Arch Dermatol 107:298, 1973

24. King LE, Rees RS: Dapsone treatment of a brown recluse bite. JAMA 250:658, 1983

25. Bettini S: On the mode of action of Lactrodectus species venom. Ann Ist Super Sanita 7:1, 1971

26. Moss HS, Binder LS: A retrospective review of black widow spider envenomation. Ann Emerg Med 16:188, 1987

27. Silvani SH, Karlin JM, DeValentine SJ, Scurran BL: Poisonous snakebites of the extremities. J Am Podiatry Assoc 70:172, 1980

28. Glass TG: Early debridement in pit viper bites. JAMA 235:2513, 1976

29. Pitts W: Snakebite. p 156. In Ravitch MM (ed): Pediatric Surgery. 3rd Ed. Year Book Medical Publishers, Chicago, 1979

30. Watt CM, Gennaro JF: Pit viper bites in South Georgia and North Florida. Trans South Surg Assoc 77:378, 1965

31. McCollough NC, Gennaro JF: Evaluation of venomous snake bite in the southern United States from parallel clinical and laboratory investigations: development of treatment. J Fla Med Assoc 49:959, 1963

32. Loprinzi CL, Hennessee J, Tamsky L, Johnson T: Snake antivenom administration in a patient allergic to horse serum. South Med J 76:501, 1983

33. Watt CN: Poisonous snakebite treatment in the United States. JAMA 240:654, 1978

34. Watt CN: Treatment of poisonous snakebite with emphasis on digit dermotomy. South Med J 78:694, 1985

10

Gunshot Wounds

Mark E. Reiner, D.P.M.

Trauma to the foot and ankle caused by gunshot wounds represents a singular aspect of podiatric care. A clear understanding of ballistics, wounding capability, wound care, and the extent of surgical treatment necessary for these injuries is important, especially for surgeons who treat these injuries infrequently.

WOUNDING CAPACITY

Three major theories exist concerning the wounding capacity of bullets,[1] the power theory, the momentum theory, and the kinetic energy theory. All have bullet weight and velocity as the outstanding variables and all relate the wounding capacity of a bullet directly to its speed at impact. The destructive effect depends on the amount of energy released by the projectile as it passes through tissue. The power theory is expressed by the equation: power = mass × velocity^3. The rate of performing work is referred to as power. Velocity, as a variable, plays an important role here since very small increments in velocity result in a large increase in work performed by the bullet and, therefore, a significant increase in its wounding potential.

The momentum theory (momentum = mass × velocity) applies to a projectile of significant weight, as mass and velocity are of equal importance. This theory applies to bullets in excess of 250 grains (7,000 grains/lb) delivered at a velocity rarely exceeding 2,600 ft/s (793 m/s). A wound created by a firearm employing this combination is rarely encountered in civilian practice.

The kinetic energy theory is described by the equation: kinetic energy = $MV^2/2$ where M = mass and V = velocity. Currently, this is the most popular concept because it places much more importance on velocity than on mass. Here, the total energy delivered by a missile upon an object will determine the amount and extent of injury. It is important to understand that the energy imparted on impact is the most important aspect of the wounding agent.[3] Therefore, if the mass is doubled, the kinetic energy is doubled; double the velocity and *quadruple* the kinetic energy. It is important to note, however, that an increase in either variable will increase the energy and consequent destructive effect.

HIGH-VELOCITY WOUNDS

Gunshot wounds are usually caused by a single metal projectile fired from a long- or short-barrel gun and are generally classified into high- and low-velocity injuries. High-velocity injuries typically result when the muzzle velocity of the bullet exceeds 2,000 ft/s (610 m/s). Low velocity is considered less than 2,000 ft/s.[1–3] Some researchers use 2,500 f/s (762 m/s) as the point of distinction.

High-velocity wounds are almost exclusively encountered on the military battlefield or as accidents sustained during big game hunting. Any wounding agent that delivers 58 ft-lbs (78.6 J) of energy is capable of producing a casualty. Demuth and Smith point out that high-velocity rifle bullets carry energies far exceeding the 58 ft-lb minimum, approaching 3,000 ft-lbs (4,068 J) at the muzzle and having a residual energy of 1,000 ft-lbs (1,365 J) at a distance of 300 yards (274 m). Commonly, military rifle bullets weigh between 140 and 200 grains and have muzzle velocities between 2,300 and 2,900 ft/s (701 to 884 m/s). The destruction created by a high-velocity bullet is directly proportional to the amount of kinetic energy produced.

The wound tract created by a high-velocity bullet can be divided into three components[1,4,5]: (1) The permanent wound tract or primary cavity; (2) the contusion zone; and (3) the concussion zone.

The permanent wound tract is the area of tissue destruction that exists after the projectile passes. The size of this tract depends on the characteristics of the adjacent tissues, bullet weight, size, and shape, and physical behaviors of the bullet such as yaw and tumble. At high velocities, over 2,000 ft/s, the missile will traverse a relatively straight course and have entry and exit ports. In high-velocity gunshot wounds, the exit wound is typically larger than the entrance wound.

A temporary cavity is created in the trail of a high-velocity projectile. Temporary cavitation is the most important effect of high-velocity wounds, becoming apparent only when missile velocity exceeds 1,000 ft/s and becoming extensive only when velocity exceeds 2,000 ft/s.[6] As the projectile penetrates, it accelerates tissue particles forward and laterally to expand the tract to a larger temporary cavity. Harvey et al.[5] demonstrated pressure pulses as high as 100 atm during the impact of high-velocity bullets. The negative force created during cavitation may be sufficient to suck clothing, outside debris, and bacterial matter into the sterile environment behind the missile. The characteristics of the temporary cavity vary according to the energy imparted by the missile on the tissue (disruptive force) and the elastic properties of the tissue involved (retentive force).[3] The explosive charac-

teristic of high-velocity bullets is largely due to the expansion of the temporary cavity. The violence of this expansion is so great that the expansile capacity of the adjacent tissue is exceeded and, hence, tissue destruction occurs. It is this cavitation phenomenon that results in significant tissue damage at a distance removed from the high-velocity bullet tract. Obviously, the greater the energy delivered, the more distant the tissue injury will be from the wound tract. The disruptive and retentive forces eventually equilibrate, and the temporary cavity collapses to become the permanent cavity.

Tissue density is a large contributor in the creation of cavitation. The damaging effect of projectiles intensifies with an increase in specific gravity of the tissue involved.[7] Bone has a specific gravity greater than water and is the most severely damaged of any body tissue.[1,3] Demuth determined the specific gravity of several body tissues and found that wound tracts produced were roughly proportional to the density of the tissue involved.[1]

Cortical bone has the greatest density, and long bones are at a higher risk for injury than are lower density flat bones in which cancellous bone predominates. When bony fracture occurs, bone fragments fly out into the temporary cavity but generally return close to the source. Therefore, it is unusual for the bone fragments to become secondary missiles effective at any significant distance.[3] In the absence of direct bone strike, the high-velocity missile produces a less severe fracture when passing near a long bone. The incidence of fracture is related to the striking energy and specific gravity of the tissue surrounding the bone.

The contusion zone is described as a thin layer of muscle tissue 5-mm wide adjacent to the temporary cavity. Enormous swelling of muscle fibers, up to four or five times normal size, and interstitial extravasation of blood are characteristic. Muscle fibers are disrupted and a "clotting" of the cytoplasm occurs, leaving areas of muscle severely damaged; these eventually become nonviable. Histologically, there is loss of striations with a large number of inflammatory cells. Connective tissue and blood vessels are also injured in the area adjacent to the wound tract. Fascial planes absorb the energy, and muscle lying next to these planes may be injured at considerable distances from the permanent wound tract.

The concussion zone lies beyond the contusion zone. There exists, however, no clear demarcation between these zones. The damaging effects of a high-velocity projectile are minimal in the concussion zone. The vascular supply remains intact, and there is no apparent soft tissue destruction or necrosis. However, a large number of inflammatory cells are present in this zone.

THE SHOTGUN BLAST

Shotgun injuries should be considered a separate class of wound. Although the shotgun is classified as a low-velocity weapon, the velocity of pelleted loads ranges from 1,220 to 1,330 ft/s (372 to 405 m/s)[2], and the gun has the destructive characteristics of a high-velocity weapon when fired at close range.

Shotgun loads contain pellets of varying number and size. When referring, therefore, to the kinetic energy equation when dealing with shotgun injuries, mass is an often overlooked variable. The weight of individual pellets has frequently been used to determine energy potentials.[1] The total kinetic energy will be the sum total mass of the individual pellets, or the total weight of shot in a given shell.[8] Pellets remain tightly clustered for a distance up to 10 feet (3 m) upon leaving the gun barrel, a phenomenon enhanced by the use of plastic shot-retainer caps. Shotgun shells are of poor design to maintain high kinetic energy at great distances from the gun muzzle.

At distances less than 10 feet, the total weight of shotgun loads is much greater than the weight of individual rifle bullets. Demuth et al. found that the wound created from a 12-gauge full charge of 00 buckshot fired at close range is equivalent to being struck by nine to ten .22 long rifle bullets simultaneously at muzzle velocities of most shotguns.[9] The impact of multiple small pellets on tissue does not permit great tissue penetration. The resistant tissue absorbs the kinetic energy and transforms it into elastic, plastic, and dissipative effects on tissue.[8] At close range, energy is completely released very near to the point of penetration. Massive injury to the area then occurs.[8–10] When relating total kinetic energy to injury, the mass of shotgun shells is the dominant factor when compared with rifle bullets. In absolute terms, the shotgun shell has the potential to do as much injury, if not more, as the high-velocity bullet.

A shotgun blast to the foot at close range usually results in severe skin and soft tissue injury with multiple bony fractures. The crushing and lacerating power of the blast can be profound. Muscle damage can be extensive, with fragmentation of fibers and frequent infiltration of clothing and wadding. Contusion can extend several centimeters peripheral to the tract of the pellets. Shepard refers to a blast injury component that is similar to the cavitation phenomenon in high-velocity bullet injuries.[8] This is caused by rapidly expanding gases of combustion striking tissue forcefully enough to cause injury. This injury should be treated as serious and given immediate and thorough debridement. Special attention should be directed at the removal of wadding, as this material is highly reactive in tissues. Wound debridement is discussed further below.

LOW-VELOCITY WOUNDS

Low-velocity injuries are caused by bullets weighing between 100 and 300 grains with muzzle velocities ranging from 700 to 1,700 ft/s (213 to 518 m/s). Consequently, with these variables, the kinetic energy delivered is much less than that of a high-velocity bullet and, therefore, the inflicting damage to the tissue is not as destructive.[2,6,11]

Laceration and crushing are the principal effects of the passage of low-velocity bullets through tissue, with the majority of damage confined to the permanent wound tract (Fig. 10-1).

Most often the permanent wound tract has only an entry port, as the energy carrying the missile

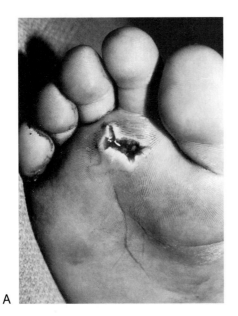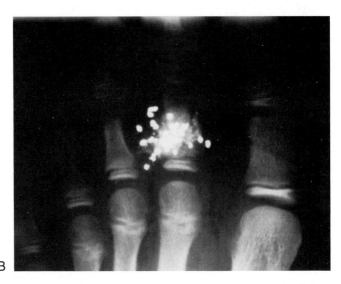

A   B

Fig. 10-1. (A) Ten-year-old boy sustained a low-velocity gunshot wound to the dorsal aspect of the second digit. Photograph reveals the exit port on the plantar aspect of the second toe sulcus. Note the irregularity and maceration of the skin edges. **(B)** Radiograph revealing direct strike of the proximal phalanx by the missile. Lead fragments have scattered, and severe comminution of the fracture is seen. Note how the injury has spared the physis. (Courtesy of Barry L. Scurran, D.P.M.)

is not sufficient for it to traverse the extremity and create an exit port. Shock waves are also generated ahead of the missile as it penetrates.

Low-velocity gunshot wounds usually occur at short ranges and produce no cavitation effects, since the expansile capacity of the surrounding tissue exceeds that of the kinetic energy delivered by the bullet. In the absence of cavitation, necrosis of tissue at a distance from the primary wound tract is not usually significant. The low-velocity missile wound, therefore, results in laceration and crushing of soft tissues with a permanent wound tract of minimal diameter.

Low-velocity bullets produce a "drill hole" defect when striking areas of bone with a high proportion of cancellous material, such as the distal tibia (Figs. 10-2 and 10-3). The .45 caliber automatic (United States) bullet produces such a wound. The method of treatment depends on the extent of tissue damage and whether the injury involves soft tissue or bony fracture or dislocation.

MANAGEMENT OF PEDAL GUNSHOT WOUNDS

Gunshot wounds to the foot are typically from projectiles of low velocity. The foot has a very high ratio of bone to soft tissue, and most pedal gunshot wounds involve fracture. Principles inherent to the management of open fractures should, therefore, be employed in the initial treatment of pedal gunshot wounds. The foot deserves particular concern because structural integrity is a most important consideration, with functional mobility being a somewhat lesser concern.

For a polytraumatized patient, resuscitation and stabilization of vital functions demand immediate attention. Any obvious hemorrhaging is controlled. Once the patient has been stabilized, further assessment of the injury is performed.

A thorough examination of the foot and ankle should be performed. The presence or absence of

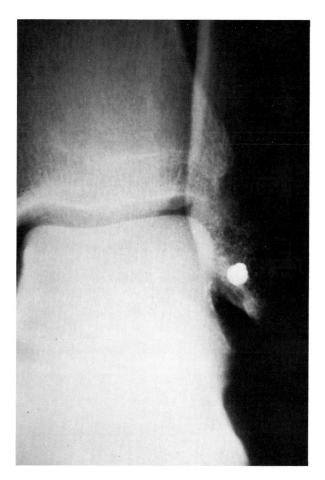

Fig. 10-2. Anterior view of the ankle joint revealing buckshot pellet lodged in the anterior surface of the distal lateral malleolus. Note the absence of bony fracture. Shot was fired from a range in excess of 30 feet.

debris may be noted in the entry port from pieces of shoe, sock, or wadding pushed or sucked into the wound. The involved extremity should be properly stabilized by splinting while radiographs in three projections are obtained.

Fractures associated with gunshot wounds, since they communicate with the external environment, are considered open. The bullet is not heat sterilized upon firing; consequently, all wounds must be considered contaminated and potentially infected.[6,12,13] Organisms can be drawn into the wound by temporary cavitation from high-velocity bullets, and bits of clothing,

all lower extremity pulses is determined, and a thorough neurologic examination is performed. Active muscle movement of the involved part is beneficial in establishing muscular and motor nerve integrity. Sensory nerve deficits can be tested by sharp/dull and two-point discrimination and vibratory sensation. The entire foot and ankle should be inspected for entrance and exit ports, lacerations, skin slough, ecchymosis, and edema. All pedal and ankle joints should be put through their ranges of motion and the presence of pain, crepitus, or gross deformity noted. The wound may exhibit powder burns, and foreign

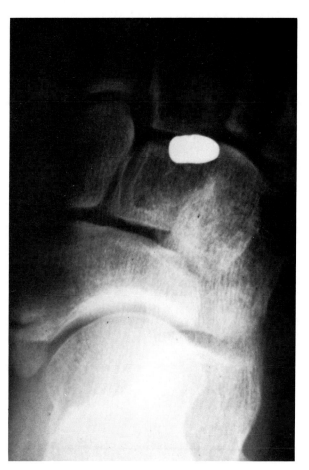

Fig. 10-3. Dorsal view of a low-velocity .22 caliber bullet, which was fired at a distance of 50 feet, lying in the capsular structures of the tarsal-metatarsal articulation. Note the absence of any fracture or dislocation.

environment, and skin contaminants are potential foci of infection.

Tetanus prophylaxis is mandatory. For those previously immunized, a passive booster of 0.5 ml of tetanus toxoid is administered. Those patients not previously immunized require a minimum of 250 units of human tetanus immune globulin and 0.5 ml of tetanus toxoid as an initial dose, followed by a series of three 0.5-ml doses at monthly intervals, and a final reinforcing dose 1 year later (see Table 3-1).

The management of gunshot wounds at this point depends largely on the degree of soft tissue and bony destruction, neurovascular compromise, and articular involvement and the level of wound contamination.

High-velocity bullets and shotgun pellets usually cause extensive soft tissue and bony destruction. It is universally agreed that these wounds require aggressive and extensive surgical debridement, antibiotic prophylaxis, and delayed closure of the wound.[3,6,14,15] Many investigators contend that low-velocity gunshot wounds

should be managed in a limited or nonsurgical manner.[6,10,11,14,16] Ziperman, however, recommends surgical exploration of all gunshot wounds because tissues must be inspected to evaluate their viability.[15] Every gunshot wound should be individually evaluated for the degree of soft tissue and bony destruction. The caliber, mass, and velocity of the projectile should be determined, if possible, to aid the treating physician in determining whether conservative treatment or surgical debridement is required.

Marcus et al. determined that low-velocity gunshot wounds with or without fracture can be managed safely and with a low rate of complication by a limited, nonoperative approach[16] (Fig. 10-4).

Bretther et al. did not attempt to debride, explore, or remove bullet fragments and found formal debridement rarely necessary.[14] Treatment routinely consisted of cleansing the wound and utilizing systemic antibiotics.

It is generally thought that a formal surgical debridement is indicated when low-velocity

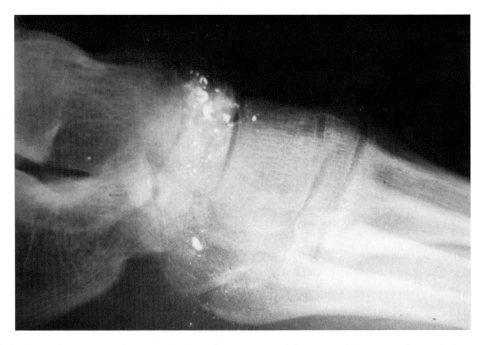

Fig. 10-4. Lateral view revealing nondisplaced comminuted fracture of the navicular with dispersion of the missile fragments. Note how the pellet fragments have penetrated into the body of the bone. Debridement was not performed on this patient.

gunshot injuries are complicated by gross necrosis and contamination, intra-articular injury, neurovascular destruction, or compartment syndromes.[6,10,14,16] Additionally, if the physician is unable to determine with certainty that the wound is low velocity in nature, formal surgical debridement is recommended.

The use of prophylactic systemic antibiotics varies among most researchers, and no established guidelines exist. Woloszyn et al. found no statistical advantage in the use of intravenous over oral antibiotic administration in the treatment of low-velocity gunshot wounds.[11] Howland et al. recorded a study of 72 patients with fractures resulting from low-velocity gunshot wounds in which the majority did not receive prophylactic antibiotics.[10] Only two of these patients suffered minor wound infections. The use of prophylactic antibiotics appears not to be essential for wounds that are not grossly contaminated.[6,11,14,16] The use of antibiotic therapy should be determined by the clinical appearance of each individual wound and the clinical judgment of the treating physician.

Initial Surgery

It is well documented that high-velocity gunshot wounds should be aggressively treated. As previously mentioned, the significant tissue damage far from the bullet tract is due to the cavitation phenomenon. These injuries are very similar to high-voltage electrical burns in which the extent of injury is not readily appreciated on initial examination. Because of inability to ascertain the limits of damaged tissue and extent of gross contamination of the wound, wide surgical debridement and excision of obviously devitalized muscle and fascia as well as delayed closure of the wound are the best guidelines for wound management (Fig. 10-5).

The majority of gunshot wounds to the foot are caused by small-caliber, low-velocity weapons. Devitalization of tissue at a distance from the primary wound tract is usually not significant and extensive debridement of soft tissues is unnecessary. The presence of bony fracture is not an indication for extensive surgical debridement.[17] Initial surgical intervention should be limited to and aimed at the prevention of infection and closing the wound as efficiently as possible. Cleansing of the wound and immobilization are usually all that is necessary.

Cleansing refers to the gentle removal of debris and skin contaminants. Copious lavage with at least 3 L of saline or 10 percent povidine-iodine-saline solution is performed at the entrance site. Exposed muscle and fascia are carefully and gingerly excised. Under local anesthesia, necrotic skin edges are excised in a conservative fashion. Under no circumstance should incisions be extended, counterincisions made, or probing of the missile tract performed. Foreign bodies are removed only if excessive dissection is not required.[15] Free floating bone fragments are excised, but fragments attached to soft tissue are retained. Periosteum is sacrificed if it is severely contaminated. Exposed tendon should be covered with soft tissue and retained. Bullets are not excised unless they are superficially located and can be palpated in the subcutaneous tissue. Complicated exploration should be avoided unless the bullet's location is threatening a vital structure. Retained bullets in the foot often become painful at a later date and require excision[10] (Fig. 10-6). Intra-articular lead missiles should be removed to prevent the destructive effects related to lead arthropathy and mechanical joint jamming. The joint is thoroughly explored and copiously irrigated to free loose foreign bodies and debris.

The wound is then properly stabilized by splinting and observed for signs and symptoms of infection. Low-velocity gunshot wounds may be complicated by significant vascular and muscular injury with excessive bleeding and hematoma formation. Excessive increase in closed compartment pressures should be relieved by emergency fasciotomy (Fig. 10-7A).

Fractures often result from direct strike of a bullet. The principle outlined by Gustillo for the management of open fractures should be strictly adhered to.[19] An open fracture is considered contaminated, and if it is more than 8 hours old, it is considered an infected wound. Most low-velocity gunshot wounds are of the type I class[19] without gross contamination, and a broad-spectrum

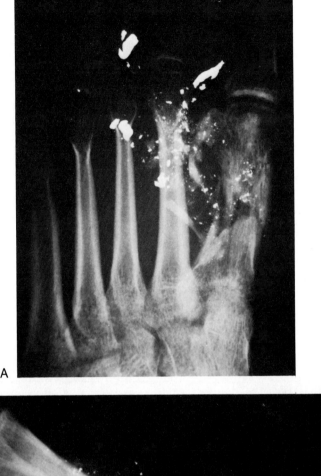

A

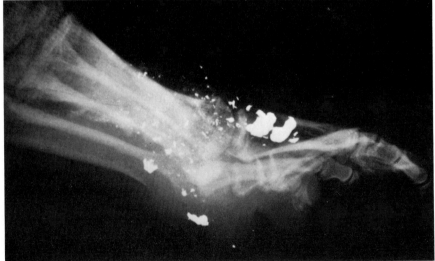

B

Fig. 10-5. (**A**) Dorsal view of a high-velocity gunshot wound of the medial foot with nondisplaced distal second metatarsal and comminuted first metatarsal diaphyseal fractures. (**B**) Lateral view showing anatomic position of the fractured first metatarsal with numerous dispersed metallic densities. (*Figure continues.*)

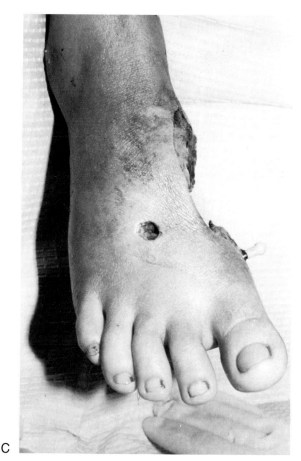

C

pins are easily used in the foot and together with plaster cast or splint immobilization help promote fracture stabilization (Fig. 10-7B–D). When large bones of the tarsus and ankle are involved, rigid internal fixation with plates and screws may be indicated.

The closure of a low-velocity gunshot wound depends on the degree of surgical intervention. Most often, these small wounds are left open and allowed to granulate and epithelialize over the defect. If formal surgical debridement is performed in a Gustillo type I or II fracture, the wound can normally be closed primarily if less than 8 hours old. If any question remains regarding the status of the wound, it should be left open and closure delayed until there is no sign of infection, which usually is evident within 3 to 7 days. When open reduction and internal fixation are performed in any type of fracture, the wound may be left open and delayed primary closure performed.

Fig. 10-5 *(Continued)*. **(C)** Postoperative photograph displaying dorsal entrance port and enlarged medial exit port after debridement. Removal of all nonviable soft tissue and bone was performed within 8 hours of injury. The Kirschner wire through the first metatarsal head provided stabilization to the fracture. The medial wound was eventually covered with a split-thickness skin graft and uneventful healing soon followed. (Photograph courtesy of Jeffrey M. Karlin, D.P.M.)

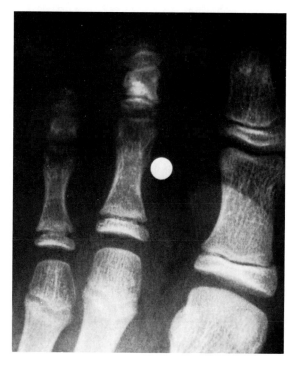

cephalosporin usually offers sufficient antimicrobial coverage. Antibiotic therapy is continued for 3 days, at which time the wound will or will not exhibit infection.

Open reduction is indicated for those fractures whose configuration requires intra-articular reconstruction or rigid internal fixation to maintain stability. Stabilization of fractures promotes conditions optimal for soft tissue healing and helps restore function. Kirschner wires or Steinmann

Fig. 10-6. Dorsal view displaying a low-velocity pellet embedded in the soft tissues adjacent to the proximal phalanx. The space-occupying effect of the foreign body produced pain that necessitated excision.

SUMMARY

Gunshot wounds to the foot and ankle can be classified as high-velocity, low-velocity, and shotgun wounds. The majority of gunshot wounds to the foot and ankle are of the low-velocity type, resulting in laceration and crushing of tissue with damage limited to the primary wound tract. Most low-velocity gunshot injuries result in Gustillo type I open fractures.[19] This is in contrast to high-velocity gunshot wounds in which temporary cavitation occurs and soft tissues and bone are extensively injured.

High-velocity wounds are considered an emergency, and radical wound debridement is often necessary. Most researchers believe low-velocity injuries can be treated in a nonoperative fashion by excision of skin margins, copious wound irrigation, and primary closure. The administration of prophylactic antibiotics in these wounds is not usually necessary.

For gross contamination, neurovascular injury, intra-articular involvement, soft tissue necrosis, compartment syndromes, and the presence of foreign bodies, formal surgical debridement for low-velocity injuries may be indicated. Strict adherence to the principles of wound care and frac-

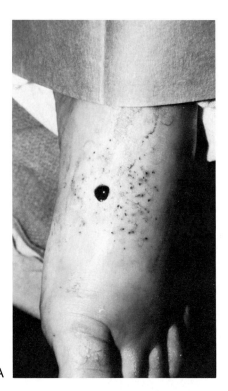
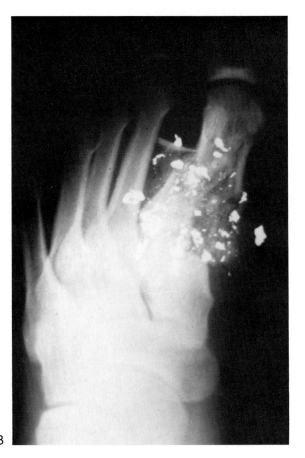

Fig. 10-7. (A) High-velocity bullet entrance port at the medial midtarsus in a 28-year-old man. Note the well-circumscribed wound with adjacent powder burns. Tautness of the skin can be seen secondary to severe hematoma formation. This patient was initially treated as an inpatient for intercompartmental decompression and debridement of the wound. **(B)** Preoperative radiograph showing that a direct strike by the bullet resulted in a displaced, comminuted midshaft fracture of the first metatarsal. (*Figure continues.*)

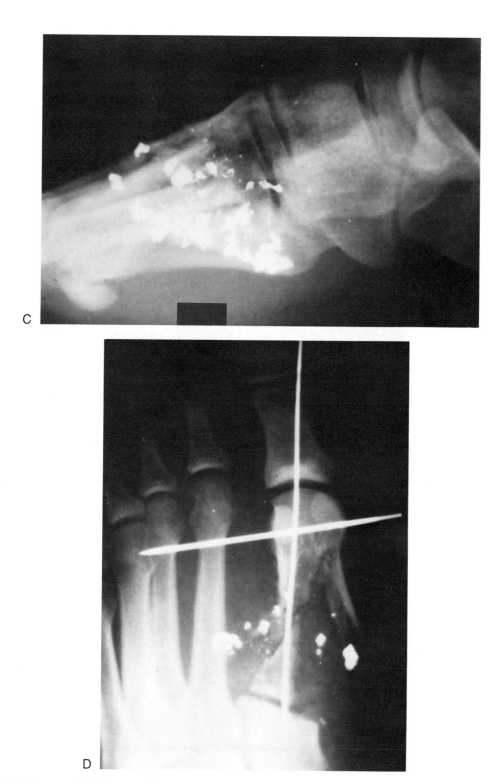

Fig. 10-7 (*Continued*). (**C**) Lateral view again displaying the first ray fracture and multiple metallic fragments in the bone and soft tissue. (**D**) Postoperative radiograph revealing two crossing Kirschner wires used to stabilize and maintain some length to the first ray after extensive bony and soft tissue debridement. In the presence of severe soft tissue and bone loss, an eventual first ray resection was performed. (Courtesy of Barry L. Scurran, D.P.M.)

ture management is mandatory. The surgeon should be well versed in the treatment of gunshot wounds to the foot and ankle. If they are managed properly, limited morbidity and disability can be expected.

REFERENCES

1. DeMuth WE, Jr: Bullet velocity and design as determinants of working capability: an experimental study. J Trauma 6:222, 1966
2. Beyer JC (ed): Wound Ballistics. Office of the Surgeon General, Department of the Army, Washington, D.C., 1972
3. Demuth WE, Smith JM: High velocity bullet wounds of muscle and bone: the basis of rational early treatment. J Trauma 6:744, 1966
4. Wang RG, Feng JX, Liv YQ: Pathomorphological observation of gunshot wounds. Acta Chir Scand, suppl., 508: 185–195
5. Harvey EN, Korr JM, Oster G, McMillen JH: Secondary damage in wounding due to pressure changes accompanying the passage of high velocity missiles. Surgery 21:218, 1947
6. Hennessy MJ, Banks HH, Leach RB, Quigley TB: Extremity gunshot wounds and gunshot fractures in civilian practice. Clin Orthop 114:296, 1976
7. Daniel RA, Jr: Bullet wounds of the limbs: an experimental study. Surgery 15:774, 1944
8. Shepard GH: High-energy, low-velocity close-range shotgun wounds. J Trauma 20:1065, 1980
9. DeMuth WE, Nicholas GG, Munger BL: Buckshot wounds. J Trauma 18:53, 1976
10. Howland WS, Jr, Ritchey SJ: Gunshot fractures in civilian practice. J Bone Joint Surg 53:47, 1971
11. Woloszyn JT, Uitulugt GM, Castle ME: Management of civilian gunshot fractures of the extremities. Clin Orthop 226:247, 1988
12. Wolf AW, Benson DR, Shoji H et al: Autosterilization in low-velocity bullets. J Trauma 18:63, 1978
13. Thoresby FP, Darlow HM: The mechanism of primary infection of bullet wounds. Br J Surg 54:359, 1967
14. Bretther D, Sedlin ED, Mendes DG: Conservative treatment of low velocity gunshot wounds. Clin Orthop 140:26, 1979
15. Ziperman HH: The management of soft tissue missile wounds in man. J Trauma 1:361, 1961
16. Marcus NA, Blair WF, Schrek JM, Omer GI, Jr: Low velocity gunshot wounds to extremities. J Trauma 20:1061, 1980
17. Hampton OP: Indications for debridement of gunshot wounds of extremities in civilian practice. J Trauma 1:368, 1961
18. Beaxley WC, Rosenthal RE: Lead intoxication 18 months after a gunshot wound. Clin Orthop 190:199, 1984
19. Gustillo RB: Management of open fractures and complications. p. 31. In Frankel VH (ed): Instructional Course Lectures, American Academy of Orthopaedic Surgeons. CV Mosby, St. Louis, 1982

SUGGESTED READINGS

Anania WC, Rosen RC, Giuffre AM: Gunshot wounds to the lower extremity: principles and treatment. J Foot Surg 3:228, 1987

Ashby ME: Low velocity gunshot wounds involving the knee joint: surgical management. J Bone Joint Surg 56A:1047, 1974

Cleveland M, Manning JC, Stewart WJ: Cause of battle casualties and injuries involving bones and joints. J Bone Joint Surg 33A:517, 1951

Cohen SM, Schulanburg CAR: Treatment of war wounds of the limbs. Lancet 239:351, 1940

DeMuth W: Velocity as applied to military rifles' wounding capacity. J Trauma 9:27, 1969

Dimond TD: M-16 rifle wounds in Viet Nam. J Trauma 7:619, 1967

Elstrom JA: Extra-articular low velocity gunshot wounds of the radius and ulna. J Bone Joint Surg 60A:335, 1978

Hopkins DAW, Marshall TK: Firearm injuries. Br J Surg 54:344, 1967

Hurst JM, Rybezynski J, Wertheimer JS: The physics, pathophysiology and management of high velocity gunshot wounds. J Foot Surg 25:440, 1986

Nuzzo JJ: Gunshot wounds of the foot. J Foot Surg 2:76, 1976

Omer GE, Reiner RE, Batch JW: Gunshot wounds of the tarsal joints. Am J Surg 90:575, 1955

Patzakis MJ, Harvey JP: The role of antibiotics in the management of open fractures. J Bone Joint Surg 56A:532, 1974

Shepard GH, Ferguson JV, Foster JH: Pulmonary contusion. Ann Thorac Surg 7:110, 1969

Tian HM, Huang MJ, Liv YQ, Wang SG: Primary contamination of wound track. Acta Chir Scand, suppl., 508: 265–269, 1982

11

Burns and Frostbite

Daniel Tuerk, M.D.

Each year between 1 million[1] and 2 million[2,3] people are burned. Approximately 100,000 to 150,000 of them are hospitalized (one-third to one-half of them in specialized burn centers), and more than 10,000 die. Those at the extremes of age are at most risk for a burn injury, with the highest incidence in young children, and those over 60 years of age next. In addition to the cost in pain and suffering, the financial cost is enormous. This includes the cost of hospitalization and professional fees, and days lost from work for both the acute injury and necessary future reconstructive procedures.

In addition to being the largest organ in the body, the skin is our interface with the external environment. As such, it is subject to, and protects the internal body structures from, all sorts of physical trauma. Thermal trauma to the skin can effect changes in all the body's organ systems and cause severe internal metabolic and physiologic derangements. These include (1) fluid loss with consequent hypovolemia and (2) a hypermetabolic state with increased catabolism and weight loss. Pulmonary injury, immunologic dysfunction, ileus, and infection can contribute in large amounts to the difficulties in bringing about a successful outcome.

EVALUATION OF THE INJURY

The depth of a burn depends on the thickness of the skin at the site of the injury, the heat of the burning agent, and the length of time the agent is applied to the skin. Burns are of either partial thickness (first or second degree) or full thickness (third degree). First degree burns are characterized by erythema without blister formulation. Second degree burns can be further subdivided into superficial and deep burns.[4] Superficial second degree burns are erythematous and have blisters present (Fig. 11-1). They are usually painful. Deep second degree burns may or may not have blisters, may be dry and anesthetic, and may appear mottled (Fig. 11-2). Third degree burns involve destruction of the full thickness of the skin and its appendages (hair follicles, sweat glands, and sebaceous glands). They are anesthetic, leathery, and whitish to dark in color and may have thrombosed vessels present (Fig. 11-3). Accurate estimation of burn wound depth is often difficult and sometimes made in retrospect.

PATHOPHYSIOLOGY

The heat from the burn causes a local tissue injury to which the body responds with both a local and a generalized reaction. The heat can denature the body's proteins (both intracellularly and extracellularly), interfere with cellular enzyme systems, lyse the cell membrane (with resultant release of potassium into the extracellular space), and cause hemodynamic changes.

On a cellular level, the response can vary from immediate cell death by coagulation necrosis to an injury that could potentially be reversed. The tissues must be protected against further

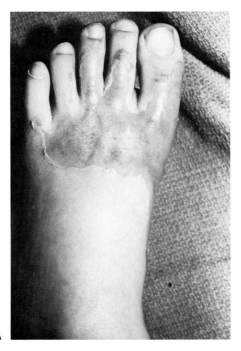
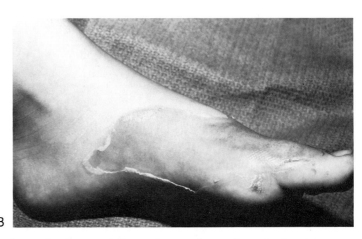

A   B

Fig. 11-1. (A & B) Dorsal and lateral view of superficial second degree burn. Blisters have broken but the erythematous base is present.

trauma (thermal or mechanical) or infection, which could kill burned cells that otherwise might survive.

The vascular response is an initial arteriolar and arteriole constriction followed by vasodilation. This results in capillary permeability with consequent leakage of intravascular protein into the extravascular, extracellular third space for 12 to 24 hours after the burn. The complex fluid and electrolyte shifts of large burns complicate the initial treatment beyond simply attending to care of the local burn wound.

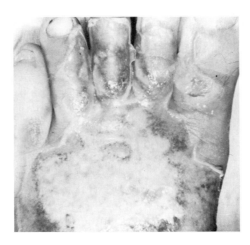

Fig. 11-2. Deeper second degree burn with characteristically mottled appearance.

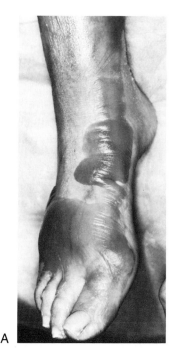
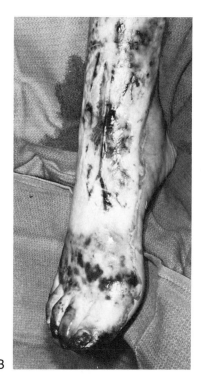

Fig. 11-3. (**A**) Early bleb formation demonstrates the difficulty often encountered in assessment of wound depth. (**B**) After demarcation, this full-thickness burn is characterized by a white-to-dark, leathery appearance with thrombosed blood vessels. The wound is anesthetic.

INITIAL MANAGEMENT OF A MAJOR BURN

At the scene of the injury, the first objective is the cessation of the burning process. Attention should be paid to the maintenance of an adequate airway and the treatment of associated injuries, such as fractures and bleeding from lacerations. The patient should be wrapped in clean linen or towels and transported to a hospital.

In a patient with a major burn, fluid resuscitation should begin as soon as possible. The purpose of fluid administration is to replenish intravascular volume to maintain tissue and organ perfusion. The burn injury results in increased capillary permeability between the endothelial cells of the capillary wall, with consequent fluid shifts into both burned and unburned tissue.

The amount of fluid necessary to maintain perfusion is proportional to the patient's size (weight in kilograms) and extent of burn (measured as a percent of total body surface area [TBSA]). During the first 24 hours postburn, crystalloid (usually plain lactated Ringer's solution without dextrose) is used. It is given in sufficient quantity to maintain an adequate urine volume and avoid tachycardia. Baxter's formula of 4 ml per percent TBSA burn per kilogram of weight is a good estimate of the amount required for the first 24 hours.[5] After the capillary leak seals, protein is given (usually as albumin) to maintain blood volume and 5% dextrose in water is given to replace insensible losses.

Initial Management of Burns of the Foot

Immediate and continuing assessment must be made of the circulatory status of the extremity.

Circumferential burns and postburn edema, particularly in the presence of a constricting eschar, can compromise the circulation to one or more digits or to the whole foot. In the presence of vascular insufficiency, an escharotomy must be done. The escharotomy should be planned anatomically to allow for release of the constriction and avoid transecting structures such as vessels, neurovascular bundles, or tendons. Often this can be done without anesthesia as the eschars are anesthetic. Tetanus prophylaxis should be considered in all patients.

A brief (3 to 5 day) course of penicillin (or erythromycin in the patient allergic to penicillin) was routinely recommended to prevent cellulitis from the streptococci that normally inhabit the skin, and it is still used in some institutions.[6] More recently, this routine treatment has not been recommended by some (except for children).[7] It is feared that more severe superinfection with yeasts and *Pseudomonas* may result. Still others use it for outpatients, but not for hospitalized patients.[8]

The burn wounds can be initially covered with sponges or towels soaked in cool (not iced) water or saline until the patient's evaluation is completed. The burns are then gently washed with a mild soap or detergent. Broken blisters should be debrided. In general, unbroken blisters are probably best left unbroken. Some recommend debriding the blisters under certain circumstances. These include patients who might not be reliable enough to care for their wounds or if there is the potential of infection of the wound.[9] Blisters are also debrided when the size and location of the blisters interfere with joint motion and exercise.

In a deep burn, below the obviously coagulated tissue exists a zone of capillary stasis. Zawacki has shown that tissue necrosis in this zone of stasis is due to wound dehydration and that prevention of wound dehydration can decrease the depth of tissue necrosis.[10] He found that stasis was reversed and necrosis was least if broken blisters were covered with porcine skin. Unbroken blisters also prevented tissue necrosis, but not as completely. The worst results, with the most necrosis, were in wounds in which broken blisters were left uncovered.

CARE OF THE BURN WOUND

The feet, along with the eyes, ears, face, hands, and perineum, are considered critical areas under the American Burn Association Severity Grading System.[11] Patients with circumferential burns of the feet or burns involving more than 5 percent of these critical areas should be managed as inpatients. A recent retrospective review of burns of the feet suggests that these injuries may require in-hospital treatment to avoid complications.[6]

In the emergency room, the wounds are covered with a topical antibiotic cream. Burn wound infection is the most common cause of morbidity and mortality in burn patients. It is not practical to maintain a sterile wound because of the inevitable contamination from endogenous (most commonly the patient's own gastrointestinal tract) or exogenous sources. Therefore, topical antibacterial agents are used to control the contamination until wound coverage is completed. Covering the burn has the added beneficial effect of decreasing the patient's pain by excluding air from contacting the wound. The most common topical antibacterial used in hospitalized patients is silver sulfadiazine.[12] Other topical agents that have been used include mafenide, 0.5 percent silver nitrate solution, gentamicin cream, and povidone-iodine ointment. Each has specific advantages and disadvantages that are beyond the scope of this chapter. As the wound flora changes or treatment side effects emerge, the topical agent must at times change.[13]

The burn wound is redressed once or twice a day. Once the patient's condition has stabilized, at least one of these dressing changes is done in a hydrotherapy setting if possible. This permits removal of the old topical antibiotic and debridement of the wound (eschar, surface fibrinous exudate, nonviable tissue, broken blisters, etc.) Second degree burns could also be treated with a medicated gauze dressing such as Xeroform, instead of an antibiotic cream. These dressings are changed every day or two. This is most easily done in a tub setting, either in the physical therapy department or at home.

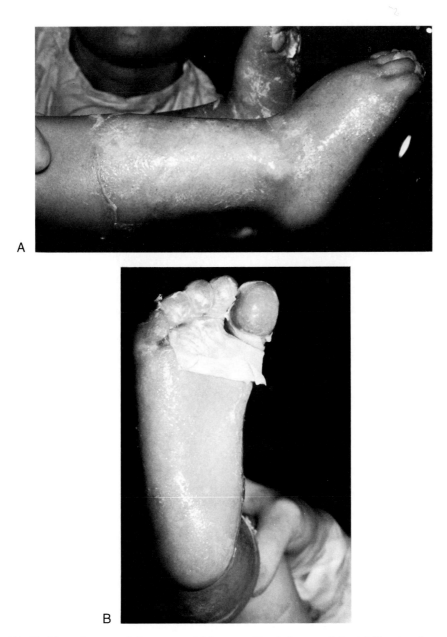

Fig. 11-4. (**A**) Child with second degree scald burns of both legs and feet following immersion in a bathtub. The blisters have broken and been debrided in the whirlpool. Notice the edema of the dorsum of the foot requiring continuing assessment of the distal circulation. (**B**) View of the plantar surface of the feet of the child in Figure A. Because the plantar skin is thicker than the skin of the instep, injuries that cause third degree burns of the instep may result in only second degree burns of the sole. (*Figure continues.*)

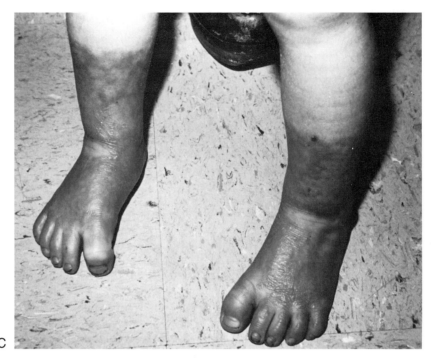

Fig. 11-4 (*Continued*). **(C)** Two months following the injury, the second degree burns have healed with the use of daily whirlpool and silversulfadiazene cream dressings. After healing, the child is measured for individually fitted pressure garments that are worn continuously to prevent burn scar hypertrophy.

Second degree burns should heal within several weeks. Some investigators believe that burns that take longer than 2 weeks to heal should be debrided and skin grafted.[4] They believe that prolonged healing by secondary intention results in a hypertrophic scar covered by unstable epithelium and will be unsatisfactory coverage for the patient in the long run. Other researchers disagree and utilize exercise, splinting, and compression during and after healing (Fig. 11-4).[14,15]

The goal of treating third degree burns is wound coverage with skin grafts. To achieve this, nonviable tissue must be removed, infection controlled, and a recipient bed established with sufficient vasculature to support a skin graft. Debridement is mechanical or enzymatic. Mechanical debridement is most often done gradually, on a daily basis in the whirlpool with scissors or as a formal operative procedure (with requisite anesthesia and attendant blood loss). Care must be used not to expose bare tendon or bare bone, neither of which without the underlying blood supply of paratenon or periosteum will support the growth of skin grafts. Wet-to-dry dressing changes are also a form of mechanical debridement, but can be quite painful and therefore should be used with some care. Travase (an inactivated derivative product of *Bacillus subtilis*) is occasionally used for enzymatic debridement. Application of Travase is sometimes painful, and the requirement for keeping the wound moist can promote burn wound infection.

There are some who advocate early excision for deep second or third degree burns (by the tangential method or by direct excision) and early grafting. But other than for small burns, this technique is probably best reserved for experienced surgeons or specialized burn centers.[16,17]

SKIN GRAFTS

To accept a skin graft, the burn wound should be free of infection and have an adequate circulation in the recipient bed. Grafts can be placed directly on paratenon, perineurium, or periosteum, but not on bare tendon, nerve, or bone. More commonly, after several weeks of wound preparation and care, a layer of granulation tissue covers the wound. At the time of the operation, the outer surface of the granulation tissue is scraped with a knife blade to remove the inevitable surface contamination. The wound is then covered with a moist gauze for hemostasis while the graft is harvested. Most commonly, an air-driven or electrically driven dermatome is used. Split-thickness grafts are usually between 0.014 and 0.016 inches thick. Donor sites are covered with Op-site dressing, which is left on for 10 to 12 days, by which time the sites are usually healed. The grafts can be placed on the wound as a sheet or meshed. The grafts are anchored with catgut sutures to obviate the need for later suture removal. Sheet grafts are dressed with N-terface gauze, fluffs, and a wrap-around bandage.

If meshed, the grafts are meshed at a 1.5-to-1 ratio, but placed on the wound unexpanded or minimally expanded. The advantage to meshing the graft is that it allows any fluid that accumulates under the graft to escape and not float the graft off its vascular bed. My policy is to moisten the meshed graft to keep the thin skin graft strips from desiccating. I use an antibiotic solution that the pharmacy prepares, consisting of one ampule (50,000 units) of bacitracin and one ampule (500,000 units) of polymyxin per liter of normal saline. The graft is moistened, without disturbing the dressing, every 4 hours for 5 to 7 days. The graft dressing is changed and the graft is inspected daily. When the antibiotic soaks are discontinued, a medicated gauze dressing (for example, Xeroflo) is used on the graft. The limb is kept elevated for 4 to 6 days postoperatively. The patients then ambulate on a progressive regimen over the next 3 to 4 days. It is important to keep the foot wrapped with an Ace bandage whenever it is dependent to prevent the accumulation of edema fluid beneath the graft. By the fifth or sixth day postgrafting, whirlpool treatment can usually be resumed.

External pressure is maintained on the healed graft to prevent hypertrophic scar formation. This is done initially with Ace bandages or Tubigrip until custom-fitted Jobst anti-burn scar garments can be obtained. This pressure is continued for 1 year or more.

OUTPATIENT TREATMENT

Although some investigators suggest that all patients with burns of the feet, at least initially,[6,18] be managed as inpatients, others believe that minor burns of this critical area can be treated on an outpatient basis.[4] Even minor third degree burns of the feet can be treated outside the hospital. However, because of the difficulties with elevation in the initial postoperative period, most grafting procedures to the feet are done on an inpatient basis.

The general principles of outpatient burn care of the feet are occlusion of the wound and elevation of the extremity to prevent edema formation. In the emergency room, the wound is cleansed with a bland soap or detergent and loose blisters are debrided. Some clinicians use Silvadene (silver sulfadiazene) on the burn wound.[11] Others think that the major therapeutic indication for Silvadene is the prevention of burn wound infection in large (>20 percent TBSA) burns and that it should not be used in minor burns because it might retard epithelialization and wound healing. Other agents that are commonly employed are polysporin or bacitracin ointments or Xeroform gauze. The wound is then wrapped in a bulky dressing. The patient is initially told not to bear weight and to elevate the foot.

The dressings are changed every 24 to 48 hours in a tub. This can be done in a physical therapy unit or office setting initially. Eventually the patient and family can be instructed in doing this at home in the bathtub. The dressings are soaked off, loose skin is trimmed, and the wounds are redressed.

By 2 weeks, a determination can be made regarding the extent of the burn. Many superficial burns will be healed or almost healed. Wounds that show no evidence of healing by 2 to 3 weeks should be considered for debridement and grafting.

LONG-TERM CARE

Most minor burns of the feet will heal without significant disability. Nevertheless, certain principles of management should be instituted before and after wound closure. Physical therapy with active range of motion should begin as early as possible to prevent joint stiffening. Elevation will promote early resolution of the edema, which can delay wound healing. Proper positioning (for example, night splints to maintain ankle dorsiflexion) can help prevent joint contracture. Some protocols stress bed rest and elevation.[6] Others begin weight bearing once the edema has subsided to help prevent heel cord shortening.[4,19,20] However, the extremity should be wrapped in an Ace bandage when dependent to prevent reaccumulation of edema. The early use of orthotics and exact-fit inserts[21] and modified postoperative shoes has been recommended to prevent the formation of joint contractures.

Hypertrophic scar formation is a common postburn complication. It is frequently seen in deep burns that have been allowed to heal secondarily and in children. Continuous pressure on the healed wound prevents or even reverses the scar hypertrophy. Custom measured anti-burn scar garments are available (Jobst Co.) for use in the postburn period. To be effective, the garments should be worn virtually 24 hours a day during the period of scar maturation (i.e., for 1 year or longer).

Patients (children in particular) should be observed periodically to assess the need for delayed reconstruction. Hypertrophic scars that interfere with the wearing of shoes or become irritated by mechanical friction may require serial intralesional steroid injection or excision and replacement with a skin graft. Linear contractures that interfere with joint range of motion may require Z-plasties or the addition of skin by further grafting procedures (Fig. 11-5).

No review of burns of the feet would be complete without a discussion on prevention. Children are at risk for burns in both the kitchen and the bathroom. A contact time with hot water of 1 second at 160°F (71°C) will cause a full-thickness burn injury; less than 5 seconds at 140°F (60°C) can cause a partial-thickness skin injury.[22] Turning hot water heater temperatures below 135°F (57°C) and proper supervision in the bathtub and around heated pots on the stove can go a long way in the prevention of potentially crippling burn injuries. Gridlike burns of the feet from floor furnace registers have been reported and can be avoided. The possibility of child abuse as a cause of burn injury, although unpleasant to think about, must never be forgotten, particularly in immersion scald burns. In some states, by law, possible child or adult abuse must be reported to the proper authorities.

COLD INJURY

Historically, the military has had the greatest experience with cold injury. However, the number of cases seen in civilian medical practice is significant, owing to the increase in outdoor winter sports[23] and the number of homeless people exposed to the elements.

The degree of cold injury depends on the environmental temperature and the length of time of exposure. Increasing wind velocity lowers the wind chill factor and can increase the severity of injury for a given ambient temperature.[24,25] Numerous other factors affect the extent of the injury and hence the eventual prognosis. Direct skin contact with an excellent heat conductor such as bare metal can cause rapid freezing and increased tissue destruction. Associated injuries, fatigue, dehydration, and panic can affect the body's heat production and conservation and can result in more severe injuries.

Cold injury can cause tissue destruction by a combination of factors. Frostbite causes ice crystal formation in the tissues. With slow freezing, which is the more common injury, crystals form in the extracellular fluid, which then becomes hyperosmotic, causing fluid to shift out of the cells.[23,24] Rapid freezing causes both intracellular and extracellular crystal formation with irreversible destruction of cell membranes and more extensive tissue damage. The vascular response to cold injury includes vasoconstriction, capillary damage, and eventual arteriolar shunting. The

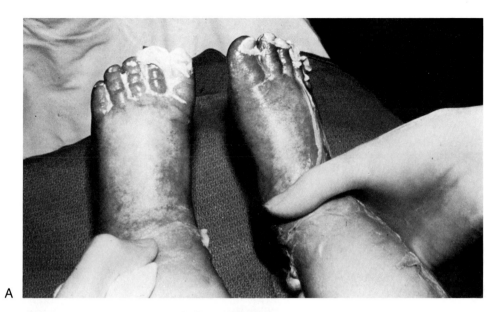

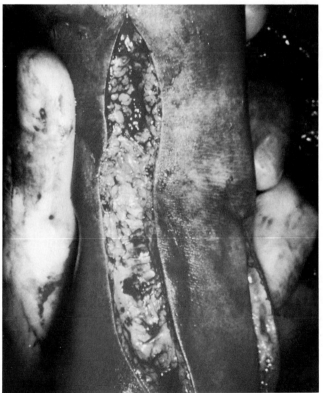

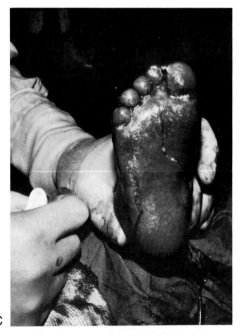

Fig. 11-5. (**A**) Child with second and third degree scald burns of both legs and feet following immersion in a bathtub. (**B**) Escharotomy was required at 24 hours because of distal circulatory compromise secondary to edema. Escharotomy was also required on the left foot. (**C**) View of the plantar surface showing the two escharotomy incisions needed to decompress the right foot. Adequacy of the escharotomy is judged by return of both the arterial pulse (by palpation or Doppler ultrasound) and capillary circulation. (*Figure continues.*)

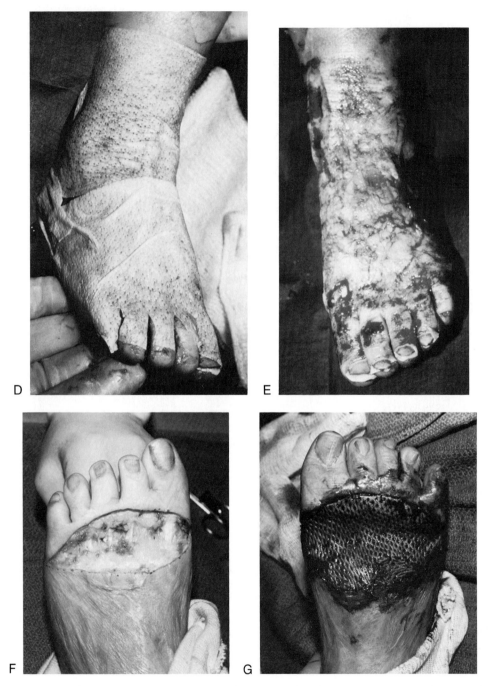

Fig. 11-5 (*Continued*). (**D & E**) Porcine xenografts were utilized to promote a vascular granular bed that would be acceptable for applications of a meshed split-thickness skin graft. (**F**) Both feet were grafted prior to discharge. Over the next several years, the child developed a contracture of the skin of the dorsum of the foot requiring secondary reconstruction. This view shows the amount of skin graft required following simple incision of the dorsal burn scar contracture of the left foot. (**G**) A meshed split-thickness skin graft has been placed on the right foot following release of the scar contracture. (*Figure continues.*)

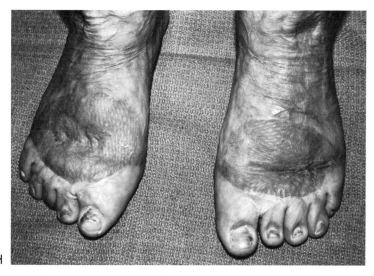

Fig. 11-5 (*Continued*). (**H**) The healed grafts following scar release. In the future further scar releases and grafting may be required with growth of the child. If necessary, burn scar contractures of the dorsal webspaces can be corrected by double opposed **Z**-plasties.

body tries to maintain its core heat by bypassing and sacrificing the limb.

Treatment

Raising the patient's core temperature and rewarming the frostbitten extremity should take place simultaneously. An important caveat is that the limb should not be thawed if the possibility exists of its being refrozen. There are documented cases of individuals walking for hours or days on frozen extremities with minimal eventual tissue loss. However, the cycle of freezing, thawing, and refreezing seems to cause more extensive tissue damage.

There is general agreement that limb rewarming should be done rapidly in water that is 38 to 44°C for 15 to 20 minutes.[23,26,27] This is often painful and requires the administration of narcotic analgesics. The administration of low-molecular-weight dextran has been advocated to decrease intravascular sludging and increase perfusion. To be effective, this must be given within 24 hours of injury. The use of surgical sympathectomy, either early or late, is also controversial. Adequate tetanus prophylaxis should be established.

Local Care

As with burn injuries, various local wound care protocols exist. McCauley et al[28] use prophylactic penicillin, aspirin, and topical aloe vera, while others use betadine. In general, the limb should be elevated to minimize edema; weight bearing and friction should be avoided; and careful attention to local wound care should be instituted to avoid infection.

It is frequently difficult to estimate accurately the depth and extent of the tissue injury. In general, it is best to avoid early surgical debridement. The necrotic tissue should be allowed to demarcate and mummify, even over several months. Amputations can then be electively performed on the mummified tissue that has clearly demarcated (Fig. 11-6). The presence of infection and wet gangrene, however, necessitate early surgical intervention for debridement or amputation.

Late sequelae of significant cold injury include premature closure of epiphyses in children, decreased resistance to recurrent cold injury in the future, chronic pain syndromes, hyperhidrosis, and late development of squamous cell carcinomas.[23,25]

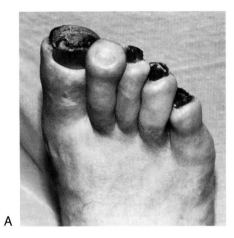

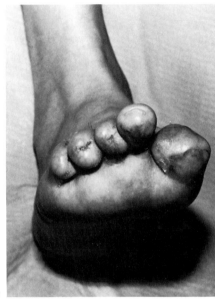

Fig. 11-6. (A) Necrotic toes following cold injury have been allowed to demarcate over a period of weeks. **(B)** Autoamputation occurred at the third, fourth, and fifth digits. Surgical amputation was elected at the great toe.

REFERENCES

1. Herndon DN, Curreri PW, Abston S et al: Treatment of burns. Curr Prob Surg 24:347, 1987
2. Silverstein P, Lack B: Fire prevention in the United States. Surg Clin North Am 67:2, 1987
3. Demling RH: Medical progress: burns. N Engl J Med 313:1389, 1985
4. Warden GD: Outpatient care of thermal injuries. Surg Clin North Am 67:147, 1987
5. Baxter C: Fluid volume and electrolyte changes of the early postburn period. Clin Probl Surg 1:693, 1974
6. Zachery LS, Heggers JP, Robson MC et al: Burns of the feet. J Burn Care 8:192, 1987
7. Dasco CC, Luterman A, Curreri PW: Systemic antibiotic treatment in burned patients. Surg Clin North Am 67:57, 1987
8. Herndon DN, Curreri PW, Abston S et al: Treatment of burns. Curr Prob Surg 24:360, 1987
9. Warden GD: Outpatient care of thermal injuries. Surg Clin North Am 67:151, 1987
10. Zawacki BE: Reversal of capillary stasis and prevention of necrosis in burns. Ann Surg 180:98, 1974
11. Hunt JL, Purdue G: Acute burns. Selected Read Plast Surg 4:2, 1987
12. Monafo WW, Freedman B: Topical therapy for burns. Surg Clin North Am 67:138, 1987
13. Herndon DN, Thompson PB, Desai MH et al: Treatment of burns in children. Pediatr Clin North Am 32:1311, 1985
14. Shuck JM: Preparing and closing the burn wound. Plast Surg Clin North Am 1:584, 1974
15. Habal MB: The burned hand: a planned treatment program. J Trauma 18:589, 1978
16. Heimbach DM: Early burn excision and grafting. Surg Clin North Am 67:93, 1987
17. Monafo WW: Tangential excision. Plast Surg Clin North Am 1:591, 1974
18. Shuck JM: Outpatient management of the burned patient. Surg Clin North Am 58:1109, 1978
19. Larson DL, Abston S, Willis B et al: Contracture and scar formation in the burn patient. Plast Surg Clin North Am 1:657, 1974
20. O'Donnell L: Control of foot contractures: a simple method. Bull Clin Rev Burn Injuries 11:26, 1985
21. Zuker RM, McLeod AME, Vaz H: Effective management of deep scald burns to the feet. J Burn Care 5:288, 1984
22. Maley MP, Achauer BM: Prevention of tap water scald burns. J Burn Care 8:62, 1987
23. Purdue GF, Hunt JL: Cold injury: a collective review. J Burn Care 7:331, 1986
24. Washburn B: Frostbite. N Engl J Med 266:974, 1962

25. House JH, Fidler MO: Frostbite of the hand. p. 1553. In Green DP (ed): Operative Hand Surgery. Churchill Livingstone, New York, 1982

26. Livingston RD, Jacobs RL: Frostbite. Orthopedics 5:1607, 1982

27. Shumacker HB: Frostbite. p. 405. In Flynn JE (ed): Hand Surgery. 2nd Ed. Williams & Wilkens, Baltimore, 1975

28. McCauley RL, Hing DN, Robson MC, Heggers JP: Frostbite injuries. J Trauma 23:143, 1983

12

General Concepts in the Management of Tendon Trauma to the Foot and Ankle

Robert Sheinberg, D.P.M.
Omar Bayne, M.D.

The structural integrity of the foot and ankle is a balance among the interrelationships of bone, ligaments, and tendons. All play a role in the intricate biomechanics of weight transfer during standing, walking, and running. Tendon injuries about the foot and ankle are relatively uncommon compared with bone or ligamentous injuries; however, tendon injuries can result in prolonged disability and late joint destruction if not diagnosed early or treated adequately.

COMPONENT

Tendons are connective tissue structures composed of three fibrous proteins; collagen, reticulin, and elastin, of which collagen is the main component estimated at 86 percent. Fibroblasts are responsible for the production of collagen and ground substance,[1] in which the collagen fibers are presumed to mature.

The strength of collagen is dependent on its cross-linkage and the surrounding environment[2] (Fig. 12-1). During the maturation of collagen, the number and quality of cross-links increase, resulting in an increase in tensile strength and a decrease in collagen solubility.[3] After maturation, when aging, collagen reaches a plateau in respect to mechanical properties. The tensile strength then begins to decrease.[4] The decrease in biomechanical parameters is correlated with a decrease in the amount of insoluble collagen and the total collagen content.[5] Tendon with its parallel collagen fibers allows flexibility, yet it maintains great tensile strength. Its flexibility enables it to be angulated around bone surfaces or deflected beneath retinacula. Its elasticity helps to resist or transmit linear forces to develop torque about a joint axes.[6] Tendons are longitudinally aligned in the line of tension. Their parallel array of fibers produces an ideal physical adaptation for tensile force transmission.[7] In tendons that have a straight course, the collagen bundles are arranged longitudinally. When abrupt changes of direction occur, spiraling of the bundles around each other occurs to prevent deformation and ensure equal distribution of tension to the whole area of insertion.[8]

At the musculotendinous junction, the perimysium becomes continuous with the endotenon and the muscle fibers are continued as collagen bundles.[1] At the osteotendinous junction, the collagen fibers continue into the bone as the perforating fibers of Sharpey and the endotenon becomes continuous with the periosteum[1,5] (Fig. 12-2). The primary tendon bundle gains attachment to bone through four characteristic zones:

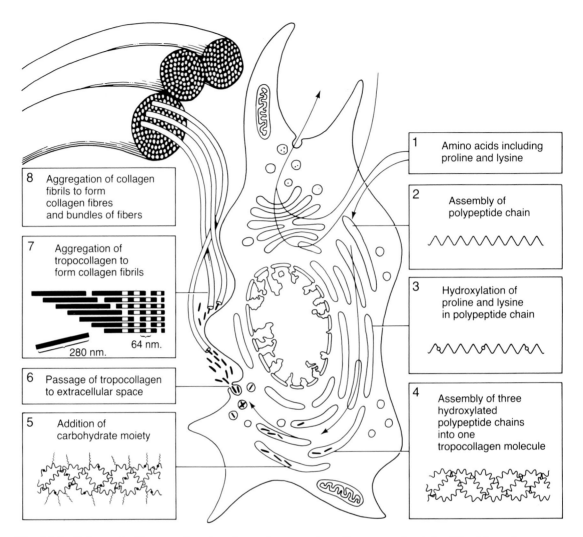

Fig. 12-1. Schematic diagram showing the major steps in collagen synthesis by fibroblasts in connective tissue. (From Warwick R, Williams PL (eds): Gray's Anatomy. 35th Br. Ed. Churchill Livingstone, Edinburgh, 1973, with permission.)

tendon, fibrocartilage, mineralized fibrocartilage, and the bone itself. Cooper and Misol found that the gradual transition to full mineralization in fibrocartilage should enhance the ability of insertions to dissipate force evenly during muscle contraction and when motion stops.[7] Increased resistance to shear by this arrangement and by the unmineralized fibrocartilage should decrease chances of failure in the entire unit.

ACTION

Tendons enable muscles to concentrate or extend their action. The long tendons of the feet exemplify the function of extending the effect of more proximal muscles. The long flexors of the fingers are of most interest to surgeons. The mechanics and physiology of these finger tendons

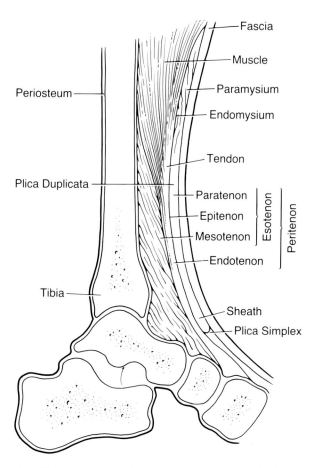

Fig. 12-2. Ideal longitudinal section through the tibialis anticus tendon and the adjacent structures. See text for description. (From Mayer,[17] with permission.)

are usually studied, but most of the generalizations are applicable to other tendons of similar design in the foot and ankle.[10]

The maximal tensile strength of a tendon is four times the isometric strength of the associated muscle.[11] Training results in increased tensile strength and collagen content in tendons. Immobilization results in a decrease in tensile strength and an increase in collagen turnover.[12] The presence of elastic fibers in tendon is postulated as having a protective function by causing the increase in tension to be gradual, thus absorbing the first shock of contraction.[13]

PARATENON AND SYNOVIAL SHEATH

During its course, a tendon may lie entirely in loose areolar tissue called paratenon, or partly in paratenon and partly in synovial sheath or bursa.[14] Whenever a tendon turns a corner or has to bend in association with neighboring joints, it is restrained under a pulley, a retinacular system, and is lubricated in this region by a synovial sheath.[10] A tendon that is traversing a straight course and that is not subject to pressure is covered with paratenon. The paratenon is multilayered[15] (Fig. 12-3) and built up of long elastic fibers and curved vessels, to allow straightening during excursion of the tendon.[1] A paratenon is not a true gliding mechanism. The tendon is not free as in a sheath but is attached to the paratenon, which is dragged with the tendon during excursion.

A tendon sheath mechanism consists of two layers of synovia: a visceral layer covering the

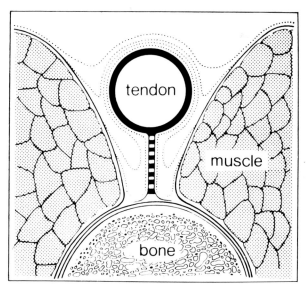

Fig. 12-3. Schematic diagram of a nonsheath tendon in cross section to show the multilayered nature of paratenon. (Modified from Colville et al.,[15] with permission.)

tendon and a parietal layer lining the fascial tunnel through which the tendon glides. The parietal layer joins the visceral layer in a double layer, the mesotenon. It is located on the convex side of the tendon away from friction and carries blood vessels to the tendon.[16] Synovial fluid exists between the two layers of synovia. The tendon glides on this thin film of synovial fluid.

BLOOD SUPPLY

Mayer was the first to clearly describe the blood supply to tendons.[17] Blood vessels to the tendon are derived from three main sources: (1) from muscular branches, (2) from vessels running in the surrounding connective tissue, paratenon, mesotenon, and vincula, and (3) from vessels of the periosteum and bone near the point of insertion of the tendon.

The circulatory pattern can be divided into an intratendinous and extratendinous arrangement. The intratendinous pattern consists of longitudinal blood vessels that course along the endotenon between tendon bundles and anastomose with transverse branches (Fig. 12-4). These intratendinous vessels are connected with its external environment in four places.[18] (1) At the musculo-tendinous junction, the vessels within the muscle continue as the interfascicular vessels. (2) At the osteotendinous junction, the interfascicular vessels anastomose with periosteal vessels. (3) Where the tendon is surrounded by paratenon, vessels in the tendon vicinity give rise to small vessels that penetrate the paratenon at frequent and regular intervals. On approaching the tendon, the vessels branch several times in the direction of the longitudinal axis of the tendon, lying in the interfascicular groove. (4) Where the tendon lies within the synovial sheath, the parietal layer of the sheath is vascularized from the surrounding tissues. The mesotenon conveys blood vessels to the visceral layer, which is also vascularized by continuity with the parietal layer.

Peacock found that blood vessels entering long tendons from the muscular origin and periosteal insertion are able to nourish the proximal and distal third of the tendon.[19] The middle one third is vascularized by vessels entering through paratenon or mesentary. Tendons also receive neovascularization through adhesions to adjacent tissue during repair. Isolation of a juncture of devascularized tendon to prevent adhesions results in its failure to unite.[20]

HEALING

There are three schools of thought with regard to tendon healing: (1) tendon heals itself by reparative cellular growth directly from the cut tendon ends; (2) tendon heals by the cellular activities of surrounding tissues that proliferate, invade the gap between the tendon, and repair it and not by any intrinsic cellular response of its own; and (3) healing occurs through both processes.[21]

Primary tendon healing occurs when sutures are used to coapt the two tendon ends. The initial stage characteristic of primary tendon healing is the *substrate* phase. An inflammatory reaction occurs, with the outpouring of fibrin and inflammatory cells. The degree of this reaction depends on the magnitude of trauma to the tendon and paratendinous structures. On the second or third

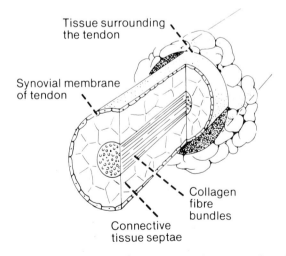

Fig. 12-4. Intrinsic tendon anatomy. (From Lindsay,[2] with permission.)

Tissue surrounding the tendon

Synovial membrane of tendon

Collagen fibre bundles

Connective tissue septae

day following tendon wounding, the *fibroplasia* phase begins. This phase is characterized by the proliferation of fibroblasts and capillaries from the extratendinous structures including the paratenon and tendon sheath. Fibroblasts synthesize collagen and various mucopolysaccharides needed for the synthesis of scars.[22] They deposit collagen between the cut tendon ends, restoring tendon continuity and tensile strength.[21] Fibroblasts continue to increase in density, and by day 21, there is a mass of granulation tissue surrounding the tendon.[23] The earliest collagen fibrils laid down are in a totally random orientation. At 2.5 to 3 weeks, the wound collagen is reoriented and, in response to tensile forces, lies parallel to the long axis of tendon. This process is one of gradual wound maturation with gradual restoration of tensile strength.[21]

During the remodeling phase, restoration of the gliding function of the tendon depends on the effectiveness of dissolution and reformation of the collagen fibers during the scar-remodeling phase.[5] With successful tendon repair, the collagen between the ends of the repaired tendon will be reorganized into almost completely polarized parallel bundles having great strength, whereas the collagen between the tendon and adjacent tissues remains randomly oriented and highly elastic or mobile.[20]

Peacock described the healing process of tendon when the cut ends are left to heal in loose connective tissue.[19] In an area where cells have the ability to synthesize new connective tissue, the wound becomes filled at first with gelatinous and then with dense fibrous scar. Following synthesis of this scar, remodeling occurs. The newly synthesized tissue is both qualitatively and quantitatively different from that found in normal tendon. There is no continuity between the end of the tendon and new connective tissue. A tendon formed in this manner seldom develops a gliding function over a substantial period.

Anchorage of Tendon to Bone

The anchorage of tendon to bone must be secure to allow healing to take place and to restore normal function. Tendon may be secured to bone in three ways. (1) It may be sutured to the outside of bone through drill holes, (2) passed into the bone, or (3) passed through the bone and anchored back on itself (Fig. 12-5).

Zinmeister and Edelman used a 4.0-mm cancellous screw with a 3.5-mm spike polyacetal resin washer for stabilization of the tibialis posterior tendon into the navicular for a Kidner procedure.[24] The ends of a pull-out suture may be passed through a transverse hole in the cortex and tied. If a tendon has sufficient length, it may be brought through the hole and tied back on itself. Gould described the use of a Michel trephine to remove a bone plug during tendon transplantation.[25] The tendon is dropped into the hole and sutured to surrounding tissue. The bone plug is then packed into the hole and firmly fixes the tendon implant into position. Large tendons may be transfixed through the medullary canal.[26] Sutures are placed in the end of the tendon, leaving two long, free strands. A trapdoor is made in the bone exposing the medullary canal at a predetermined point of attachment. Two drill holes are made distal to the exposed medullary canal, and the free ends of the suture are passed through the trapdoor and out through the two holes. The sutures are tied after removing all the slack in the tendon, and the trapdoor is replaced en toto or used as small broken fragments packed into the osseous defect.

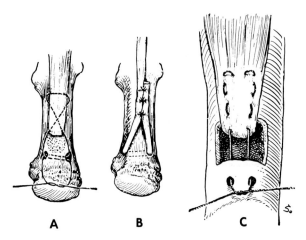

Fig. 12-5. Fixation of tendon to bone. (From Crenshaw,[26] with permission.)

A pull-out wire suture may be placed in the end of a tendon and pulled into or through a drill hole in the bone.[27-29] The sutures in the tendon end are placed on long straight needles and are drawn out through the skin on the opposite side. They are tied over gauze or a padded button. Cast immobilization is used until the parts heal (Fig. 12-6).

Tendon-to-bone healing has been described well.[30,31] A proliferation of immature connective tissue occurs at the entrance of tendon to bone. This tissue becomes organized over a 2 to 3 week period, forming a secure attachment between the tendon and periosteum. At 4 weeks, a progressive deposition of new bone is seen between the collagen fibers of the tendon. These collagen fibers become attached directly to the bone and resemble Sharpey's fibers seen in normal tendon-to-bone insertions. The bony attachment is extensive in cancellous bone and the progress is slower in cortical bone, making it important to remove or elevate cortex over a large enough area to allow implantation of tendon into bone. At 3 months, the union between the collagen fibers and osseous tissue appears similar to that seen in the normal insertion of tendon to bone.

There is disagreement as to the time of immobilization. Kernwein recommends immobilization of this attachment for a maximum of 3 weeks because prolonged immobilization will retard the tensile strength of the union.[30] Forward and Cowan found that unrestricted use after 3 weeks allowed separation of the tendon to bone ends, making a prolonged immobilization necessary.[31] Immobilization for 4 to 6 weeks will provide protection to the repair. Gentle active motion may be commenced in or out of the cast at 4 weeks. This is followed by a gradual return to a painless full range of motion. The patient can start to bear weight at 6 weeks. Guarded use over the next 2 to 4 weeks follows.

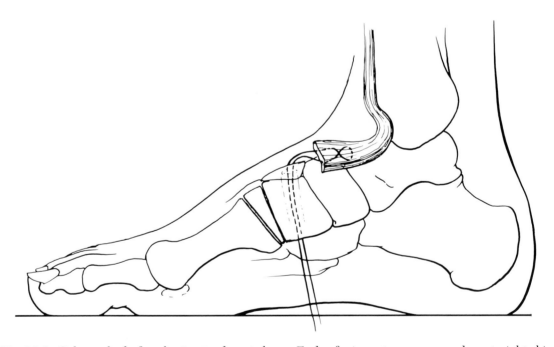

Fig. 12-6. Cole method of anchoring tendons to bone. Ends of wire suture are passed on straight skin needle through hole drilled in bone. Needle is drawn through skin on opposite side. Wire sutures are anchored over rubber tube or button. To prevent necrosis of skin when suture is under considerable tension, ends of wire may be passed through bottom of cast. Subsequently wire is anchored over button on outside of cast. (From Blum CE: Dorsal bunion. In Evarts CM: Surgery of the Musculoskeletal System. 2nd Ed. Churchill Livingstone, New York, in press.)

Suture Material

The ideal suture material should be nonreactive, nonrigid, of small caliber, strong, easy to handle, and able to hold a good knot.[32]

Following pedal tendon repair, immobilization is necessary for a minimum of 3 weeks before gentle active motion may be commenced. Up to about 10 days postoperatively, the tensile strength of the union is almost totally dependent on the technique of inserting the suture and the material used.[33] Therefore, the material chosen should be nonabsorbable to prevent gapping of the repair during this time.

Synthetic absorbable suture materials such as Vicryl and Dexon loose approximately 80 percent of their original tensile strength at 3 weeks.[34] This rapid decrease in strength may permit possible early tendon rupture at the site of repair.

Synthetic nonabsorbable suture materials used may be nylon, polypropylene, or polyester. Monofilament stainless steel may also be used as a pull-out suture. It produces the greatest resistance against gapping and eventual rupture,[35] has the greatest tensile strength before and after knotting,[36] and causes the least tissue reaction. The tensile strength of stainless steel decreases by 50 percent at 3 weeks. At 1 month, it is not significantly different from synthetic suture materials.[37] Its difficulty in handling and knotting, inelasticity, and brittleness have caused it to fall into disfavor as the newer synthetics emerge.

Many types of synthetic nonabsorbable suture materials are available to surgeons for tendon repair. The size of the tendon will determine the size of the suture used. Ketchum found Supramid to be the strongest of the synthetic materials[35] (Fig. 12-7). At 3 weeks, its ability to withstand

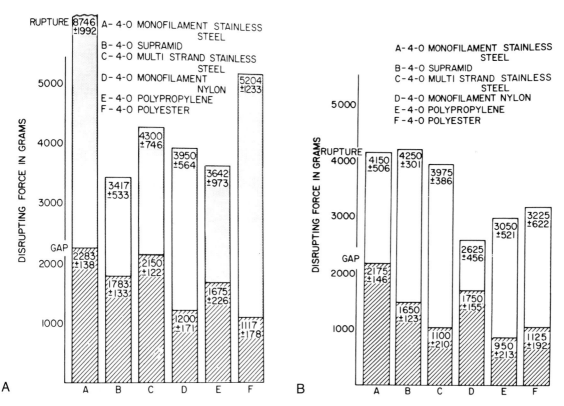

Fig. 12-7. **(A)** Abilities of tendon repairs with various suture materials to withstand gap-producing and rupture-producing forces at the time of the tendon repair. **(B)** Abilities of tendon repairs with various suture materials to withstand gap-producing and rupture-producing forces at 3 weeks after the repair. (From Ketchum et al.,[33] with permission.)

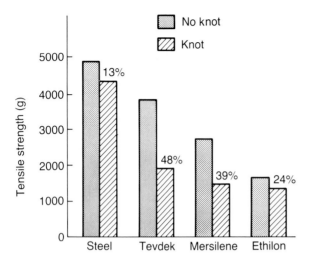

Fig. 12-8. Tensile strength of two strands of the 4-0 suture materials tested. Stainless steel was the least affected by knotting. (From Urbaniak,[36] with permission.)

gap- and rupture-producing forces was greater than that of monofilament stainless steel. It is composed of caprolactam, which is the chemical composition of some nylons. It is similar to monofilament nylon except that its polyfilament construction improves strength and handling while eliminating the problems of springiness and knot slippage. Urbaniak found Tevdek to be the strongest synthetic suture material before and after knotting[36] (Fig. 12-8).

Suture Techniques

Attempts have been made to suture tendons in such a manner that early guarded active motion may take place without tendon gap formation. Gap formation occurs when the suture ruptures or pulls out of the tendon. A proportional in-

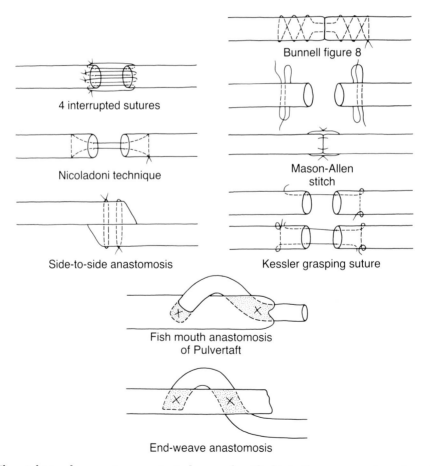

Fig. 12-9. The eight tendon anastomoses tested were classified into three groups based on the strength of their union. (From Urbaniak,[36] with permission.)

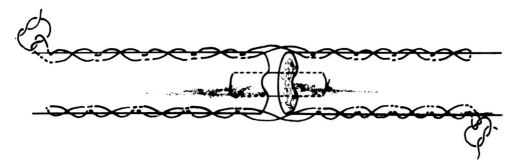

Fig. 12-10. The lateral trap suture was designed after the Oriental finger trap, to grip the lateral part of the tendon and avoid constricting the microcirculation in the central area of the tendon. The mattress suture at the repair site may be removed after the lateral trap suture is finished; before then it is used to avoid continuous forcep manipulation of the tendon as the lateral trap suture is put in. (From Ketchum et al.,[33] with permission.)

crease in the number of adhesions may be expected if gapping occurs during the repair process. Maintenance of the tendon repair depends on the suture material, suturing technique, and postoperative management.

Various suturing techniques have been studied experimentally.[37–44] The orientation of the suture and the direction of transmitted forces across the tendon repair will affect the final result. The strongest union occurs when sutures are placed perpendicular to both the collagen bundles of the tendon and the stress applied to repair. Urbaniak found this to occur with the Pulvertaft and end-weave anastomoses.[36] The Bunnell, Kessler, and Mason-Allen stitches were of intermediate strength because the longitudinal pull of these sutures is converted to an oblique or transverse compressive force on the tendon. The weakest repair occurred with the interrupted circumferential suture, the Nicoladoni, and side-to-side anastomoses. These techniques allow the suture to apply a shearing force to the tendon ends parallel to the longitudinal collagen bundles of the tendon (Fig. 12-9). Ketchum found that the greatest resistance to rupture was achieved by the lateral trap technique[35] (Figs. 12-10 and 12-11).

Early guarded active motion of tendon repairs may be beneficial in decreasing the number and quality of adhesions affecting the repair process.[38–43] Motion allows adhesions to stretch in the direction of the tendon gliding, thus allowing a freer range of excursion. In the repair of large

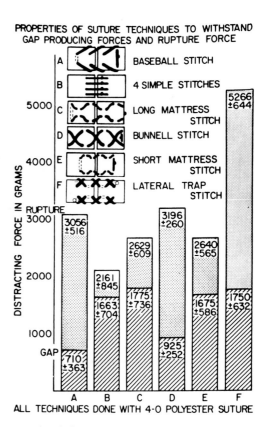

Fig. 12-11. Abilities of tendon repairs after various suture techniques to withstand gap-producing and rupture-producing forces. (From Ketchum et al.,[33] with permission.)

pedal tendons, early active motion may be undesirable because the stress generated by the muscle may be too high for the repair to withstand. The tendon anastomosis should be relaxed by flexing the joints with splinting instead of relying on the strength or type of suture repair. Guarded active motion is begun after 3 weeks.[29] Six weeks of protection from excessive strain should be maintained.

Gapping, bulkiness of repair, damage to the intrinsic or extrinsic blood supply of the tendon, inappropriate suture size or material, and poor postoperative treatment will all lead to a poor surgical result. Before the tendon ends are approximated, and ends must be debrided of necrotic tissue to allow quicker revascularization to take place.

TENDON RUPTURE

When a tendon is extended beyond its point of elasticity, which is approximately 8 percent extension of its total length, overstretching and rupture of some or all of the collagen fibers occurs, accompanied by cell damage.[45] Sudden application of a stretching force to a muscle that was contracting strongly is the most common mechanism causing tendon rupture (Fig. 12-12).

McMaster proved experimentally that tendons are the strongest link in the muscle–tendon unit.[46] When subjected to severe strain, normal tendon does not rupture. Rupture may occur at the insertion of tendon to bone, musculotendinous junction, through the muscle belly, or at the muscle origin. Disease processes in the tendons predispose to their spontaneous rupture, often from only slight strain.

Several causative factors have been suggested to contribute to tendon rupture. Usually a combination of factors are present. Structural foot, ankle, and leg deformities, advanced age, occupation, vascular impairment, corticosteroid use, infections, arthritis, tendonitis, tenosynovitis, and tendon calcification have all been implicated. These processes weaken tendon enough to allow rupture from minimal trauma.

Tibialis Anterior

The tibialis anterior muscle takes its origin from the lateral condyle and lateral shaft of the tibia and the interosseous membrane. It courses beneath the superior and inferior extensor retinaculum to insert on the medial and plantar aspect of the first cuneiform and base of the first metatarsal. It acts as a dorsiflexor of the ankle and invertor at the subtalar and midtarsal joints.

Rupture of this tendon is rare. It is reported in middle-aged to elderly persons whose foot is forced plantarly by a sudden single strong force that is greater than the power of the suddenly contracted muscle.[47–54] Several episodes of pain in the region of the tendon may precede the final rupture.[54]

Tendon rupture usually occurs 1 to 2 cm proximal to the insertion,[50,55] with the proximal tendon stump retracting and forming a bulbous enlargement above the anterior medial ankle.[48,50,51,54,55]

The patient usually presents with a history of a direct or twisting injury in which the foot was caught in a plantar flexed position. Pain and swelling will be present along the course of the tendon. Active dorsiflexion is diminished and passive plantar flexion may be painful. As the patient attempts to actively contract the muscle, no prominence of the tendon is palpated. A variable degree of footdrop and a slapping gait may be observed. The patient will have difficulty walking on the heels, but as a rule, the ability to walk is not lost.[50] Electromyography may confirm the diagnosis when needed.

Conservative treatment with below-knee casting for 4 to 6 weeks may return the foot to complete function.[47,53] The foot should be casted in a dorsiflexed, inverted position. Weakness of the tendon will be compensated by the digital extensors.

Many investigators consider operative repair to be the procedure of choice in young and middle-aged patients.[41,50,51,53,54,56] An attempt should be made at debriding any necrotic tendon edges, and an end-to-end repair should be performed with nonabsorbable suture material. Lipscomb reported good results in 8 of 12 patients treated in this manner, with follow-up of 1 to 15 years.[56] He followed the surgery by immobilizing the foot in

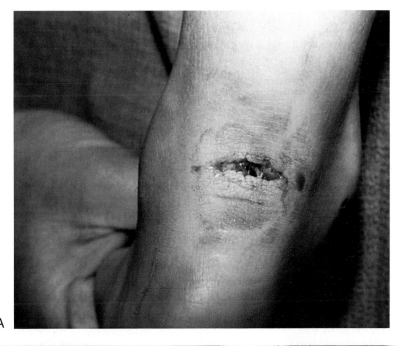

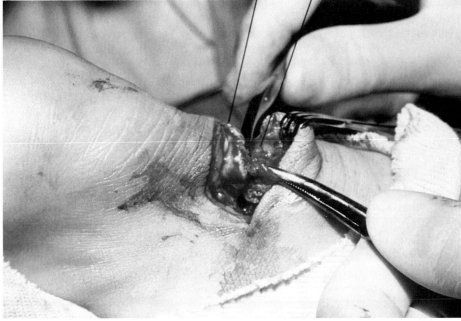

Fig. 12-12. (A) Lacerated achilles tendon following a kick to a glass shower door. (B) Bunnell-type repair shown here was reinforced with circumferential simple interrupted sutures. (Courtesy of Barry L. Scurran, D.P.M.)

plaster for 4 to 6 weeks. If this is not possible and the tendon is ruptured close to its insertion, the proximal tendon stump may be tied to a point just behind the original insertion.[51,54] A gap between the tendon stumps may be filled with a free tendon graft of the extensor digitorum longus to the fifth toe or with a split half of the tibialis anterior tendon proximal stump.[55] The alternative is to divide the extensor hallucis longus at the base of the first metatarsal and to suture the proximal tendon stump to the insertion of the tibialis anterior. The ruptured tendon stumps are sutured side to side onto the extensor hallucis longus. The distal extensor hallucis longus stump may then be sutured to the extensor digitorum longus tendon to the second toe. The phasic activities of the anterior muscle groups are approximately the same, making the procedure almost physiologic. Postoperatively, a below-knee non-weight-bearing cast with the foot in dorsiflexion and inversion is used for 6 weeks. This is followed by a weight-bearing below-knee cast with the foot in neutral position for 2 to 4 weeks.

Tibialis Posterior

The tibialis posterior muscle originates from the tibia, fibula, and interosseous membrane. The tendon arises in the distal one-third of the leg, courses behind the medial malleolus in its groove, and inserts into the foot. The major insertion of the tendon is to the navicular tuberosity, with small slips of tendon inserting into all the tarsal bones except the talus. Small intermetatarsal slips of tendon insert into the base of the middle three metatarsals.[57] The muscle plantar flexes the foot at the ankle and supinates the subtalar and midtarsal joints.

Spontaneous rupture of the posterior tibial tendon is uncommon. Rupture may be due to acute or chronic stress on an already degenerated tendon. Tenosynovitis may be present prior to the disruption.[58] Avascularity in a critical zone just posterior to the medial malleolus may be a precipitating factor.[59] An association between pes planus foot types and ruptures has been made. Rheumatologic conditions, most commonly rheumatoid arthritis, may cause progressive degeneration of the tendon, leading to rupture.

Patients will present with a history of pain along the course of the posterior tibial tendon from the medial malleolus to its insertion into the navicular. An inciting injury may be recalled. Activity and stance will aggravate the pain. The patient will relate a history of progressive lowering of the longitudinal arch.

Disruption of the tendon can be palpated as the patient attempts active inversion. As the patient attempts heel rise, the subtalar joint fails to invert. The calcaneus will assume an increased valgus position when viewed from behind. With chronicity, the unapposed action of the peroneals will abduct the forefoot, causing a reverse C-shaped foot. The talus will bulge medially with lack of medial soft tissue support. The foot will remain pronated throughout the gait cycle.

Standing anteroposterior and lateral radiographs should be evaluated. Early changes will be minimal in acute tears. Untreated cases may show progressive pronatory changes. The lateral radiograph view will demonstrate plantar flexion of the talus and an increase in the talocalcaneal angle. The anteroposterior view shows abduction of the forefoot at the midtarsal joint leaving the medial half of the talar head uncovered. An increase in the talocalcaneal angle will also be present. Changes seen on radiographs are best appreciated when a comparison is made with the unaffected side.

When clinical examination is undefinitive and surgery is contemplated, tenography[60] and magnetic resonance imaging[61–63] may be helpful in confirming the diagnosis of a rupture.

The most common site of a posterior tibial tendon rupture is between the navicular and medial malleolus. A tendon stump of 1 to 2 cm is usually left attached to the navicular. If untreated, the tendon stumps will fibrose to the adjacent soft tissue.

Conservative treatment consists of a below-knee non-weight-bearing cast with the foot in maximum plantar flexion, adduction, and inversion for 6 weeks. This is followed by a below-knee weight-bearing cast with the foot in neutral position for an additional 2 to 4 weeks. Following cast removal, orthotics should be used for continued longitudinal arch support. Aggressive physical therapy after the period of immobilization is used to attempt to regain power, strength, and endurance of the muscle–tendon. Conservative care should be reserved for the elderly patient with a sedentary lifestyle. All other patients should undergo surgical repair in an attempt to restore inversion power and protect against severe disabling pes planovalgus deformity, which may later necessitate a triple arthrodesis.

Surgical repair techniques differ according to the anatomic location of the rupture, the extent of the rupture, and the time at which tendon repair is considered. The proximal tendon stump will retract, making primary repair difficult after 6 weeks. Midsubstance tears should be sutured end to end if tendon length is available. Most often this is not possible, and a Z-plasty lengthening of the proximal fragment, tendon graft, or tendon transfer is necessary. Various clinicians have used the flexor digitorum longus tendon in their surgical repairs. Mann and Thompson passed the tendon dorsally through a drill hole in the navicular and sutured it under maximum tension back on itself with the foot in maximum plantar flexion and inversion.[64] At follow-up (average, 31 months), excellent results were obtained in 11 of 14 patients. Funk et al. interposed the flexor digitorum longus tendon between the posterior tibial tendon stumps and found five of five subjects with subjective improvement, noting pain relief and the ability to do single limb heel rise.[65] Wrenn reported satisfactory results in 12 of 12 patients by suturing the proximal segment of the posterior tibial tendon to the flexor digitorum longus tendon proximal to the medial malleolus, and then sectioning the flexor digitorum longus distal to the medial malleolus, and suturing this proximal segment to the posterior tibial expansion.[66]

The best results in the treatment of posterior tibial tendon rupture can be expected with flexor digitorum longus transfer (Fig. 12-13). The flexor digitorum longus tendon is transected at the level of navicular. The distal tendon stump is tied into the flexor hallucis longus to allow function of the digital flexors. The proximal stump is then tied into the navicular through drill holes or into the

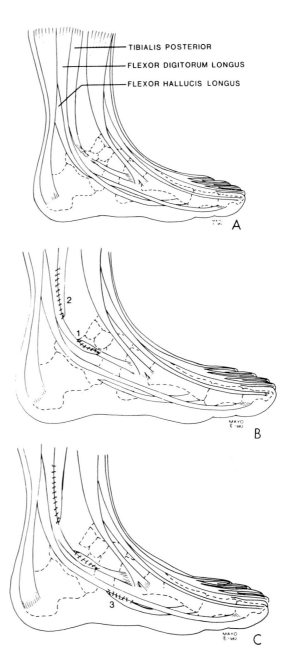

Fig. 12-13. (A) Common site of tibialis posterior tendon separation. **(B)** After appropriate transection of the adjacent flexor digitorum longus, tenodesis is completed to remaining tibialis posterior both (1) distally and (2) proximally. **(C)** Optional tenodesis of the distal segment of the flexor digitorum longus to (3) the flexor hallucis longus. (From Johnson KA: Tibialis posterior tendon rupture. Clin Orthop 177:140, 1983, with permission.)

posterior tibial tendon expansion plantarly. Side-to-side anastomoses of the posterior tibial tendon stumps to the proximal segment of the flexor digitorum longus are performed proximally and distally with the foot in plantar flexion, inversion, and adduction. Available tendon sheath is used to surround the tendon without constricting normal gliding. Postoperatively, a non-weight-bearing below-knee cast is used for 6 weeks with the foot in plantar flexion, inversion, and adduction. This is followed by a weight-bearing cast for 4 weeks with the foot in a neutral position. After cast removal, a longitudinal arch support is used along with aggressive physical therapy.

When failure of nonoperative and soft tissue procedures to restore alignment and function occurs, the patient will need an arthrodesis to restore function. A triple arthrodesis will provide better structural alignment of the tarsal bones and improve function of the remaining pedal tendons that might otherwise attempt to compensate for the deformity.

Peroneal Tendons

The peroneus longus originates from the upper half of the fibula and adjacent soft tissue. The peroneus brevis origin is anterior to the longus from the lower two-thirds of the lateral fibula surface. The brevis lies deep to the longus as they both course in the malleolar groove of the fibula. The peroneus longus courses around the peroneal groove in the cuboid to insert into the base of the first metatarsal (90 percent) and medial cuneiform (10 percent). The peroneus brevis inserts into the lateral base of the fifth metatarsal.[57] They are weak plantar flexors of the ankle joint and strong pronators of the subtalar joint.

Closed ruptures of the peroneal tendons are most commonly due to a violent eversion tendon contraction against an actively inverting foot as seen with a lateral ankle sprain.[67–70] Munk and Davis described a longitudinal rupture of the peroneus brevis.[71] They hypothesized that the peroneus longus acts as a wedge, cutting through the peroneus brevis tendon as the brevis gets caught between the malleolus and peroneus longus in forceful dorsiflexion. Burman associated the peroneus longus tear with an enlarged peroneal trochlea from pressure of the peroneus longus in a varus foot.[67] Rupture of the peroneus longus has been associated with fractures of the os peroneum.[70] Peroneal tendon injuries have long been associated with calcaneal fractures. Impingement of fracture fragments from the calcaneus may lead to tenosynovitis and eventually tendon rupture.

Patients may present with acute or chronic lateral foot, ankle, and leg pain. Without the protective eversion role of the lateral tendons, recurrent inversion ankle sprains may be an initial complaint.

Swelling in the dorsolateral foot may be present. An enlarged peroneal trochlea[67] may be palpated. Pain will be present as the patient attempts active eversion. Forceful inversion will cause symptoms laterally. It is important to differentiate between peroneus brevis and peroneus longus ruptures. As the patient actively everts, the examiner should palpate the course of the tendons to test their continuity. Plantar flexion of the first metatarsal will be lost with peroneus longus rupture, and the examiner can easily push up against the first metatarsal head without resistance.

Anteroposterior, lateral, medial oblique, and calcaneal axial films should be taken to rule out impingement of fracture fragments of the calcaneus or fibula, enlarged peroneal trochlea, or fractured os peroneum. Tenograms may show blockage of flow in the peroneal sheath distal to the inferior peroneal retinaculum.[68] In indeterminate cases, magnetic resonance imaging should be used. Large gaps within the substance of the tendon will be visualized.[62]

Little has been written on the subject, leading us to believe this injury goes unrecognized in many instances and possibly without any significant disability. If the injury is recognized early, we recommend a below-knee weight-bearing cast for 6 to 8 weeks in the nonathletic or recreational athletic individual. In the highly competitive athlete, surgical repair should be instituted. If primary apposition of the tendon ends cannot be performed, the stumps of the peroneus brevis should be sutured to the peroneus longus if the peroneus brevis is ruptured, or the peroneus longus stumps sutured to peroneus brevis tendon if peroneus longus is ruptured.

In a limited number of reported cases, these researchers have found good results with surgical repair followed by a below-knee weight-bearing cast for 6 weeks.[67–71]

Flexor Hallucis Longus

The flexor hallucis longus muscle takes its origin from the distal two-thirds of the posterolateral aspect of the fibula. Its tendon arises in the distal posterior portion of the leg. It travels in the fibro-osseous canal in the posterior aspect of the

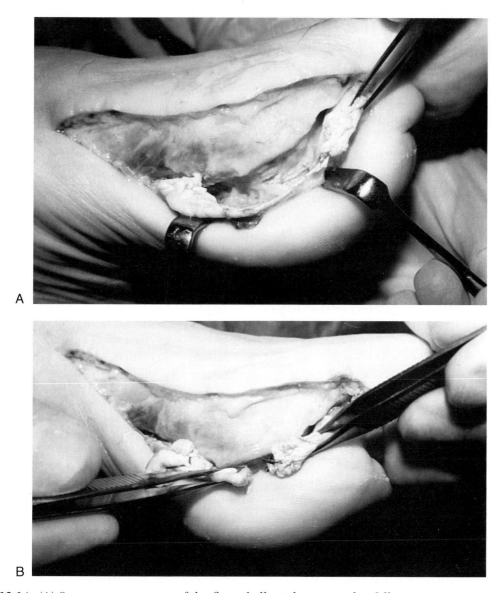

Fig. 12-14. (A) Spontaneous rupture of the flexor hallucis longus tendon following tennis serve push-off. Note severely frayed tendon ends. (B) Frayed ends are individually repaired using a circumferential long mattress stitch. (*Figure continues.*)

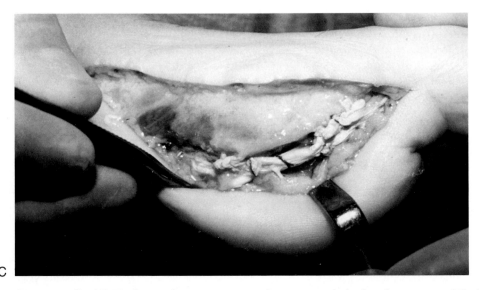

Fig. 12-14 (*Continued*). (**C**) End-to-end anastomosis is then accomplished utilizing a modified Bunnell-type stitch. (Courtesy of Barry L. Scurran, D.P.M.)

talus and beneath the sustentaculum of the talus as it courses to its insertion on the plantar aspect of the base of the distal phalanx of the hallux. In the non-weight-bearing foot, the tendon flexes the hallux interphalangeal joint. It also assists in plantar flexion of the hallux at the metatarsal phalangeal joint, supination of the foot at the subtalar joint, and plantar flexion of the foot at the ankle joint.

Rupture of the flexor hallucis tendon is extremely rare (Fig. 12-14). Kracow reported on one acute traumatic rupture in a diver.[72] The mechanism of injury was violent dorsiflexion of the foot, ankle, and great toe. Sammarco and Miller reported four cases of partial rupture of the tendon's central fibers in the posteromedial ankle compartment.[73]

Subjective symptoms with this rupture may be minimal. The patient may complain of weakness during propulsion or instability as an attempt is made to stand on the toes.

With stabilization of the first metatarsal phalangeal joint, active interphalangeal joint flexion is lost. Sammarco and Miller noted fusiform enlargement of the tendon just distal to the flexor canal in the posteromedial ankle compartment.[73] This was due to the central rupture of the tendon fibers. A popping sensation may be felt in the compartment with flexion and extension of the hallux. Triggering of the hallux may occur if the enlarged portion of the tendon is proximal to the retinaculum with the foot in a neutral position.

Radiographs should be taken in at least two planes to rule out an avulsion fracture of the base of the distal phalanx.

Localization of the tendon stumps is important so that the proper skin incision is planned for primary tendon repair. Repair of the tendon will allow active interphalangeal joint flexion of the great toe and reduction of the risk to hallux elevatus from the unapposed action of the extensor hallucis longus. Kracow performed primary repair utilizing a pull-out wire suture since the rupture was 0.5 cm from the insertion.[72] Frenette and Jackson reported on 10 traumatic lacerations.[74] Primary repair was performed on six patients. Four of the six patients lost active interphalangeal joint flexion. They concluded that the tendon was bound in scar tissue and that an intact flexor hallucis longus tendon is not essential for good push-off and balance in running sports. Following primary repair, the tendon should be immobilized for 3 weeks. Because of tendon size, mobilization may be commenced at the end of 3 weeks so that active motion will be restored. Weight bearing at 5 to 6 weeks as tolerated is permitted. When partial rupture and triggering is suspect, releasing of the flexor retinaculum portion overlying the ruptured tendon fibers permits smooth gliding.[73]

INFLAMMATORY DISORDERS OF TENDON

Inflammatory conditions affecting tendons with or without involvement of their corresponding paratenon or synovial sheath may be divided into tendinitis, paratendinitis, tenosynovitis, or tendovaginitis. Depending on the time frame over which deforming forces are present, tenosynovitis may be further divided into acute, chronic, or stenosing. Varying degrees of tendovaginitis is usually present and will be discussed here.

Early in the disease process, fragmentation of collagen within the substance of the tendon may be present.[75] If the process continues, the tendon pathology may be characterized by thinning and flattening at sites of constriction with bulbous thickening beyond the constriction sites. Nodules may be present within the substance of the tendon.[76,77] They may be sequels to partial tendon ruptures, and adhesions may be greatest where the nodules exist.[78] The tendon usually lacks its normal shining color and frequently appears yellow and dull.

The paratenon and synovial sheath are characterized by brown or reddish discoloration[77] with excess fluid contained within them.[76,79,80] They may become inflamed and heal with thickening,[77-81] adhesions, and constriction.[77] This thickening will restrict normal gliding of the tendon.

Peroneal Tendons

Tendovaginitis of the peroneal tendons and their sheaths may occur at the three locations: (1) the lateral malleolus, where they share a common sheath; (2) the peroneal tubercle, where the tendons are contained within their own sheath;

and (3) the peroneal groove in the cuboid where the peroneus longus courses plantarly to insert into the base of the first metatarsal and medial cuneiform.

These inflammatory conditions may be nonspecific or related to static foot deformities,[77] inversion injuries,[82] enlarged peroneal tubercle,[82] soft tissue mass,[83] infection,[84] multipartite os peroneum,[82,84] or direct trauma. It is most commonly due to acute or prolonged use of the involved tendon.[77,81-84]

The condition is characterized by pain with active eversion and passive inversion. Pain and fusiform swelling are localized along the course of the tendon where the restriction to tendon gliding exists. Dorsiflexion of the first metatarsal may cause pain from the cuboid to the insertion of the peroneus longus plantarly.

Treatment is directed toward identifying the cause of the inflammatory process. Tendovaginitis and acute tenosynovitis will usually respond to conservative care, whereas chronic and stenosing tenosynovitis often require surgery to allow pain-free tendon function. Mild cases of tenosynovitis due to prolonged unaccustomed activity may respond to resting the foot. If static deformities exist, orthotics may be necessary to decrease the functional demand of the tendon. Whirlpools, contrast baths, and ultrasound may be an adjunct in the treatment plan. Nonsteroidal anti-inflammatory drugs or injections of cortisone directly into the tendon sheath or both may be of benefit. Immobilization in more severe cases for 2 to 6 weeks will put the tendon to rest and decrease the local inflammation. Gradual return to full tendon function is then resumed.

When conservative measures fail, surgery may be necessary to allow normal pain-free function. Attention must be directed toward the tendon and synovial sheath. A longitudinal incision is made through the peroneal retinaculum and tendon sheath. All inflamed, hypertrophic synovium is excised. Release of the constricting portion of the sheath is necessary to allow smooth tendon gliding without entrapment. If poststenotic enlargement of the tendon exists, a longitudinal wedge of tendon is resected to allow the diameter to approximate that of the uninvolved part. Any local bony exostosis or soft tissue mass, if present, must be removed to decompress the area. Postoperatively, non-weight-bearing early range of motion is essential for 4 weeks to decrease the formation of new adhesions. A slow return to activity then follows.

Posterior Tibial Tendon

Tendovaginitis of the posterior tibial tendon can occur anywhere along its course from the medial malleolus to its major insertion into the navicular. It is most commonly present in its groove behind the medial malleolus. Pronated foot types have been implicated as the cause by some investigators.[77,79,85] This produces mechanical strain on the posterior tibial tendon and its sheath. Over time, this strain may cause posterior tibial tendon dysfunction. Fractures of the medial malleolus, talus, calcaneus, or navicular may impinge on the tendon and its sheath. Ghormley and Spear described an accessory posterior tibial tendon causing mechanical irritation.[79] Eversion injuries may produce symptoms, but the condition is most likely caused by acute or prolonged use of the tendon in a person who is unaccustomed to the activity involved.

This inflammatory disorder is characterized by pain anywhere along the course of the tendon. Pain increases with active inversion and passive eversion that put undue tension on the tendon. Running uphill will similarly heighten the symptoms. Fusiform swelling may be seen and palpated along the course of the tendon.

Rest, ice, and nonsteroidal anti-inflammatory medication will alleviate the symptoms in acute cases. Arch supports will benefit the foot that pronates excessively. If no response is achieved, one or two cortisone injections over a 1-month period may be injected directly into the sheath. Cast immobilization may be necessary for 2 to 6 weeks to put the tendon to complete rest. It is important to assess the posterior tibial tendon function. Trevino et al. found partial or complete rupture of the tendon in 6 to 8 patients treated surgically for tenosynovitis.[86] Williams achieved relief in 40 of 52 patients with conservative care.[80] He attained relief in 11 of 12 patients treated surgi-

cally by simple division of the sheath. Ghormley and Spear obtained relief in three patients after the accessory posterior tibial tendon had been excised.[79]

Anterior Tibialis Tendon

The anterior tibialis tendon and its sheath may become inflamed in the anterior ankle compartment as the tendon passes beneath the superior and inferior extensor retinaculum.

Lipscomb found it to be the most commonly affected tendon in the foot.[77] Inflammation was often due to irritation by shoes and boots. Trauma and overuse syndromes may also cause inflammatory changes in the tendon and its sheath. An increase in the functional demand of the tendon may be present in patients with gastrocsoleus equinus as the tendon attempts to dorsiflex the foot for ground clearance in gait. Downhill running will likewise increase the demand on the tendon as it attempts to decelerate the foot to avoid foot slap.

Pain is usually present in the anterior ankle. Active dorsiflexion and passive plantar flexion will both reproduce symptoms. As the patient attempts to walk on the heels, pain and weakness are noted. During the physical examination, it is important to check for equinus of the posterior leg muscle group.

Most patients in Lipscomb's series responded to rest. Occasionally he released the synovial sheath in front of the ankle. This condition usually responds to rest and nonsteroidal anti-inflammatory medication when needed. After the acute phase of inflammation has passed, stretching tight posterior muscles and modification of shoegear or training methods will prevent recurrence.

Flexor Hallucis Longus Tendon

Tendovaginitis of the flexor hallucis longus may occur at three locations: (1) the posterior aspect of the talus as the tendon passes between the medial and lateral talar tubercles; (2) beneath the sustentaculum of the talus; and (3) between the sesamoids and the insertion of the tendon into the base of the distal phalanx of the hallux.

This inflammatory process is commonly found in ballet dancers in the fibro-osseous groove in the posterior aspect of the talus.[87] Gould described nine cases of stenosing tenosynovitis of the flexor hallucis longus as the tendon passes through its sheath between the sesamoids and its insertion.[76] He thought mechanical factors were responsible. Damage to the fibro-osseous canal may also interfere with smooth gliding of the tendon.

Patients will complain of pain anywhere along the course of the tendon from the posterior ankle to its insertion. Active flexion of the interphalangeal joint or passive dorsiflexion of the hallux will reproduce symptoms in the area of constriction to gliding. If stenosis is present, a snapping sensation will be felt and limitation of hallux dorsiflexion will be seen.

In acute or chronic cases, rest, ice, and nonsteroidal anti-inflammatory medications may be of benefit. Orthotics in a stiff-soled shoe will limit active metatarsal phalangeal motion. Gould forcibly injected lidocaine into the tendon sheath to inflate the sheath and break adhesions.[76] He achieved relief in three of nine patients. Six patients required tenolysis for relief. Conservative care of stenosing tenosynovitis is usually unsuccessful. Surgical release of the sheath and possibly the flexor retinaculum may be necessary to allow free hallux motion.

LACERATIONS OF TENDONS

The time of wounding, type of wound, and location are important factors in considering primary versus secondary repair of tendon lacerations. The best period in which primary repair may be performed is approximately 6 hours after wounding, but clinical judgment as to the wound status should be made. A simple incised wound with a tendon laceration from sharp cutting objects may be closed after 6 hours if the local wound environment is clean and little tissue re-

action is expected. If primary healing of the skin is expected to take place, the tendon is sutured at the same time as skin closure (Fig. 12-15).

A lacerated crushed wound with skin avulsion or skin loss should not be closed within the first 6 hours if a large amount of tissue damage is present. These wounds show a greater propensity toward inflammation and infection. Healing takes place with edema and fibrosis. Secondary closure may be performed in 3 to 5 days if initial wound cultures are negative and local inflammation has diminished.

If there is any doubt about the advisability of primary closure, a conservative approach is taken. It is safe and better for the patient to undergo a secondary closure than to develop an infection after primary closure. End-to-end suture, tendon grafting, or tendon transfer may be necessary in the reparative process. Skin coverage over the tendon repair is mandatory.

A history of tetanus immunization should be obtained. Gram stains, cultures, and sensitivities of organisms taken from the wound should be obtained on initial presentation before prophylactic or therapeutic antibiotics are administered. The use of antibiotics depends on the local wound environment and the host.

Surgical debridement is the essential first step in removing gross contamination and nonvital tissue. This is best performed in the operating room with local sedation or general anesthesia. Tourniquets will provide a bloodless field. The wound is prepared and draped for evaluation. Damage to the tendon and other underlying structures is identified (Fig. 12-13). Pulsatile irrigation with saline will aid in removing any clotted blood, nonvital tissue, foreign bodies, dirt, and other debris. The ends of the tendon are picked up with Adson tissue forceps and a through-and-through box-type suture with nonabsorbable material is inserted near the tip of the tendon for use in handling and later in reanastomosing. If the ends of the tendon have retracted, a hemostat may be placed through the tendon sheath in an attempt to retrieve the stump. If this cannot be achieved, small incisions should be made at the points where the surgeon expects to find the tendon stumps. The incisions should be placed in the

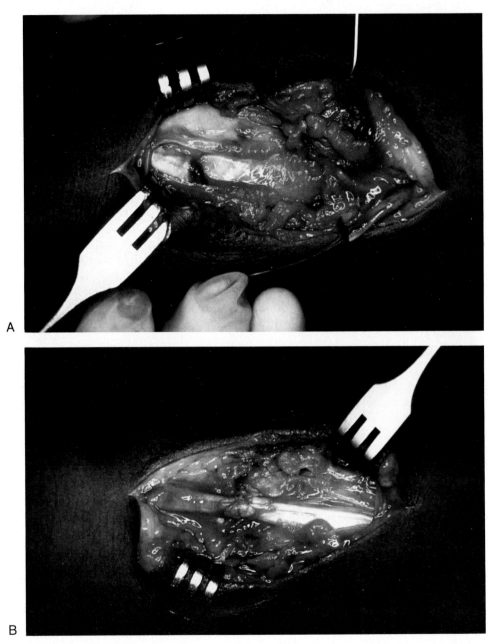

Fig. 12-15. **(A)** Traumatic laceration of extensor hallucis longus tendon. **(B)** Primary repair utilizing a modified Kessler stitch. (Courtesy of Nicholas Daly, D.P.M.)

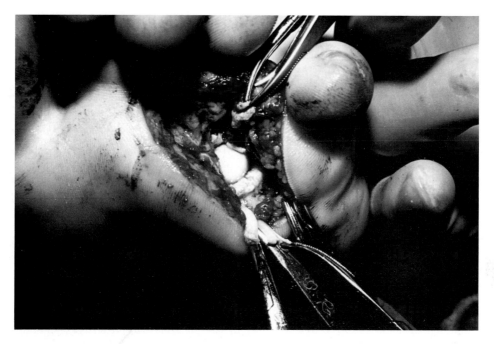

Fig. 12-16. Multiple tendon lacerations are identified during inspection of this contaminated open fracture. (Courtesy of Barry L. Scurran, D.P.M.)

proper skin lines. After the stumps have been found and tagged with sutures, a probe is passed through the tendon sheath or paratenon in the original wound and the tendon stumps are retrieved. The tendon ends are debrided of crushed tendon ends and then coapted. Buried sutures should be kept to a minimum. A small drain may be used for 24 to 48 hours to prevent hematoma. A compression dressing and elevation of the extremity will aid in healing by decreasing swelling. The tendon repair should be protected with 4 to 6 weeks of immobilization in a short leg cast.

REFERENCES

1. Van Der Meulen JC, Leistikow PA: Tendon healing. Clin Plast Surg 4:439, 1977
2. Lindsay WK: Tendon healing: a continuing experimental approach. p. 35. In Verdan C (ed): Tendon Surgery of the Hand. Churchill Livingstone, Edinburgh, 1979
3. Piez KA: Cross-linking of collagen and elastin. Ann Rev Biochem 37:574, 1968
4. Yamada H: Strength of biological materials. In Evans FG (ed): Williams & Wilkins, Baltimore, 1970
5. Carlsedt CA: Mechanical and chemical factors in tendon healing. Acta Orthop Scand 58: suppl 224, 1987
6. Miller SJ: Principles of muscle tendon surgery and tendon transfers. In McGlamry ED (ed): Comprehensive Textbook of Foot Surgery. Williams & Wilkins, Baltimore, 1987
7. Cooper RR, Misol S: Tendon and ligament insertion. J Bone Joint Surg 52A:1, 1970
8. Field PL: Tendon fibre arrangement and blood supply. Aust NZ J Surg 40:298, 1971
9. Edwards DAW: The blood supply and lymphatic drainage of tendons. J Anat 80:147, 1946
10. Semple C: The design of tendons and their sheaths. In Owen R, Goodfellow J, Bullough P (ed): Scientific Foundations of Orthopaedics and Traumatology. WB Saunders, Philadelphia, 1980
11. Harkness RD: Mechanical properties of collagenous tissues. In Gould BS (ed): Treatise on Collagen. Academic Press, Orlando, FL, 1968
12. Amiel D, Woo SLY, Harwood FL, Akeson WH:

The effect of immobilization on collagen turnover in connective tissue. A biochemical-biomechanical correlation. Acta Orthop Scand 53:325, 1982

13. Elliot DH: Structure and function of mammalian tendon. Biol Rev 40:392, 1965
14. Crockford DA: Reconstructive Plastic Surgery. Vol. 1. p. 271. WB Saunders, Philadelphia, 1977
15. Colville J, Callison JR, White WL: Role of mesotenon in tendon blood supply. Plast Reconstr Surg 43:53, 1969
16. Boyes JH: Tendons. In Boyes JH (ed): Bunnell's Surgery of the Hand. 4th Ed. JB Lippincott, Philadelphia, 1964
17. Mayer L: The physiological method of tendon transplantation. Surg Gynecol Obstet 22:182, 1916
18. Edwards DA: The blood supply and lymphatic drainage of tendon. J Anat 80:147, 1946
19. Peacock EE: Research in tendon healing. In Tubiana R (ed): The Hand. WB Saunders, Philadelphia, 1981
20. Beasley RW: Tendon injuries. In Beasley RW (ed): Hand Injuries. WB Saunders, Philadelphia, 1981
21. Potenza AD: Tendon and ligament healing. In Owen R, Goodfellow J, Bullough P (ed): Scientific Foundations of Orthopaedics and Traumatology. WB Saunders, Philadelphia, 1980
22. Peacock EE: Tendon. In Peacock EE (ed): Wound Repair. 3rd Ed. WB Saunders, Philadelphia, 1984
23. Ketchum LD: Primary tendon healing: a review. Hand Surg 2:428, 1977
24. Zinmeister B, Edelman R: A new technique for tenodesis of the tibialis posterior in the Kidner procedure. Foot Surg 24:442, 1985
25. Gould N: Trephining your way. Orthop Clin North Am 4:157, 1973
26. Crenshaw AH: Surgical techniques. In Campbell's Operative Orthopaedics. 7th Ed. CV Mosby, St. Louis, 1987
27. Cole WH: The treatment of clawfoot. J Bone Joint Surg 22:895, 1940
28. Key JA: Fixation of tendons, ligaments and bone by Bunnell's pullout wire suture. Ann Surg 123:656, 1946
29. Boyles JH: Tendons. In Boyes JH (ed): Bunnell's Surgery of the Hand. 5th Ed. JB Lippincott, Philadelphia, 1970
30. Kernwein GA: A study of tendon implantation into bone. Surg Gynecol Obstet 75:794
31. Forward AD, Cowan RJ: Tendon suture to bone. J Bone Joint Surg 45A:807, 1963
32. Leddy JP: Flexor tendons: acute injuries. In Green DP (ed): Operative Hand Surgery. Churchill Livingstone, New York, 1982
33. Ketchum LD, Martin NL, Knappel DA: Experimental evaluation of factors affecting the strength of tendon repairs. Plast Reconstr Surg 59:708, 1977
34. Yu GV, Cavaliere R: Suture materials. J Am Podiatry Assoc 73:57, 1983
35. Ketchum LD: Suture materials and suture techniques used in tendon repair. Hand Clin 1:43, 1985
36. Urbaniak J: Tendon suturing methods: analysis of tensile strength. In AAOS Symposium of Tendon Surgery in the Hand. CV Mosby, St. Louis, 1975
37. Mangus DJ, Brown F, Byrnes W, Habel A: Tendon repairs with nylon and a modified pullout technique. Plast Reconstr Surg 48:32, 1971
38. Kessler I: The "grasping" technique for tendon repair. The Hand 5:253, 1973
39. Kessler I, Nissim F: Primary repair without immobilization of flexor tendon division within the digital sheath. Acta Orthop Scand 40:587, 1969
40. Pennington DG: The locking loop tendon suture. Plast Reconstr Surg 63:648, 1979
41. Becker H, Orak F, Duponselle E: Early active motion following a beveled technique of flexor tendon repair: report on fifty cases. Hand Surg 4:454, 1979
42. Tsuge K, Ikuta Y, Matsuishi Y: Repair of flexor tendons by intratendinous tendon suture. Hand Surg 2:436, 1977
43. Becker H, Davidoff M: Eliminating the gap in flexor tendon surgery. The Hand 9:306, 1977
44. Pulvertaft RG: Suture materials and tendon junctures. Am Surg 109:346, 1965
45. Williams IF: Cellular and biochemical composition of healing tendon. In Jenkins HR (ed): Ligament Injuries and Their Treatment. Aspen, Rockville, MD, 1985
46. McMaster PE: Tendon and muscle ruptures. J Bone Joint Surg 15:705, 1933
47. Burman M: Subcutaneous strain or tear of the dorsiflexor tendons of the foot. Bull Hosp Jt. Dis Orthop Inst 4:44, 1943
48. Moskowitz E: Rupture of the tibialis anterior tendon simulating peroneal nerve palsy. Arch Phys Med Rehab Sept: 431, 1971
49. Scheller AD, Kasser JR, Quigley TB: Tendon injuries about the ankle. Orthop Clin North Am 2:801, 1980
50. Moberg E: Subcutaneous rupture of the tendon of the tibialis anterior muscle. Acta Chir Scand 95:455, 1947

51. Dooley BJ, Kudelka P, Menelaus MD: Subcutaneous rupture of the tendon of tibialis anterior. J Bone Joint Surg 62B:471, 1980

52. Meyn MA: Closed rupture of the anterior tibial tendon. Clin Orthop 113:154, 1975

53. Burman MD: Subcutaneous rupture of the tendon of the tibialis anticus. Ann Surg 100:368, 1934

54. Mensor MC, Ordaway GL: Traumatic subcutaneous rupture of the tibialis anterior tendon. J Bone Joint Surg 35A:675, 1953

55. Lapidus PW: Indirect subcutaneous rupture of the anterior tibial tendon. Bull Hosp Jt Dis Orthop Inst 2:119, 1941

56. Lipscomb PR: Injuries to the extensor tendons in the distal part of the leg and in the ankle. J Bone Joint Surg 37A:1206, 1955

57. McCarthy DJ: Anatomy. In McGlamry ED (ed): Fundamentals of Foot Surgery. Williams & Wilkins, Baltimore, 1987

58. Kettelkamp DB, Alexander HH: Spontaneous rupture of the posterior tibial tendon. J Bone Joint Surg 51A:759, 1969

59. Frey CC, Shereff MJ: Tendon injuries about the ankle in athletics. Clin Sports Med 7:103, 1988

60. Jahss MH: Spontaneous rupture of the tibialis posterior tendon: clinical findings, tenographic studies and a new technique of repair. Foot Ankle 3:158, 1983

61. Alexander IJ, Johnson KA, Berquist TH: Magnetic resonance imaging in the diagnosis of disruption of the posterior tibial tendon. Foot Ankle 3:144, 1983

62. Beltran J, Noto AM, Herman LJ, Lubbers LM: Tendons: high field strength, surface coil MR imaging. Radiology 162:735, 1987

63. Resnick D, Niwayama G: Magnetic resonance imaging. p. 203. In: Diagnosis of Bone and Joint Disorders. 2nd Ed. Vol. 1. 1988

64. Mann RA, Thompson FM: Rupture of the posterior tibial tendon causing flatfoot. J Bone Joint Surg 67A:556, 1985

65. Funk DA, Cass JR, Johns KA: Acquired flat foot secondary to posterior tibial tendon pathology. J Bone Joint Surg 68A:95, 1986

66. Wrenn RN: Isolated ruptures of the posterior tibial tendon. J Bone Joint Surg 57A:1035, 1975

67. Burman M: Subcutaneous tear of the tendon of the peroneus longus. Arch Surg 73:216, 1956

68. Abraham E, Stirnaman JE: Neglected rupture of the peroneal tendons causing recurrent sprains of the ankle. J Bone Joint Surg 61A:1247, 1979

69. Evans JD: Subcutaneous rupture of the tendon of peroneus longus. J Bone Joint Surg 48B:507, 1966

70. Peacock KC, Resnick EJ, Thoder JJ: Fracture of the os peroneum with rupture of the peroneus longus tendon. Clin Orthop 202:223, 1986

71. Munk RL, Davis PH: Longitudinal rupture of the peroneus brevis tendon. J Trauma 16:804, 1976

72. Krackow KA: Acute traumatic rupture of the flexor hallucis longus tendon. Clin Orthop 150:261, 1980

73. Sammarco GJ, Milerr EH: Partial rupture of the flexor hallucis longus tendon in classical ballet. J Bone Joint Surg 61A:149, 1979

74. Frenette JP, Jackson DW: Lacerations of the flexor hallucis longus in the young athlete. J Bone Joint Surg 59A:673, 1977

75. Gould N, Korson R: Stenosing tenosynovitis of the pseudosheath of the tendoachilles. Foot Ankle 1:179, 1980

76. Gould N: Stenosing tenosynovitis of the flexor hallucis longus tendon at the great toe. Foot Ankle 2:46, 1981

77. Lipscomb PR: Nonsuppurative tenosynovitis and paratendinitis. p. 254. In: Instructional Course Lectures, American Academy of Orthopaedic Surgeons. Vol. 7. CV Mosby, St. Louis, 1950

78. Kvist H, Kvist M: The operative treatment of chronic calcaneal paratenonitis. J Bone Joint Surg 62B:353, 1980

79. Ghormley RK, Spear IM: Anomalies of the posterior tibial tendon. Arch Surg 66:512, 1953

80. Williams R: Chronic non-specific tendovaginitis of tibialis posterior. J Bone Joint Surg 45B:542, 1963

81. Parvin RW, Ford LT: Stenosing tenosynovitis of the common peroneal tendon sheath. J Bone Joint Surg 38A:1352, 1956

82. Burman M: Stenosing tendovaginitis of the foot and ankle. Arch Surg 67:686, 1953

83. Webster FS: Peroneal tenosynovitis with pseudotumor. J Bone Joint Surg 50A:153, 1968

84. Lapidus PW, Seidenstein H: Chronic nonspecific tenosynovitis with effusion about the ankle. J Bone Joint Surg 32A:175, 1950

85. Gilula LA, Oloff L, Caputi R et al: Ankle tenography: a key to unexplained symptomatology. Radiology 151:581, 1984

86. Trevino S, Gould N, Korson R: Surgical treatment of stenosing tenosynovitis at the ankle. Foot Ankle 2:37, 1981

87. Hamilton WG: Foot and ankle injuries in dancers. Clin Sports Med 7:133, 1988

88. Boyes JH: Wounds, burns and amputations. In Boyes JH (ed): Bunnell's Surgery of the Hand. 5th Ed. JB Lippincott, Philadelphia, 1970

13

Management of Achilles Tendon Trauma

John M. Schuberth, D.P.M.

Injuries to the Achilles tendon complex occur frequently and are often the cause of prolonged disability and morbidity. The vast majority of these injuries involve a disruption of the continuity of the tendon elements. Therefore, this chapter focuses on that entity.

ANATOMY

Before one can adequately assess and treat injuries to the Achilles tendon, a thorough understanding of the anatomy is essential. The Achilles tendon complex is composed of three distinct muscles collectively known as the triceps surae.

Gastrocnemius

The gastrocnemius is the largest of the triceps surae. It originates by two heads, medial and lateral, from the respective posterior aspects of the femoral condyles. Fibers also arise from the aponeurosis on the posterior aspect of the muscle. As the fibers course distally, they form an aponeurosis of insertion on the anterior aspect of the muscle. This aponeurosis of insertion courses distally and forms a tendon that unites with a portion of the soleus tendon to form the Achilles tendon (Fig. 13-1). The gastrocnemius like the plantaris is a triarticular muscle in that it crosses the knee, ankle, and subtalar joints. The position of each of

these articulations will have a profound influence on the tension placed across the muscle-tendon unit.

Soleus

The soleus originates from the posterior aspect of the tibia and fibula. There is also a tendinous arch between the tibia and fibula from which fibers arise posteriorly. Fibers unite inferiorly to form an aponeurosis of insertion that courses distally to form the tendon, which converges with the gastrocnemius tendon to form the Achilles tendon (Fig. 13-2). The tension on the muscle-tendon unit of the soleus is only influenced by the articulations of the subtalar and ankle joints.

Plantaris

The plantaris is a small muscle that originates primarily from the lateral condyle of the femur. The muscle, which is 7 to 10 cm long, forms a long thin tendon that passes obliquely between the gastrocnemius and soleus to the medial side of the Achilles tendon. It inserts directly into the calcaneus. Its insertion can vary greatly in both location and morphology. An indeterminate percentage of the population does not exhibit a plantaris tendon. Both anatomic and intraoperative surveys report the presence of a plantaris tendon 91.8 to 93.8 percent of the time.[1–3] Recently, how-

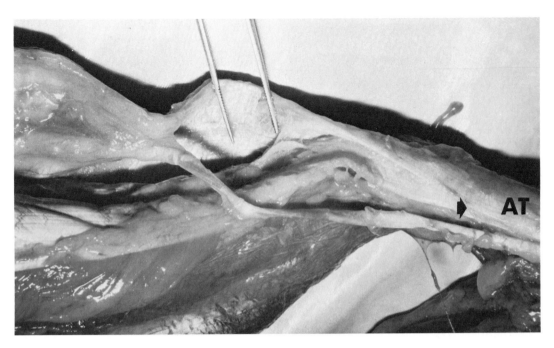

Fig. 13-1. Cadaver specimen of gastrocnemius-soleus complex. The forceps indicate the gastrocnemius contribution to the Achilles tendon (AT). Arrow indicates the point of confluence.

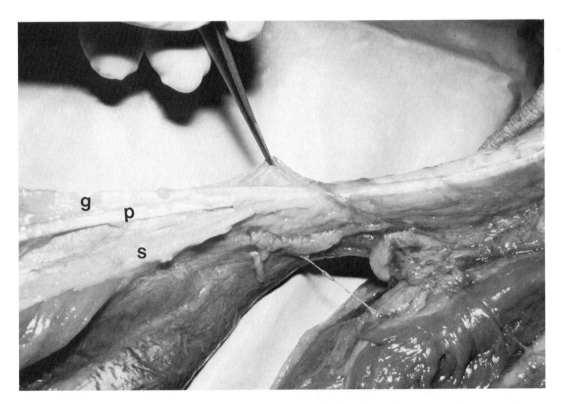

Fig. 13-2. Cadaver specimen of gastrocnemius-soleus complex. The plantaris (p) is shown here between the gastrocnemius (g) and soleus (s) aponeuroses. The forceps holds the paratenon encompassing the entire complex.

ever, Incavo and associates reported the presence of a plantaris tendon in only 40 percent of 40 cases of achilles tendon ruptures.[4] My experience with over 150 open repairs fails to confirm this low incidence of occurrence. Review of the 50 most recent operations in which the plantaris was specifically sought demonstrated a distinct plantaris tendon in 47 cases.

Achilles Tendon

The Achilles tendon itself courses distally to insert into the central one-third of the posterior surface of the calcaneus. It articulates with the smooth superior one-third of the posterior calcaneus when the foot is dorsiflexed at the ankle. There is usually a retrocalcaneal bursa between the tendon and the calcaneus.

Careful inspection of the Achilles insertion will show that the tendon is intimately associated with the plantar fascia as the fascia inserts inferiorly on the tuber of the calcaneus. In fact, some of the fibers of the Achilles tendon are continuous with the plantar fascia as it courses distally. This association allows the plantar fascia and Achilles tendon to function as a unit.

The question of whether or not the fibers of the Achilles tendon twist in the long axis as they proceed distally is controversial. The literature tends to support the existence of such a longitudinal torque.[5,6] Fortunately, in the situation of trauma, this phenomenon is irrelevant. I believe that there is no torque of the tendon fibers.

Anomalous Muscles

Anomalous muscles occur with some frequency in the posterior aspect of the leg. These are well discussed in standard anatomic textbooks.[7,8] The accessory soleus arises from the anterior surface of the normal soleus with is fibers coursing distally.[9,10] The insertion merges with

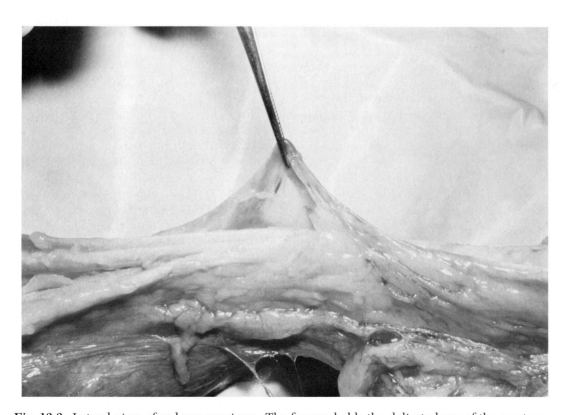

Fig. 13-3. Lateral view of cadaver specimen. The forceps holds the delicate layer of the paratenon.

the normal Achilles tendon or inserts in one of several ways directly into the calcaneus, anterior to the usual tendon.[11] The accessory soleus is a relatively frequent finding in patients with posterior leg pain. It is frequently mistaken for tumor and often biopsies are done.[12] Histologic studies of these and other anomalous muscles are universally normal.

The flexor accessorius longus is found in approximately 12 percent of the population[13] in the posteromedial aspect of the ankle. It exhibits a great deal of variation.[13] It usually originates in the lower leg structures, but deep or anterior to the deep crural fascia, thus not traversing through the superficial posterior compartment. Whether these anomalies affect the vulnerability of the Achilles complex to injury has not been determined. However, the practitioner should be cognizant of their presence to avoid confusion if they are encountered in the traumatic setting.

Peritendinous Structures

The peritendinous structures, comprising the paratenon and the paratendinous structures, are important relative to injuries in this area. The Achilles tendon does not possess a true synovial sheath, but is encased in a triple layer of tissue. The most superficial layer and the most durable is synonymous with the deep fascia. It is the posterior boundary of the superficial posterior compartment. The next layer is the mesotenon, which is typified by its rich red color. This is the major source of blood supply to the central portion of the Achilles tendon. The third or deepest layer is thin filmy tissue that is quite delicate (Fig. 13-3). However, it can always be isolated from the most superficial layer of the tendon itself, the epitenon.

Blood Supply

The blood supply to the Achilles tendon comes principally from three sources. The muscular and myotendinous junctional branches supply the proximal portion of the tendon. Nutrient branches emanate directly from muscle and nourish the proximal aspect of the tendon and the distal aspect of the gastrocnemius aponeurosis.[14]

The tendon-bone junction supplies the distal aspect or insertion of the Achilles tendon. Here anastomotic branches form between the periosteal vessels and the tendon vessels. There are also a few branches that pierce the cortical bone of the calcaneus and pass directly into the center of the tendon.

The mesotenon or the central layer of the paratendinous structures provides the major blood supply to the bulk of the Achilles tendon. The vessels enter the tendon segmentally through the fine connections of the deepest paratendinous layer. They come off radially and enter the tendon perpendicular to the long axis and then course both distally and proximally. There are few of these radially arranged vessels along the posterior aspects and many along the anterior aspect of the tendon. This is because of the presence of friction supplied by the overlying structures and externally applied forces and the relative lack of friction mediated by the largely adipose posterior triangle tissues.

Sural Nerve

The sural nerve is formed by contributions from the medial sural cutaneous nerve branch of the tibial nerve and from the peroneal anastomotic branch of the lateral sural cutaneous branch of the common peroneal nerve. It runs along the lesser saphenous vein in the posterior midline of the leg in the central third. They then course laterally as they descend distally. They are located in the subcutaneous layer superficial to the superficial posterior compartment. In the lower third of the leg, they are lateral to the Achilles tendon (Fig. 13-4). The sural nerve is purely a sensory nerve and supplies the skin on the posterior and lateral aspect of the leg. Distal to the ankle, it is the lateral dorsal cutaneous nerve and supplies the skin on that edorsolateral aspect of the foot. Occasionally, it can supply skin plantar to the fifth ray, increasing the significance if it becomes lacerated.

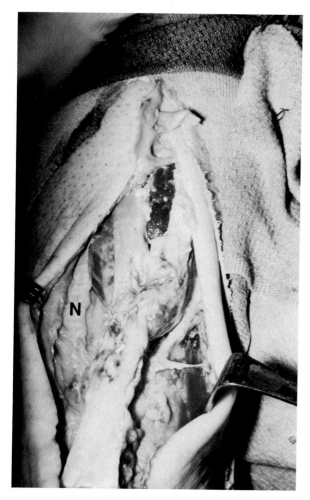

Fig. 13-4. Intraoperative photograph of Achilles tendon repair. Note the large sural nerve (N) in the subcutaneous layer lying lateral to the tendon.

ETIOLOGY

The precise etiology of Achilles tendon ruptures has been debated in the literature since the first report of this injury by Ambroise Paré over 400 years ago. The fundamental question is whether there is some predisposing factor(s) within the tendon itself that intrinsically weakens it.

The literature is biased toward the theory that there is almost always some degenerative pro-

cess at the site of rupture. Cronkite,[15] McMasters,[16] Ralston and Schmidt,[17] and Arey[18] have all demonstrated the enormous tensile strength of normal tendon. DiStefano and Nixon have stated that during normal fast running the forces across the Achilles tendon exceed 900 kg.[19] It can be theorized that when the Achilles tendon is histologically normal, then it is not the weak link in the system and failure would rather occur at the muscle, myotendinous junction, tendo-osseous junction, or bone. Therefore, the forces necessary to rupture a healthy tendon cannot be generated by normal human movement and function. Davidsson and Salo have demonstrated that examination of the excised tissue procured during primary repair showed that there were pathologic changes that could not be accounted for by the rupture alone.[20] Degeneration and necrobiotic changes as well as inflammatory and reparative processes were found. Since all of the specimens were obtained the same day of the rupture and since there were histologic changes representative of the various stages of tendon healing, they postulated that these changes were the cumulative result of repeated microtrauma and the respective reparative processes. Specimens obtained during surgical treatment for chronic Achilles tendonitis have confirmed a degenerative process in the tendon substance.[21,22] Although these patients had not yet sustained complete disruptions, it is believed that the chronic inflammatory condition incites the microtraumatic and reparative processes responsible for these changes. The histologic changes observed in both groups of patients were virtually identical (Fig. 13-5).

The area of rupture is usually at the area of poorest blood supply. Arner and Lindholm found that this is the area of tendon 2 to 6 cm proximal to the calcaneal insertion.[23] This corresponds exactly to the anatomic studies of Lagergren and Lindholm.[24] Here microangiographic studies indicated that the area of poorest blood supply was indeed the area 2 to 6 cm proximal to the calcaneal insertion. The consequence of regional ischemia may be the local necrobiotic process. In addition, as the tendon is subjected to microtrauma, the undernourished segment may be

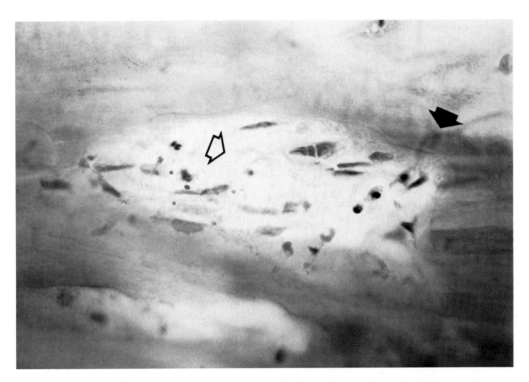

Fig. 13-5. Histologic section of a ruptured Achilles tendon. Note the osseous metaplasia (arrow) with central degeneration (open arrow).

more susceptible to injury, thereby enhancing the entire cycle.

Ruptures at the tendo-osseous and myotendinous junctions occur much less frequently. This can be linked to better blood supply in these areas.

Age has also been linked to the pathogenesis of rupture. Vascularity of the Achilles complex has been shown to decrease with increasing age.[25] This is corroborrated by excellent correlation of increased incidence of rupture with advancing age.

Intralesional steroids have been implicated in the pathogenesis of Achilles rupture.[26–29] Balasubramaniam and colleagues have described a direct effect of steroid on the tendon fibers.[30,31] This effect was essentially a weakening of the fibers secondary to loss of organized structure and the decrease of periodic banding. The collagen ultimately became a structureless mass. Bloom and Fawcett contend that cortisone lowers the protein polysaccharide content of

ground substance.[32] It is these same ground substance constituents that diminish friction and wear between collagen fibrils. This lends further support to the theory of the attenuated tendon.

Phelps et al.[33] and Mackie et al.[34] countered this by showing that no deleterious effects occurred when steroids were injected into healthy tendons. Perhaps the effects of steroids are more pronounced on the Achilles tendon because of the lack of a true synovial sheath. The production of synovial fluid may act as a continuous diluent in a true synovial sheath, thereby diminishing the deleterious effects of steroids. Certainly the solubility of the various injected clinical preparations will also affect the local concentration.

The presence of some systemic diseases has been shown to predispose individuals to spontaneous rupture of the Achilles tendon. There are reports of patients sustaining tendon ruptures with gout,[35] hyperparathyroidism[36,37] systemic lupus erythematosis (SLE),[38–40] ochronosis,[41] syphilis,[42] and tuberculosis.[42,43] Although spontaneous tendon rupture in patients with rheumatoid arthritis is common, it is unlikely to see a spontaneous Achilles rupture in these patients. This is because the paratenon is not true synovial sheath, the target tissue of rheumatoid arthritis. However, patients with rheumatoid arthritis or any other collagen vascular disease are treated with oral steroids, the incidence of Achilles rupture rises precipitously.[44,45] Whether or not systemic steroids in these patients have their deleterious effect through the healing response to the already altered tendon or through some collagenolytic activity is relevant only when treatment is concerned. However, the presence of concomitant collagen-type disease and oral corticosteroid use is not a prerequisite for tendon rupture. I have observed several steroid-dependent asthmatics who have sustained spontaneous tendon ruptures.

Ossification and calcification have been implicated as causes of spontaneous rupture.[46,47] Whether the ossification is the cause or just an exuberant response to the reparative process of the unhealthy collagen is debatable. Metaplastic bone formation in tendon is uncommon, and yet the presence of the same does not necessarily produce symptoms. Its main implication is in treatment.

MECHANISMS OF INJURY

There are a variety of mechanisms that result in disruptions to the continuity of the Achilles tendon complex. These are divided into two distinct groups: direct and indirect trauma. The overwhelming majority of Achilles tendon injuries are the result of indirect trauma.

Indirect Trauma

The common denominator of ruptures of the Achilles tendon is a force across the tendon fibers that exceeds the tensile strength of the tendon. This force may be applied to a tendon that is histologically normal or, as is usually the case, a tendon that has become attenuated for a variety

of reasons. There is usually some physiologic pertubation. Therefore, it is common to see a ruptured tendon in the face of a seemingly minor traumatic event.

The force required to exceed the tensile strength of the tendon can be generated by either forceful distraction of the tendon elements of forceful contraction of the triceps surae. Most indirect ruptures probably result from a combination of the two mechanisms. Distraction occurs either when the knee is extended with the ankle and foot fixed or when the foot is forcibly dorsiflexed at the ankle while the knee is locked in extension. Again, combinations of these mechanisms may occur, resulting in an accumulation of forces. It is no accident that the two tendons ruptured most in the body, the patellar and Achilles tendons, both cross two major joints. This reinforces the concept that force synergism may play the important role in the generation of sufficient energy for rupture. The position of the subtalar joint will also affect tension of the Achilles tendon. When the subtalar joint is pronated, it creates a relative laxity in the Achilles tendon, whereas in the supinated position the tendon is relatively taut. The position of the midtarsal joint can also influence the tension across the Achilles tendon at any given moment. If this joint is not loaded through the forefoot, then the stabilizing action of the plantar fascia on the calcaneus cannot be realized and again a relative laxity of the Achilles tendon is observed. The exact position of each of these joints is important at the exact moment of maximal tension across the Achilles tendon.

The most common mechanism for disruption in the indirect manner usually involves athletic events. For example, eccentric contraction of the tendon results when the victim's heel is anchored to the ground by another athlete. This usually occurs while the patient is running forward.

Acute contraction of the triceps surae can also generate sufficient force to cause a rupture. The same biomechanical considerations relative to joint position also apply here. Active contraction can be mediated volitionally or reflexively.

Stretching injuries during racquetball or tennis are infrequent causes of Achilles tears. Jumping maneuvers are infrequently implicated because usually the jump is a conscious rather than an unexpected event. Falls from a height are unusual causes of Achilles injuries because the nature of most falls make a dorsiflexion moment at the ankle with a fully extended knee an unlikely event. Unless the knee is almost fully extended, it is unlikely that enough tension across the tendon elements would be realized to cause failure.

During the actual rupturing process, the posterior fibers are the first to fail because these fibers sustain the most stretch for any given position of the ankle joint. The lever arm of the calcaneus is the longest at the most posterior aspect and therefore the tension here is the highest. This notion is confirmed by multiple intraoperative observations that the anterior fibers are frequently not completely disrupted but attenuated and stretched to varying degrees (Fig. 13-6). In addition, it is not uncommon to find an intact plantaris tendon in the patient with a spontaneous tear. This is also because the plantaris inserts at the anterior aspect of the Achilles tendon insertion, which affords it too a shorter lever arm and the resultant lesser tension.

Direct Trauma

Direct trauma to the Achilles tendon is the result of sharp or blunt objects coming into contact with the posterior aspect of the leg. Direct blunt trauma is a rare cause of Achilles disruption. If this is thought to play a role in the injury, the wary clinician should suspect an indirect mechanism, but realize that considerably more soft tissue damage may have ensued. Appropriate precautions should then be taken. Viability of the skin should be of major concern, and watchful waiting is indicated before any aggressive therapy or constrictive bandages are applied. As with all crush injuries, the initial damage appears to be of much less magnitude than has actually occurred.

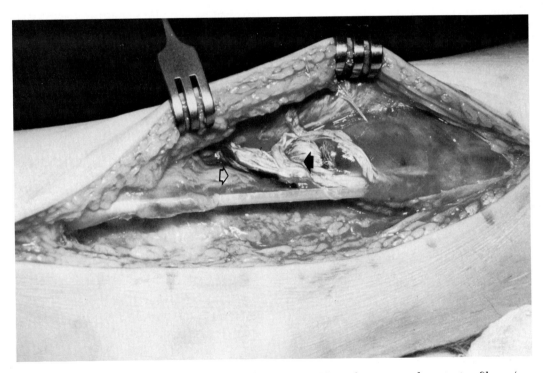

Fig. 13-6. Intraoperative view of Achilles tendon rupture. Note the ruptured posterior fibers (arrow) and the intact but attenuated anterior fibers (open arrow). The plantaris tendon is also intact.

Lacerations of the Achilles tendon complex are uncommon but not rare. When they do occur it is almost always the result of a broken plate of glass that has fallen on the patient or the patient somehow placing the leg tangentially along the edge of glass. The mechanism can usually be determined by the pattern of the skin laceration. If the skin flap is based superiorly, the latter mechanism has probably occurred. If the skin flap is based inferiorly, the sharp object has usually fallen from above (Fig. 13-7). Complete disruptions are rare because the density of the tissue of the posterior aspect of the leg prevents complete laceration.

Gunshot wounds are also infrequent causes of Achilles tendon disruptions. These are discussed in Chapter 10.

HISTORY AND PHYSICAL FINDINGS

The history of patients sustaining spontaneous Achilles tendon ruptures is fairly typical. There is usually an association with some seemingly trivial event that places stress on the Achilles tendon complex. The patient often relates a feeling of being "clubbed in the back of the leg" or "shot in the calf," with surprisingly little pain at the exact moment of failure.[42,48] There is usually an audible pop or snap heard by the patient that can take on various pitches. Less frequently, with the slower eccentric type of mechanisms, the patient relates a feeling of a searing, burning pain experienced during the traumatic event.

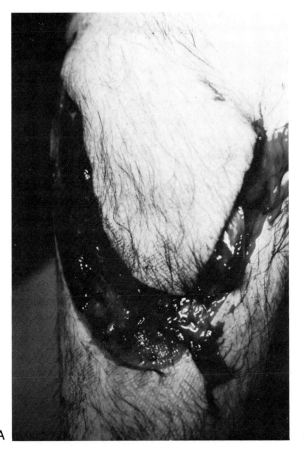
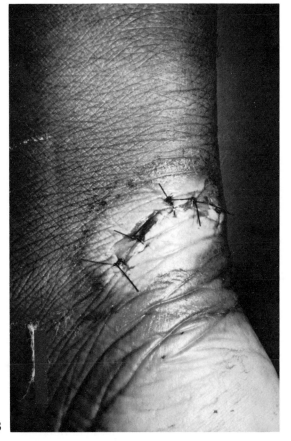

A   B

Fig. 13-7. (A) Photograph of patient with superior based skin flap created by gastrocnemius laceration. (B) Photograph of another patient with inferiorly based skin flap from Achilles tendon laceration.

In the majority of cases, the history alone is sufficient to make the diagnosis because it is such a common feature. Often there is so little post-injury pain that the patient will be able to finish the sporting event, although there is usually some persistent subjective weakness. The prolongation of weakness often prompts the patient to seek medical attention.

Prodromal symptoms in the involved tendon are usually not elicited. The vast majority of patients will deny any history of symptoms of Achilles tendinitis or Achilles tendon pain even when specifically prompted. Other investigators have related that some preinjury diathesis was present.[49] Most of the patients with pre-existing symptoms were athletically inclined.[22,50–52]

The literature has described the typical patient who suffers an Achilles tendon rupture as a male between the ages of 30 and 40 years who only occasionally engages in strenuous activity.[48] In the past 5 years, I have treated over 150 patients, and in this group, most of the patients were self-described athletes. The activities during which the injury was sustained were rarely of different intensity than the patient was usually accustomed to on a routine basis.

Physical findings are quite consistent. In the acute setting, there is usually swelling that is concentrated around the posterior ankle but can often extend bimalleolarly. Ecchymosis is usually present in the same distribution, but its absence should not be misleading. The clinician should not be fooled by the patient who presents with a complaint of a weak ankle, especially if an insufficient history was elicited. The pattern of ecchymosis and edema may so resemble that of an acute ankle sprain or fracture that palpation of the Achilles tendon is omitted.

A palpable gap along the course of the triceps surae complex is a highly reliable diagnostic finding. In the acute setting, despite the presence of edema, this deficit can almost always be identified. However, it is not always possible to determine the exact percentage of the loss of continuity of the tendon substance. If the rupture is old or neglected and sufficient time has elapsed for defect fill, then the palpable gap may be subtle if present at all.[53]

When the patient is observed in the prone position with the feet and ankles free over the end of the examining table, the injured extremity will exhibit less ankle equinus than the uninjured leg. This is due to the lack of physiologic tension usually mediated by the triceps surae.

The most reliable clinical diagnostic test for an acute rupture of the Achilles tendon is the Thompson test.[54] With the patient in the prone position, the examiner squeezes the calf muscle just distal to its maximal girth. A reciprocal plantar flexion of the foot at the ankle is indicative of at least some integrity of the Achilles tendon at a physiologic tension. This is defined as a negative Thompson test or normal response. A lack of reciprocal plantar flexion with this maneuver is diagnostic of the loss of integrity of the Achilles tendon and is defined as a positive Thompson test. False-negatives can be observed with the patient who has a partial tear of the tendon or in the patient with accessory muscles in the leg that can reciprocate lateral compression of the calf with plantar flexion.[9–13,55] It is extremely rare to have a false-positive test, and in fact this has not been reliably reported. Extremely tense patients may exhibit a positive test owing to voluntary splinting, but the lack of other physical findings usually steers the practitioner away from the diagnosis. Other false-positives may be obtained if the patient is not in the prone position with the foot free of support. Careful adherence to proper technique will minimize erroneous results.

Diagnosis should not be based on the ability of the patient to plantar flex the foot.[53,56] The posterior and lateral muscle groups are quite capable of plantar flexion of the foot in an open kinetic chain situation and can mask the insufficiency of the Achilles tendon. In some patients, these muscles are developed to the point that the patient may be able to rise on the toes. However, this test is clearly not recommended because it may accentuate the amount of rupture and cause further damage.

Deliberate examination of the patient's gait is also not recommended for the same reasons. However, observations of patients with complete ruptures or old neglected ruptures show a gait pattern consistent with marked flexor substitution, particularly of the posterior tibial tendon. There is exaggeration of dorsiflexion in stance with a marked supinatory moment about the subtalar joint during push-off. Push-off is typically weak. An increase in knee flexion during stance is also observed. Difficulty in negotiation of stairs can be observed or reported by the patient.

DIAGNOSTIC AIDS

Although the diagnosis of an acute Achilles tendon rupture is usually made on the basis of history and physical alone, imaging modalities can often supply additional information. The questionable or delayed rupture may be confirmed or denied on the basis of this information when physical findings are obscure, and the exact nature of the injury may be ascertained.

Conventional Radiographs

Radiographs are usually taken to rule out other pathologic conditions rather than to confirm a rupture. Radiographs are indicated in certain instances. When the rupture appears to occur distally, it is important to ascertain whether there are any bony injuries to the calcaneus. Avulsion fractures at the calcaneal insertion are rare and have a different treatment scheme. Films are also indicated whenever there is suspicion of calcific changes or there is a history of repository steroid injection into the tendon sheath (Fig. 13-8).

The acute Achilles tendon rupture has unique radiographic findings. On the normal lateral projection, a border is formed by the shadows of the anterior aspect of the Achilles tendon, the deep posterior muscles, and the superior surface of the calcaneus. This is referred to as Kager's triangle (Fig. 13-9). When the Achilles tendon is ruptured, there is blunting of the superior angle owing to proximal retraction of the Achilles tendon. Adjunctively there may be some soft tissue swelling in this triangular area.

Xerography

Xerography can confirm the diagnosis or delineate pathology owing to its excellent imaging of soft tissue. However, because of its limited availability and replacement with more versatile modalities, its use is becoming obsolete.

Ultrasound

Ultrasound is a noninvasive, nonradiating imaging technique that is useful in the diagnosis and treatment of injuries to the Achilles tendon complex. It is particularly useful in determining incomplete rupture and in assessing the required amount of equinus in closed treatment. It should be used routinely when there is any question as to the amount of disruption of the tendon. If, however, this information is not going to dissuade the examiner from closed treatment, then the test may be forgone. Sagittal plane scanning in real time is more useful than transverse plane scanning (Fig. 13-10).

If the rupture is complete and the patient is going to be treated nonoperatively, then ultrasound is recommended to assess the adequacy of approximation of the tendon ends.[57] The foot is passively manipulated in the sagittal plane to visualize the exact moment of approximation of tendon ends. The angle of ankle plantar flexion is measured, and the initial cast is set at that position. This maneuver will be described in detail below.

False-negatives for ruptures can occur when there is a large hematoma in the void created by the separation. Although tendon and hematoma have different echogenicities, they can be confusing to the experienced and nonexperienced ultrasonographer alike. It is also difficult to obtain an accurate estimation of tendon end approximation in the face of hematoma. The longer the hematoma has had a chance to organize, the greater the chance for a false-negative result. Ultrasound is not very useful in the old neglected rupture as the void is likely to be filled with scar tissue with a similar echogenicity as normal tendon. However, the contour of the tissue filling the void may be determined.

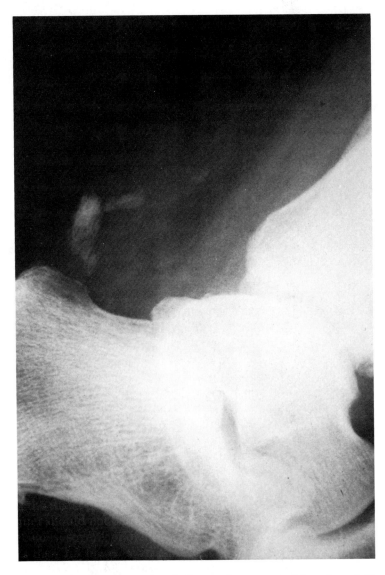

Fig. 13-8. Lateral radiograph of patient with Achilles tendon rupture. Note the calcific deposits secondary to steroid injections.

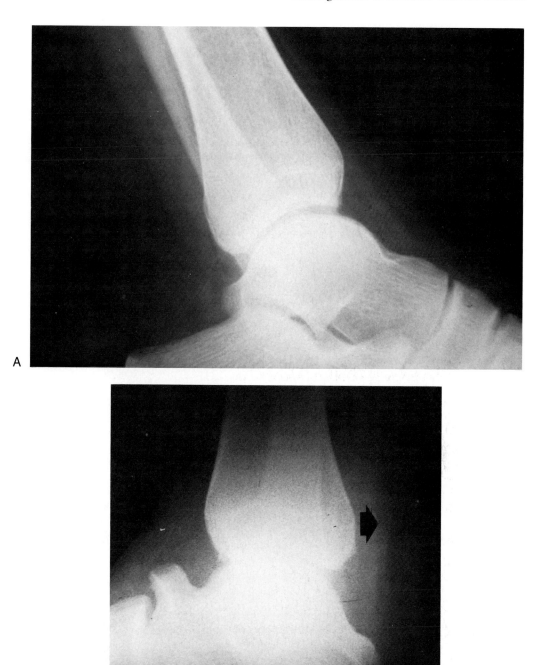

Fig. 13-9. (**A**) Lateral radiograph in a patient who did not sustain an Achilles tendon rupture. Note the sharp definition of the superior aspect of Kager's triangle. (**B**) Lateral radiograph of a patient sustaining an Achilles tendon rupture. There is loss of definition of the superior angle of Kager's triangle (arrow).

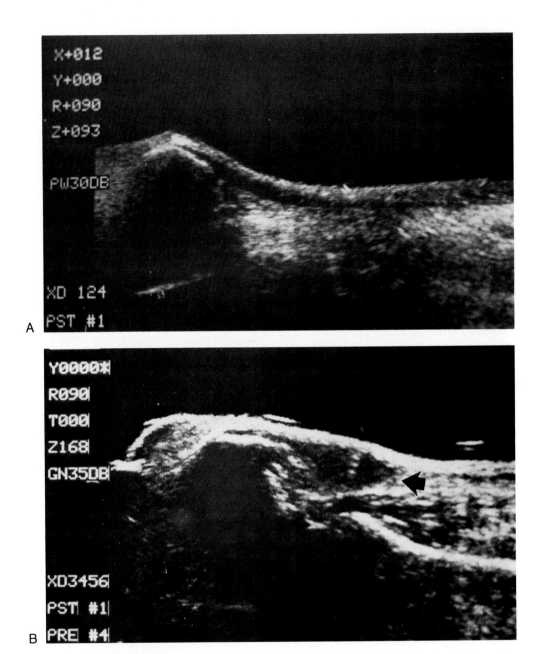

Fig. 13-10. (A) Sagittal plane ultrasonograph of normal Achilles tendon. (B) Sagittal plane ultrasonograph of patient with an Achilles tendon rupture. There is a large void (arrow) created by the proximal retraction of the tendon.

TREATMENT OF ACUTE RUPTURES

There are several factors that determine the best form of treatment for each patient. Generally patients fit into the conservative or surgical treatment category based primarily on age and activity level. However, the literature abounds with papers touting both sides of the argument regardless of the patient's age or functional level.[58–64] There is not much controversy when dealing with older sedentary individuals.

Although there is no absolute age cutoff before excluding a patient from consideration of surgical repair, a good general guideline is 50 years old. Unless one is dealing with an extremely athletic individual, then surgical repair is better forgotten. Conservative management will give satisfactory results without the altered risk of surgical or anesthetic complications. In the athletic or younger patient, primary surgical repair should be offered. The immobilization period is somewhat shorter than with the conservative scheme with all other factors being equal.

The most significant and frequent complication regardless of the form of treatment is rerupture. Tensile forces are likely to exceed the tensile strength of the tendon if the damaged tendon has healed with residual equinus.[65] Therefore, every effort should be made to minimize the equinus condition regardless of the treatment chosen.

There are two popular philosophies relative to the conservative treatment of acute Achilles tendon tears. The basic difference between the two is the use of a long leg cast. Lea and Smith have popularized the method of a below-the-knee walking cast with the foot in gravity equinus for 8 weeks.[66,67] No interim manipulation was advocated. Their rerupture rate was relatively low.

Patients who cannot tolerate an above-the-knee cast or crutch ambulation should be offered conservative treatment in a similar manner. These patients are usually the elderly and those with steroid-dependent pulmonary or rheumatic disease. Fiber glass-type casting material should be used to ensure immediate ambulation with minimal additional effort.

For these patients an ultrasound examination is done first to determine the exact amount of equinus to ensure tendon end apposition. The patient's leg is then casted in that position. This may necessitate forced equinus, but extreme forced equinus is poorly tolerated and should be avoided. This position is maintained for 4 weeks, at which time the cast is changed and the equinus gradually reduced. The patient returns at 2-week intervals with gradual reduction of the equinus at each visit. The casting must be supervised, and the reduction of the equinus is predicated on the ability to palpate continuity of the tendon along its course. The amount of reduction is determined by the ability to dorsiflex to resistance. Care must be taken, particularly in early episodes, not to disrupt the healing process with overzealous dorsiflexory force. This process is continued at 2-week intervals until the foot is at neutral dorsiflexion. After the patient has spent 2 weeks at neutral dorsiflexion in a non-weight-bearing cast, the cast is converted to a walking cast and left on for an additional 2 weeks. The minimum total casting time is usually 12 weeks. However, small deviations from this are usually well tolerated. The clinician should be aware of the total amount of ankle joint dorsiflexion of the opposite uninjured side. It is important not to be satisfied with attainment of dorsiflexion of the injured side equal to that of the opposite side if there is any pre-existing equinus. This can predispose to rerupture if the injured tendon heals in the equinus attitude. Because immature collagen has the best potential for remodeling, the clinician should reduce equinus during this opportune period. Occasionally, some residual equinus occurs. The patient should be apprised of this and the appropriate precautions taken.

The goal of this technique in this group of patients is a plantigrade foot with an intact Achilles tendon. Strength and power are usually compromised, but this is seldom clinically significant owing to the decreased functional demands of these patients.

In the young athletic patient who is treated conservatively, the casting regimen is modified. Ultrasonic examination is again done. However, the amount of ankle equinus that results in tendon end approximation is determined with the knee flexed 25 to 30 degrees. This will usually allow the foot to be positioned in 5 more degrees of dorsiflexion that would occur if the knee were fully extended. The patient is then placed in an above knee cast with the knee and ankle positioned as described above. The initial cast is left in place for 4 weeks. The cast is then changed with the equinus at the ankle reduced using the above guidelines. Two weeks later (6 weeks total time), the cast is converted to a non-weight-bearing short leg cast, again with ankle equinus manipulation. When ankle neutrality is obtained and maintained for 2 weeks, the patient is allowed to bear weight in a short leg cast. The cast is removed after a 2-week period of weight bearing at neutral position.

Again, the range of motion of the opposite side ankle should not discourage the clinician from achieving more in terms of dorsiflexion. The goal again is an intact Achilles tendon that will not rerupture under the same stresses and strains. The reduction of equinus is paramount in deceasing the chance of rerupture. Strength and power are initially compromised, but will be regained with an aggressive physical therapy program (described below). The disadvantages of not bearing weight in terms of patient convenience are overshadowed by the attainment of a predictable result. The release of the gastrocnemius in the initial period by knee flexion allows for the commencement of casting with much less equinus. The precise apposition of tendon fibers is important to avoid bridging of the gap with nontendinous tissue, which does not have the same consistency as normal tendon.[68] In the weight-bearing regimen, active contraction of the gastrocnemius is expected and will result in proximal retraction of the proximal stump, thereby diminishing the quality of the repair. This possibility is avoided with the non-weight-bearing treatment. The initial long leg cast allows earlier mobilization of the ankle because the precise approximation of tendon ends allows them to become mutually adhesed. If there is the proximal retraction of tendon ends, then the tendon ends will take longer to become sticky enough to tolerate mobilization.

Surgery

Surgical treatment of an acute rupture should be reserved for those patients who are very athletic and aspire to return to their previous level of activity. Patients who are poorly motivated are poor candidates for surgery.

In the literature, the principal reason for disfavoring surgery is the difficulty in achieving a satisfactory repair in the face of the ragged appearance of the tendon ends. It has been likened to "nailing a custard pie to the wall." Evolvement of techniques over the last 5 years have led a physiologic and anatomic approach to primary repair.

The patient is placed in the prone position on the operating table with the feet just over the end of the table. Tourniquet control is optional but advised. The approach to the Achilles tendon is designed to minimize scar contracture. It must also be designed to allow for complete access to the plantaris tendon and the proximal structures if necessary. The incision is S-shaped and fashioned so that the central transverse limb is centered over the palpable defect or site of rupture. The distal limb is placed medially to allow for access to the plantaris tendon. The proximal limb parallels the posterior midline of the calf (Fig. 13-11). The transverse limb is slightly oblique to the transverse plane. This minimizes scar contracture of the skin along the direction of the tendon. The incision is deepened through the subcutaneous level without any underscoring whatsoever of the skin. Care should be exercised proximally not to injure the sural nerve and lesser saphenous vein, which lie in the posterior midline in the middle third of the leg.

The skin and subcutaneous tissues are reflected as a single layer off of the deep fascia. Most if not all of the subcutaneous tissue should be taken off of the deep fascia to ensure vascularity to the skin and prevent wound slough. The sural nerve and lesser saphenous bundle are reflected with the lateral skin flap if encountered. Only skin hooks or hand-held retractors are used throughout the procedure. Self-retaining retractors are inappropriate in this area.

The deep fascia and paratendinous tissues are

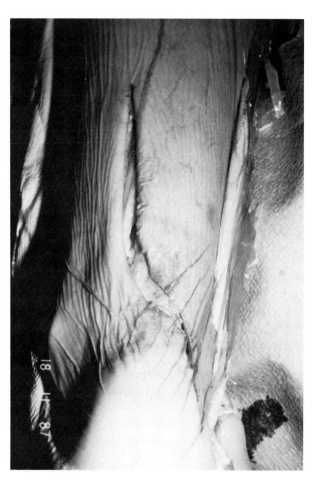

Fig. 13-11. Intraoperative photograph demonstrating approach to the ruptured Achilles tendon.

incised directly in the middle of the tendon itself. The incision should be made through all three layers. This includes the deep fascia, the mesotenon or vascular layer, and the thin filmy layer closest to the tendon. All three layers are dissected off of the Achilles tendon tissue. It is remarkable that the paratendinous layer is almost always intact despite injury to the tendon itself. The injured tendon is then in full view after evacuation of the usual hematoma.

At this point, the quality and extent of the damage are assessed. The posterior aspect of the tendon is invariably separated. The anterior aspect is often intact, but attenuated. The plantaris ten-

don should be located. It is usually within a separate fascial compartment within the confines of the paratendinous compartment. The foot is then plantar flexed to approximate the tendon ends. Any redundant strands of tendon should be debrided and discarded.

Two modified Kessler sutures are used to maintain the end-to-end approximation. This stitch has excellent holding power and interferes little with intrinsic tendon blood supply. Suture material is variable but should be nonabsorbable and of 0 caliber or greater. I utilize 0 braided nylon because of its strength and knot-holding ability. These sutures are placed to avoid central strangulation of the tendon elements (Fig. 13-12). The sutures are tied on the side to avoid interference with the gliding function of the tendon within the paratendinous sheath. The sutures are tightened to the point of approximation only. The amount of equinus should be minimized and compared with that of the opposite side. The repair is checked for strength by allowing the foot to suspend naturally off the end of the operating table.

Closure of the paratendinous structures is the most critical step in the repair of the Achilles tendon rupture because the mesotenon is a major source of blood supply to the tendon in the midsubstance. The healing potential of the repair is greatly enhanced by the integrity of the mesotenon blood supply. The integrity of the paratendinous structures also functionally isolates the tendon from the subcutaneous layer, thereby reducing the tendency for adhesions. If this layer was dissected with meticulous care, then its repair and restitution will not be difficult. Only occasionally will reapproximation be impossible. A fine-caliber absorbable suture with knots placed on the superficial side of the deep fascia will minimize the formation of adhesions. The subcutaneous layer is then closed with absorbable sutures. The skin is closed with nonabsorbable sutures with gentle handling of the skin.

Once the wound is dressed, the short leg portion of the long leg cast is applied while the patient is still in the prone position on the operating table. The ankle is casted with the foot in gravity equinus. Once the plaster has hardened, the pa-

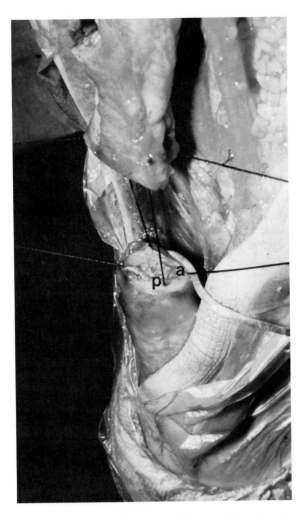

Fig. 13-12. Intraoperative photograph showing scheme of suture placement. Two Kessler stitches are placed. The first is in the anterior portion of the tendon (a). The second is in the posterior aspect of the tendon (p). Note that each suture is tied on the side.

tient is placed on the gurney in the supine position and the remainder of the long leg cast is applied. The knee is positioned at 25 degrees of flexion.

The first cast change is between 12 and 14 postoperative days. The wound is checked and the sutures are usually replaced with Steri-Strips. The cast is changed and the ankle equinus is reduced. The foot is dorsiflexed to resistance. The knee remains flexed at 25 degrees. This process is repeated 4 weeks postoperatively. At 6 postop-

erative weeks the cast is converted to a short leg cast without manipulation of the ankle. Two weeks later, the cast is changed again with manipulation of the equinus. I usually find that the foot is able to dorsiflex to a level of 90 degrees to the leg at this time. At 10 postoperative weeks the ankle is placed in neutral dorsiflexion and a short leg walking cast is applied. Three months after the time of surgery, the patient is taken out of immobilization and given 0.5-inch (1.25 cm) heel lifts bilaterally. These are reduced to 0.25-inch (0.6 cm) elevation 6 weeks later and worn for an additional 6 weeks. All elevation is discontinued 6 months postoperatively.

Dorsiflexion to 90 degrees may be impossible. It is permissible to permit weight bearing at the end-range motion provided that the cast is modified with a posterior elevation to prevent excessive stretch at the repair site.

The philosophy of periodic manipulation is predicated on the goal of graduated increase in physiologic tension across the repair site and optimal organization of collagen. It would be ideal to mobilize the adequately repaired tendon after a very short period of immobilization (3 weeks). However, patient compliance cannot be ensured and one misstep on the freshly repaired tendon is certain to result in reinjury. The increase in tension should be gradual to avoid ischemia and tension at the suture line. Even though it is certain that adhesions will form, as long as the tendon is mobilized at 2-week intervals they will be elongated. However, mobility does diminish the chance of "spot-weld" adhesions that might significantly inhibit gliding function.

When the patient who has sustained an acute rupture is initially examined, the amount of dorsiflexion of the uninjured extremity is assessed. If there is an exaggerated amount of gastrocnemius equinus, then an intraoperative lengthening procedure should be considered to minimize the change of rerupture.[65] The equinus should be minimized to reduce the development of excessive tension across the healed tendon in the future. This is impossible when the repaired tendon has healed in marked equinus.

In the acute setting, the gastrocnemius recession is preferred because it is (1) a local procedure, (2) it results in end-to-end approximation of analogous tissue, and (3) it does not disrupt the primary blood supply of the tissue being mobilized. The tongue-and-groove recession of Fulp and McGlamry is utilized most frequently.[69] However, any of the other gastrocnemius tendon recessions can be used.[70–72] All of these techniques are designed to mobilize the proximal portion of the tendon and the gastrocnemius aponeurosis distally to reduce the gap created by placing the foot in the desired position of dorsiflexion. This position ideally should be one of less plantar flexion than the opposite side. Attachments of the underlying soleus muscle belly should be as undisturbed as possible to maintain an adequate blood supply to the repair site. Only when translocation is difficult should additional dissection be performed. Postoperative management is the same as for the uncomplicated primary repair.

TREATMENT OF NEGLECTED RUPTURES

Old or neglected ruptures of the Achilles tendon present a different challenge to the treating physician. Despite sophisticated diagnostic techniques that are available today, there are still patients in whom either the original diagnosis was missed or who never sought acute medical care. Ambulation in these patients is usually resumed after the acute discomfort dissipates. This results in elongation of the gap and atrophy of the tendon ends. If left alone for a long enough period, the resultant gap in the tendon will fill in with fibrovascular tissue that is poorly organized and of poor tensile strength. More importantly, the length–tension relationship of the gastrocnemius-soleus complex is altered.

When these patients finally present for treatment, the options are more limited. Neglected ruptures must be approached for different reasons. (1) The tendon ends may be hypertrophied because of fibroblastic proliferation. (2) Scar tissue will heal poorly compared with acute ruptures. (3) Shredded friable ends of tendon may become enmeshed in scar tissue or degenerate. (4) Retraction of the tendon ends will be accentu-

ated by ambulation. (5) The resultant gap may fill in with fibrovascular tissue that is poorly organized and has poor tensile strength. For these reasons, end-to-end approximation of the ruptured tendon ends is difficult whether conservative or surgical treatment is utilized. The treatment goal, however, remains the same: restoration of tendon continuity with as normal as possible length–tension relationship.

Most researchers recommend surgical treatment if the repair is more than a few days old.[73–75] Only in the poorest surgical candidate should conservative treatment be entertained. One cannot achieve the stated goal without elimination of the pathologic tissues and the pathomechanics caused by the gap. Surgeons in the past have recognized these difficulties and have devised plastic surgical procedures to circumvent them. These techniques were directed toward providing a gliding action between the overlying skin envelope and bridging the deficit in tendon continuity. Christensen[76] and later Gebhardt[77] used a distally based flap of the gastrocnemius aponeurosis to reinforce the suture line of a primary end-to-end repair. Silfverskiold modified this technique by turning the flap 180 degrees at its attached base to improve gliding function.[78] Lindholm[79] and Kirschenbaum and Kelman[80] devised similar procedures by taking two smaller flaps and rotating them in the manner of Silfverskiold[78] and again using them to reinforce an end-to-end repair. These smaller flaps were used to avoid bulk at the site of rotation and diminish disruption of their blood supply.

All of these techniques are predicated on being able to use an end-to-end repair. With the neglected rupture, this is not always possible or even desirable because of poor quality of the tissues, a gap in tendon continuity, or both. This requires the fashioning of a graft from other tendon or fascial structures or performing a lengthening procedure to reposition appropriate tendinous tissue across the deficit.[81,82]

Gastrocnemius Recession

The preferred technique for gap reduction in the treatment of neglected ruptures is the gastrocnemius recession.[69] The basic preoperative preparation and surgical approach are identical to that of the acute primary repair. Once the paratendinous layer is entered, the typically sclerotic tendon ends must be trimmed to remove the edges of scar tissue (Fig. 13-13). The resultant gap is measured while the foot is held at a position equal to that of the opposite side.

A gastrocnemius recession is performed by elevating the gastrocnemius aponeurosis from the underlying soleus muscle belly. The medial and lateral thirds of the aponeurosis are grasped and transected at the proximal aspect of the structure. The central third is then transected at a more

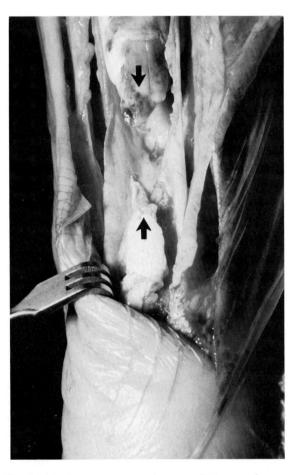

Fig. 13-13. Intraoperative photograph 1 year after neglected rupture of the Achilles tendon. Note the proximal and distal components with the sclerotic atrophic stumps (arrows).

distal level. The distance of separation between the proximal and distal cuts should be governed by the desired mobilization distance. In contradistinction to gastrocnemius recessions for tight triceps surae, the recession incisions must frequently be connected by sharp dissection instead of relying on a sliding function. This is because of the presence of scar tissue caused by the injury. It is helpful to encourage distal mobilization by placing the surgeon's index finger into the surgically created groove and pulling the proximal portion distally with manual pressure. This will negate the need to place clamps or other crushing instruments on the already compromised tendon.

When mobilization is sufficient for end-to-end approximation, the modified Kessler stitches are used to maintain apposition. Closure is in layers as in the acute repair. If there was a sufficient time lapse between injury and delayed repair, one may have difficulty with skin closure owing to reestablishment of the tension of the tendon. If this is the case, adequate relaxation of the tissues can be obtained with relaxing incisions[82] or Z-plasty (Fig. 13-14). The postoperative regimen is similar to that of the acute repair, keeping in mind that the tendon is likely to heal more slowly. Therefore, longer periods of immobilization may be required.

If conservative treatment is chosen, it is imperative to realize that the casting period is likely to be much longer at each respective stage. Ultrasound is indicated to assess the composition of tissue in the gap, if any. If there is a great deal of fibrous tissue in the gap, conservative treatment is deemed to failure. Ultrasound will also indicate the amount of equinus necessary for tendon apposition. It is not uncommon to have a resultant void even with forced maximal equinus. This poor approximation of tendinous tissue is expected to result in a larger portion of the healed tendon being composed of collagenous tissue with a microstructure different from normal tendon. Tendon resiliency will be affected.

Once the appropriate level of initial ankle equinus is determined, the patient is placed in a long leg cast with the knee at 25 degrees. The first cast period is extended to 4 weeks. Subse-

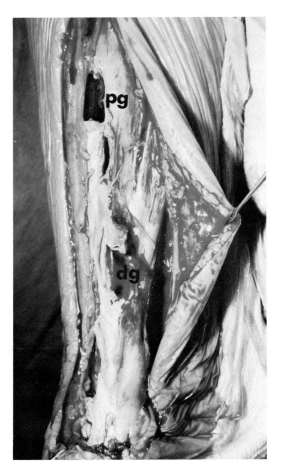

Fig. 13-14. Intraoperative specimen showing gastrocnemius recession. The resultant length is measured by the proximal gap (pg) or the distal groove (dg).

quent manipulative intervals are 3 weeks apart. The long leg cast is converted to a short leg cast when tendon continuity is ensured. This is usually 7 to 10 weeks after commencement of treatment. The short leg cast is changed and manipulated every 2 weeks according to the scheme for nonoperative fresh repairs.

In rare instances, the patient with a neglected rupture may be treated with benign neglect. Many patients have surprising plantar flexing power even after many months without treatment. Elderly patients and those with appreciable fibrous tissue in the rupture site are the usual recipients of this form of treatment.

RERUPTURES

Most patients who sustain reruptures of the Achilles tendon do so shortly after the cessation of immobilization regardless of the method of treatment. It is extremely rare to encounter a patient who has reruptured the tendon more than 4 months after the previous injury.[50,65,82,83] This can be attributed to several factors. First, the resultant scar tissue that spans the two ruptured ends becomes more fibrotic with time. The tensile strength of this more mature tissue equals or exceeds that of tendon but is compromised by lack of elasticity and resiliency.[84] Early during healing the tissue has not had sufficient time for its collagen to organize and it is of lesser strength.[68]

The rerupture should be treated as was the original injury. However, more clinicians favor surgical treatment of the rerupture even if the initial regimen was cast immobilization.[50] The immobilization period should be prolonged if the treatment is identical to that for the initial injury or if casting is chosen for treatment of the failed surgically repaired primary rupture. If surgical treatment is initiated with the second injury, the postoperative period can be similar to that of a primarily repaired injury.

LACERATIONS

Lacerations of the Achilles tendon are relatively uncommon. Despite the lack of experience in any one center, the treatment of this injury is not complicated. The usual precautions for wound care are taken and tetanus prophylaxis is administered if necessary. The primary contrast in the treatment of lacerations versus spontaneous ruptures is the condition of the tendon itself. The zone of injury in lacerations is quite narrow compared with the wide area of attenuation in spontaneous ruptures. With lacerations, the cut surface is usually smooth compared with the friable mop-ended appearance of the ruptured tendon.

The patient should be examined for concomitant injuries by wound exploration. This can usually be done in the emergency room or, rarely, in the operating room. If the laceration is in the middle of the calf, then injury to the sural nerve and lesser saphenous vein would be suspected. Sensory deficits in the expected distribution indicate nerve laceration. If this denervated area encompasses a large area of plantar skin, primary nerve repair should be considered. In skiving-type injuries, the nerve is vulnerable to dual lacerations, which may complicate the repair (Fig. 13-15). Nerve grafts may be necessary.

Once the extent of injury to other tissues is determined, the extent of Achilles tendon disruption must be established. When the site of injury is purely within the tendon proper, many lacera-

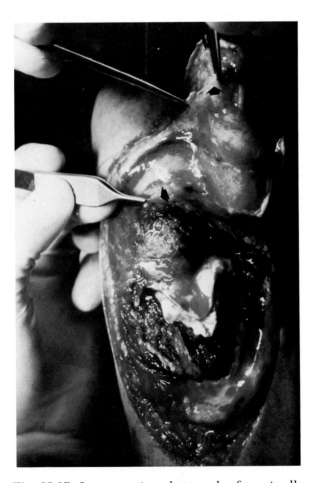

Fig. 13-15. Intraoperative photograph of proximally based flap from a gastrocnemius laceration. The flap has been turned proximally. The sural nerve has been lacerated twice (arrows).

tions may be handled conservatively. If 50 percent or less of the tendon is disrupted, then primary repair is not necessary. After appropriate wound management, a long leg cast is applied with the knee at 25 degrees of flexion and the foot in relaxed equinus. This is converted to a short leg non-weight-bearing cast at 3 weeks. After six total weeks of immobilization, unprotected weight bearing with heel elevation is utilized for an additional 6 weeks. Gradual return to full activity then ensues. If there is more than 50 percent but less than 100 percent tendon disruption, then conservative care is again indicated. However, longer periods of immobilization are necessary. Each of the periods is extended to 4 weeks, followed by a weight-bearing short leg cast after the 8 weeks of non-weight bearing.

The main consideration for advocating conservative treatment in the incomplete laceration is that end-to-end approximation and preservation of the length–tension relationship is ensured. Operative intervention is unlikely to improve the result in most cases. In addition, periodic mobilization and reduction of equinus is not necessary for the same reasons. Adhesions are usually not a problem but if so can effectively be dealt with in a later operative session.

When the laceration encompasses 100 percent of the cross-sectional area of the tendon, then operative treatment should be considered. Wound exploration and manipulation of ankle equinus will determine the degree of tendon end approximation. If approximation is adequate, the patient can be treated conservatively.

However, in most cases primary surgical repair of the completely lacerated tendon is the treatment of choice. This affords additional strength to the tendon ends and decreases the immobilization time. It also allows for earlier mobilization during the casting period.

Surgical exposure is much less extensive than with ruptures, but creative incisional approaches are often necessary to avoid crossing the laceration with a vertically oriented surgical incision. It is preferable to incorporate the wound into the surgical approach. This is usually done by increasing vertical exposure through incisions placed at either end of the transverse laceration. Deeper exposure is identical to that previously discussed. Simple end-to-end suture with a non-absorbable material is acceptable, as are other tendon sutures. However, it is best not to over extend exposure for the sake of a fancier suture technique.

Once repair is accomplished, a long leg cast is placed and left for 2 weeks. Manipulative reduction of equinus is done at that time, and the replaced long leg cast is removed at 4 weeks. A short leg cast is applied, and manipulative reduction of equinus is done 2 weeks later. At this time, the ankle position should equal that of the opposite side. Rapid reduction of the equinus is facilitated by the optimal length–tension relationship and security of the surgically stabilized injury. After 2 weeks of casting with the ankle at 90 degrees, the last 2 weeks are in a short leg walking cast. The cast is followed by protection with heel lifts.

PHYSICAL THERAPY

Physical therapy begins immediately after the final cast is removed regardless of the type of injury or treatment. Modalities designed to improve range of motion and flexibility are initiated and continued for 4 weeks. This is followed by strengthening techniques with gradual increase in resistance over the next several months. Full activity is allowed no sooner than 4 months after the injury and should be discouraged until 6 months postinjury.

EVALUATION OF RESULTS

Conflicting reports regarding the functional deficits in patients sustaining Achilles tendon ruptures abound.[58,85] The most controversial issue is what treatment modality gives the best functional results. Although it is not the purpose of this chapter to resolve the issue, the most compelling arguments are presented here.

There are four basic parameters that have been utilized to assess functional results. They are (1) return to preinjury activity level; (2) calf circum-ference; (3) strength and power; and (4) dorsiflexion of the ankle. Nistor in his multicenter study measured plantar flexion strength on the Cybex dynamometer.[85] He found no significant difference between surgically and nonsurgically treated groups. He did discover that there was reduction in plantar flexion strength, especially in the plantar flexed position, but that this was independent of treatment.

Inglis et al. found contrary results.[50] They found a significant decrease in strength in the nonsurgically treated group. Power of the injured leg was also significantly reduced in this group when compared with that of the opposite leg. Haggmark et al. showed that there was a significant difference between calf muscle cross sectional area in the nonoperatively treated Achilles tendon and that in the contralateral limb.[57] In this group, the calf muscle on the injured side was significantly smaller. This correlated with a statistically significant decrease in work load for the nonoperated leg, again compared with the opposite side. The measured differences in the surgically treated group were not significant for both parameters.

Many reports discuss increased dorsiflexion of the injured extremity following treatment. This is attributed to muscle activity and the lack of perfect apposition of the tendon ends as well as the failure to reestablish the optimal length–tension relationship.[86] Results in this institution have not corroborated this. In fact, I have observed increased dorsiflexion only rarely. Rather, dorsiflexion is almost always comparable to that of the uninjured leg. Although several parameters have been used to evaluate results, the most important factor is the ability of the patient to return to preinjury levels of activity. This includes the community ambulator to the competitive athlete. The most reliable prognostic indicator is the amount of ankle joint dorsiflexion. Presumably, the reestablishment of the optimal length enables more efficient muscular contraction.

Observations of over 120 ruptures at my facility show consistent calf atrophy. Functional limitations correlate poorly with calf size. My finding of consistent atrophy and the rare occurrence of overlengthening can be attributed to the relatively long immobilization period. However, in my patient sample, over 95 percent of the injured returned to the preinjury activity levels within 8 months after rupture despite rather marked calf atrophy.

COMPLICATIONS

There are several complications of Achilles tendon injuries regardless of the form of treatment.[87] Weakness, pain, limp, and, most significantly, rerupture have been discussed at length. When considering rerupture alone, most investigators report a higher incidence of rerupture for conservatively treated patients.[85] However, many of the reports show a markedly shorter immobilization period than is recommended here. Perhaps the rerupture rate would drop precipitously if longer immobilization periods were utilized.

Surgical repair has decreased the incidence of rerupture. However, careful analysis of those reports shows casting periods that certainly were no shorter than those for nonoperatively treated patients. Second, surgeons tend to be more "protective" of their work and may prolong casting periods, with serendipitous benefits. Finally, patients who have had surgery are more likely to appreciate the seriousness of their injury and may tolerate longer periods of immobilization.

The incidence of wound dehiscence and infection can often dissuade even the aggressive surgeon from performing surgical repair. These complications are often devastating to the patient in terms of the functional result, and complete loss of the Achilles tendon can be the end result. However, the occurrences of these disasters are minimized with careful selection of patients and careful, meticulous technique. Primary repair in patients with significant systemic disease, advanced age, or other physiologic dysfunctions is to be avoided. It is critical not to underscore the skin edges during the dissection. Traumatic forceps and self-retaining retractors should not be used. I have had no incidences of even minor wound problems or infections by following these guidelines in over 150 open repairs.

Adhesions of the tendon to the overlying skin are uncommon in the surgically treated patient and rare to nonexistent in the conservatively treated patient. If this does occur, the area of adherence is almost always in the line of repair at the level of rupture. This is where reestablishment of the sheath is sometimes impossible. Treatment of these adhesions other than an explanation to the patient is seldom necessary. At the patient's request, they are easily handled with surgical lysis followed by early immobilization.

Sural nerve damage is also an infrequent complication of primary surgical repair. It is more likely to occur in the delayed rupture in which the surgical incision is higher, but in any case is minimized by careful separation of the subcutaneous layer with the skin off of the deep fascia. The usual strategies for nerve entrapment are used if symptoms warrant.

SALVAGE TECHNIQUES

When the practitioner is faced with massive tissue deficits secondary to infection or failure of another technique, alternative procedures are indicated (Fig. 13-16). Procedures that create a substitute for the deficient Achilles tendon are usually used but only in the most functionally impaired patients.

Tendon Transfers

Tendon transfers are useful for the purpose of preventing the accentuation of a calcaneal position. As a rule, they cannot and should not be expected to provide much in the way of plantar flexion power.

Two muscles are readily available for transfer. The peroneus brevis is easily accessible and its transfer is relatively easy to perform (Fig. 13-17). It is an in-phase transfer, and therefore little retraining is necessary.[88]

Transfer of the tibialis anterior is an out-of-phase transfer and is more difficult to perform. The axis of pull is at a poorer mechanical advantage than that of the peroneus brevis. It cannot be

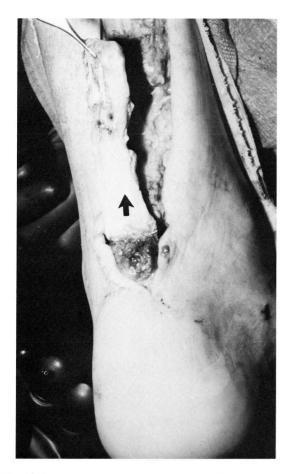

Fig. 13-16. Intraoperative photograph of a patient sustaining loss of Achilles tendon continuity secondary to postoperative infection. Here a large homograft of gastrocnemius aponeurosis (arrow) is used to replace the tendon.

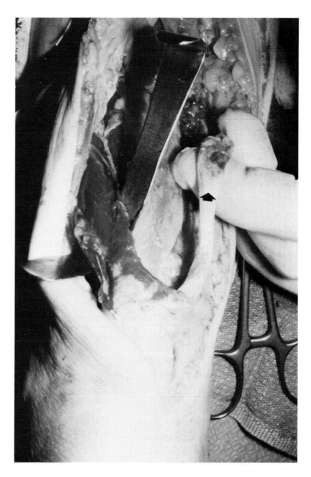

Fig. 13-17. Intraoperative photograph of peroneus brevis transfer. The malleable retractor is under the muscle belly, which extends all the way to the calcaneus. The redundant tendon (arrow) can be excised or used to anchor the muscle to the calcaneus via a drill or trephine hole.

expected to convert phase or provide much plantar flexion power. We have had no experience at this institution with this transfer other than with patients with neuromuscular disease.

Several investigators have attempted to induce neotendinous tissue in the gap created by the loss of tendon substance. These techniques essentially employ synthetic materials. Carbon fiber, polyester fibers, or polygalactin mesh[89–91] have all been placed into the deficit, with gradual replacement of the synthetic tissue with autogenous neotendon. Although reported results are mixed, the principle of inductive substitution remains an intriguing concept.[92,93]

Finally, restoration of plantar flexion power can be attained by a free muscle transfer. These techniques are best left to plastic surgeons, but practitioners dealing with Achilles tendon injuries should be aware of their availability.

REFERENCES

1. Daseler EH, Arson BJ: The plantaris muscle. An anatomical study of 750 specimens. J Bone Joint Surg 25:822, 1943

2. Harvey F, Chu G, Harvey PM: Surgical availability of the plantaris tendon. J Hand Surg 8:243, 1983

3. Pilcher R: Repair of herniia with plantaris tendon grafts. Arch Surg 38:16, 1939

4. Incavo SJ, Alvarez RG, Trevino SG: Occurrence of the plantaris tendon in patients sustaining subcutaneous rupture of the Achilles tendon. Foot Ankle 8:110, 1987

5. Cummins EJ, Anson BJ, Carr BW et al: The structure of the calcaneal tendon (of Achilles) in relation to orthopedic surgery with additional observations on the plantaris muscle. Surg Gynecol Obstet 83:107, 1946

6. White JW: Torsion of the achilles tendon. Its surgical significance. Arch Surg 46:784, 1943

7. Bardeen CR: Development and variation of nerves and musculature of the inferior extremity and neighboring regions of the trunk in man. Am J Anat VI:259, 1907

8. Le Double AF: Traites des Variations du Systeme Musculaire de l'Homme. Schleicher Freres, Paris, 1897

9. Gordon SL, Matheson DW: The accessory soleus. Clin Orthop 97:129, 1973

10. Johansen BE, Flintholm J: A case study: the accessory soleus. J Orthop Sports Phys Ther Sept:84, 1983

11. Bonnell J, Cruess RL: Anomalous insertion of the soleus muscle as a cause of fixed equinus deformity. A case report. J Bone Joint Surg 51A:999, 1969

12. Dunn AW: Anomalous muscles simulating soft tissue tumors in the lower extremity. A report of three cases. J Bone Joint Surg 47A:1397, 1965

13. Nathan H, Gloobe H, Yosipovitch Z: Flexor digitorum accessorius longus. Clin Orthop 113:158, 1975

14. Schatzker J, Brånemark PI: Intravital observation of the microvascular anatomy and microcirculation of tendon. Acta Orthop Scand, suppl., 126, 3, 1969

15. Cronkite AE: The tensile strength of human tendon. Anat Rec 64:173, 1935

16. McMaster PE: Tendon and muscle ruptures; clinical and experimental studies on the causes and location of subcutaneous ruptures. J Bone Joint Surg 15:705, 1933

17. Ralston EL, Schmidt ER: Repair of the ruptured achilles tendon. J Trauma 11:15, 1971

18. Arey LB: Human Histology. 3rd Ed. WB Saunders, Philadelphia, 1968

19. DiStefano VJ, Nixon JE: Achilles tendon rupture; pathogenesis, diagnosis, and treatment by a modified pullout wire technique. J Trauma 12:671, 1972

20. Davidsson L, Salo M: Pathogenesis of subcutaneous tendon ruptures. Acta Chir Scand 135:209, 1969

21. Clancy WG, Neidbart D, Brand RL: Achilles tendonitis in runners. A report of five cases. Am J Sports Med 4:46, 1976

22. Fox JM, Blazina ME, Jobe FW et al: Degeneration and rupture of the Achilles tendon. Clin Orthop 107:221, 1975

23. Arner O, Lindholm A, Orell SR: Histologic changes in subcutaneous rupture of the Achilles tendon. A study of 74 cases. Acta Chir Scand 116:484, 1959

24. Lagergren C, Lindholm Å: Vascular distribution in the Achilles tendon. An arteriographic and microangiographic study. Acta Chir Scand 116:491, 1958/1959

25. Håstad K, Larsson HG, Lindholm Å: Clearance of radiosodium after local deposit in the Achilles tendon. Acta Chir Scand 116:251, 1958/1959

26. Cowen MA, Alexander S: Simultaneous bilateral rupture of Achilles tendons due to triamcinalone. Br Med J 1658, 1961

27. Goforth P, Gudas CJ: Effects of steroids on wound healing: a review of the literature. J Foot Surg 19:22, 1980

28. Kapetanos G: The effect of the local corticosteroids on the healing and biomechanical properties of the partially injured tendon. Clin Orthop 163:170, 1982

29. Lee HB: Avulsion and rupture of the tendo calcaneus after injection of hydrocortisone. Br Med J 395, 1957

30. Balasubramaniam P, Prathap K: The effect of injection of hydrocortisone into rabbit calcaneal tendons. J Bone Joint Surg 54B:729, 1972

31. Balasubramaniam P, Chong KL: The effect of hydrocortisone injections into calcaneal tendons: an electron microscopal study in rabbits. J Bone Joint Surg 56B:583, 1974

32. Bloom W, Fawcett DW: A Textbook of Histology. 9th Ed. WB Saunders, Philadelphia, 1968

33. Phelps D, Sonstegard DA, Matthews LS: Corticosteroid injection effects on the biomechanical properties of rabbit patellar tendons. Clin Orthop 100:345, 1974

34. Mackie JW, Goldin B, Foss ML et al: Mechanical properties of rabbit tendons after repeated anti-inflammatory steroid injections. Med Sci Sports 6:198, 1974

35. Mahoney PG, James PD, Howell CJ et al: Sponta-

neous rupture of the Achilles tendon in a patient with gout. Ann Rheum Dis 490:416, 1981

36. Cirincione RJ, Baker BE: Tendon rupture with secondary hyperparathyroidism. J Bone Joint Surg 57A:852, 1975

37. Preston ET: Avulsion of both quadriceps tendons in hyperparathyroidism. JAMA 221:406, 1972

38. Cruickshank B: Lesions of joint and tendon sheaths in SLE. Ann Rheum Dis 18:111, 1959

39. Potasman I, Bassan HM: Multiple tendon rupture in systemic lupus erythematosus: case report and review of the literature. Ann Rheum Dis 43:347, 1984

40. Twining RH, Marcus WY, Garey JL: Tendon rupture in systemic lupus erythematosus. JAMA 189:123, 1964

41. Abell JM: Bilateral Achilles tendon rupture secondary to ochronosis. Orthop Rev 14:91, 1985

42. Christensen I: Rupture of the Achilles tendon; analysis of 57 cases. Acta Chir Scand 106:50, 1953–1954

43. Goldberg I, Avidor I: Isolated tuberculous tenosynovitis of the Achilles tendon. A case report. Clin Orthop 194:185, 1985

44. Haines JF: Bilateral rupture of the Achilles tendon in patients on steroid therapy. Ann Rheum Dis 42:652, 1983

45. Melmed EP: Spontaneous rupture of the calcaneal tendon during steroid therapy. J Bone Joint Surg 47B:104, 1965

46. Fisher TR, Woods CG: Partial rupture of the tendo calcaneus with heterotopic ossification. Report of a case. J Bone Joint Surg 52B:334, 1970

47. Mallinson FB: Ossification of both Achilles tendons with traumatic fracture of one. Br Med J ii:836, 1929

48. Hooker C: Rupture of the tendo calcaneus. J Bone Joint Surg 45B:360, 1963

49. Leach RE, James S, Wasilewski S: Achilles tendinitis. Am J Sports Med 9:93, 1981

50. Inglis AE, Scott WN, Sculco TP et al: Ruptures of the tendo Achillis. An objective assessment of surgical and nonsurgical treatment. J Bone Joint Surg 58A:990, 1976

51. Kvist H, Kvist M: The operative treatment of chronic calcaneal paratenonitis. J Bone Joint Surg 62B:353, 1980

52. Puddu G, Ippolito E, Postacchini F: A classification of Achilles disease. Am J Sports Med 4:145, 1976

53. Kitting RW: Some observations on repairing rupture of the Achilles tendon. J Am Podiatry Assoc 64:97, 1974

54. Thompson TC, Doherty JG: Spontaneous rupture of tendon of Achilles: a new clinical diagnostic test. J Trauma 2:126, 1962

55. Ger R, Sedlin E: The accessory soleus muscle. Clin Orthop 116:220, 1976

56. Livingston VG, Stockey LR, Lepow GM et al: Rupture of the tendo Achillis. J Am Podiatry Assoc 65:19, 1975

57. Haggmark T, Liedberg H, Eriksson E, Wredmark T: Calf muscle atrophy and muscle function after non-operative and operative treatment of Achilles tendon ruptures. Orthopedics 9:160, 1986

58. Jacobs D, Martens M, VanAudekercke R et al: Comparison of conservative and operative treatment of Achilles tendon rupture. Am J Sports Med 6:107, 1978

59. Lawrence GH, Cave EF, O'Connor H: Injury to the Achilles tendon. Experience at the Massachusetts General Hospital. Am J Surg 89:795, 1955

60. Lynn TA: Repair of the torn Achilles tendon using the plantaris tendon as a reinforcing membrane. J Bone Joint Surg 48A:268, 1966

61. Percy EC, Conochie LB: The surgical treatment of ruptured tendo Achillis. Am J Sports Med 8:244, 1980

62. Quigley TB, Scheller AD: Surgical repair of the ruptured Achilles tendon. Analysis of 40 patients treated by the same surgeon. Am J Sports Med 8:244, 1980

63. Skeoch DU: Spontaneous partial subcutaneous rupture of the tendo Achillis. Review of the literature and evaluation of 16 involved tendons. Am J Sports Med 9:20, 1981

64. Stein SR, Leukens CA: Methods and rationale for closed treatment of Achilles tendon ruptures. Am J Sports Med 4:162, 1976

65. Kuwada GT, Schuberth JM: Evaluation of Achilles tendon rerupture. J Foot Surg 23:340, 1984

66. Lea RB, Smith L: Rupture of the Achilles tendon. Nonsurgical treatment. Clin Orthop 60:115, 1968

67. Lea RB, Smith L: Non-surgical treatment of tendo Achillis rupture. J Bone Joint Surg 54A:1398, 1972

68. Ketchum LD, Martin NL, Kappel DA: Experimental evaluation of the factors affecting tendon gap and tendon strength at the site of tendon repair. Plast Reconstr Surg 59:708, 1977

69. Fulp MJ, McGlamry ED: Gastrocnemius tendon recession: tongue in groove procedure to lengthen gastrocnemius tendon. J Am Podiatry Assoc 64:163, 1971

70. Abraham E, Pankovich AR: Neglected rupture of the Achilles tendon. Treatment by V-Y tendinous flap. J Bone Joint Surg 57A:253, 1975

71. Baker LD: A rational approach to the surgical needs of the cerebral palsy patient. J Bone Joint Surg 38A:313, 1956

72. Strayer LM: Gastrocnemius recession: five year report of cases. J Bone Joint Surg 40A:1019, 1956

73. Bosworth DM: Repair of defects in the tendo Achillis. J Bone Joint Surg 38A:111, 1956

74. Bugg EI, Boyd BM: Repair of neglected rupture or laceration of the Achilles tendon. Clin Orthop 56:73, 1968

75. Fish JB: Ruptured Achilles tendon. A method of repair. Cont Orthop 5:21, 1982

76. Christensen RE: To tilfgelde af subcutan achillesseneruptur. Dansk Kirurgisk Selskabs Forhandlinger 75:39, 1931

77. Gebhart K: Zur Wiederherstellungschirugie versorgung des Achillessehnenrisses. Arch Klin Chir 189:681, 1937

78. Silfverskiold N: Uber die subkutane totale Achillessehnenrupture und deren Behandlung. Acta Chir Scand 84:393, 1941

79. Lindholm A: A new method of operation in subcutaneous rupture of the Achilles tendon. Acta Chir Scand 117:261, 1959

80. Kirschenbaum SE, Kelman C: Modification of the Lindholm procedure for the plastic repair of ruptured Achilles tendon: a case report. J Foot Surg 19:4, 1980

81. Parker RG, Repinecz M: Neglected rupture of the Achilles tendon. Treatment by modified Strayer gastrocnemius recession. J Am Podiatry Assoc 69:548, 1979

82. Schuberth JM, Dockery GL, McBride RE: Recurrent rupture of the tendo Achillis. Repair by free tendinous autograft. J Am Podiatry Assoc 74:157, 1984

83. Scott WN, Inglis AE, Sculco TP: Surgical treatment of reruptures of the tendo Achilles following nonsurgical treatment. Clin Orthop 140:175, 1979

84. Hattrup SJ, Johnson KA: A review of ruptures of the Achilles tendon. Foot Ankle 6:34, 1985

85. Nistor L: Surgical and non-surgical treatment of Achilles tendon rupture. J Bone Joint Surg 63A:394, 1981

86. Nystrom B, Holmlund D: Separation of tendon ends after suture of Achilles tendon. Acta Orthop Scand 54:620, 1983

87. Gilles H, Chalmers J: The management of fresh ruptures of the tendo Achillis. J Bone Joint Surg 52A:337, 1970

88. Teuffer AP: Traumatic rupture of the Achilles tendon: reconstruction by transplant and graft using the lateral peroneus brevis. Orthop Clin North Am 5:89, 1974

89. Amis AA, Campbell JR, Kempson SA et al: Comparison of the structure of neotendons induced by implantation of carbon or polyester fibres. J Bone Joint Surg 66B:131, 1984

90. Howard CB, Winston I, Bell W et al: Late repair of the calcaneal tendon with carbon fibre. J Bone Joint Surg 66B:206, 1984

91. Roberts JM, Goldstrohm GL, Brown TD et al: Comparison of unrepaired, primarily repaired, and polylactin mesh-reinforced Achilles tendon lacerations in rabbits. Clin Orthop 181:244, 1983

92. Andreef IV, Dimoff G, Metschkarski ST: A comparative experimental study on transplantation of autogenous tissue and homogenous tendon tissue. Acta Orthop Scand 38:35, 1967

93. Mendes DG, Angel D, Grishkan A et al: Histologic response to carbon fibre. J Bone Joint Surg 67B:645, 1985

14

Management of Neurologic Trauma

Michael S. Downey, D.P.M.

The literature, including this text, is replete with descriptions of the anatomy, classification, treatment, and sequelae of most soft tissue and osseous injuries. Only recently have similar attempts been made toward the assessment and management of neurologic trauma. Indeed, the physician dealing with trauma to the foot and ankle will frequently be faced with direct or concomitant trauma to vital neural and neurovascular structures. If these injuries are not properly assessed and appropriately treated, the resulting sequelae may remain long after satisfactory healing of associated soft tissue and osseous trauma. Awareness of the long-term effects of nerve trauma should modify our initial approach to the injured lower extremity to include immediate evaluation of the peripheral nervous system in virtually any injury.

ANATOMY

Although gross vascular injury in most cases will be apparent, subtle ischemic compromise may go unnoticed. This traumatic ischemia may further compromise any neural injury present. A complete understanding of the gross neurovascular anatomy is prerequisite to the proper diagnosis of these injuries. Further, the ability of the traumatologist to recognize and treat peripheral nerve injuries depends on a working knowledge of the microscopic anatomy and physiology of the peripheral nerve trunk and an understanding of the relationship of the nerve to its local environment.

The peripheral nerve trunk is composed of functional neural fibers surrounded by several different layers of supportive connective tissue. The surgeon must have an appreciation of the layers, including the nerve fiber, endoneurium, fasciculus, perineurium, and epineurium, as the optimal methods of nerve repair are based on the arrangement of these microscopic and macroscopic structures (Fig. 14-1).

The nerve fiber, or axon, is the smallest functional unit within the nerve trunk. It varies from 0.5 to 20 μm in diameter and from 0.5 mm to 1 m in length. Nerve fibers can be classified as myelinated or unmyelinated, with fibers smaller than 2 μm in diameter generally being unmyelinated. Conduction rates are directly related to fiber size; thus, unmyelinated axons conduct at a slower rate than myelinated axons. When present, myelin is produced and laid down along the axon by the Schwann cell, which wraps itself circumferentially around the axon. Between the Schwann cells, spaces or nodes are present that are bare of myelin. The internodal distance is the space between two adjacent nodes. The action potential of the myelinated fiber passes rapidly along the axon by saltatory conduction from node to node[1] (Fig. 14-2).

The endoneurium is a loose connective tissue layer, consisting of primarily longitudinally oriented collagen fibers, that intimately surrounds

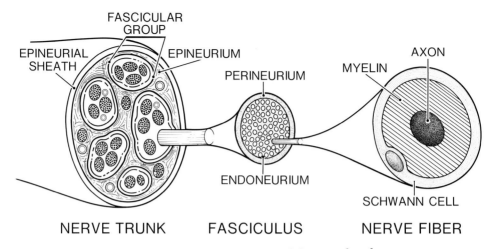

Fig. 14-1. Main structural elements of the peripheral nerve.

each nerve fiber or axon. The endoneurium is a relatively permeable structure allowing exogenous chemicals such as bacterial toxins, steroid compounds, local anesthetics, and noxious substances to reach the axon.[2,3] Extravasated large plasma proteins in the endoneurium may alter the oncotic pressure and effect intraneural edema.

Groups of nerve fibers within their individual endoneurial sheaths are gathered together to form a bundle called a fasciculus or funiculus. Nerve fibers within each fasciculus can be sen-

sory, motor, or autonomic in nature. However, only one or two of these types is usually present within any particular fasciculus.[4] The fasciculus is the smallest surgical unit of the peripheral nerve.

Perineurium is the tissue that encloses the fasciculi. It is formed by several collagenous layers with fibers oriented in oblique, circular, and longitudinal directions. These fibers are very closely linked together, and their arrangement affords the perineurium unique diffusion properties. The perineurium, because of these characteris-

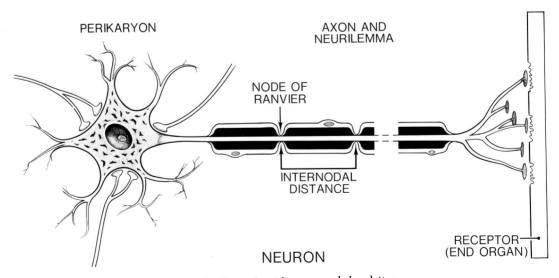

Fig. 14-2. Neuron with axon and dendrites.

tics and unlike the endoneurium, acts as a selective barrier between external noxious substances (e.g., bacterial toxins and plasma proteins) and the enclosed nerve fibers.[2,3] Thus, the perineurium forms a sheath that contains the fasciculi and maintains intrafascicular pressure.[5,6]

The epineurium consists of thick areolar connective tissue that surrounds the perineurium-enclosed fascicles. Approximately 30 to 75 percent of a peripheral nerve's cross-sectional area is made up of epineurium.[7] The epineurium is condensed at the nerve's surface to form a definite encasing sheath, the epineurial sheath. The epineurial sheath thus defines the outer margin of a peripheral nerve. In addition, the epineural sheath has a loose attachment to the surrounding connective tissue, which is well demonstrated by the relative mobility of the peripheral nerve as it courses through the extremity.

The microvascular supply to the peripheral nerve, the vasa nervorum, consists of an extrinsic (perineural) blood supply and an intrinsic (intraneural) vascular network.[8] The interrelationship of the extrinsic and intrinsic blood supplies provides a wide margin of safety to the peripheral nerve in most instances. However, ischemia plays an important role in many traumatic neur-

opathies and can independently produce a severe neuropathy.[9,10] Temporary ischemia (e.g., following inflation of a pneumatic tourniquet) may also produce neural dysfunction.[8]

Extrinsic blood supply to a peripheral nerve arises from regional perineural vessels located in surrounding tissues. The vessels are of small diameter and penetrate the epineurial sheath segmentally along the course of the nerve. The vessels are suspended about the nerve and are somewhat coiled about themselves. This coiled configuration allows the extrinsic blood supply to uncoil and elongate as the peripheral nerve moves with limb motion. Excessive traction or stretching of a nerve trunk may overextend this coiled reserve, causing constriction or disruption of the extrinsic blood supply (Fig. 14-3).

The intrinsic blood supply is a microvascular network consisting of anastomotic small arteries and arterioles running longitudinally within the nerve trunk and a rich capillary network oriented perpendicular to the anastomotic vessels. The anastomotic vessels are located within the perineurium and epineurium, while the capillary beds course through the endoneurium (Fig. 14-4). The intrinsic blood supply possesses a significant reserve capacity, as seemingly dormant

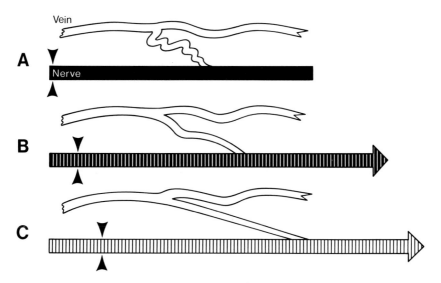

Fig. 14-3. Illustration of extrinsic system of vasa nervorum demonstrating the segmental or "coiled" reserve length. (**A**) Nerve trunk at rest. (**B**) Nerve placed under stretch as extrinsic reserve uncoils. (**C**) Maximal stretch of extrinsic reserve. Any further tension would disrupt the extrinsic vascular supply.

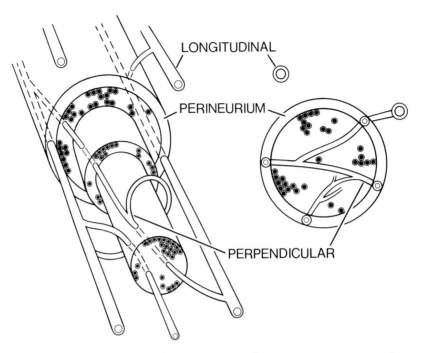

Fig. 14-4. Illustration of intrinsic system of vasa nervorum demonstrating microcirculation with longitudinal vessels in the epineurium and perineurium and the perpendicular highly anastomotic cross network of capillaries located within the endoneurium.

capillaries respond to local injury or increased temperature by vasodilation and reactive hyperemia.

Clearly, the peripheral nerve trunk is a complex functional unit. Knowledge of the nerve trunk's functional anatomy and physiology provides the basis for an understanding of the pathologic effects of trauma to the structure. The type of therapy, whether conservative or surgical, will be based on the nature of the anatomic and functional damage to the nerve itself.

CLASSIFICATION

A classification scheme of nerve injury can be initiated based on a thorough understanding of the surgical anatomy and physiology of the nerve trunk. Such a classification will permit a unified assessment of the functional severity of the pathologic condition, aid in the formulation of the

prognosis, and serve as a guide to rational therapy. Since nerve injuries have only recently been regularly studied, a classification system provides the traumatologist who infrequently sees nerve injuries basic guidelines for treatment.

During World War II, Seddon defined the three classic nerve injuries based on the degree of injury to the axon.[11,12] He classified lesions as (1) neurapraxia, (2) axonotmesis, and (3) neurotmesis. The injuries are each caused by specific types of trauma (Table 14-1). The lesions generally progress in severity, with neurapraxia being least severe and neurotmesis being most severe.

Neurapraxia is considered to be a conduction deficit without axonal destruction. It is generally a minor injury involving a contusion or mild compression to a peripheral nerve resulting in physiologic but not anatomic disruption to the nerve fiber. The injurious force causes distortion of the myelin sheath, and the transmission of nerve impulses by saltatory conduction is temporarily interrupted. Larger and more heavily myelinated

Table 14-1. Causes of the Three Main Types of Nerve Injury[a]

Cause of Injury	Neurapraxia	Axonotmesis	Neurotmesis
Cuts and lacerations	−	±	+
Fractures	−	+	±
Missiles	+	+	+
Traction	+	+	+
Compression	+ (momentary)	+ (prolonged)	−
Thermal	+	+	−
Ischemia	+	+	+

[a] +, frequent; ±, occasional; −, infrequent.

fibers are thus more susceptible to neurapraxia. Recovery from neurapraxia is usually complete and occurs over several hours to several weeks.

Axonotmesis is defined as axonal disruption without destruction of the endoneurial tubes. In this condition, there is anatomic disruption of the axon and its myelin sheath, but no disruption of the endoneurial tube. Various amounts of distal wallerian degeneration (i.e., degeneration of the axon distal to the point of injury) will result, and nerve conduction will be absent. Although there is total distal degeneration of the axon and its myelin sheath, there is spontaneous regeneration and total functional recovery because the intact endoneurial tubes guide the outgoing streams of proximally generated axoplasm to their proper peripheral connections.

The major pathologic catastrophe facing the peripheral nerve trunk is neurotmesis. Neurotmesis is complete nerve disruption, which may occur with or without gross disruption of the epineurium. However, the axon, Schwann cell, and endoneurial tubes are completely disrupted. Unlike neurapraxia and axonotmesis, recovery from neurotmesis is always imperfect (Table 14-2).

Seddon's classification was a useful one, but with the recent advances in surgical therapy, a further breakdown is frequently necessary. Sunderland classified nerve injuries into five degrees that incorporate neurapraxia, axonotmesis, and neurotmesis[13] (Fig. 14-5).

A first degree injury corresponds to neurapraxia and is a conduction deficit without axonal degeneration. Again, the injury is followed by

Table 14-2. Differentiating Features of the Three Main Types of Nerve Injury

Feature	Neurapraxia	Axonotmesis	Neurotmesis
Pathologic			
Anatomic continuity	Preserved	Preserved	May be lost
Essential damage	Myelin sheath distortion	Wallerian degeneration with endoneurial tube preservation	Complete disorganization
Clinical			
Motor paralysis	Complete	Complete	Complete
Muscle atrophy	Very little	Progressive	Progressive
Sensory paralysis	Usually spared	Complete	Complete
Autonomic paralysis	Usually spared	Complete	Complete
Recovery			
Quality	Perfect	Perfect	Imperfect
Rate of recovery	Rapid; days to weeks	1–2 mm/d	1–2 mm/d (if surgically repaired)
March of recovery	No order	According to order of innervation	According to order of innervation
Treatment			
Surgical repair	Not necessary	Usually not necessary	Essential

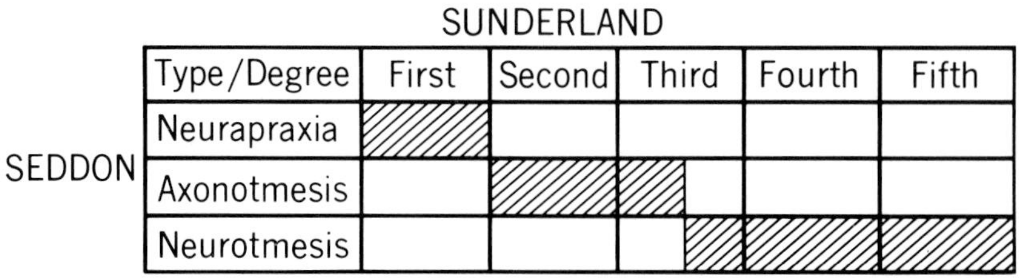

SUNDERLAND

SEDDON	Type/Degree	First	Second	Third	Fourth	Fifth
	Neurapraxia	////				
	Axonotmesis		////	////		
	Neurotmesis				////	////

Fig. 14-5. Correlation of two major classifications of nerve injuries.

rapid recovery (hours to weeks). Predictive factors in the recovery rate include the nature, intensity, and duration of the injury or disruptive forces. When first degree injury results from brief nondestructive blunt trauma, undisplaced fractures, tourniquet use, or mild hematoma formation, rapid recovery is usual but not certain.[14]

Second degree injury corresponds to axonotmesis and consists of axon disruption without endoneurial disruption. Wallerian degeneration occurs. The recovery rate depends on axonal regeneration, which occurs at 1 to 2 mm/day from the point of disruption.

Third degree injury can be considered a form of axonotmesis or neurotmesis and involves sectioning of the axons with disruption of the endoneurial tubes. This results in disorganization of the internal arrangement of the fascicles. Regeneration is irregular, with interfascicular and intrafascicular fibrosis. This disorganization leads to predictable residual deficits, and as soon as this pattern of nerve injury is identified, surgical intervention should be contemplated.

Fourth degree injury consists of physical disruption of the fascicles and perineurium with an intact epineurium. Thus, it may be considered a form of neurotmesis. The fascicles become disorganized and are no longer sharply demarcated from the epineurium. Damage from this injury is irreversible and will lead to imperfect recovery in the form of a neuroma-in-continuity. This injury will require surgical intervention to minimize permanent dysfunction.

Fifth degree injury is true neurotmesis or complete physical disruption of the nerve trunk. Laceration or rupture from severe stretch may produce this injury. Symptoms may be indistinguishable from those of a fourth degree injury if

the continuity of the epineurial sheath is not fully visualized. Obviously, this injury will require surgical repair.

Mixed nerve injuries may occur with variations of the degrees mentioned above. Classification of nerve injuries enables the traumatologist to determine the prognosis of the injury and the possible need for surgical intervention to achieve the best functional result.

DIAGNOSIS

Diagnosis of the patient with suspected peripheral nerve injury should include a complete history and physical examination. The history should include the usual parameters: nature, location, duration, onset, course, aggravating factors, and past treatment. The physical examination should include evaluation of the central, autonomic, and peripheral sensorimotor nervous systems. The peripheral examination can be divided into sensibility testing, skeletal motor testing, and electrodiagnosis. Evaluation may be performed in several different circumstances including (1) as a diagnostic aid to determine the presence or absence of various nerve injuries; (2) to assess objectively the clinical and functional results of neurorrhaphy or nerve grafting; and (3) to determine the extent of suspected nerve entrapment and the need for neurolysis.

Sensibility Testing

The distribution of sensibility loss is important to the determination of specific nerve injury and to evaluation of that nerve's recovery. Primary sensory qualities that may be evaluated include pain or sharp-dull distinction, light touch-pressure, two-point discrimination, vibration, temperature, and proprioception. The distribution of the abnormalities of these sensations is important since it may provide evidence of a specific nerve lesion. The examination should always compare the involved lower extremity with the uninvolved contralateral limb. Since virtually all sensibility tests are subjective, whenever possible, the quantity and quality of the sensations should be noted. The British Medical Research Council has introduced a system for grading sensibility that can be used (Table 14-3). Accurate documentation is necessary as subtle changes over time can mean the difference between the progression or regression of recovery.

Pain (Sharp-Dull)

Pain is the key diagnostic parameter used to assess recovery following nerve trunk injury. Dysesthesia, hypoesthesia, and hyperesthesia may be present. Palpation and percussion of the traumatized nerve will allow observation for tenderness, swelling, and the presence of Tinel's sign (distal tingling on percussion [DTP]).

Tinel's sign is an important monitor of sensory nerve regeneration and may be considered the earliest clinical indicator of axonal regeneration. The regenerating ends of axons are very sensitive to pressure, and the level of regeneration may be accurately determined by tapping over the nerve distally and progressing proximally until paresthesias appear (Tinel's sign). As regeneration occurs, the level of the Tinel's sign should move distally at the rate of 1 to 2 mm/day. Reinnervation of muscles and skin to that level will also be seen. Absence or unusually slow progression of Tinel's sign 2 to 3 months after nerve injury indicates that regeneration, even of fine fibers, is not occurring.

Sharp-dull or pain distinction can be easily evaluated with a simple pin, sharp on one end and dull on the other. The skin area to be examined is identified symmetrically on both lower extremities. The test compares the sensitivity to the pin prick versus that to a dull surface (the pin head). The uninvolved extremity is compared with the involved extremity.

Light Touch and Pressure

Light touch and pressure can be evaluated but are frequently difficult to quantitate. von Frey initially attempted to standardize the stimuli for testing the subjective sense of light touch. He accomplished this by using horsehairs of various thickness and stiffness, and attempts at objective testing in this manner typically bear his name. The Weinstein-Semmes esthesiometer is a more modern instrument that may be helpful in von Frey pressure testing. The instrument consists of several lucite rods, each with a monofilament nylon fiber mounted in it like a single-fiber brush. The monofilaments are of varying thickness, and each will bend at a specific pressure when applied perpendicular to the skin surface. The rods are marked from 1.65 to 6.65 with the number representing the logarithm of 10 times the force in milligrams required to bow the monofilament. The calculated pressure of the monofilaments ranges from 3.25 to 439 g/mm^2. von Frey pressure testing should begin on the uninvolved limb. The patient's view of the area is blocked, and the smallest monofilament is applied to an area in one motion until it bends (Fig. 14-6). If the patient feels the pressure, the patient identifies the area touched. If the patient does not feel the monofilament or if the area touched is not localized, the next larger monofilament is se-

Table 14-3. British Medical Research Council Scale for Grading Nerve Sensibility

S0	Absence of sensibility
S1	Recovery of deep cutaneous pain sensibility within the autonomous area
S2	Return of some degree of superficial cutaneous pain and tactile sensibility within the autonomous area
S3	Return of superficial cutaneous pain and tactile sensibility throughout the autonomous area with disappearance of any previous over-reaction
S3+	Some recovery of two-point discrimination within the autonomous area
S4	Complete recovery

(From Omer,[15] with permission.)

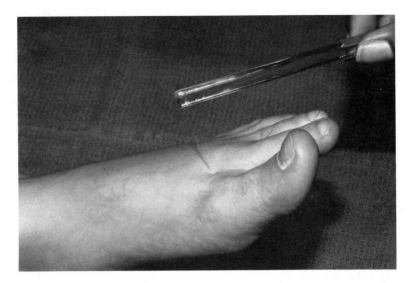

Fig. 14-6. Demonstration of use of one rod in von Frey pressure testing.

lected and the procedure repeated. After the patient's normal sensibility is determined and the patient is familiar with the testing procedure, the test is performed on the contralateral injured extremity. The test may be repeated at a later time

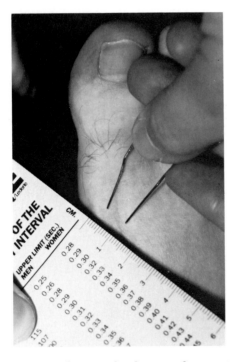

Fig. 14-7. Use of paper clip for test of two-point discrimination.

in a similar objective manner. Thus, light touch and pressure can be accurately measured quantitatively and charted to aid in determination of nerve regeneration or degeneration.

Two-Point Discrimination

Two-point discrimination similarly can be quantitated. The instrument for two-point discrimination can be a Boley gauge, blunt-eye caliper, two pins, or even an ordinary paper clip (Fig. 14-7). The test is begun distally, and the pressure applied should be firm but should not produce blanching of the skin. The initial distance should be far enough apart that the patient distinguishes two points of contact. The distance can then be systemically decreased (usually in 5-mm increments) until the two-point sensation is lost or becomes one-point sensation. Normal two-point discrimination just below the knee is 40 to 50 mm. Two-point discrimination can be said to be diminished if lost at a distance of 50 to 80 mm and absent if not felt above 80 mm.[15] Decreased two-point discrimination is an early finding of entrapment neuropathy.[16] Edema or callosities can alter these sensibility values, and the two-point discrimination distance is much smaller more distally (i.e., in the foot).

Vibration

Vibration is assessed with a tuning fork (Fig. 14-8). A set of tuning forks with various frequen-

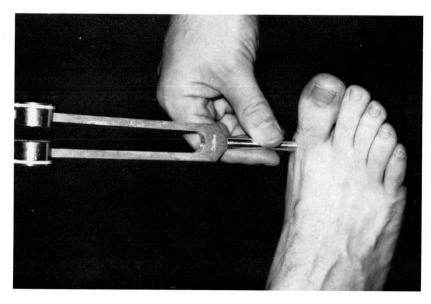

Fig. 14-8. Testing vibratory sense with a tuning fork. A 256-cps tuning fork evaluates the pacinian corpuscles or corpuscles of pressure. A 30-cps tuning fork evaluates the Meissner's corpuscles or corpuscles of tactile touch.

cies (i.e., cycles per second [cps]) may be used to test different end organs. For example, a 30-cps tuning fork can be used to evaluate the Meissner's corpuscles (corpuscula tactus or corpuscles of tactile touch), whereas a 256-cps tuning fork evaluates the pacinian corpuscles (corpuscula lamellosa or corpuscles of pressure). One should choose the appropriate tuning fork and apply it from distal to proximal until the patient feels the vibration. The test should first be performed on the uninjured extremity. Comparison should be then made between the injured extremity and the uninjured extremity with the patient asked whether the vibration intensity is more, less, or the same on the injured side.[17]

Temperature

Hot-cold sensation and discrimination can also be tested, but are more difficult to assess accurately. The two sensations may be confused by the hypersensitive patient, and accurate determination of temperature requires an instrument with calibrated thermometers that can produce a cold temperature of approximately 4 to 5° C (40° F) or a hot temperature of approximately 46 to 48° C (115 to 120° F).[17] Test progression proceeds

from distal to proximal with care taken to avoid thermal trauma in a suspected area of denervation.

Proprioception

The precision of sensibility for body position and movement is the reverse of that of cutaneous sensibility. Whereas cutaneous sensibility is greater distally, proprioception is greater proximally. Therefore, a digital interphalangeal joint may require 5 to 10 degrees of motion in the normal foot to be perceived by the patient, while only 1 to 2 degrees of ankle motion will be noticed (Fig. 14-9). This test can only be performed as a comparison between the uninjured limb and the injured limb and is very difficult to quantitate.

Sympathetic Testing

Abnormal sympathetic functions that may be observed in the patient include (1) vasomotor—abnormal skin color, generally bluish or mottled; (2) pilomotor—loss of the piloerection response; (3) trophic—changes in skin texture, delayed dermal healing, slowed nail and hair growth, and atrophy or tapering of the digits; and (4) sudomotor—loss of innervation to the sweat glands. Of

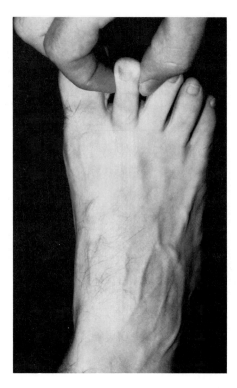

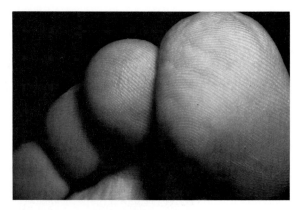

Fig. 14-10. Patient with denervated second digit. Wrinkle test demonstrates lack of skin wrinkling owing to loss of sudomotor function. Note normal wrinkling of skin on the hallux and adjacent toes.

Fig. 14-9. Testing for proprioception at the lesser metatarsophalangeal joint.

these tests, those for sudomotor function are considered the most reliable.

Sudomotor recovery is a hallmark of nerve regeneration. Sweat proliferation and skin wrinkling are both good indicators of autonomic sensibility, and many tests exist for the evaluation of sudomotor function.[17] Since sudomotor function cannot be influenced by the patient, these are the only true objective tests in the battery of sensibility tests. The easiest of these tests to perform is

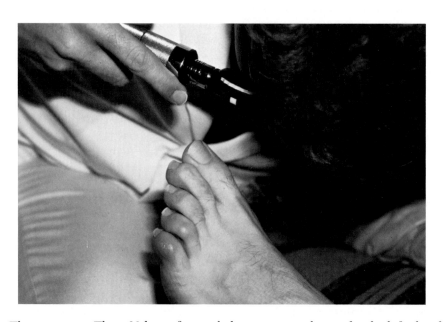

Fig. 14-11. The sweat test. The +20 lens of an opthalmoscope may be used to look for beads of sweat.

the wrinkle test described by O'Riain.[18] Normal skin will wrinkle or shrivel when immersed in warm water (40° C) for 30 minutes. This may fail to occur in a denervated area (Fig. 14-10). In a similar manner, an area may be tested for sweat production. An area placed under a heat lamp for several minutes should produce sweat. Absence of sweat gland function in an area that normally produces sweat may indicate denervation (Fig. 14-11).

Motor Testing

Muscle weakness or paralysis may be present in cases of motor branch laceration or disruption. Motor changes will generally be seen later in less severe injuries. Muscles should be evaluated individually and compared with those of the contralateral extremity. Each muscle should be assessed for mass, tone, and strength. The muscle should also be palpated for any fibrosis or painful areas.

Electrodiagnosis

Electrodiagnosis may be helpful when subjective and objective clinical examination are not definitive. Electrodiagnosis may also be used to help confirm a diagnosis. Sensory evoked potentials may reveal a decreased conduction velocity through the injured nerve, and electromyography may aid in the evaluation of motor deficits.

In summary, the combination of a complete history and neurologic physical examination (with electrodiagnosis as indicated) is a necessity in the consistent evaluation of nerve trauma and pathology.

TREATMENT

The successful treatment of peripheral nerve injuries depends on several factors including patient age, location and degree of severity of the injury, condition of the injured nerve endings including vascularity, delay between the time of injury and treatment, and the skill and training of the surgeon. Initial treatment of a nerve injury should attempt to assess the level of the injury and prevent further compromise. Protection of the injured part with appropriate splinting will allow inspection and testing for neural function. Any concomitant vascular compromise should also be assessed and treated. Further, the mechanism of injury may afford valuable clues to the severity of the neural pathology. In an open wound with a peripheral nerve injury, it is important that the wound be thoroughly cleansed and debrided of any necrotic tissue or foreign debris, so that proper assessment can be made. Severe localized crush injuries, blunt injuries, and missile injuries (e.g., gunshot wounds) pose specific problems including delayed necrosis and damage to adjacent soft tissues. The necessity for further debridement can be predicted in these traumatic instances. Once examination has been completed, a determination can be made whether surgical intervention is necessary.

Conservative Management

Conservative management is most likely indicated in first and second degree nerve injuries (i.e., neurapraxia and axonotmesis with endoneurial tube preservation). Initial management will consist of supportive measures to control any associated edema. Splinting and rest will provide an environment for peripheral nerve recovery. Physical modalities such as massage, passive stretching, heat, ultrasound, and galvanic stimulation can then be instituted to aid in the rehabilitation of the peripheral nerve injury and to prevent muscular atrophy. Regular evaluation should be performed to assess the progression of nerve recovery. Prolonged conservative observation should not be a substitute for surgical intervention when surgery is indicated, as irreversible intraneural and end organ damage may occur.

Surgical Management

When an immediate nerve deficit follows trauma, neural disruption must be suspected (third, fourth, and fifth degree injuries) and surgical intervention is usually indicated. Immediate surgical repair might consist of primary nerve suture (primary neurorrhaphy) or nerve reapproximation for later nerve suture (secondary neurorrhaphy) or nerve grafting. In any degree of nerve injury, significant scarring may occur over time, resulting in significant symptomatology or a conduction deficit. This scarring may be internal or external to the nerve's epineurial sheath and may require resection (neurolysis). Finally, in some nerve injuries, resulting sequelae (e.g., neuroma formation) and symptomatology may require nerve resection to afford relief. Thus, surgery may consist of nerve suture (neurorrhaphy), nerve grafting (nerve reconstruction), nerve scar tissue resection (neurolysis), or nerve resection (neurectomy).

As with any surgical procedure, proper preoperative planning is the key to success. Whenever

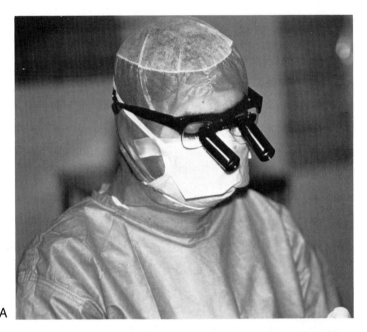

A

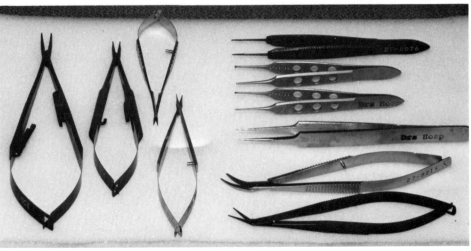

B

Fig. 14-12. (**A**) Loupes. (**B**) Microsurgical instruments.

possible, surgery should be performed utilizing loupes or an operative microscope. Indeed, optimal repair may necessitate the use of a ×10 to ×25 operating microscope and microsurgical instrumentation (Fig. 14-12A and B). The surgeon should plan to approach the region of nerve injury from normal tissue, so that uninjured nerve can be identified proximal and distal to the traumatized site. Any fractures present in the area should be appropriately reduced and stabilized. Careful anatomic dissection with accurate anatomic reapproximation of the injured nerve segments under minimal tension is necessary to produce the optimal surgical result.

Neurorrhaphy

If a significant nerve laceration is identified, immediate primary repair is preferred if at all possible. The repair should be performed with the limb in the extended position, so that the nerve is repaired in the position in which it will be placed under maximal tension. The success of neurorrhaphy is greatest if performed within the first 3 to 7 days following injury. Repairs performed after the first 7 days virtually always require debridement of the nerve ends to eliminate fibrosis and to provide viable fascicles. This debride-

ment will increase the tension needed for primary apposition. Approximately 15 to 20 percent of peripheral nerve lacerations are partial lacerations with essentially complete distal neural deficits.[19] These injuries are also amenable to primary repair. Primary nerve repair (neurorrhaphy) can consist of epineurial (nerve trunk) repair, group fascicular (bundle) repair, or perineurial (fascicular) repair. Debate continues as to which repair is preferable, although theoretically, perineurial neurorrhaphy should provide a superior functional result owing to more accurate anatomic alignment.[4,20]

In epineurial neurorrhaphy, the severed nerve is exposed and loose areolar tissue is dissected away from the circumferential epineurium. Loupes or an operating microscope greatly enhance the accuracy of this procedure. If necessary, the nerve ends are then freshened by sharp dissection. If the nerve ends are under tension when coapted, retraction or stay sutures may be placed to allow neurorrhaphy under minimal tension. The epineurium is then repaired with nonabsorbable sutures (usually 9-0 or 10-0 gauge) in simple interrupted fashion (Figs. 14-13 to 14-15).

In perineurial (fascicular) neurorrhaphy, an operating microscope is necessary. While the nerve

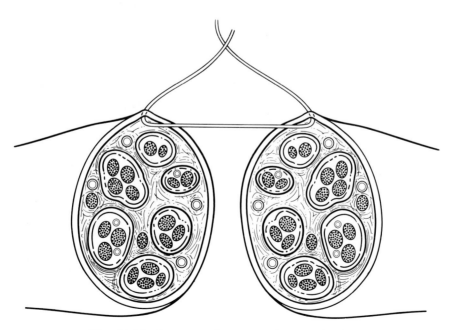

Fig. 14-13. Diagram of epineurial neurorrhaphy.

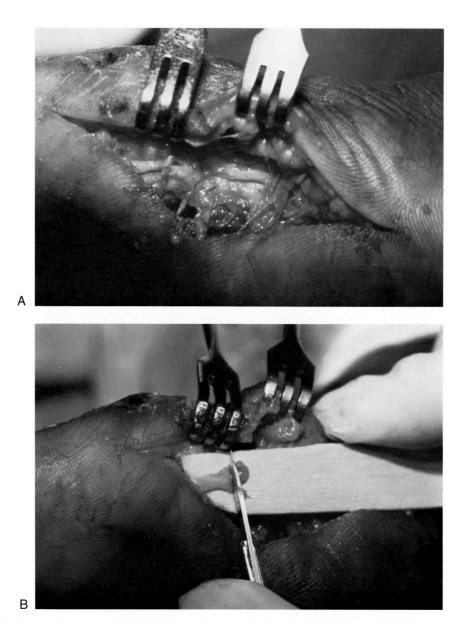

Fig. 14-14. Gross demonstration of epineurial neurorrhaphy in lacerated medial digital nerve of the hallux. **(A)** Lacerated nerve on medial aspect of hallux. **(B)** Freshening nerve ends. (*Figure continues.*)

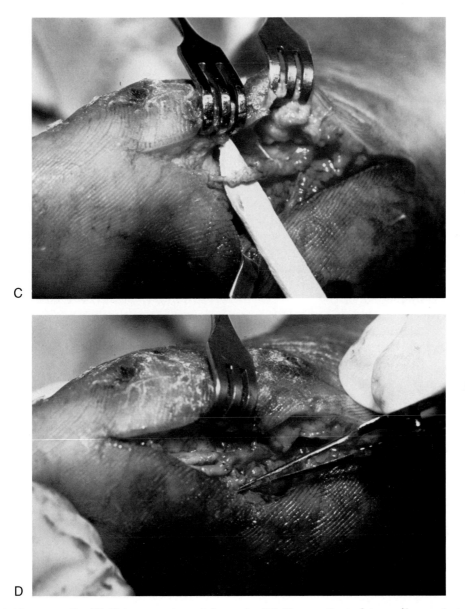

Fig. 14-14 (*Continued*). (**C**) Primary epineurial repair. (**D**) Nerve situated in well-vascularized soft tissue bed.

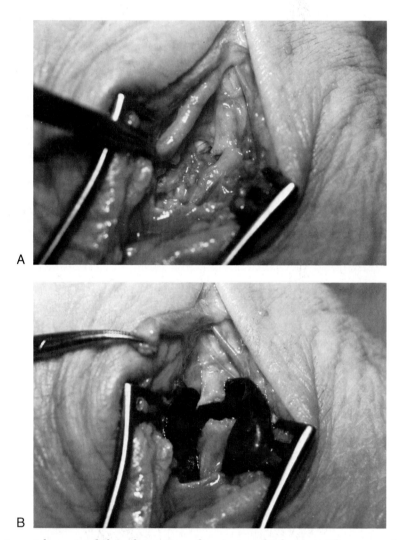

Fig. 14-15. Epineurial repair of clean laceration of posterior tibial nerve. The neurorrhaphy was performed while using loupes for improved visualization. (**A & B**) Laceration identified. (*Figure continues.*)

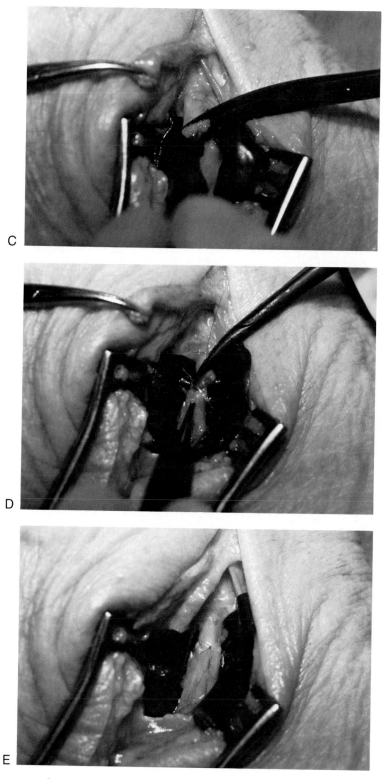

Fig. 14-15 (*Continued*). (**C**) Nerve ends freshened. (**D & E**) Primary epineurial neurorrhaphy.

is visualized through the microscope, the epineurium is incised longitudinally on both sides of the laceration and reflected 1.0 to 1.5 mm to expose the underlying perineurium. The fasciculi are then isolated and trimmed. The surgeon then matches the fasciculi according to size and location and reapproximates them with 10-0 or 11-0 gauge nonabsorbable suture in simple interrupted fashion (Figs. 14-16 and 14-17). The sutures may pass through the epineurium to afford additional strength. If this is not done, the epineurium is closed as a separate layer with nonabsorbable sutures in simple interrupted fashion.

Group fascicular (bundle) repair is similar, with groups of fascicles isolated, matched, and repaired. The bundles or groups of fasciculi are embedded in epineurium. Group fascicular repair involves suturing the epifascicular epineurium around the matched groups of fasciculi together (Fig. 14-18). This can usually be done under magnification with 10-0 nonabsorbable suture. Group fascicular repair is generally less traumatic and less time consuming than perineurial (fascicular) repair.

Following primary neurorrhaphy, the limb is immobilized for 3 weeks, after which active motion and physical therapy are begun.

It is of the utmost importance that primary neurorrhaphy be performed only when the nerve ends can be reapproximated under minimal tension and preferably with the extremity extended.

In some instances, length needed for primary neurorrhaphy may be gained by nerve mobilization, nerve transposition, permanent joint flexure (e.g., by arthrodesis), or removal of bone to effectively shorten the nerve's course. In all instances, it is important that the nerve be protected from further trauma and be maintained in a well-vascularized area away from contact with overlying skin. If there are any suspicions regarding the integrity of the nerve bed, repair should be delayed. This may be the case in the management of severe localized crush or blunt injuries or after missile injuries (e.g., gunshot wounds). In these injuries, the wound is debrided and the injured nerve ends are grossly reapproximated with epineurial sutures to prevent retraction. Definitive nerve repair is delayed until the wound bed is found to be well vascularized and free of necrotic tissue and infection.

If it is not possible to bring the nerve ends completely together, they should be reapproximated as close as possible with epineurial sutures. The nerve ends should not be brought together by repositioning a joint. A nerve should be reapproximated with all joints positioned to create maximal tension on a nerve unless joint function is to be sacrificed by arthrodesis. If this is not done, the initial repair will be disrupted when the joints are allowed to move. The repair will suffer from biomechanical stress, and the growing axons will be injured. One of the most com-

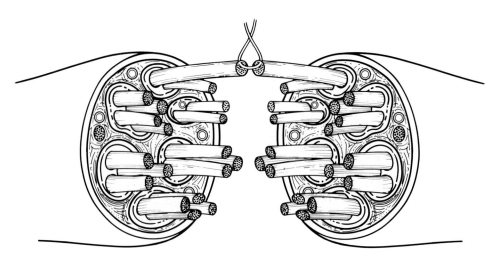

Fig. 14-16. Diagram of perineurial or fascicular neurorrhaphy.

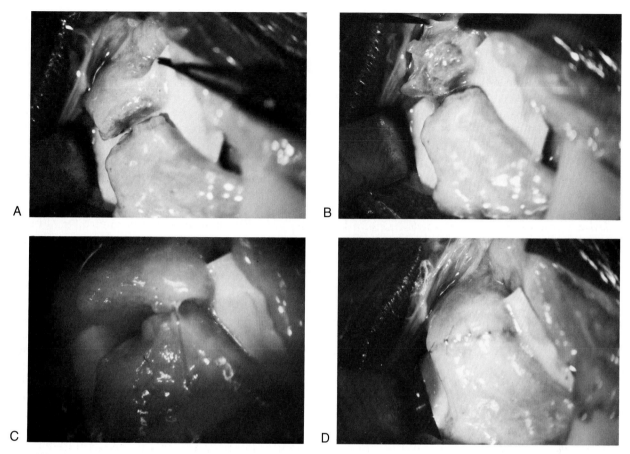

Fig. 14-17. Demonstration of fascicular alignment and repair of lacerated posterior tibial nerve under operative microscope. (**A**) Laceration identified. (**B**) Epineurial sheath reflected. (**C**) Fasciculi matched and reapproximated. (**D**) Epineurial sheath closed.

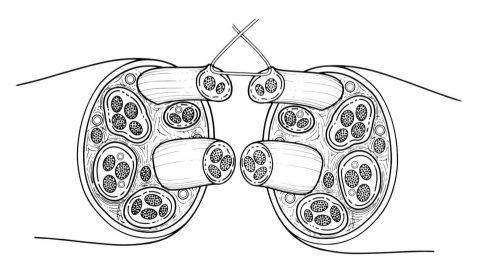

Fig. 14-18. Diagram of group fascicular (bundle) repair.

mon causes of failure of nerve regeneration is too much tension during primary neurorrhaphy of a lacerated nerve.

If primary neurorrhaphy is not possible, secondary neurorrhaphy may be performed later if the wound environment improves and nerve reapproximation can be achieved without tension.

Nerve Reconstruction

Nerve reconstruction may be necessary in instances in which there has been loss of nerve substance or a delay in nerve repair causing retraction of the nerve or scar tissue formation. Experimental and clinical evidence suggests that regenerating axons can cross two suture lines through a nerve graft under minimal tension more easily than they can one suture line with tension.[21,22] Millesi et al. popularized the technique of interfascicular grafting in the forearm.[23] Using their work as a foundation, Hattrup and Wood have recently described their results of interfascicular grafting in the lower extremity.[24] In their series, they utilized the sural nerve from the contralateral uninjured extremity as a group fascicular nerve graft or cable autograft. In practice, any "pure" sensory nerve may be utilized as a graft when a gap must be bridged. The nerve is generally harvested from the contralateral limb to minimize additional sensory loss in the injured extremity. As with primary neurorrhaphy, experi-

ence in a microvascular laboratory is essential before the surgeon can perform the procedure with a reasonable chance of success.

Under magnification, the injured nerve ends are identified and freshened to remove all scar tissue and neuroma formation. The major fascicular groups of the nerve are then identified, and the gap between the nerve ends is assessed. The donor sensory nerve to be used (e.g., sural nerve from the opposite extremity) is then harvested with enough length obtained to create from two to five grafts that are roughly 15 percent longer than the gap distance. The major fascicular groups of the nerve ends are then matched and connected with the donor grafts. The nerve grafts are implanted in a reverse direction. This will reduce axon dissemination through the small branch exits in the nerve. The grafts are sutured in place with 10-0 nonabsorbable suture connecting the epineurium of the graft to the epifascicular epineurium of the fascicular group. Postoperatively, the extremity is immobilized for 3 weeks. Thus, the donor grafts act as cables bridging the gap in the injured nerve and reuniting the fascicles in the proximal and distal nerve segments (Figs. 14-19 and 14-20).

Interfascicular nerve grafting is not a substitute for primary neurorrhaphy and should only be utilized when primary neurorrhaphy is not possible. The technique is difficult and the results are unpredictable. Millesi et al. reported a large series,

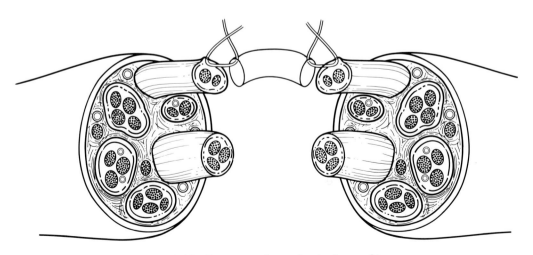

Fig. 14-19. Diagram of interfascicular grafting.

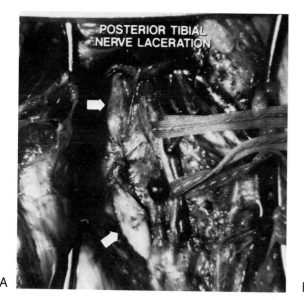

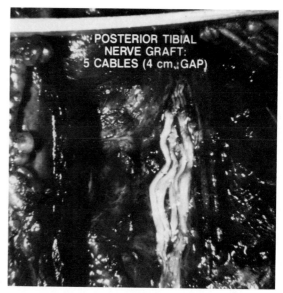

Fig. 14-20. **(A)** Laceration of posterior tibial nerve identified at surgical exploration 3 months after injury. **(B)** Interfascicular nerve grafting of 4-cm gap in nerve with five grafts. (From Hattrup and Wood,[24] with permission.)

but only 16 cases involved a nerve of the lower extremity.[23] Follow-up on three procedures was too short to be evaluated for the return of nerve function. In the remaining 13 procedures, 12 resulted in regeneration of the distal nerve segment. The functional results were good in 10 procedures and were not reported in 2 instances. Hattrup and Wood reported on 13 cases in the lower extremity.[24] They reported five good results (normal motor strength or active motor excursion against mild resistance, no brace or orthosis required; differentiation of deep pain, touch, and temperature with absence of neurotrophic ulceration; and no pain with usual activities or standard footwear), five fair results (active motor excursion with gravity present or eliminated, gait aided by a brace, orthosis, or special shoe; able to detect touch or deep pain but insufficient sensibility to prevent neurotrophic ulceration; hyperpathia improved but still requiring protection or special footwear), and three poor results (trace or no motor function with assisted gait; anesthesia or hypoesthesia identical to the preoperative state in the zone of the nerve distribution; hyperpathia unchanged). In both series, it was concluded that the results were less satis-

factory than primary neurorrhaphy and that the larger the gap site (i.e., the longer the graft), the poorer the expected result.

Neurolysis

Neurolysis involves freeing the nerve trunk or fasciculi from scar tissue and constrictive adhesions that are preventing physiologic nerve conduction, inhibiting the anatomic regeneration of axons, or obstructing the nerve's blood supply. If a previous first degree injury (neurapraxia) or second degree injury (axonotmesis) is not demonstrating satisfactory improvement, exploration with neurolysis may be indicated to facilitate the nerve's recovery. Neurolysis is generally not indicated in third, fourth, or fifth degree injuries unless these have been previously surgically repaired and are demonstrating unsatisfactory recovery.[7] Neurolysis may be either external or internal. External neurolysis involves freeing the entire nerve trunk, while internal neurolysis involves freeing the individual fasciculi from interfascicular scar tissue within the confines of the expineurial sheath.

In 1927, Babcock reported the use of neurolysis in World War I, with noted improvement of nerve function and the relief of pain following external neurolysis.[25] External neurolysis is most frequently needed in injuries that lead to post-traumatic entrapment of the injured nerve. Any open injury may lead to such a result. In external neurolysis, the nerve trunk is separated from the surrounding scar tissue by careful anatomic dissection (Fig. 14-21). Any impinging structures should be addressed. A displaced fracture, joint dislocation, or local hematoma or infection formation are immediate causes of exogenous nerve compression. Excessive soft tissue scarring and bone callus following fracture, malunion, nonunion, or local reaction to a foreign material are frequent residual causes of external nerve pressure.

External neurolysis is performed by approaching the nerve through an incision that allows complete exposure of the nerve in the injured

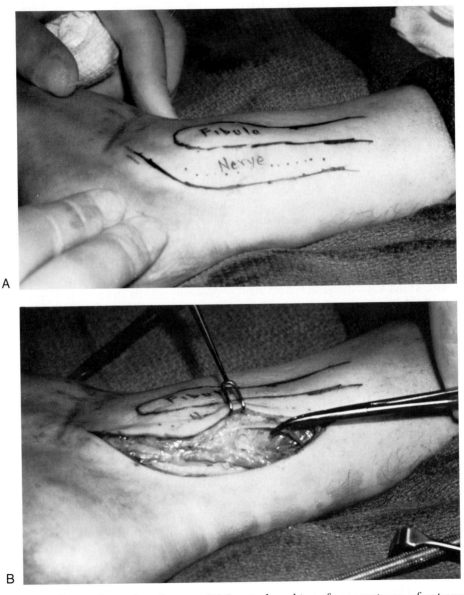

Fig. 14-21. External neurolysis of sural nerve. **(A)** Surgical marking of apparent area of entrapment. **(B)** Sural nerve entrapped in scar tissue. (*Figure continues.*)

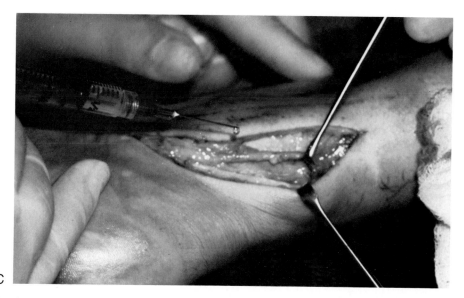

Fig. 14-21 (*Continued*). (**C**) Sural nerve after external neurolysis. Soluble steroid being infiltrated.

area. In most instances, it is preferable to approach the injured area from an area of normal anatomy. Loupes are generally preferred to aid in the visualization of the fine structures composing the adventia of the nerve trunk, especially the segmentally arranged nutrient cords providing vascularity to the nerve trunk. Uninvolved portions of the nerve should be identified proximal and distal to the injured area. Intraoperative direct nerve stimulation may be necessary to assess the degree of nerve fiber function for lesions in continuity. Direct nerve stimulation is useful for mixed nerves with skeletal motor innervation (e.g., the posterior tibial nerve). If indicated, it should be performed prior to nerve mobilization since mild mechanical deformation may result in a transient conduction block (neurapraxia). Active contraction of distal musculature when the nerve is stimulated proximal to the injured segment demonstrates satisfactory regeneration of the nerve. In this instance, external neurolysis (perhaps combined with transposition) should provide adequate facilitation of additional nerve recovery. If distal contraction is absent, intraoperative evoked nerve action potentials (NAPs) may be measured across the injured portion of the nerve. The presence of operative NAPs generally indicates that regeneration of

the nerve is occurring and that only external neurolysis is needed. The absence of operative NAPs suggests the need for internal neurolysis, neurectomy, or resection of the nonconductive nerve segment with primary neurorrhaphy or grafting. Obviously, if the nerve under investigation does not innervate skeletal muscle, direct nerve stimulation would only be useful when NAPs were being measured. In such instances, the decision as to the value of either external or internal neurolysis is primarily based on a visual and palpatory assessment of the nerve trunk. After nerve stimulation or intraoperative clinical assessment, the nerve is carefully mobilized from surrounding scar tissue. Penrose drains may be placed loosely around the nerve to assist in nerve manipulation and to minimize nerve trauma. Care must be taken to avoid damage to the extrinsic vascular system.

Following external neurolysis, the nerve bed should be evaluated. If a tourniquet has been used, it should be deflated. The injured segment of nerve should be maintained in a well-protected, vascularized soft tissue site. If this is not the case, nerve transposition should be considered if the nerve can be mobilized to a more suitable area (Fig. 14-22). Meticulous hemostasis is then obtained, and closed suction drainage may

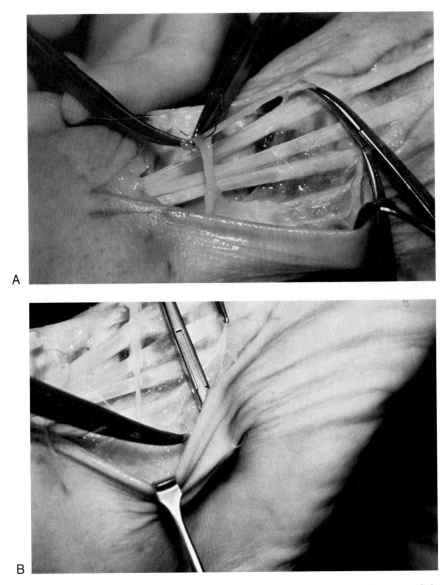

Fig. 14-22. Transposition of intermediate dorsal cutaneous nerve. **(A)** Identification of the nerve. **(B)** Transposition and suture of nerve into a more lateral position and more vascular soft tissue environment.

be used to aid in decreasing postoperative hematoma formation. Prior to wound closure, a small amount of soluble steroid may be infiltrated along the mobilized portion of the nerve trunk to decrease the recurrence of fibrosis. Anatomic wound closure is then performed, leaving the fascia open if there is a significant chance that it might impinge on the healing nerve. Great care

must be taken to support dermal approximation in cases in which the deep fascia is not primarily closed in an effort to avoid dehiscence.

As external neurolysis removes scar tissue from the external area of the nerve, internal neurolysis or endoneurolysis attempts to remove scar tissue from within the nerve. Loupes, or preferably an operating microscope, are mandatory for satisfactory visualization. Internal neurolysis consists of interfascicular (perineurial) scar tissue eradication but does not release intrafascicular (endoneurial) scar tissue.

Internal neurolysis should only be attempted when palpation of the in-continuity nerve trunk reveals induration indicative of intraneural scar formation and the surgeon believes that external neurolysis alone was inadequate. Operative evoked NAPs may have previously been performed and found to have been absent, suggesting the need for internal neurolysis. It is often helpful to inject a small amount of normal saline without preservatives under the epineurial sheath to allow differentiation between normal intraneural architecture and scarred fasciculi that adhere to the epineurial sheath. Care must be taken to avoid injection of saline into the perineurial sheath, as this could result in further damage to the intrafascicular nerve fibers. The injection of saline is no substitute for careful internal neurolysis and will not produce satisfactory internal neurolysis alone.[26] The epineurial sheath is then incised, and the fascicles are gently teased apart with microscissors. Care is taken to preserve the perineurial sheath and anastomosing interfascicular bundles and to minimize damage to the intrinsic microvascular system. Breaching the perineurial tubes or excessive damage to the interfascicular branches or to the microvascular network will induce further hemorrhage, ischemia, and scarring. Microdissection continues until each fascicle is freed from constriction. If a fascicle has been damaged severely enough to preclude satisfactory recovery following internal neurolysis, it may be resected or reconstructed.

Prior to closure, a small amount of soluble steroid may be introduced. As with external neurolysis, transposition of the nerve trunk should be considered if a new and more favorable soft tissue bed can be found. Hemostasis is obtained, and a closed suction drain is used as needed. The epineurial sheath is left open. The remaining layers are closed in anatomic fashion.

Postoperatively, the limb is immobilized for as short a period as possible. Generally, the use of a compression dressing for 7 to 10 days will allow the maximal benefit of decreased postoperative hematoma formation and yet allow early mobility.

Recently, surgical entubation of the injured nerve segment has been suggested as a possible beneficial adjunct.[27] Ideally, such ensheathment of the nerve would prevent further entrapment or scar adherence to the nerve's soft tissue bed. At the same time, it would be hoped that loose areolar and well-vascularized soft tissue would fill the pseudosheath, creating a satisfactory environment for continued nerve regeneration. Malay has specifically discussed the use of 0.02-inch-thick silicone elastomer (Silastic) for nerve trunk entubation in cases of recurrent tarsal tunnel syndrome[28] (Fig. 14-23). He described mixed results, with the main complications being impingement of the nerve trunk by the ensheathing material and the relative nonvascularity of the nerve trunk within the synthetic sheath. Both would certainly be considered major complications in the treatment of the regenerating peripheral nerve, and it remains to be seen whether synthetic or biologic entubation materials will dramatically aid postneurolysis recovery.

Neurectomy

Major peripheral nerve lacerations should be primarily repaired whenever possible. Regretfully, many major peripheral nerve injuries and almost all minor peripheral nerve lacerations are left untreated. Painful entrapment neuromas may result from any nerve injury that is left untreated (Fig. 14-24). The most common method used to prevent painful neuromas in the acute injury is by placing traction on the nerve lesion and sharply cutting it. Hopefully, this would allow the freshly cut end of the nerve to retract into a more protected, untraumatized, and well-vascularized area away from the area of injury and subsequent scar formation. The same basic principle is used for the excision of an intermetatarsal or Morton's neuroma.

Unfortunately, this is not always successful, and additional surgical treatment may be necessary. Such treatment for traumatic neuromas has included operative techniques to inhibit axonal regrowth and transposition away from painful stimuli (Table 14-4). Simple neurectomy, neurectomy with absolute alcohol stump infiltration,[29]

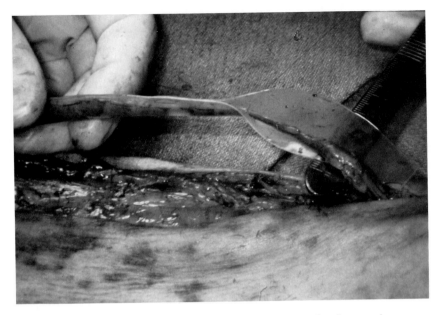

Fig. 14-23. Entubation of posterior tibial nerve with silicone sheet.

neurectomy with nerve transposition,[30,31] and neurectomy with silicone capping[32] have been associated with a high rate of recurrence, with success rates (determined by minimal postoperative pain or tenderness) ranging as low as 25 percent.[33] More recent suggestions including neurectomy with electrocoagulation, neurectomy with laser cautery, or neurectomy with phenol or steroid stump infusion would seem to offer only similar expected results.

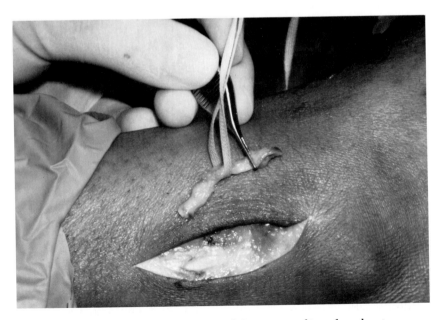

Fig. 14-24. Excised post-traumatic neuroma of the intermediate dorsal cutaneous nerve.

Table 14-4. Surgical Treatment of Traumatic Neuromas

Inhibition of axonal regrowth
   Physical containment (chemical treatment, ligation, cautery)
   Synthetic containment (capping with inert materials)
   Physiologic containment (neurorrhaphy or grafting techniques)

Translocation away from painful stimuli
   Excision and retraction
   Implantation into muscle
   Implantation into bone
   En bloc translocation

Alternatively, en bloc transfer of an intact neuroma[34] or neuroma resection with primary neurorrhaphy or grafting[35] offer considerably higher success rates. Herndon et al. reported 72 percent minimally painful or tender results following en bloc transfer of the intact neuroma with its fibrous scar tissue encapsulation to an adjacent area that was more protective and free from scar tissue.[34] This soft tissue bed may consist of muscle, fatty tissue, or cancellous bone. As mentioned earlier, Hattrup and Wood reported that 77 percent (10 of 13) of their patients had diminished symptomatology following neuroma resection with interfascicular grafting.[24]

Ideally, neurectomy alone should not be a substitute when nerve reconstruction is feasible. Since many different causes exist for peripheral nerve entrapment,[16] it remains to be seen which form of treatment will be most appropriate for post-traumatic nerve entrapment.

SUMMARY

The long-term sequelae of nerve injuries have been studied and described in detail following virtually every war period. Awareness of this frequently debilitating form of trauma should cause the traumatologist to increase the index of suspicion for nerve injury when managing any soft tissue or osseous trauma. With recent advances in microsurgical technique, more accurate anatomic reapposition and reconstruction of neural elements is possible. Although still a developing science, the proper management of peripheral nerve injuries will frequently be the determining factor in the successful recovery from virtually any traumatic injury.

ACKNOWLEDGEMENT

I thank Larry Stein for his assistance in medical illustration.

REFERENCES

1. Battista AF, Lusskin R: The anatomy and physiology of the peripheral nerve. Foot Ankle 7:65, 1986
2. Thomas PK: The connective tissue of peripheral nerve: an electron microscope study. J Anat 97:35, 1963
3. Olsson Y, Kristensson K: Permeability of blood vessels and connective tissue sheaths of the peripheral nervous system to exogenous proteins. Acta Neuropathol, suppl., V: 61–69, 1971
4. Urbaniak JR: Fascicular nerve suture. Clin Orthop 163:57, 1982
5. Krajevic K: The connective tissue sheath of the frog sciatic nerve. Q J Exp Physiol 39:55, 1954
6. Ochoa J, Fowler TJ, Gilliatt RW: Anatomical changes in peripheral nerves compressed by a pneumatic tourniquet. J Anat 113:433, 1972
7. Sunderland S: Nerve and Nerve Injuries. 2nd Ed. p. 12. Churchill Livingstone, New York, 1978
8. Lundberg G: Ischemic nerve injury: experimental studies on intraneural microvascular pathophysiology and nerve function in a limb subjected to temporary circulatory arrest. Scand J Plast Reconstr Surg, suppl., 6: 1–106, 1970
9. Benjamin HA, Nagler W: Peripheral nerve damage resulting from local hemorrhage and ischemia. Arch Phys Med Rehabil 54:263, 1973
10. Lundborg G: Limb ischemia and nerve injury. Arch Surg 104:631, 1972
11. Seddon HJ: Classification of nerve injuries. Br Med J 2:237, 1942
12. Seddon HJ: Three types of nerve injuries. Brain 66:237, 1943
13. Sunderland S: A classification of peripheral nerve injuries producing loss of function. Brain 74:491, 1951

14. Lusskin R, Battista A: Evaluation and therapy after injury to peripheral nerves. Foot Ankle 7:71, 1986

15. Omer GE: Sensibility testing. p. 3. In Omer GE, Jr., Spinner M (eds): Management of Peripheral Nerve Problems. WB Saunders, Philadelphia, 1980

16. Malay DS, McGlamry ED, Nava CA: Entrapment neuropathies of the lower extremities. p. 668. In McGlamry ED (ed): Comprehensive Textbook of Foot Surgery. Vol. 2. Williams & Wilkins, Baltimore, 1987

17. Waylett-Rendall J: Sensibility evaluation and rehabilitation. Orthop Clin North Am 19:43, 1988

18. O'Riain S: New and simple test of nerve function in the hand. Br Med J 3:615, 1973

19. Kline DG: Operative experience with major lower extremity nerve lesions, including the lumbosacral plexus and the sciatic nerve. p. 607. In Omer GE, Jr., Spinner M (eds): Management of Peripheral Nerve Problems. WB Saunders, Philadelphia, 1980

20. Tupper JW, Crick JC, Matteck LR: Fascicular nerve repairs: a comparative study of epineurial and fascicular (perineurial) techniques. Orthop Clin North Am 19:57, 1988

21. Terzis JK, Faibisoff B, Williams HB: The nerve gap: suture under tension vs. graft. Plast Reconstr Surg 56:166, 1975

22. Yoshihiro M, Watari S, Tsuge K: Experimental studies on the effects of tension on intraneural microcirculation in sutured peripheral nerves. Plast Reconstr Surg 63:398, 1979

23. Millesi H, Meissi G, Berger A: The interfascicular nerve-grafting of the median and ulner nerves. J Bone Joint Surg 54A:727, 1972

24. Hattrup SJ, Wood MB: Delayed neural reconstruction in the lower extremity: results of interfascicular nerve grafting. Foot Ankle 7:105, 1986

25. Babcock WW: A standard technique for operations on peripheral nerves with special reference to the closure of large gaps. Surg Gynecol Obstet 45:364, 1927

26. Brown BA: Internal neurolysis in traumatic peripheral nerve lesions in continuity. Surg Clin North Am 52:1167, 1972

27. Mackinnon SE, Dellon AL, Hudson AR, Hunter DA: Nerve regeneration through a pseudosynovial sheath in a primate model. Plast Reconstr Surg 75:833, 1985

28. Malay DS: Update: peripheral entrapment neuropathy. p. 153. In McGlamry ED (ed): Reconstructive Surgery of the Foot and Leg. Update '88. Podiatry Institute Publishing Company, Tucker, GA, 1988

29. Pinto VADC, Junqueira LCU: A comparative study for the methods of prevention of amputation neuroma. Surg Gynecol Obstet 99:492, 1954

30. Mackinnon SE, Dellon AL, Hudson AR, Hunter DA: Alteration of neuroma formation by manipulation of its microenvironment. Plast Reconstr Surg 76:345, 1985

31. Mass DP, Ciano MC, Tortosa R et al: Treatment of painful hand neuromas by their transfer into bone. Plast Reconstr Surg 74:182, 1984

32. Swanson AB, Boere NR, Biddulph SL: Silicone-rubber capping of amputation neuromas—investigational and clinical experience. Int Clin Inform Bull 11:1, 1972

33. Tupper JW, Booth NM: Treatment of painful neuromas of sensory nerves in the hand: a comparison of traditional and newer methods. J Hand Surg 1:144, 1976

34. Herndon JH, Eaton RG, Littler JW: Management of painful neuromas in the hand. J Bone Joint Surg 58A:369, 1976

35. Kline DG, Nulsen FE: The neuroma in continuity: its preoperative and operative management. Surg Clin North Am 52:1189, 1972

15

Management of Vascular Trauma

Nicholas Daly, D.P.M., M.S.

Acute injuries to the anterior tibial, posterior tibial, and peroneal arteries account for approximately 2 to 3 percent of all civilian acute arterial injuries.[1] The vast majority of these injuries reported in the literature involve injuries to the leg and not the foot and ankle. Consequently, the diagnosis and treatment of vascular trauma at or below the ankle has been only briefly mentioned or completely overlooked in the literature. Extrapolation of the principles of management of vascular trauma in the leg to include vascular trauma at or below the ankle may be assumed by some investigators but has never been demonstrated. Therefore, the guidelines for treatment in this chapter are drawn almost exclusively from those formulated for management of acute vascular trauma to the leg.

ANATOMY

The posterior tibial, anterior tibial, and peroneal arteries supply the foot and ankle. The anterior tibial artery becomes the dorsalis pedis artery as it passes the ankle joint line. The dorsalis pedis gives off the anterior medial and lateral malleolar arteries and lateral and medial tarsal arteries and terminates in the first dorsal metatarsal and arcuate arteries as it passes from proximal to distal. It runs with the deep peroneal nerve and is usually palpable between the extensor hallucis longus and extensor digitorum longus tendon as it courses over the navicular and second cuneiform. The dorsalis pedis may be absent or greatly attenuated in 12 percent of the population, leaving the perforating branch of the peroneal artery to supply the dorsum of the foot.[2]

The posterior tibial artery passes the ankle joint line from the leg in the fourth compartment of the tarsal tunnel. The fourth compartment also contains two accompanying veins and the posterior tibial nerve, which runs lateral to the artery. As it passes behind the medial malleolus, the neurovascular bundle lies posterior to the tunnel of the flexor digitorum longus and superficial and medial to the tendon of the flexor hallucis longus. The artery and vein continue medial to the nerve. At or approaching the sustentaculum tali, the posterior tibial artery divides into the medial and lateral plantar arteries, dividing above and below, respectively, the transverse intermuscular septum. The transverse intermuscular septum originates from the fascia of the abductor hallucis and inserts into the inferior border of the flexor hallucis longus.

Prior to bifurcating, the posterior tibial artery gives off an anastomotic branch to the posterior peroneal artery, the posteromedial malleolar artery, calcaneal rami to the medial heel of calcaneus, and the artery of the tarsal canal.

The lateral plantar artery is usually the largest of the two terminal divisions of the posterior tibial artery and remains posterolateral to the lateral plantar nerve as it courses obliquely across the foot. The artery then divides into the superficial and deep branches. The deep transverse portion curves medially and inosculates with the deep plantar branch of the dorsalis pedis artery to form the deep plantar arch. The superficial branch contributes to the superficial plantar arch by anastomosing with the superficial branch of the medial plantar artery. The medial plantar artery continues anteriorly in the medial compartment of the foot under the abductor hallucis muscle and then divides into superficial and deep branches. The superficial branch contributes to the superficial plantar arch. The deep branch divides into a tibial and lateral branch that usually anastomose with the first plantar metatarsal artery and the tibial segment of the deep plantar arch, respectively.[3]

In the leg, the peroneal artery divides into posterior and anterior branches. The anterior or perforating branch pierces the interosseous membrane and passes anteriorly over the anterior aspect of the distal tibiofibular syndesmosis behind the peronus tertius tendon. It anastomoses with the anterior lateral malleolar artery and contributes to the lateral malleolar vascular anastomotic network. Huber found that the perforating peroneal continued as the dorsalis pedis in 3 percent of his specimens.[2] He also described an anastomotic artery between the anterior tibial and perforating peroneal arteries about 5 cm above the ankle joint in 50 percent.

The posterior peroneal artery continues distally in the compartment of the flexor hallucis longus and gives off two anastomotic branches, the medial and lateral. The medial transverse branch anastomoses with a similar branch from the posterior tibial artery. The anterolateral branch runs transversely to anastomose with the anterolateral malleolar artery, thereby contributing to the formation of the transverse perimalleolar arterial circle.

ETIOLOGY

Vascular trauma can be divided into two broad categories, blunt and penetrating. Most series reporting on civilian trauma since 1980 have shown a 57 to 86 percent incidence of penetrating wounds as the cause of injury to the lower ex-

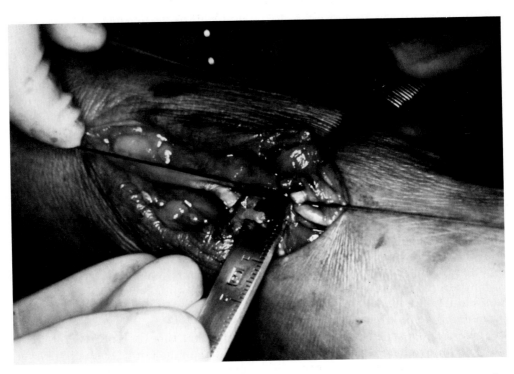

Fig. 15-1. Concomitant laceration of the dorsalis pedis artery and extensor hallucis longus tendon. The dorsalis pedis artery (under scalpel) was ligated and the tendon was repaired.

tremity.[4–9] In the foot, these injuries can range from a small puncture wound or laceration to a high-velocity gunshot wound.

Blunt trauma in civilian injuries most commonly results from automobile or motorcycle accidents. The artery and surrounding tissues are crushed or contused, resulting in hemorrhage or arterial thrombus. Hemorrhage may cause compartment syndrome requiring decompression. The surrounding soft tissue may become nonviable, presenting difficulties with infection, soft tissue coverage, or bone healing. For these reasons, blunt trauma may be a more difficult management problem.

Figure 15-1 illustrates penetrating trauma involving laceration of the dorsalis pedis artery and a concomitant laceration of the extensor hallucis longus tendon. A 1.5-cm laceration caused by a piece of glass had been sustained to the dorsum of the midfoot. The patient was able to stop the bleeding at home with direct pressure prior to coming to the emergency room. A patent posterior tibial pulse was noted, and laceration of the dorsalis pedis artery had not caused vascular compromise. At surgery, the dorsalis pedis artery was ligated and the extensor hallucis longus tendon was repaired. There was no involvement of the deep peroneal nerve.

DIAGNOSIS

Immediate management consists of stopping active bleeding by gentle manual compression. Most researchers do not advocate the use of a tourniquet as this may further compromise ischemic tissue.[1,10,11] One should also avoid clamping the bleeding vessel if contemplating later surgical repair as this will cause further injury. Embedded objects are rarely, if ever, removed in the emergency room since they may be preventing further bleeding. The injured extremity should be kept horizontal as elevation may further compromise an ischemic foot. Once hemostasis has been obtained, a thorough history and physical examination should be performed to identify any life-threatening or other associated injuries.

A complete physical examination of the foot

and ankle should then be performed. If there is a wound in the vicinity of one of the major pedal blood vessels, the physician must assume that a vascular injury has occurred.[11] The pedal pulses should be palpated, and a Doppler examination should be performed if none are found. A palpable pulse does not ensure the absence of a proximal arterial injury.[1,4,8] An ankle brachial index is obtained to assess perfusion pressure and allow intraoperative and postoperative monitoring of the vascular repair. Even if pulses are present, the foot should be observed for signs of compartment syndrome as a venous laceration or arterial bleeding from a branch of one of the main pedal arteries may cause vascular compromise. These changes may not appear immediately but rather may appear hours or even days later.

A thorough neurologic examination must be performed. The dorsalis pedis and posterior tibial arteries run in close proximity to the deep peroneal and posterior tibial nerve, respectively, which may also have been traumatized. Loss of sensitivity is one of the earliest signs of compartment syndrome.[12]

The skin, too, must be completely inspected. If the injury is a laceration, assess the level of contamination. If blunt trauma was involved, assess the amount of skin that may become nonviable and require some form of soft tissue coverage.

Obtain at least anteroposterior and lateral radiographs and update the patient's tetanus prophylaxis as necessary. Prophylactic antibiotic therapy should be instituted in the emergency room if necessary after the wound has been initially assessed.

If there is any question about the viability of the foot, obtain a vascular surgery consultation immediately. Angiography may be necessary to assess the extent of vascular trauma.

CONSERVATIVE MANAGEMENT

Forefoot vascular injuries are rarely surgically repaired. A possible exception would be complete amputation of a digit or larger portion of the forefoot in a child.[13] Unlike the hand, in which digital neurovascular structures are often repaired to restore adequate function to a finger, the function of the foot is not severely compromised by the loss of a digit. In fact, the hallux is sometimes removed and used to replace the thumb in hand reconstruction. Basic principles of wound irrigation, debridement, and primary, delayed primary, or secondary closure described elsewhere should be followed.

With trauma to one of the major pedal arteries in the rear foot, most clinicians believe that conservative treatment may be employed if the foot is viable and that collaterals will eventually develop.[14–17] This is especially true with penetrating trauma. Blunt trauma, however, may require more aggressive care.

Shah et al. studied the outcome of largely blunt trauma resulting in an isolated tibial artery injury.[18] They treated 29 patients, 25 of which had blunt trauma. Nine of these injuries were immediately and successfully reconstructed because of acute ischemia or bleeding. The remaining 20 patients were deemed to have viable feet and their injuries were not immediately reconstructed. Of these 20 patients, 3 required primary amputation. Fifteen of the remaining 17 required further radiographic evaluation for arterial reconstruction 2 to 12 months later for nonhealing of wounds, malunion of fractures, and soft tissue defects. These delayed reconstructions were more difficult to perform and required autogenous vein bypass surgery. Eventually, 13 of the feet were made viable. Shah et al. noted that blunt trauma injuries to the tibial arteries behave differently from low-velocity penetrating injuries because of loss of compartmental blood supply and associated injuries.[18] They concluded that in blunt arterial trauma injuries, a single anterior or posterior tibial artery should be repaired immediately. If only the peroneal artery is injured, it may be safer to observe. Two or more injured tibial vessels must be repaired immediately irrespective of how the foot looks.

SURGICAL MANAGEMENT

As mentioned previously, penetrating trauma causing injury to one of the three major pedal arteries is almost always treated nonsurgically or, if surgery is elected to repair other structures, by ligation. However, the dorsalis pedis artery is very small or absent in 12 percent of the cases and the posterior tibial artery may be hypoplastic in some cases.[2] Consequently, even after an isolated penetrating trauma to one of the three arteries, the foot should be observed very closely for signs of ischemia.

Surgical repair may be elected in cases of blunt, isolated tibial artery injury and is required in instances of injury to two or more of the pedal arteries.[18] In these situations, consultation with a vascular surgeon should be obtained immediately. In most cases a preoperative angiogram is performed. However, this may take a minimum of 2 hours and may be foregone if the foot is in immediate danger.

Method of Repair

Options for surgical repair at the pedal level include end-to-end anastomosis and autogenous vein grafting.[8,10] At the level of the midfoot and rear foot the average diameter of the dorsalis pedis artery is 2 to 3 mm with an average diameter at the upper limit of the extensor retinaculum of 2.79 mm.[3] The posterior tibial artery is slightly larger (2.3 to 3 mm), and the peroneal artery is slightly smaller (1.9 mm). Arteries of this size may be repaired without the aid of optical magnification devices such as loupes or microsurgical instruments, although these devices are very helpful.[19] Monofilament polypropylene suture of size 6-0 or 7-0 is usually sufficient. Most investigators recommend interrupted rather than continuous sutures in vessels under 5 mm diameter to avoid the purse-string effect.[10,20] After the vessel ends are identified, atraumatic vascular clamps are applied. The vessel ends are debrided and then irrigated with heparinized saline to remove thrombi.

The technique of anastomosis begins with the placement of two sutures placed anteriorly 120 degrees from each other in relationship to the circumference of the vessel wall (Fig. 15-2). This allows the posterior wall of the vessel (240 degrees) to fall away and not be accidentally caught much difference in large vessels but becomes more important as the vessels get smaller. One end of each of these "stay" sutures is left long. Interrupted sutures are then placed between these stay sutures. The long ends of the stay sutures are then used to rotate the vessel, exposing the posterior wall. A third stay suture is then placed between the first two, and one end of this suture is cut long. Interrupted sutures are then placed between the three stay sutures, and all ends are cut short.

When the anastomosis is complete the vascular clamps are released. Doppler studies may be used to document flow if the vessel is large enough.

If, after adequate debridement of the vessel ends, an end-to-end anastomosis is not possible, then autogenous saphenous vein grafting is usually employed. The vein on the opposite leg is commonly used to preserve superficial venous flow on the injured side. The saphenous vein near the ankle is often recommended because the more proximal part may be needed later to provide a sufficiently long segment for remote bypass or proximal venous repair.[10]

Sequence of Repair

There is disagreement whether fractures should be stabilized before or after vascular repair. The recent trend has been toward revascularization before fracture fixation if the bony fragments are not grossly displaced.[5,6,8,15,21] The choice of fixation depends on the type of wound and the surgeon's preference. When applied to the long bones of the leg, external fixation (Fig. 15-3) might offer some advantages in wounds with extensive soft tissue damage including less tissue destruction, ease of wound care, and shorter operative time. However, neither fixation technique seems detrimental to ultimate healing.[8] The advantages of vascular repair prior to fracture stabilization are that restoration of flow to ischemic tissue is not further delayed and that the vascular repair can be performed without interference from fixation devices.[10]

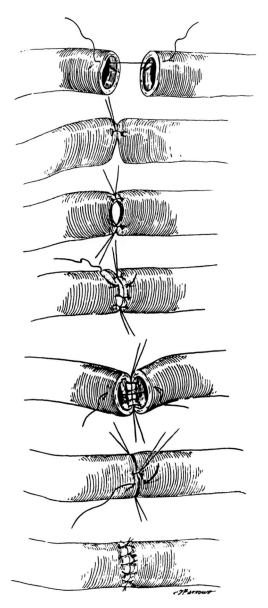

Fig. 15-2. Steps in the end-to-end anastomosis of small arteries and microarteries. (From Silber,[20] with permission.)

with any of the subsequent stitches. Silber emphasizes the point as being no different from that originally suggested by the Nobel prize-winning Alexis Carrel in 1905 but states that many surgeons neglect this advice and place their first two sutures at 180 degrees.[20] This does not make

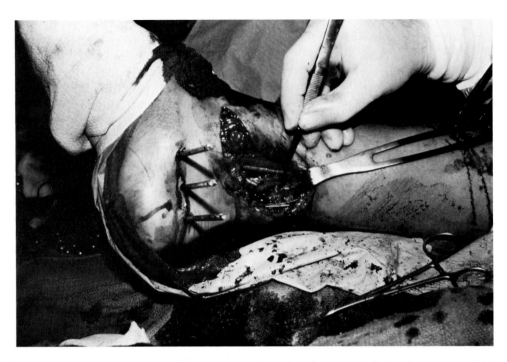

Fig. 15-3. Laceration of the posterior tibial artery. Note the placement of pins for an external fixation device. The external fixator was applied after vascular repair was performed. (Courtesy of Barry L. Scurran, D.P.M.)

Postoperative Management

The principles of soft tissue injury management should be followed. Early and possibly frequent debridement as well as early soft tissue coverage may be necessary when there is significant soft tissue damage. A plastic surgeon should be consulted if any extensive reconstruction is planned. The use of porcine xenografts for temporary coverage followed by split-thickness skin grafting, ideally within 4 to 5 days, is an approach advocated by several researchers.[8,15,18,22,23] Most investigators do not believe that postoperative heparinization is necessary; however, the extremity should be observed closely for any signs of ischemia.

COMPARTMENT SYNDROME

Acute compartment syndrome is a well-described clinical entity resulting from increased pressure within an osseofascial compartment. In the leg, compartment syndrome is commonly encountered after either blunt or penetrating trauma, and fasciotomy is liberally used for compartmental decompression. However, there have been few reports of pedal compartment syndrome and little has been written about the proper technique for decompression. Failure to recognize and promptly decompress the affected compartments may lead to acute ischemia with myoneural necrosis. In the foot this could result in a clawfoot deformity with permanent loss of function, contracture, weakness, and sensory disturbances.[24–27]

Kamel and Sakla divided the foot into four compartments (Fig. 15-4)—central, medial, lateral, and interosseous.[28] The central compartment is bounded superficially by the central segment of the plantar aponeurosis, laterally and medially by the lateral and medial intermuscular septae, and dorsally by the tarsometatarsal skeleton and interosseous fascia. This compartment contains the flexor digitorum brevis muscle, the

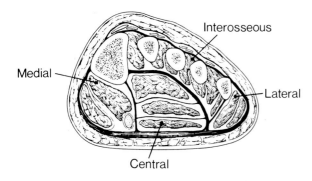

Fig. 15-4. Compartments of foot illustrated with their muscular contents through a coronal section at level of base of metatarsals. (From Myerson,[49] with permission.)

flexor digitorum longus tendons and the four lumbricals, the quadratus plantae muscle, the adductor hallucis muscle, the peroneus longus tendon, and the plantar segment of the tibialis posterior tendon.

The medial compartment is bounded superficially and medially by the medial segment of the plantar aponeurosis, laterally by the medial intermuscular septum, and dorsally by the inferior surface of the first metatarsal shaft. The space contains the abductor hallucis and flexor hallucis muscles and the flexor hallucis longus tendon. The terminal portions of the peroneus longus and tibialis posterior tendons are also in this compartment.

The lateral compartment is bounded superficially and laterally by the lateral segment of the plantar aponeurosis and medially by the lateral intermuscular septum. The space contains the abductor, short flexor, and opponens muscles of the little toe.

The interosseous compartment is limited below by the interossei fascia and above by the central metatarsals and contains the interossei muscles.

Pathophysiology

Increased compartment pressure resulting in myoneural necrosis usually results from muscle

edema and not hemorrhage.[29] Causes of muscle edema include direct trauma, proximal venous occlusion, or reperfusion of ischemic muscle. The precise mechanism of the compartment syndrome at the cellular level is still poorly understood. Several factors including increased capillary permeability, cellular swelling, and production of oxygen-derived free radicals may be involved.

Perry noted that although hemorrhage may abruptly raise the compartment pressure, more often compartment syndromes are delayed and follow a period of ischemia.[29] The resistance of different tissues to ischemia becomes an important factor in determining which structures are most affected by the compartment syndrome. It appears that skeletal muscle and peripheral nerves do not tolerate ischemia well, while skin and subcutaneous tissue fare better.[12,30,31]

Studies of skeletal and cardiac muscle have demonstrated that red and white blood cells become swollen after a period of ischemia.[32,33] Other workers have found that the capillary becomes narrower secondary to compression by swollen blood cells and formation of intravascular blebs of injured capillary endothelium.[34,35] The combination of capillary narrowing and cellular swelling can lead to trapping of red and white blood cells in the narrow capillaries and play an important role in tissue damage and irreversibility.[36–39]

Willerson et al. demonstrated that mannitol infusion could reduce cell swelling in myococardium and perhaps preserve capillary patency.[39] Recent studies have demonstrated that mannitol is a scavenger of oxygen-derived free radicals.[33] These free radicals are thought to damage cell membranes, leading to increased capillary and cell membrane permeability and thereby increasing compartmental pressure.[32] Shah and coworkers demonstrated a fivefold reduction in the need for fasciotomies in patients with blunt arterial trauma by decreasing the muscle edema that results from reperfusing ischemic muscle with mannitol.[16] An intravenous bolus of 100 ml of 20 percent mannitol was given immediately before flow was restored, followed by a constant infusion of 10 g of mannitol per hour for 6 to 24 hours.

Etiology

Compartment syndrome is usually associated with trauma, either direct or indirect. Mubarak and Hargens state that fractures are the leading cause of compartment syndrome.[12] Indirect injuries that result in the ischemia-reperfusion syndrome may also cause compartment syndrome.[12,30] Perry states that the true incidence of compartment syndrome or its complications is unknown, partly because of the inconsistencies in the criteria used to establish the diagnosis, and also because prophylactic fasciotomies are sometimes performed to prevent ischemia.[29]

Diagnosis

The "six Ps" have classically been used to diagnose compartment syndrome.

Pain
This is described as out of proportion to that expected from a particular type of injury and is usually described as a deep, throbbing, unrelenting pressure. If pain is absent, an overlying neural deficit is usually involved.

Pressure
A swollen, tense compartment is often the earliest objective finding. This tenseness may be masked by subcutaneous edema.

Pain with Stretch
When one of the muscles in the involved compartment is stretched, pain may be noted. This is not a very specific test since all patients with fractures or contusions will have pain. Additionally, some patients with compartment syndrome may not have any pain owing to nerve ischemia.

Paresis
Muscle weakness is also very difficult to assess and may result from guarding secondary to pain, primary muscle ischemia, or nerve involvement.

Paresthesia
Sensory deficit is the most reliable physical finding provided the patient is conscious. As compartment pressure increases, anesthesia will result.

Pulses Present
An increased compartment pressure will usually not be enough to compress a major artery. Additionally, in the foot, the posterior tibial pulse is palpated just posterior to the medial malleolus and before the artery enters the compartments involved, so unless there is a more proximal arterial injury the pulse will usually be palpable (even if there is a more proximal arterial injury, the pulse may still be palpable.)

Measurement of Intracompartmental Pressure

A variety of techniques have been utilized for the measurement of intracompartmental pressure including the needle technique, infusion technique, wick catheter, and slit catheter.[40–45] The wick and slit catheters are presently the two most widely used methods. The slit catheter is a modification of the wick catheter and has the advantage of being less prone to coagulation, and of more uniform manufacture. Both the wick and slit catheters can be used for continuous monitoring. The recent development of solid-state transducers that have been placed into catheter tips has simplified the measurement of compartment pressure. There is less artifact, greater reproducibility, and ease of repeated measurement.[31]

Mubarak and Hargens have identified three groups of patients in whom measurement of intracompartmental pressure is especially indicated.[12] These include (1) uncooperative or unreliable patients, including children who may be frightened, making a careful neurologic examination difficult, or adults under the influence of alcohol or other drugs; (2) unresponsive patients; and (3) patients with a nerve deficit attributable to other causes. It may be hard to differentiate a neuropraxia secondary to stretch or contusion from neurologic deficits resulting from increased intracompartmental pressures. Mubarak and Hargens also recommend the measurement of intracompartmental pressures whenever clinical signs and symptoms are absent or confusing.

Indications for Fasciotomy

If the surgeon is clinically uncertain whether a compartment syndrome exists, then intracompartmental pressures should be measured. Mubarak and Hargens recommend fasciotomy if the intracompartmental pressure is greater than 30 mmHg combined with other positive clinical findings.[12] Rorabeck et al., using the slit catheter technique, also recommend decompression with pressure at or above 30 to 40 mmHg.[45] Matsen and colleagues noted that there was great individual variance in tolerance of increased tissue pressure and recommended fasciotomy above 45 mmHg assuming normal peripheral vasculature, adequate blood volume, and normal blood pressure.[30] Perry concluded that there is no unanimity to the absolute levels above which fasciotomy should be performed and below which it should not.[29] He concluded that near 40 to 45 mmHg, with appropriate clinical findings, fasciotomy is indicated but higher than normal pressures in a totally asymptomatic, alert, and cooperative patient may be safely observed.

Technique of Pedal Fasciotomy

Grodinski in 1929[46] and later Loeffler and Ballard[47] advocated a long plantar medial incision for decompression of deep pedal infections (Fig. 15-5). Mubarak and Hargens proposed two dorsal longitudinal incisions over the metatarsals (Fig. 15-6).[48] Utilizing cadaver specimens, Myerson attempted to test the efficacy of both these methods.[49] He concluded that the medial approach decompressed the tissues more rapidly and was preferable in the absence of fractures requiring stabilization. The dorsal procedure was preferred when there were metatarsal or tarsometatarsal fractures to be reduced or if the surgeon felt uncomfortable with the anatomy of the plantar aspect of the foot.

In their case report of an isolated compartment syndrome of the foot, Bonuti and Bell used the plantar medial approach.[50] Their patient was a 66-year-old woman who sustained a crush injury of the left foot in a motor vehicle accident. On initial examination, positive physical findings included weakness of dorsiflexion and plantar flex-

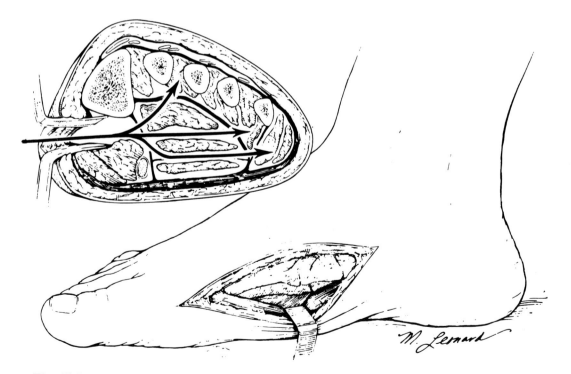

Fig. 15-5. Fasciotomy via medial longitudinal incision. (From Myerson,[49] with permission.)

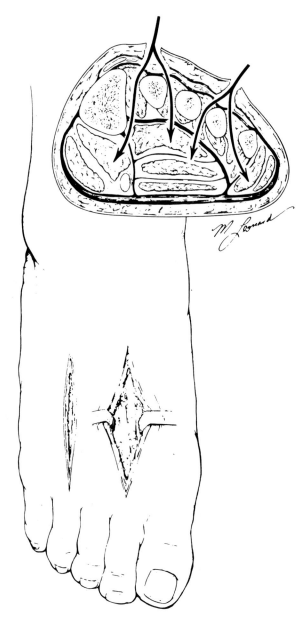

Fig. 15-6. Fasciotomy via double incision, dorsal approach. (From Myerson,[49] with permission.)

ion of the toes and a pale appearance of the toes. Dorsalis pedis and posterior tibial pulses and sensory examination were normal.

Subsequently, severe, rapidly increasing pain and increased swelling of the plantar aspect of the foot developed, with loss of motor function to the toes. Sensation to the forefoot and toes was decreased and a plantar intracompartmental pressure of 60 mmHg developed. The patient was immediately taken to the operating room and decompressed by the plantar medial approach. The wound was packed open, a split-thickness skin graft was subsequently applied, and the patient had an uneventful postoperative course.

LATE SEQUELAE OF VASCULAR TRAUMA

Late sequelae associated with vascular injuries include false aneurysms and arteriovenous fistulas.

False aneurysms occur when vessel wall disruption is walled off but not surgically repaired. The vessel wall may become weak, enlarge in this area, and possibly spontaneously rupture.

An arteriovenous malformation secondary to trauma is shown in serial angiograms of a woman who had stepped on a piece of glass 24 months prior to presentation (Fig. 15-7). Subsequently, an arteriovenous malformation developed between the medial branch of the posterior tibial artery and the medial marginal vein that diverted blood prematurely into the greater saphenous vein. The arteries and veins involved in the malformation were surgically ligated.

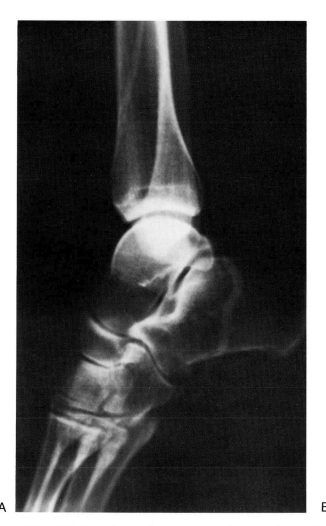
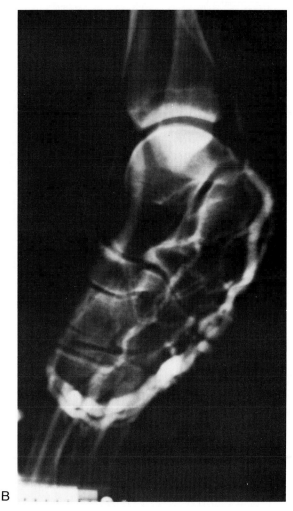

A

B

Fig. 15-7. (A–C) Serial angiograms showing the medial plantar aspect of the arch viewed 14 months after patient stepped on a piece of glass. Note filling of the posterior tibial artery followed by the medial marginal and saphenous veins. (Courtesy of Michael Petersen, M.D.) (*Figure continues.*)

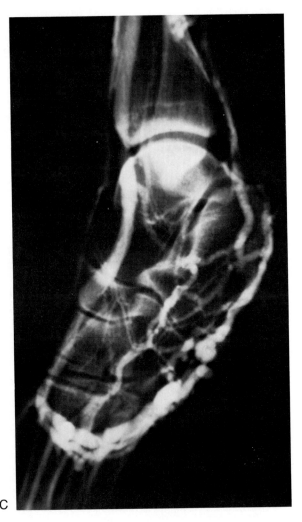

C

Fig. 15-7 (*Continued*). (**C**)

SUMMARY

While there is a large body of literature addressing vascular trauma of the leg, there are very few references investigating the morbidity and management of vascular trauma at the level of the foot and ankle. Therefore, any guidelines for management of pedal vascular trauma are drawn to a great degree from experience above the ankle level and should be interpreted with caution.

With an isolated, penetrating injury to one of the major pedal arteries, most clinicians agree that surgical intervention is not necessary if the artery is thrombosed and the foot appears well perfused clinically. If surgery is being performed for another reason the vessel may be ligated at that time. If, however, there is evidence of ischemia with an isolated arterial injury, then the artery should be repaired.

In a blunt, isolated arterial injury there is now some support for repair of the artery owing to the higher incidence of nonunion, soft tissue loss, and infection in these injuries.

When two arteries are disrupted, they should be repaired regardless of whether or not the foot appears ischemic. Options for repair include end-to-end anastomosis and reversed saphenous vein grafting.

There is no agreement whether fractures should be stabilized before or after vascular repair, although the trend is toward repairing the vascular structures first. Fasciotomy should be performed if necessary from either a dorsal or medial plantar approach.

Postoperatively, the basic principles of soft tissue wound management including debridement and early soft tissue coverage should be followed. The patient should be observed for late sequelae of vascular trauma including pseudoaneurysms and arteriovenous malformation.

REFERENCES

1. Rich NM, Spencer FC: Vascular Trauma. p. 549. WB Saunders, Philadelphia, 1978
2. Huber JF: The arterial network supplying the dorsum of the foot. Anat Rec 80:373, 1941
3. Sarrafian SK: Anatomy of the Foot and Ankle. p. 261. JB Lippincott, Philadelphia, 1983
4. Keeley SB, Snyder WH, Weigett JA: Arterial injuries below the knee: fifty one patients with 82 injuries. J Trauma 23:285, 1983
5. Lim LT, Muchada MS, Flanigan DP et al: Popliteal artery trauma. Arch Surg 115:1307, 1980
6. Snyder WH: Vascular injuries near the knee: an updated series and overview of the problem. Surgery 91:502, 1982
7. Feliciano DV, Herskowitz K, O'Gorman RB et al: Management of vascular injuries in the lower extremities. J Trauma 28:319, 1988
8. Ashworth EM, Dalsing MC, Glover JL, Reilly MK: Lower extremity vascular trauma: a compre-

hensive, aggressive approach. J Trauma 28:329, 1988

9. Pasch AR, Bishara RA, Lim LT et al: Optimal limb salvage in penetrating civilian vascular trauma. J Vasc Surg 3:189, 1986

10. Snyder WH: Popliteal and shank arterial injury. Surg Clin North Am 68:787, 1988

11. Lim RC, Raviola CA: Vascular emergencies. p. 387. In Mills J, Ho MT, Trunkey DD (eds): Current Emergency Diagnosis and Treatment. Lange Medical Publications, Los Altos, CA, 1983

12. Mubarak SJ, Hargens AR: Acute compartment syndromes. Surg Clin North Am 63:539, 1983

13. McCO'Brien B, Franklin JD, Marrison WA, Macleod AM: Replantation and revascularization surgery in children. The Hand 12:12, 1980

14. Holleman JH, Killebrew LH: Tibial artery injuries. Am J Surg 144:362, 1982

15. Menzolan JO, Doyle JE, Cantelino NL et al: A comprehensive approach to extremity vascular trauma. Arch Surg 120:801, 1985

16. Shah DM, Narayhsingh V, Leather RP et al: Advances in the management of acute popliteal vascular blunt injuries. J Trauma 25:793, 1985

17. Snyder WH, Thal ER, Perry MO: Peripheral and abdominal vascular injuries. p. 460. In Rutherford RB (ed): Vascular Surgery. WB Saunders, Philadelphia, 1984

18. Shah CM, Corson JD, Karmody AM et al: Optimal management of tibial arterial trauma. J Trauma 28:228, 1988

19. Olinsky DI, Lieberman JA, Shader AF: Anastomosis of small vessels in the foot. J Foot Surg 24:209, 1985

20. Silber SJ: Microsurgery. p. 16. Williams & Wilkins, Baltimore, 1979

21. Roberto RM, Strinas ST: Arterial injuries in extremity shot-gun wounds: requisite factors for successful management. Surgery 96:902, 1984

22. Ledgewood AM, Lucas CE: Biological dressings for exposed vascular graft. A reasonable alternative. J Trauma 15:569, 1975

23. Menzolan JO, Loberto FW, Doyle JE et al: Management of vascular injuries to the leg. Am J Surg 144:231, 1982

24. Chuinard ET, Baskin M: Clawfoot deformity. J Bone Joint Surg 55A:151, 1973

25. Cole WH: The treatment of clawfoot. J Bone Joint Surg 22A:895, 1980

26. Jones R: An address on Volkman's ischemic contracture with special reference to treatment. Br Med J 2:639, 1928

27. Tsuge K: Treatment of established Volkman's contracture. J Bone Joint Surg 57A:925, 1975

28. Kamel R, Sakla BF: Anatomical compartments of the sole of the human foot. Anat Rec 140:57, 1961

29. Perry MO: Compartment syndromes and reperfusion injury. Surg Clin North Am 68:853, 1988

30. Matsen FA, Winquist RA, Krugmire RB: Diagnosis and management of compartmental syndrome. J Bone Joint Surg 62:286, 1980

31. Russel WL, Burns RP: Acute upper and lower extremity compartment syndromes. p. 203. In Bergen JJ, Yao JST (eds): Vascular Surgical Emergencies. Grune & Stratton, Orlando, FL, 1987

32. Bulke GB: Pathophysiology of free radical mediated reperfusion injury. J Vasc Surg 5:512, 1987

33. McCord JM: Oxygen-derived free radicals in post ischemic tissue injury. N Engl J Med 313:154, 1985

34. Ames A, Wright RL, Kowada M et al: Cerebral ischemia: the no-reflow phenomenon. Am J Pathol 52:437, 1968

35. Fischer EG, Ames A: Studies on mechanisms of impairment of cerebral circulation following ischemia: effect of hemodilution and perfusion pressure. Stroke 3:538, 1972

36. Bagge V, Amundson B, Lauvitzen C: White blood cell deformability and plugging of skeletal muscle capillaries in hemorrhagic shock. Acta Physiol Scand 108:159, 1980

37. Ernst E, Hammerschmidt DE, Bagge V, et al: Leukocytes and the risk of ischemic diseases. JAMA 257:2311, 1987

38. Flores J, Dibona DR, Beck CH et al: The role of cell swelling in ischemic renal damage and the protective effect of hypertonic solution. J Clin Invest 51:118, 1972

39. Willerson JT, Powell WJ, Guiny TE: Improvement in myocardial function and coronary blood flow in ischemic myocardium after mannitol. J Clin Invest 11:2981, 1972

40. Reneman RS: The Anterior and the Lateral Compartment Syndrome of the Leg. Morton, The Hague, 1968

41. Whitesides TE, Jr., Haney TC, Hirada H et al: A simple method for tissue pressure determination. Arch Surg 110:1311, 1978

42. Matsen FA, III, Mayo KA, Sheridan GW et al: Monitoring of intramuscular pressure. Surgery 79:702, 1976

43. Scholander PF, Hargens AR, Milley SL: Negative pressure in the interstitial fluid of animals. Science 161:321, 1968

44. Rorabeck CH, Castle P, Hargens A et al: The slit catheter: a new technique for measuring intracompartmental pressures. Orthop Trans 5:324, 1981

45. Rorabeck CH, Castle GSP, Hardie R et al: Com-

partment pressure measurements: an experimental investigation using the slit catheter. J Trauma 21:446, 1981

46. Godinski M: A study of fascial spaces of the foot. Surg Gynecol Obstet 49:739, 1929
47. Loeffler RD, Ballard A: Planatar fascial spaces of the foot and a proposed surgical approach. Foot Ankle 1:11, 1980
48. Mubarak SJ, Hargens AR: Compartment Syndrome and Volkman's Contracture. WB Saunders, Philadelphia, 1981
49. Myerson MS: Experimental decompression of the fascial compartments of the foot—the basis for fasciotomy in acute compartment syndromes. Foot Ankle 8:308, 1988
50. Bonuti PM, Bell GR: Compartment syndrome of the foot: a case report. J Bone Joint Surg 68A:1449, 1986

16

Marine-Related Foot Injuries

John H. Walter, Jr., D.P.M., M.S.
Mark Burton, D.P.M.

Physicians who live, work, or vacation near saltwater habitats should be familiar with marine creatures that can prove harmful to humans. Numerous species are capable of inflicting injuries of varying degrees of severity, some of which are deadly.

The most common mechanisms of injury are envenomation and tearing. Envenomation occurs directly through a sting or bite. The toxin, or venom, enters the victim, who may suffer only a minor skin irritation with burning and itching at the puncture site, or who may have a severe enough reaction to cause paralysis, shock, and even death. Biting injuries may serve as a portal of entry for toxins; in many cases, however, nonvenomous biting injuries are the ones most frequently encountered off the coasts of North America. Poisonous creatures that have a deleterious effect on humans only when ingested are not discussed in this chapter.

INVERTEBRATES

Coelenterates are a group of invertebrates that number greater than 9,000 species. Many of them are frequently encountered during marine-related activities.[1] Members of the Cnidaria, a subgroup of coelenterates, with approximately 70 species, possess nematocysts capable of inducing venom through human skin. Nematocysts, or stinging cells, usually found on tentacles, inject their large molecular toxins through the skin with the slightest contact (Fig. 16-1). The venom of coelenterates is composed of various concentrations of histamine, histamine activators, catecholamines, and serotonin.[1]

Portuguese Man-of-War

The Portuguese man-of-wars, with tentacles from 30 to over 90 feet long, float aimlessly across the seas, influenced only by currents and wind, which blows on the carbon monoxide- and nitrogen gas-filled bag, or sail. Each tentacle's outer surface (and mouth, in some cases) bears more than 750,000 nematocysts. These nematocysts are discharged when the tentacle comes in contact with a foreign body or victim. The severity of the injury is directly related to the toxicity of the venom and the number of stinging cells that have been discharged, which sometimes reaches hundreds of thousands.

When mildly envenomated, the victim will experience immediately a severe burning pain, and pruritic hivelike lesions will erupt in the areas of contact for 3 to 7 days. The urticarial response may last several hours and, in some cases, is followed by a second erythematous papular lesion pattern, localized edema, and superficial skin sloughing. If skin necrosis occurs in severely envenomated patients, ulceration and infection usually precede hypertrophic scar formation. Systemically, the victim may experience weak-

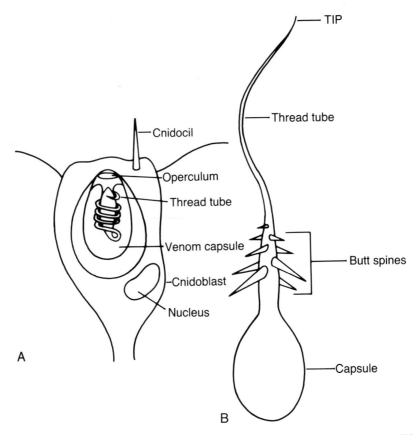

Fig. 16-1. **(A)** A coiled nematocyst ready to discharge its toxic contents upon contact. **(B)** A nematocyst after discharge.

ness, dizziness, shortness of breath, and nausea. Occasionally in the most severe man-of-war stings, convulsions may occur, along with cardiac arrest or coma.[2]

Jellyfish

The sting from a jellyfish is one of the more common injuries experienced by ocean bathers. Changing the pH of the skin will deactivate the toxin released by the jellyfish. This is best achieved by applying ammonia or meat tenderizer directly onto the involved skin. Nematocysts remaining in the skin eruptions, or wheals, should be removed by rubbing a coarse material such as sand aggressively over the wound. For more severe or acute dermatologic reactions, an-

tihistamines, topical steroids, and analgesics are recommended.[3]

Fire Coral

Fire coral, although not true coral, possess razor sharp exoskeletons of lime carbonate, which branch out 3 to 7 feet. These white to yellow-green tropical sea creatures, also called stinging coral, bear their nematocysts on very small surface tentacles that cover the coral (Fig. 16-2). Concentrated formic acid is responsible for the typical coelenterate-type lesion, which is red, tender, and produces a burning sensation. Ammonia will neutralize the formic acid, although superficial dermal lesions produced by fire coral usually resolve without treatment. Deeper

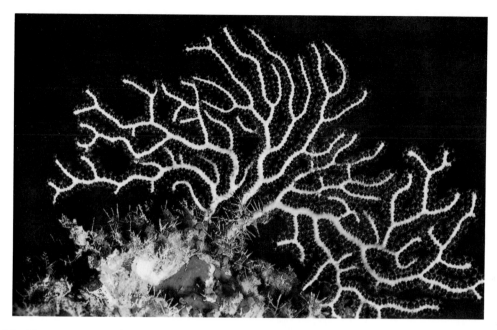

Fig. 16-2. Nematocysts on the tentacles of the fire coral produce the fiery sting experienced on contact. (From Cousteau,[16] with permission.)

wounds generated by fire coral are called "coral cuts" and may ulcerate and become secondarily infected. Local wound care should consist of debridement of devitalized tissue, frequent copious irrigation, and appropriate systemic antibiotics.[4]

Cone Shell

Cone shells, from the class Gastropoda and phylum Mollusca, are small but deadly marine animals found along the California coast. Averaging only 4 inches (10.3 cm) in length, the beautiful shells of these nocturnal feeders are an attraction that night divers find difficult to resist.

Venom contained on the cone shell's extendable proboscis is strong enough to be lethal to small children as a result of its curarelike effect, which disrupts neuromuscular transmission (Fig. 16-3). More significant envenomations may progress beyond the local cyanotic and ischemic changes into generalized paresthesias, paralysis, and respiratory failure. Less severe symptoms associated with cone shell stings may include weakness, blurred vision, and dysphagia.

Immersing the injured part in the hottest water tolerated by the patient (45 to 50°C) helps to reduce pain. Local anesthetics can also be used for nerve blocks or local infiltrations.[5] When necessary, supportive therapy in the more serious envenomation should include the administering of naloxone-reversible narcotics.

Sea Urchin

The most familiar and largest number of sea urchins are nonvenomous types, possessing long, sharp spines that protrude from a round shell. Venomous sea urchins (approximately 80 out of 6,000 species) have much shorter spines. These creatures store the venom in jawlike organs, called pedicellariae, located along the spines. When the spines puncture the foot, severe burning pain and significant bleeding may result. If the spines protrude from the skin, they should be extracted promptly.[6] Smaller spines may break off beneath the skin and be reabsorbed within 3 weeks. Soft tissue radiographs may be helpful in locating spines composed of calcium carbonate[7]

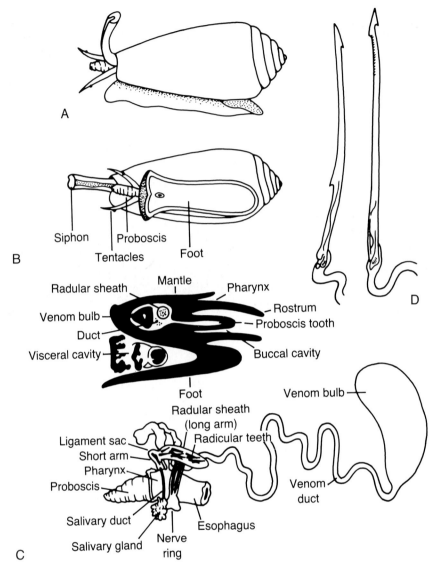

Fig. 16-3. (A) Located beneath the cone shell conus is the dangerous venom-containing proboscis. **(B)** A cross section of venom apparatus. **(C)** The venom bulb houses the venom until an attack. **(D)** Rodular teeth of the venomous cone shell penetrate the skin and allow envenomation of the skin. (From Halstead,[5] with permission.)

(Fig. 16-4). Reckless probing is rarely warranted, and surgical exploration significantly increases the chance of fracturing these hollow, fragile spines.

Venom from the pedicellariae can produce severe and intense pain in the immediate area of envenomation, followed by local swelling, bleeding, and numbness. Systemically, the victim may feel faint, experience paralysis, have difficulty breathing, and become hypotensive. Support therapy for the systemic problems is crucial. Hot water soaks should relieve the intense burning pain.[8] Secondary bacterial infections may be encountered, and appropriate antibiotics and local wound care are utilized when appropriate. Foreign body reactions inducing granulomas and sarcoidlike granulomatous lesions may develop in 2 to 12 months.

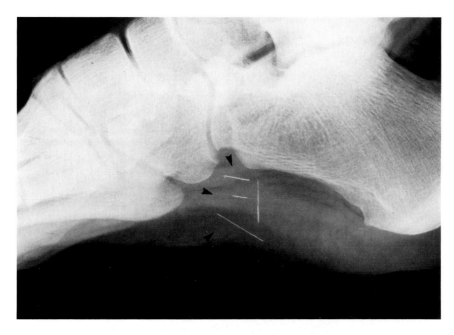

Fig. 16-4. Sea urchin spines (arrows) can be seen on standard radiographs; however, soft tissue studies may be more helpful.

Sea Anemone

Like all coelenterates, the beautifully colored sea anemones have stinging cells on their numerous fingerlike tentacles (Fig. 16-5). A true coral and member of the Anthozoa class, the sea anemone produces a cutaneous rash when touched. Burning sensations develop instantly at the points of contact and are followed by erythematous and edematous changes. To reduce these symptoms, alcohol or meat tenderizer (papain) may be applied immediately to the skin, even if loose tentacles remain attached.[9]

True Coral

Hard coral organisms, sensu strictu, of the phylum Cnidaria produce hard razor-sharp external skeletons of calcium carbonate, which after many years of growth may appear as fields of large rocks or perhaps as the horns of a deer. Coral cuts like a razor, almost painlessly, and quickly causes reddened, pruritic, weltlike lesions. Initial therapy consists of wound irrigation and local debridement of foreign material and nonviable tissue. Local tissue necrosis may occur if preceded by secondary infection. The effervescence of hydrogen peroxide may prove helpful in mechanical debridement of the wound. Continued aggressive local wound care is necessary as well as antibiotic therapy appropriate for the myriad of potentially virulent marine organisms.[10]

Sea Cucumber

Appearing as short fat wormlike creatures scattered over the ocean floor, sea cucumbers defend themselves by excreting a visceral liquid toxin called holothurin (Fig. 16-6). Following exposure to this toxin, contact dermatitis and severe conjunctival irritation are common. Lavaging the eyes with saline and applying acetic acid or isopropyl alcohol to the skin help to counteract the irritating effects of the toxin.[11]

Sponges

Anchored to the ocean floor, sponges possess an elastic exoskeleton of spongin, which is composed of calcium carbonate or silicon dioxide

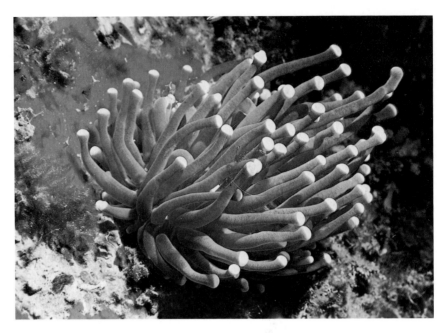

Fig. 16-5. The sea anemone's fingerlike projections house the nematocysts. (From Cousteau,[16] with permission.)

spicules incorporated into compressible connective tissue. Some sponges are capable of producing a significant contact dermatitis by a yet-to-be identified toxin introduced into the skin through abrasions resulting from handling the sponge.

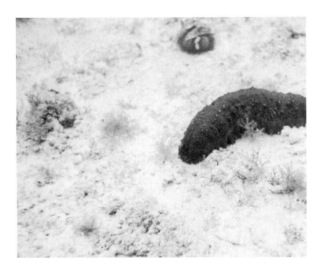

Fig. 16-6. This harmless-looking sea cucumber can excrete a liquid toxic to humans.

Fire sponges (*Tedania ignis*), which are generally found in Hawaii and the Florida Keys, produce a typical burning pain and intense itching, hence their name.[12] The toxin of this particular sponge, however, has the potential to cause acute eczematous dermatitis, local joint swelling, and stiffness. These symptoms tend to resolve in 2 to 3 days with appropriate local supportive treatment.

Anaphylactoid reactions and erythema multiforme have been associated with the brilliant and beautiful yellow-orange fire sponge.[13] Initial therapy for the immediate relief of the dermatitis consists of the application of a weak acetic acid solution (5 percent), such as vinegar, or the less effective isopropyl alcohol. Systemic corticosteroids and antihistamines may also be considered in more severe cases. Meticulous local wound care and systemic antibiotics are indicated if sloughing or necrosis of skin occurs at contact points. Adhesive tape can be very helpful in retrieving the calcium carbonate or silicon dioxide spicules that have become embedded in the skin.

VERTEBRATES

Shark

Shark attacks are relatively rare injuries; the annual report of shark attacks off North America totals 1 in 5 million people. Although 24 of 225 species of shark have been implicated in attacks on humans worldwide, the great white shark, blue shark, hammerhead shark, Mako shark, and gray reef shark are the most common offenders in the coastal waters of the United States. Most victims never see the attacking shark, which may intentionally bump the human prey just prior to the first strike.[14] Biting, tearing, and ripping of flesh from the victim create various degrees of blood loss as well as soft tissue and osseous damage.

Hypovolemic shock is the most immediate threat to life, and therefore, fluid replacement measures must be considered of primary importance. Direct pressure is immediately indicated to control hemorrhaging. Judicious use of torniquets should only be considered if major arteries have been violated, as tissue perfusion may be further compromised. Volume replacement is achieved with crystalloid solutions or other appropriate blood products. Transport to the nearest emergency medical facility is required.

Military antishock trousers or similar devices provide pneumatic compression to the lower extremities. This aids in control of bleeding from the extremities and also serves to increase cardiac filling and peripheral vascular resistance necessary to sustain vital organ perfusion until blood volume can be restored. Wounds should only be evaluated in appropriate facilities with surgical capabilities necessary for wound exploration, copious lavage, and debridement.

Pencillin prophylaxis remains generally accepted. Appropriate antitetanus therapy as described in Chapter 30 must be considered.[8]

Moray Eels

Holes and crevices amid rocks and coral reefs serve as the habitat for moray eels. These crea-tures are generally harmless to humans unless provoked or cornered in their small dwellings. Severe lacerations and punctures, usually of the hand and less often of the foot, are created by the vicelike grip of the moray eel's narrow and pointed jaws, which possess caninelike fangs. Closed space infections are possible, necessitating incision and drainage, irrigation, and appropriate antibiotic therapy. Fatal encounters have been postulated in cases in which the eel appeared strong enough to maintain its grasp on the diver, causing eventual drowning.[9]

Scorpion Fish

The scorpion fish is responsible for over 250 yearly injuries or fatalities in the coastal waters

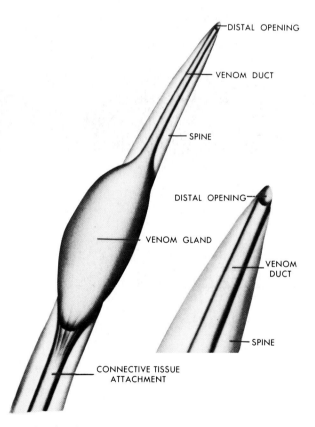

Fig. 16-7. The spine of the scorpion fish houses the venom gland. (From Halstead,[5] with permission.)

off North America. Trapped in nets by divers or fishermen, the scorpion fish, in most cases, envenomates its unsuspecting victims while being removed from the net. Intense pain, swelling, the formation of blisters, and necrosis occur at the site of venom injection (Fig. 16-7). Diaphoresis and shortness of breath may occur. The victim may also exhibit symptoms of hyperactivity.[5] Cyanosis, shock, coma, and death have been reported. Supportive hospital therapy is indicated for survival.

Barracuda

A common sight around piers, docks, and coral reefs, the barracuda often swims alone. A long, sleek body enables the barracuda to be extremely quick, and with its caninelike teeth it is capable of inflicting deep V-shaped lacerations. Weighing, in some cases, 50 to 100 lbs (23 to 45 kg) and approaching 9 feet (2.7 m) in length, the barracuda has been known to attack humans in waters of poor visibility. The fish seems attracted to the

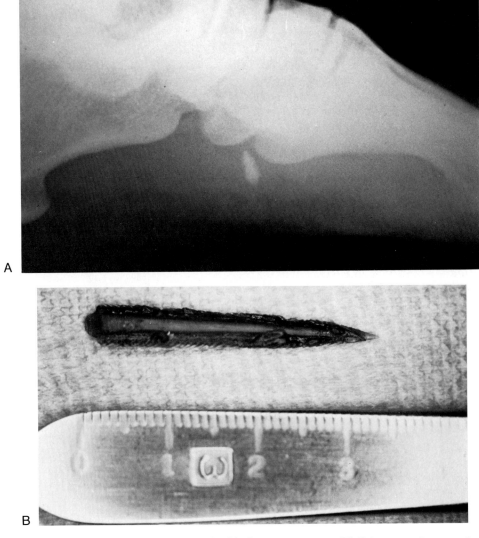

Fig. 16-8. **(A)** Preoperative radiograph of embedded stingray spine. **(B)** Stingray spine specimen after removal. (Courtesy of Robert Cooke, D.P.M.)

reflections from swimmers' jewelry, which might appear to the barracuda as similar to the reflection from a fish it desires to feed upon. Local wound care, control of hemorrhage, tetanus prophylaxis, and indicated antibiotics constitute appropriate management of barracuda bites.[1]

Stingray

Most human envenomations that occur along the coastal waters of the United States are attributed to six families of stingrays. As many as 1,460 stingray injuries have been reported in 1 year. Stingray-inflicted wounds occur usually to the wading swimmer or diver who steps on the animal while it is partially submerged in sand or mud. With a whiplike motion, the long tail moves upward and forward to meet the intruder's foot or leg (Fig. 16-8). Serrated spines on the stinger located at the base of the stingray's tail penetrates the victim's skin. Venom is instantaneously released by glandular epithelia immediately surrounding the stinger. Significant pain is generated at the site of laceration or puncture in 3 to 15 minutes but may increase in intensity up to 1 to 2 hours after envenomation. Edematous changes contribute to the cyanosis of the wound, and subsequent necrosis of the wound edges occurs frequently. High-molecular-weight polypeptides contained in the venom produce various systemic reactions such as nausea, vomiting, cardiac dysrythemias, muscle spasm, and respiratory depression; death, however, is rare.

Initial treatment includes prompt removal of the stinger, immediate irrigation of the wound with fresh or salt water, and immersion of the foot in the hottest water tolerated by the victim to deactivate the heat-labile venom. Local wound care should continue to be aggressive throughout the healing period. Tetanus prophylaxis and therapeutic antibiotics are recommended.[15]

Of course, foreign body penetration by any object in or near marine environments may be encountered. Unless the specific foreign body requires a specialized treatment, for example, stingray spines, the general principles of foreign body management as described in Chapter 8 should be adhered to.

REFERENCES

1. Auerback PS: Emergency Clinics of North America. 1st Ed. Vol. 2. WB Saunders, Philadelphia, 1984
2. Banner AH: Poisonous marine animals—a synopsis. J Forensic Sci 12:10, 1967
3. Arnold RE: What to do about bites and stings of venomous animals. Fed Proc 26:1206, 1967
4. Manowitz NR, Rosenthal RR: Cutaneous-systemic reactions to toxins and venoms of common marine organisms. Cutis 23:450, 1979
5. Halstead BW: Poisonous and Venomous Marine Animals of the World. Revised Ed. Darwin Press, Princeton, NJ, 1978
6. Baden HP, Burnett JW: Injuries from sea urchins. South Med J 70:459, 1977
7. Warin AP: Sea-urchin granuloma. Clin Exp Dermatol 2:405, 1977
8. Halstead BW: Dangerous Marine Animals That Bite, Sting, Shock, and Are Non-edible. Maritime Press, Centreville, MD, 1980
9. Rosco MD: Cutaneous manifestations of marine animal injuries including diagnosis and treatment. Cutis 19:507, 1977
10. Auerback PS, Geehr EC: Management of Wilderness and Environmental Emergencies. Macmillan, New York, 1983
11. Baslow MH: Marine toxins. Annu Rev Pharm 11:447, 1971
12. Fisher AA: Atlas of Aquatic Dermatology. Grune & Stratton, Orlando, FL, 1978
13. Yaffee HS, Stargardter F: Erythema multiforme from Tedania ignis. Arch Dermatol 87:601, 1963
14. Baldridge AD, Williams J: Shark attack: feeding or fighting? Milit Med 134:130, 1969
15. Bitseff EL, Garoni WJ, Hardison CD et al: The management of stingray injuries of the extremities. South Med J 63:417, 1970
16. Cousteau J: The Ocean World. Abrams, New York, 1979

17

Dislocation Injuries of the Foot

Thomas F. Smith, D.P.M.   *Stephen V. Corey, D.P.M.*
Thomas Cain, D.P.M.   *Bradley D. Castellano, D.P.M.*
Richard DiNapoli, D.P.M.   *Robert Tupper, D.P.M.*
Marc Bernbach, D.P.M.

Dislocations represent injury, not to osseous joint structures or the tendons that move them, but to the soft tissues that bind them. The capsular and ligamentous soft tissues paradoxically provide the strength for joint stability and yet permit the freedom for joint motion. When the end range of motion for a joint is reached, the joint soft tissues limit further excursion. Limitation of joint motion is further aided by joint biomechanics, osseous contours, and active muscular agonist and antagonist function. Sprains or strains represent stresses to joints beyond the ability of the soft tissues to maintain osseous congruity, and subluxation ensues. Soft tissue disruption of some degree must be present to have permitted the dislocation to occur.

The capsular and ligamentous soft tissues can be compromised by several different means. They may become stretched in a plastic fashion, maintaining some degree of structural continuity. There may be complete disruption of the tissue. The tissue may be pulled directly from the bone. None of the above means are radiographically evident. The ligament may have pulled away a fragment of bone. Small fracture fragments about joints may be the only radiographic evidence of severe joint compromise. Any combination of the above patterns may be present.

Occult dislocations are radiographically evident by the incongruity of the osseous compo-nents. Postreduction radiographs or spontaneously reduced dislocations may appear "normal" because no osseous compromise or fracture has occurred. The diagnostic challenge of pedal dislocations is thus apparent. Plain radiographs may provide minimal diagnostic help. Careful clinical evaluation is critical. Contralateral comparison radiographs can be very helpful. Stress radiography to test the invisible ligaments can be performed at any joint level. These techniques, coupled with an appreciation of the joint anatomy, enable the podiatric physician to assess the severity of the soft tissue injuries present.

The old saying, "well, at least nothing is broken," demonstrates a lack of understanding for ligamentous injury, its complexity, and the potential sequelae for serious complications. The multiplicity and complexity of the pedal joints challenge the physician to apply these principles to a specific anatomic area.

GENERAL PRINCIPLES

The general history and physical evaluation are vitally important in any trauma situation and must not be overlooked. Healthy, debilitated, and compromised patients may all find themselves victims of traumatic episodes. The treatment plan must be tailored to each individual pattern of injury as it applies to the general health status of a particular patient.

The specific history of the particular injury is vitally important. The exact history of the injury or the mechanism of injury will help predict the degree of ligamentous compromise present. It also aids in predicting possible associated injuries common to the dislocation present. Any prior history of injury or surgery on the lower extremity should likewise be assessed to aid in understanding factors that may affect the reduction and prognosis.

Once the history has been established, the affected extremity can be evaluated. The part is visually examined for lacerations, contusions, and abrasions. Localization of soft tissue edema and erythema and other physical signs are assessed and charted. Areas of potential tissue compromise and loss are noted. Open dislocations present the possibility of serious joint infection complications. The neurovascular status must be carefully examined to help assess tissue viability. Muscle function is tested to rule out tendinous injury. All joints are palpated for pain, range of motion, and stability. The contralateral lower extremity is a useful standard for comparison.

Only now should radiographs be considered. A minimum of three views of the foot or ankle is needed to accurately assess dislocation or fracture. Comparison contralateral radiographs are essential in subtle difficult situations. Stress radiographs of any pedal joint can be performed to assess capsular and ligamentous stability. Anesthesia, either local or general, may be required for accurate assessment. Such measures reduce pain and prevent muscular guarding of the injured joint. False-negative stress testing can then be avoided.

An accurate diagnosis of a pedal dislocation has two important facets. The first is to establish the exact joint or joints involved or the particular anatomy affected. These injuries can be extremely subtle compared with the clinical presentation. The second facet is to establish how the particular injury occurred or to formulate the mechanism of injury. The mechanism of injury helps to identify associated injuries that occur in predictable injury patterns. Also, as a general

principle, to reduce dislocations maneuvers represent an exaggeration, distraction, and reversal of the mechanism of injury.

The prognosis following reduction is based on the location of the injury within the lower extremity and the severity of soft tissue compromise present. Healing of capsular and ligamentous structures to preinjury levels of function is never guaranteed under optimal conditions of care. The ligament-scar complex that replaces preinjury ligament may never function at the preinjury level. Surgical reinforcement may be needed. Immediate primary repair may be indicated in certain situations. Arthrodesis may be the only final solution to joint instability and pain following any pedal dislocation regardless of the severity.

The individual pedal joints are reviewed in terms of diagnosis, treatment, and prognosis of dislocation injury. Figures and illustrations demonstrate the visual nature of these injuries. The podiatric physician has a vital role in the management of pedal dislocations. They are certainly a more common presenting complaint than is reported. These patients commonly present with problems some time after the original injury has occurred. To manage these sequelae, requires a thorough understanding of these injuries as they originally present and an appreciation for the anatomy that is affected.

SUBTALAR JOINT DISLOCATIONS

Subtalar joint dislocation is an uncommon injury with simultaneous dislocation of the talocalcaneal and talonavicular joints. The incidence of this dislocation is estimated to be approximately 1 percent of all dislocations.[1,2] This injury has appeared in the literature under many titles including luxatio pedis subtalo, subastragalar dislocation, and peritalar dislocation. The most descriptive term is talocalcaneonavicular dislocation; but the most utilized term is subtalar joint dislocation.[3] The distinguishing feature of this injury is simultaneous disruption of both the subtalar and talonavicular joints with a grossly intact ankle and calcaneocuboid joint.

Classification

The most common type of subtalar joint dislocation reported in the medical literature is the medial dislocation.[1,4–7] The medial subtalar joint dislocation is so named for the gross direction the foot assumes clinically following the injury (Fig. 17-1). The clinical presentation has been described as the basketball foot[8] or acquired clubfoot owing to the appearance of the foot following injury.[9,10] Larsen described the mechanism for medial subtalar joint dislocation as a forceful in-version of the foot.[9] The initial joint to dislocate is the talonavicular joint. This is followed by a rotatory subluxation of the talocalcaneal joint as the calcaneus proceeds medially under the talus with the remainder of the foot (Fig. 17–2). The talus remains intact as part of the leg. The ankle joint is weakened, with rupture of the calcaneo-fibular ligament and superficial deltoid liga-ment[11] (Fig. 17-3). Further inversion force can produce total ankle subluxation. Leitner described subtalar joint dislocation as the primary stage of total dislocation of the tarsus and ankle.[12]

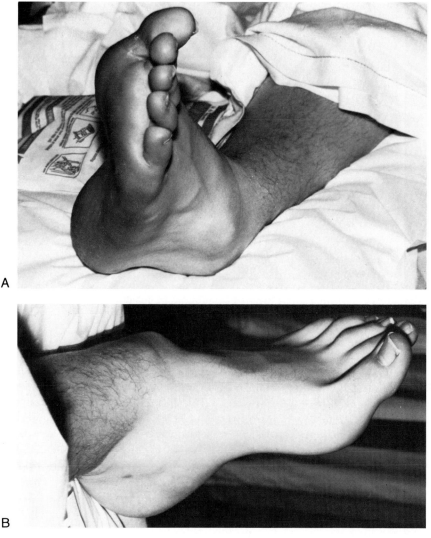

A

B

Fig. 17-1. Clinical presentation of medial subtalar dislocation. (**A**) Prereduction on anterior perspective of the foot and leg. (**B**) Prereduction medial perspective of the foot and leg.

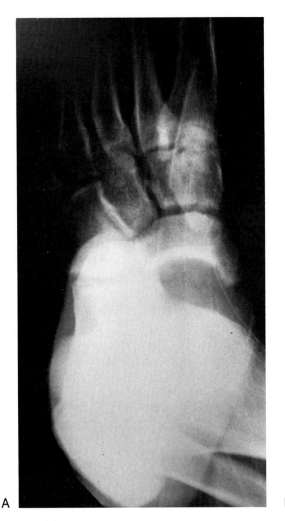

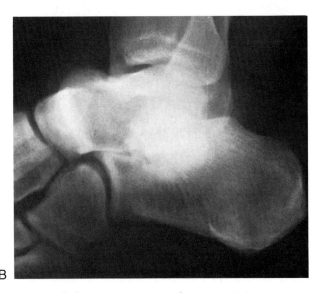

Fig. 17-2. Radiographic presentation of the foot in subtalar dislocation. **(A)** Prereduction anteroposterior view. **(B)** Prereduction lateral view.

The medial swivel dislocation of the midtarsal joint as described by Main and Jowett[13] may in fact represent the first stage of this injury not progressing through talocalcaneal joint involvement.[14] Christensen and associates have summarized the associated injuries and their incidences.[4] Avulsion and rupture injuries occur along the lateral column of the foot and ankle. Crushing type injuries occur more frequently along the medial column secondary to the forces involved to create the injury.

Lateral subtalar joint dislocation results from forceful eversion of the foot. The talar head is forced through the talonavicular joint capsule medially. The calcaneus along with the remainder of the foot is forced laterally from beneath the talus, leading to disruption of the talocalcaneal joint (Fig. 17-4). Again, the talus remains congruent within the ankle mortis as part of the leg. The calcaneocuboid joint and ankle joint remain intact as in medial subtalar dislocation.

Posterior and anterior subtalar joint dislocations are extremely rare.[8] These injuries are considered variants of medial or lateral subtalar dislocations. Posterior subtalar dislocation results from falls from a height with the foot in a plantar-

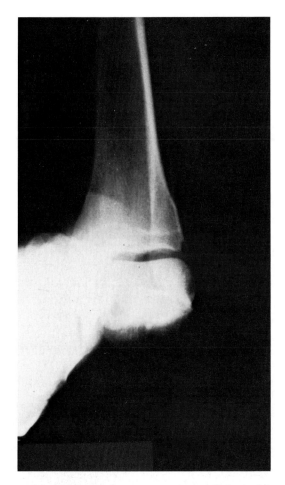

Fig. 17-3. Radiographic presentation of the ankle in medial subtalar dislocation. Prereduction anterioposterior view. (From Smith,[14] with permission.)

flexed position.[9] The posterior tubercle of the talus is usually fractured in these injuries. Anterior dislocations occur in falls from a height with the foot in a dorsiflexed position[9] (Fig. 17-5).

Anatomy

The subtalar joint is reinforced by its joint capsule. Thickenings of this capsule medially and laterally are known as the medial and lateral talocalcaneal ligaments. The strong osseous talocalcaneal ligament occupies the sinus tarsi. The talocalcaneal ligament is composed of thickenings of the anterior aspect of the subtalar joint capsule and the posterior aspect of the talocalcaneonavicular joint capsule. The ligamentum cervicus lies at the lateral aspect of the sinus tarsi, traversing the neck of the talus and the calcaneus.[15] These ligaments are all disrupted by subtalar joint dislocation.

The talocalcaneonavicular joint complex is supported by the talonavicular ligament and the joint capsule. The talonavicular ligament, after surrounding the joint, blends into the deltoid ligament. These are the two major supporting ligaments of the talonavicular joint. During the initial phase of the injury, the talar head punctures the talonavicular ligament. The bifurcate ligament and the spring ligament are the only two ligaments of the subtalar and talocalcaneonavicular complex that are not disrupted in this injury. Attachments of these ligaments do not include the talus directly. All the osseous relationships and ligamentous attachments between the calcaneus and the cuboid and between the cuboid and the navicular joints remain intact.

The complexity of this injury includes not only anatomic disruption of the subtalar and talonavicular joints but also portions of the ankle joints as well. Buckingham created medial and lateral subtalar dislocations on cadaver specimens to assess the extent of ankle ligament injury.[11] He concluded that the extent of ankle injury was the same whether creating a medial or lateral subtalar joint dislocation. The superficial portions of the deltoid ligament and the calcaneofibular ligament were ruptured in both injuries. Anatomically, both of these ligaments cross the subtalar joint. They therefore must rupture in these injuries. A portion of the superficial deltoid extends from the medial malleolus to the sustentaculum tali of the calcaneus and anteriorly to the navicular. The calcaneofibular ligament extends from the fibula to the midportion of the lateral surface of the calcaneus. Ankle instability, stiffness, and pain are all potential sequelae of subtalar joint dislocations.

Clinical Presentation

The medial subtalar joint dislocation presents clinically with the foot medially displaced on the leg (Fig. 17-1). The head of the talus is palpable on the dorsum of the foot. The talar head is disarticulated from the navicular and may be positioned between the extensor hallucis longus and the extensor digitorum longus. The head of the talus is usually sitting dorsally on either the navicular or the cuboid.[3] The skin overlying the talar head may be extremely taut and blanched. If reduction is delayed, skin necrosis can result. The lateral border of the foot appears long in relation to the shorter medial border. The digits may appear dorsiflexed.[3] The sustentaculum tali and navicular are palpable medially, while the medial malleolus is not visible.

Radiographic examinations must include multiple studies of both the foot and ankle (Fig. 17-2). The anterior ankle radiograph demonstrates the medial displacement of the foot through the subtalar joint with the talus intact in the ankle mortise (Fig. 17-3). The lateral radiographs of the foot and ankle demonstrate no clear subtalar joint space with an overlap of the talus with the other tarsal bones (Fig. 17-2B). The dorsoplantar view exhibits a nonarticular talonavicular joint with a medially displaced navicular (Fig. 17-2A). Inversion-type ankle fractures and associated pedal fractures must be ruled out.

Clinically, in the lateral subtalar joint dislocation, the foot is laterally positioned to the leg (Fig. 17-4A and B). The medial border appears lengthened, whereas the lateral border of the foot appears shortened. The talar head is palpable medially. The fibular malleolus is not visible laterally. The digits appear plantar flexed because of the stretch of the tarsal canal structures.

Radiographic evaluation must include studies of both the foot and ankle. The anterior ankle radiographs reveal a laterally displaced foot

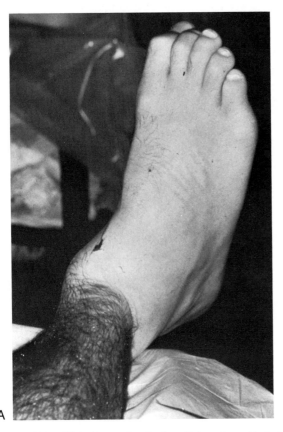
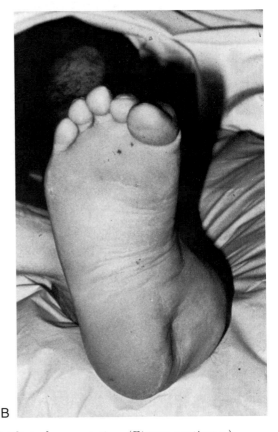

A   B

Fig. 17-4. Lateral subtalar dislocation. (**A & B**) Clinical presentation. (*Figure continues.*)

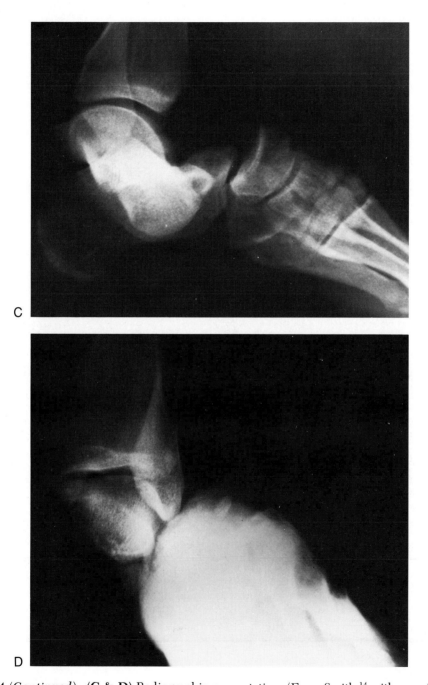

Fig. 17-4 (*Continued*). (**C & D**) Radiographic presentation. (From Smith,[14] with permission.)

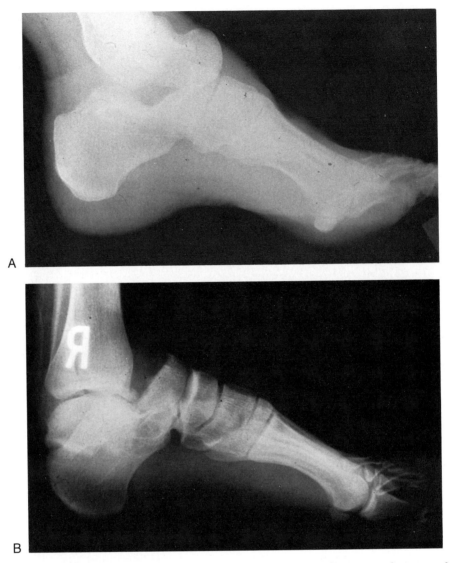

Fig. 17-5. (A) Posterior subtalar dislocation. **(B)** Hawkins type II talar fracture with intact talonavicular joint and lateral dislocation of subtalar joint.

through the subtalar joint, with the talus fixed in the ankle mortise (Fig. 17-4D). Lateral radiographs of the foot and ankle demonstrate no clear subtalar joint space, with overlap of the tarsal bones (Fig. 17-4C). The dorsoplantar radiograph of the foot reveals a lateral displacement of the navicular on the talus, with the calcaneocuboid joint intact. The radiographs must be inspected for associated ankle and foot eversion injuries. Lateral dislocations of the subtalar joint are more likely to accompany fractures of the talus than medial subtalar dislocations (Fig. 17-5B).[5]

Management

Reduction of subtalar joint dislocations should not be delayed. Pressure on vital structures and relaxation of skin tension over bony prominences should be relieved quickly. General or spinal anesthesia is usually required to obtain reduction of these injuries. Intravenous muscle relaxants or muscle-paralyzing agents may be necessary to reduce muscle spasm and splinting around the ankle and tarsal joints. The principles of reduction involve reversing the original mechanism of injury.[15] A thorough understanding of joint anatomy and the mechanism of the injury producing the dislocation is therefore necessary to affect adequate reduction.

A medial subtalar dislocation is reduced by first applying a forceful inversion force through the subtalar joint from the foot; this is followed by distraction of the subtalar joint and finally by an eversion force through the subtalar joint to return the foot to a neutral position. Distal traction is applied to the heel, with countertraction applied to a flexed knee. This maneuver helps relax the gastrocnemius muscle to facilitate reduction.[14] The subtalar joint component is thus reduced first, reversing the mechanism of injury. This joint was dislocated last during the injury episode. The talonavicular joint is reduced second, as the talonavicular joint was the first component of the injury episode. The talonavicular component is then reduced by pressing downward on the head of the talus with the foot in a plantar-flexed position. The midtarsal joint is dorsiflexed, relocating the head of the talus with the navicular.

There are certain obstacles that can prevent the successful reduction of these injuries. These obstacles include abutment of the navicular on the head of the talus and buttonholing of the head of the talus through either the extensor retinaculum or extensor digitorum brevis muscle belly and peroneal tendons encircling the head of the talus.[1] Leitner outlined closed reduction techniques to overcome these obstacles.[1] Open reduction may be necessary if closed reduction is unsuccessful. The incision is placed laterally over the head of the talus in a proximal to distal orientation. This provides access to possible impaction of the head of the talus on the navicular or to soft tissues that may encircle the head of the talus. Any structure binding the head of the talus can be effectively released this way.

The principles for reducing lateral subtalar joint dislocations are the same as those for medial dislocations. Distal traction is placed on the calcaneus with the knee in a flexed position. The foot is then forcefully everted and distracted, and an inversion force is applied through the subtalar joint, returning the foot to a neutral position. Reduction of the talonavicular joint follows by applying pressure to the head of the talus with the foot held in a pronated position. The tibialis posterior tendon,[1,16] long flexor tendons,[3] or impaction fractures of the navicular and talus[11] may prevent closed reduction. Open reduction may be accomplished by an incision lateral to the head of the talus permitting access to release any structures binding the talus.

A bulky compressive dressing is applied following the reduction. The dressings will be continued until edema is controlled and vascular status is ensured. Generally, these dressings are maintained for 3 to 5 days. Internal fixation or percutaneous pinning is generally unnecessary for subtalar joint dislocations alone. Fixation may be required for any associated pedal or ankle injuries. Kenwright and Taylor reported an unstable reduction of subtalar joint dislocation requiring fixation associated with a fracture of the sustentaculum tali.[17] Postreduction radiographs should be obtained to review the quality of reduction. Examination for fractures should be repeated. Subtle fractures may become more evident without the osseous overlap present in prereduction radiographs.

Complications

The most common immediate complication in subtalar dislocation is skin necrosis. Christensen and associates describe 3 cases of skin necrosis out of 30 subtalar dislocations.[4] One case of skin necrosis progressed, necessitating skin grafts. The importance of monitoring skin blisters was fully described by Sharit and Cole.[18]

Long-term complications resulting from subtalar joint dislocations include postural deformities, ankle instability, avascular necrosis of the talus, arthritis, and pain.[4] Avascular necrosis of the talus is not a common complication of isolated subtalar joint dislocations.[4,6,19,20] Damage to the posterior talus, however, may compromise an already damaged circulation from the sinus tarsi, increasing the risk of avascular necrosis. Subtalar joint dislocations in combination with ankle dislocation greatly increase the incidence of avascular necrosis of the talus.[4,6]

Stiffness of the subtalar joint is a consistent finding following subtalar joint dislocations. However, pain and disability are not directly proportional to the stiffness present.[5,6,11] If the pain and disability cannot be controlled, the patient may require manipulation under general anesthesia. This procedure has proved helpful in selected cases. Those not responding to manipulation may require triple arthrodesis. Isolated subtalar joint arthrodesis has not proved helpful in relieving the arthrosis complications of subtalar joint dislocation. The most common radiographic change following subtalar joint dislocation is degeneration of the posterior facet of the subtalar joint. Amazingly, the long-term disabilities are less than the degree of injury suggests.[4,6,9,11,17,19,21]

Traditionally, subtalar joint dislocations have been treated with non-weight-bearing below-the-knee cast immobilization for 4 to 6 weeks. Interestingly, patients treated with prolonged periods of immobilization had longer periods of subjective pain following the injury.[4,11] Current trends include earlier ambulation with the protecton of a below-the-knee cast.[22] This supports the findings reported by McKeever in 1963 that early guarded ambulation reduces subtalar joint stiffness and pain.[23] Presently, a non-weight-bearing below-the-knee cast is applied for 2 weeks, followed by 4 to 6 weeks of weight-bearing, below-the-knee casting. We have seen six cases of medial subtalar joint dislocations and one of lateral subtalar joint dislocation. Early immobilization left these patients with little residual pain; however, stiffness has been a common finding. Aggressive physical therapy should be instituted for a minimum of 3 months following removal of the cast. This may include hydrotherapy, ultrasonic therapy, and range of motion and muscle-strengthing exercises.

MIDTARSAL JOINT DISLOCATIONS

The midtarsal joint divides the rear foot from the forefoot and is composed of the talonavicular and calcaneocuboid joints. Dislocation injuries at this level are fairly infrequent. The common "foot sprain" that frequently occurs following minor injury forces probably represents injury to the midtarsal joint. Delayed diagnoses and misdiagnoses are common.[3,13,24] The importance of adequate radiographic evaluation cannot be overemphasized. Most researchers stress the need for a minimum of three views of the foot, including dorsoplantar, oblique, and lateral views.[13] Small avulsions or chip fractures about the talonavicular or calcaneocuboid joints may be the only indication of the injury. Even gross dislocations can be missed if the radiographic evaluation is improperly performed.[24,25] The hypermobile foot can commonly present as a false-positive-dislocated midtarsal joint on lateral radiographs. Contralateral radiographs are of vital importance in this injury.

Anatomy

The talonavicular joint is the first articulation of the medial longitudinal arch. It is usually described as condyloid. The talonavicular ligament combined with the superficial deltoid ligament represent the major ligamentous reinforcements of this joint. The joint capsule surrounds the articulation and provides further strength. The joint is further supported by the strong tendinous attachments of the tibialis posterior. Any of these structures can have a significant influence on the reducibility of this injury. All may become impacted within the talonavicular joint, preventing reduction. Avulsion injuries frequently occur when traumatic subluxation is sufficiently violent.

The calcaneocuboid joint is described as a saddle joint, with both concave and convex surfaces proximally and distally. The cuboid articulation is concave transversely and convex vertically. The motions about this joint are limited more by bone-to-bone abutment than by ligamentous reinforcement.[26] Supination causes the inferomedial beak of the cuboid to collide with the coronoid fossa of the calcaneus. Extreme pronation is blocked superiorly by the anterosuperior beak of the calcaneus. This explains the frequently encountered chip fracture seen at this level. Ligamentous structures about the calcaneocuboid joint include the lateral band of the bifurcate ligament, the dorsolateral calcaneocuboid ligament, and the inferior calcaneocuboid ligaments, including the long and short plantar ligaments. These strong fibrous attachments are common sites of avulsion fractures.[3,13,24]

Classification

Midtarsal joint fracture-dislocation has received little attention in the literature. Main and Jowett continue to be the major contributors on this subject.[13] They classify these injuries based on the mechanism of injury. The force vector and the resulting displacement are used to describe each injury type. The treatment plan is based on the type of dislocation which is present. The injuries are classified into five major groups:

1. Medial forces.
2. Longitudnal forces.
3. Lateral forces.
4. Plantar forces.
5. Crushing forces

Medial Forces
These injuries result from a force directed from lateral to medial in the transverse plane at the midtarsal joint level. They are subdivided into fracture-sprains, fracture-dislocations, and swivel dislocations. Fracture-sprains are the mildest form of medial force injury. Flake fractures of the talus, navicular, calcaneus, or cuboid all may occur dorsally, plantarly, medially, or laterally. These are among the most frequent midtarsal joint injuries. Fortunately, they have a good prognosis with simple immobilization treatment (Fig. 17-6).

Fracture-dislocations are more severe injuries and can be challenging to reduce by closed techniques if soft tissue imposition occurs. Radiographically, the midfoot and forefoot appear medially displaced on an intact rear foot. Chip or small avulsion fractures may occur about the midtarsal joint. Treatment consists of rapid reduction and cast immobilization. Failed closed reduction warrants open reduction since continued symptoms and later arthrodesis are inevitable if the injury is left untreated.

Swivel dislocations of the midtarsal joint result most often from falls from a height or from motor vehicle accidents. They are extremely rare injuries. An intact talocalcaneal relationship distinguishes this injury from a medial subtalar dislocation. Anteroposterior ankle radiographs are necessary to make this determination. Treatment involves early reduction with cast immobilization. A good prognosis follows adequate reduction. Failure to reduce the dislocation results in persistent deformity and arthrosis, necessitating triple arthrodesis.

Longitudinal Forces
Longitudinal force injury of the midtarsal joint represents forces directed at the digits distally toward the rear foot (Fig. 17-7). Such a force can be likened to striking a football or soccer ball with the foot. When such forces are transmitted longitudinally along the metatarsals while the ankle is in a plantar-flexed position, compression injury at the midtarsal joint occurs. Midtarsal fracture-dislocations occur when the cuneiforms provide longitudinal compression and shear forces significant enough to fracture the navicular. A more medial force results in varying degrees of navicular comminution and displacement with calcaneocuboid compression. A more lateral to medial force vector may result in variable degrees of calcaneocuboid joint dislocation and crushing of the lateral pole of the navicular when it is caught between the lateral cuneiform and the talar head.

A significant increase in less favorable outcomes is seen in this group of injuries. The degree of comminution of the navicular and cuboid affects the prognosis. Multiple interarticular fractures can result in significant arthrosis of the midtarsal joint. Open reduction was reported to give only fair results in three patients treated by Main and Jowett.[13]

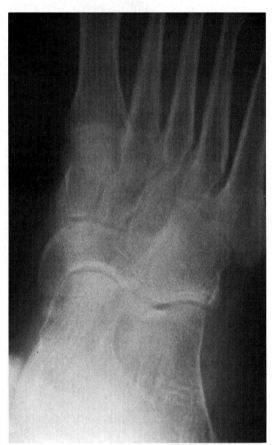

A

Fig. 17-6. Medial force fracture-sprains. Case 1: (**A**) Anteroposterior and (**B**) lateral radiographs demonstrating avulsion flake fractures from the navicular and cuboid. (*Figure continues.*)

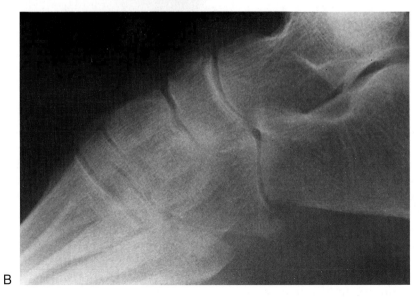

B

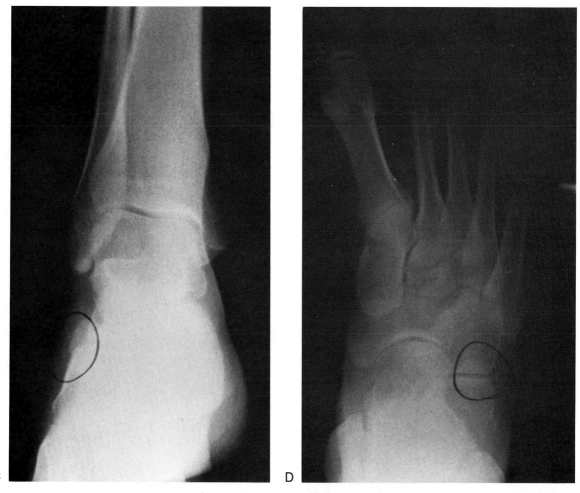

Fig. 17-6 (*Continued*). Case 2: (**C**) Anteroposterior ankle and (**D**) anteroposterior foot radiographs demonstrating flake avulsion fractures of the cuboid. (From Smith,[22] with permission.)

Lateral Forces

As in medial midtarsal dislocation, lateral force midtarsal dislocations are subdivided into fracture-sprains, fracture-dislocations, and swivel-dislocations. Fracture-sprains represent a forefoot forcefully directed laterally on the rear foot through the midtarsal joint. Avulsion fracture of the plantar aspect of the navicular can be caused by the strong attachment of the bifurcate ligament. Dorsal flake fractures resulting from ligamentous and capsular avulsion may be present as well. Impaction of the calcaneocuboid joint will result as the force continues laterally. The nut-cracker fracture,[27] or cuboid excursion dislocation,[25] represents a more severe degree of lateral force midtarsal injury.

The mechanism of lateral fracture-subluxations is similar; however, significant collapse of the calcaneocuboid articulation results in displacement of the navicular laterally on the head of the talus. These injuries are reported to have a poor prognosis with closed reduction and casting.[24] Most cases progress to triple arthrodesis or isolated calcaneocuboid fusion. This may be explained by the rigidity needed within the lateral column to permit ambulation. Any compromise

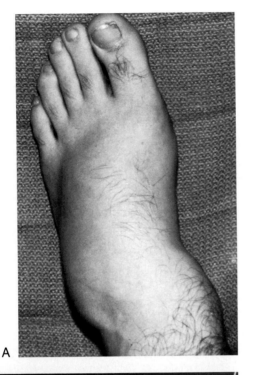

A

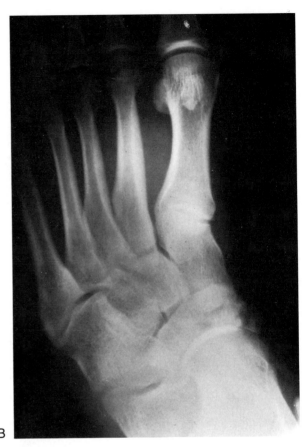

B

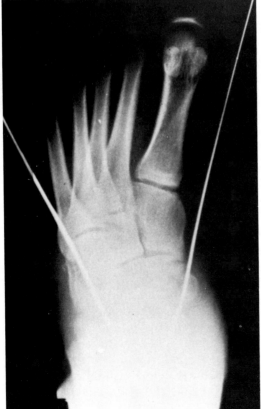

C

Fig. 17-7. Longitudinal force injury of the midtarsal joint. (**A**) Prereduction clinical representation. (**B**) Prereduction and (**C**) postreduction anteroposterior radiographs. (*Figure continues.*)

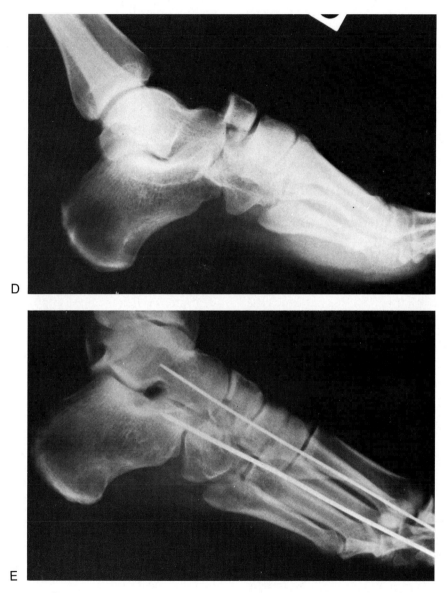

Fig. 17-7 (*Continued*). (**D**) Prereduction and (**E**) postreduction lateral radiographs. (From Smith,[22] with permission.)

in this rigidity can result in arthrosis and discomfort. The more mobile medial column of the midtarsal joint may permit a further degree of laxity or compromise in healing, presenting with less discomfort following reduction.

Swivel-dislocation injuries result as the midfoot and lateral rear-foot column twist laterally on an intact talocalcaneal ligament of the subtalar joint. Avulsion of the insertion of the tibialis posterior tendon from the navicular may occur. The prognosis for this injury is somewhat improved owing to lack of injury to the calcaneocuboid joint.

The pediatric or adult patient presenting with lateral force midtarsal joint injury and apparent fractures of the navicular presents an interesting diagnostic dilemma. The differential diagnosis of os tibiale externum or bifurcate navicular and fractures of the navicular or disruptions of ossicles can be difficult. The os tibiale externum is a well-formed round ossicle within the tibialis posterior tendon. A bifurcate navicular appears as an enlarged tuberosity with a radiolucent zone (Fig. 17-8). A determination of whether an injury has occurred to an os tibiale externum or a fracture

has occurred in the navicular can generally be made. A significantly enlarged navicular with an apparent fracture generally represents a bifurcate navicular with disruption of the nonunion zone within the navicular. Regardless of whether a navicular fracture has occurred or a bifurcate navicular or os tibiale externum has disrupted, casting and immobilization are used as treatment if alignment is satisfactory. Continued pain and discomfort in this area may necessitate removal of the fracture fragment or excision of the ossicle. Extremely large avulsion fractures of the navicular involving the articular surface of the talonavicular joint may necessitate open reduction and internal fixation to maintain joint contours and congruity. Disruption of a bifurcate navicular junctional area generally heals without difficulty. Follow-up support of the longitudinal arch after casting and immobilization greatly facilitates early mobilization.

Plantar Forces

Plantar force injuries to the midtarsal joint represent plantar flexory forces applied to the forefoot on a fixed rear foot through the midtarsal joint.

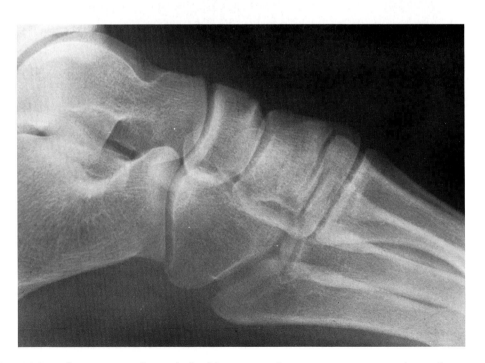

Fig. 17-8. Bifurcate navicular with double osseous density onto anterior calcaneal process.

These injuries are frequently associated with motorcycle accidents. Forward falls from stairs can result in such injury patterns. These injuries are subdivided into fracture-sprains and fracture-dislocations.

Avulsion fractures from the dorsum of the navicular are generally present. Anterior process fractures of the calcaneus represent plantar force injury through the midtarsal joint. The strong bifurcate ligament inserts into this area of the calcaneus. With a plantarly directed force from the navicular and cuboid, avulsion of this process through an intact bifurcate ligament can occur. These injuries are usually associated with long-term disability. Nonunion of the large osseous fragments will sometimes warrant surgical exci-

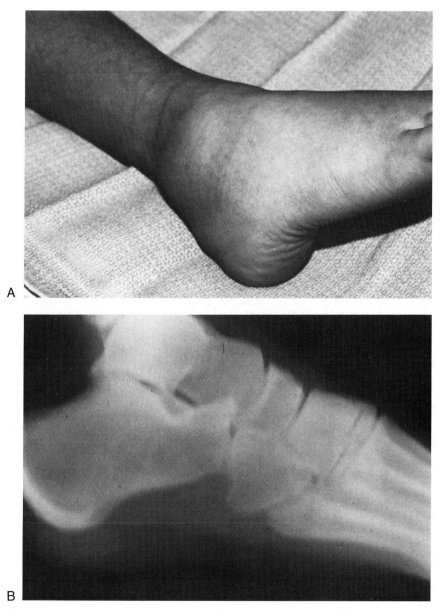

Fig. 17-9. Plantar force fracture-subluxation. (**A**) Clinical presentation. (**B**) Prereduction radiograph.

sion. Open reduction and internal fixation of any major fracture fragments may be required immediately following the injury.

More violent plantar flexion injuries may result in impaction fracture of the inferior aspect of the calcaneocuboid joint. Simple dislocations without fracture of the entire midtarsal joint can occur. These have a good prognosis if early reduction is obtained (Fig. 17-9). The strong plantar ligaments generally remain intact, lending stability to the relocated joints.[28]

Crush Injuries

Crush injuries to the midtarsal joint represent devastating fracture-dislocation patterns for the foot. These interarticular disruptions and fractures have a poor prognosis for adequate reduction and healing following the injury. Soft tissue compromise after crushing can result in significant soft tissue loss. In any crush injury to the midtarsal joint, adequate evaluation and monitoring for soft tissue injury and the presence of open injury are necessary.

Of interest is the absence of a dorsiflexory force injury pattern to the midtarsal joint.[11] No such injury has ever been reported. Studies involving dorsal forces through the midtarsal joint have demonstrated that injury with this type of force will occur at the Lisfranc's joint level.[29,30] Dorsal dislocation has been proved clinically impossible at the midtarsal joint. The strong plantar ligaments and bifurcate ligament prevent dorsal injury at the midtarsal joint level. The force is transmitted distally to the weaker Lisfranc's joint where disruption occurs.

LISFRANC'S DISLOCATION*

The tarsometatarsal joints form a bony arc from medial to lateral across the foot similar to a stone arch. This osseous configuration combined with

---

* Reprinted with permission from: Dinapoli RD, Cain TD: Lisfranc fracture-dislocation: update 1988. p. 198. In McGlamry ED (ed): Reconstructive Surgery of the Foot and Leg: Update '88. Podiatry Institute Publishing, Tucker, GA, 1988.

an extensive ligamentous support network and the "keystone" nature of the recessed second metatarsal base provide a significant amount of stability to the midfoot joint complex (Fig. 17-10). The reported incidence of dislocation and fracture of the Lisfranc's joint is less than 1 percent of all fractures.[31–37] The severity may range from an occult subluxation to a grossly malaligned fracture-dislocation.

Fracture-dislocation of the Lisfranc's joint complex is reportedly misdiagnosed approximately 20 percent of the time.[38] The morbidity associated with this injury is great. Severe edema and hematoma frequently form following the injury and necessitate the use of Doppler ultrasound for identification of pedal arteries. Damage to the perforating vessels and arterial spasms leading to circulatory compromise and amputation have been reported.[39] Other complications include severe post-traumatic degenerative arthritis, reflex sympathetic dystrophy, and painful osseous prominences. Prevention of these complications requires accurate diagnosis and prompt treatment.

Anatomy

Full knowledge of the regional anatomy is essential for appreciation of the osseous and soft tissue damage that occurs. The mechanism of this injury, the injury patterns, and the technique for reduction are fully dependent on the osseous and ligamentous relationships.

The metatarsals are bound to one another by a series of transverse dorsal and plantar ligaments as well as intermetatarsal ligaments.[29,40] The one exception is the lack of ligamentous attachment between the first and second metatarsals. This anatomic fact is responsible for the injury pattern in which the four lesser metatarsals dislocate laterally as a unit, leaving the first metatarsal unaffected.[41] It has been proposed that the pattern of dislocation of the first metatarsal does not depend on the lesser four metatarsals.[39,42]

The ligaments that tether the metatarsus to the lesser tarsus are disrupted during this injury. The ligaments are stronger plantarly than dorsally. The dorsomedial ligament attaching the medial

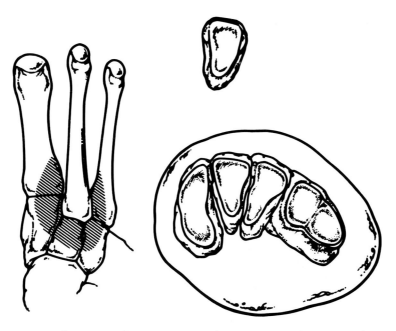

Fig. 17-10. Tarsometatarsal joint configuration is similar to stone arch. Recessed position of second metatarsal confers added stability to this point.

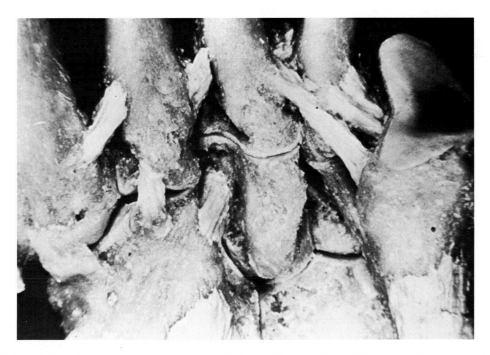

Fig. 17-11. Lisfranc's ligament attaches to medial cuneiform and medial aspect of second metatarsal base.

cuneiform to the first metatarsal is the largest ligament at this level. During open repairs of this injury, it is often possible to primarily repair this ligament. Probably the most significant ligament of the tarsometatarsal joint is the interosseous ligament that attaches the medial cuneiform to the second metatarsal base. This structure is commonly designated as Lisfranc's ligament.[29,43] It is responsible for the production of an avulsion fracture of the medial aspect of the second metatarsal[41,44–46] (Figs. 17-11 and 17-12). The remaining ligaments are either disrupted or avulsed

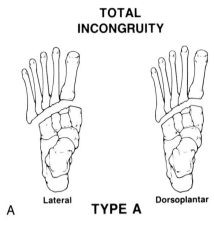

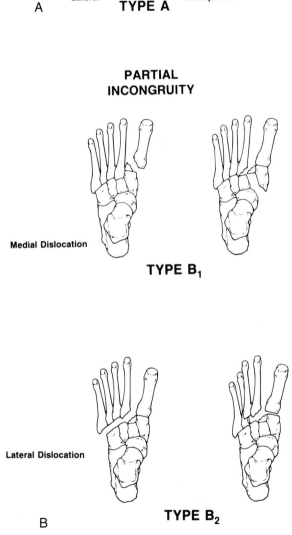

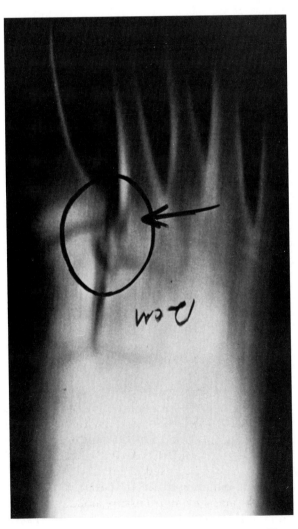

Fig. 17-12. Avulsion fracture of medial aspect of base of second metatarsal is generated by Lisfranc's ligament. Also shown is fracture of medial cuneiform.

Fig. 17-13. (A–C) Artist's interpretation of Hardcastle and associates'[36] classification of Lisfranc's joint injuries. (*Figure continues.*)

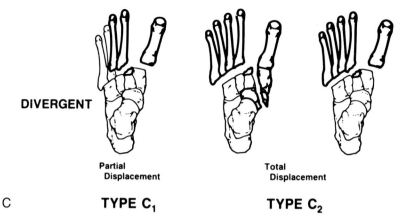

DIVERGENT

Partial
Displacement

Total
Displacement

C   **TYPE C₁**   **TYPE C₂**

Fig. 17-13 (*Continued*). **(C)**

from their attachments, creating multiple small flake fractures.

The inherent osseous stability of the tarsometatarsal joint was previously mentioned. The convex shape formed by the metatarsal-lesser tarsus articulations from medial to lateral combined with the dorsal to plantar wedge shape of the articulations creates added stability in both the transverse and sagittal planes.

Classification

Numerous classifications of this injury have been proposed in the literature based on mechanics of injury,[29,41,46,47] direction of force,[35] and resultant injury pattern.[36,48] No particular study has specifically addressed the injury pattern in light of surgical repair and end results. Hardcastle and associates describe a comprehensive classification that was based on the injury pattern of metatarsal displacement[36] (Fig. 17-13). They reported that the amount of displacement will influence the degree of fixation and prognosis. The classification system is simple to apply and is based on the radiographic appearance.

Type A—total displacements involve total incongruity of the entire tarsometatarsal joint. The displacement may occur in the sagittal or transverse planes.

Type B—partial displacements involve partial incongruity of the joint complex in either sagittal or transverse planes, or both. Partial injuries of two types may exist. *Medial displacement* affects the first metatarsal either in isolation or combined with displacement of one or more of the second, third, or fourth metatarsals. *Lateral displacement* involves one or more of the four lesser metatarsals while the first is unaffected.

Type C—divergent displacements may involve partial or total incongruity of the joint. The first metatarsal is displaced medially and any combination of the lateral four metatarsals is displaced laterally in either the sagittal or transverse planes or both.

Two mechanisms of tarsometatarsal joint injury have been postulated—direct and indirect.[35] The direct mechanism involves a crushing force concentrated at the dorsum of the foot with a variable pattern of load, direction, and velocity, resulting in a variety of fracture-dislocation patterns.

The indirect mechanism is the least understood and most variable. Wiley in 1971 performed cadaver studies and proposed that there were two main forces associated with the indirect mechanism, forefoot abduction and forced forefoot plantar flexion.[29] The foot is usually injured while in a plantar-flexed or equinus position. A traumatic abductory force is applied to the forefoot that produces an excessive amount of shear stress at the second metatarsal base. This results in either a transverse base fracture of the second metatarsal or an avulsion fracture of the medial aspect of the second metatarsal base. The avulsion fragment is usually attached to Lisfranc's ligament. If the abduction force continues, the lesser metatarsals may shift laterally as the lateral tarsometatarsal ligaments fail and rupture. Occasionally, the severe abductory force will result in a distal cuboid compression fracture.

Clinical Presentation

The diagnosis of tarsometatarsal fracture-dislocation requires little insight with obvious clinical and radiographic evidence. This is contrasted to the diagnosis of an occult, reduced fracture-dislocation, which requires a high index of clinical suspicion because of the long-term sequelae of a missed diagnosis.[49,50]

Often the patient recalls an audible snap or pop after experiencing a forced plantar flexion or direct injury mechanism. The patient may relate stepping off of a curb, slipping on the stairs, or stepping in a hole. The indirect mechanism more often occurs in a motor vehicle accident in which the plantar-flexed foot sustains a longitudinal force against the floor board.[34,36,51]

In both, physical examination will reveal gross edema over the entire forefoot and midfoot region. There will be marked palpatory tenderness over the tarsometatarsal joints. Pedal pulses must be identified. If the dorsalis pedis and posterior tibial artery cannot be palpated, Doppler ultrasound must be used. Excessive range of motion at the tarsometatarsal joint may be present.

Standard diagnostic radiographs should be obtained for the foot and ankle, and comparison views may also be warranted. If initial radiographs appear superficially normal, careful scrutiny may discern the pathognomonic sign of a relocated tarsometatarsal joint fracture-dislocation. Attention should be directed to the first metatarsal base, which may reveal a slight diastasis between the first and second metatarsals. Careful examination of the second metatarsal base may highlight a small avulsion fragment diagnostic of dislocation at this level. One should also follow the cortical margins of the metatarsals and their adjacent tarsal bones. The most consistent relationship appears to be the medial cortical margin of the second metatarsal and the medial edge of the second cuneiform (Fig. 17-14).[51] A compression fracture of the cuboid may also be diagnostic of the lateral displacement type of tarsometatarsal fracture-dislocation.

If standard radiographs prove negative but clinical symptoms persist, stress radiographs should be obtained.[38] Stress radiographs in the transverse or sagittal plane may be performed under local anesthesia or general anesthesia for a more accurate diagnosis (Fig. 17-15).

Management

The literature concerning appropriate treatment combines all injuries under the heading of Lisfranc's dislocation regardless of the injury pattern. Some researchers have noted differences among the injury patterns and the type of treat-

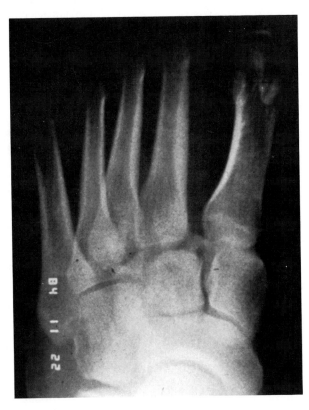

Fig. 17-14. Dorsoplantar radiograph of type C injury. Careful scrutiny of medical cortical margin of second metatarsal and cuneiform will reveal a diastasis and avulsion fracture.

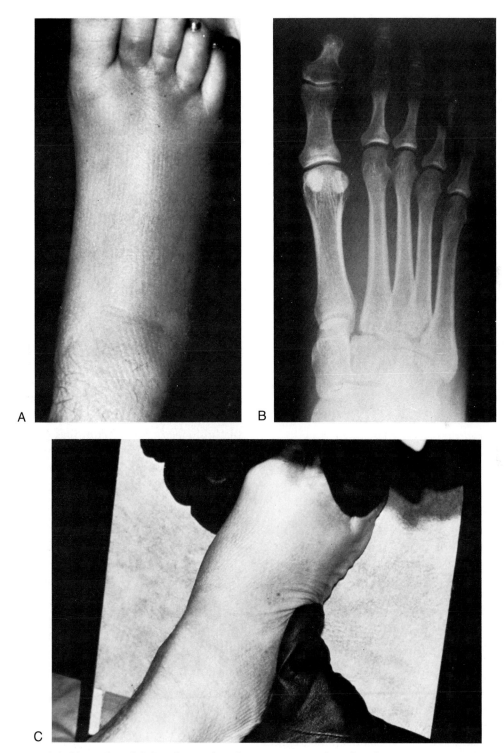

Fig. 17-15. (A) Clinical and (B) radiographic demonstration of Lisfranc's injury type C with marked edema and pathognomonic diastasis of first and second metatarsal. (C) Excessive motion is present clinically at the tarsometatarsal articulation. (*Figure continues.*)

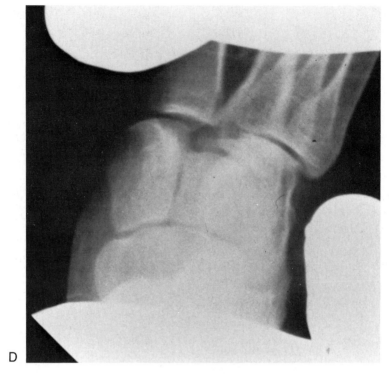

D

Fig. 17-15 (*Continued*). (**D**) Abduction stress radiograph reveals gross dislocation.

ment that was rendered.[36] The best functional results are provided through accurate anatomic alignment whether open or closed.[30,34,35,52,53] Wire fixation will maintain alignment following reduction.[34,36,54] Closed reduction with casting of the unstable joints has not proved effective.[34,36,38] Factors that will influence the outcome of the injury are delay in diagnosis, amount of displacement, local soft tissue injury, and quality and maintenance of the initial reduction.

We treat this injury initially with closed reduction.[22] Anesthesia combined with muscle relaxation is usually required. Distal forefoot traction is applied against countertraction of the heel. The forefoot is suspended from the operating room table by finger traps and tape, with countertraction weights applied to the heel. Manipulation may then be attempted to reposition the second metatarsocuneiform articulation. Once relocation is verified radiographically, percutaneous wire stabilization may be utilized.

Soft tissue interposition between osseous segments or even fracture comminution may prevent

anatomic reduction. The tibialis anterior and peroneus longus may interpose between osseous articulations and prevent anatomic realignment.[41,55–57]

Should closed reduction methods fail, open reduction is indicated. Open reduction is also indicated for inspection of pedal blood vessels if circulatory compromise is present.[36,39] The operative approach employs longitudinal curvilinear incisions to help prevent further compromise. The first incision is usually placed medially over the first metatarsocuneiform joint with adequate distal exposure. Recent experiences have demonstrated that the dorsal medial ligament of this joint can be separated from the joint capsule during the dissection process. A second dorsal incision is commonly placed just over the articulation of the second and third metatarsal bases and articulating cuneiforms. The second metatarsocuneiform joint must be inspected and any osseous fragments found within the joint excised. A similar approach is utilized for the fifth metatarsocuboid joint.

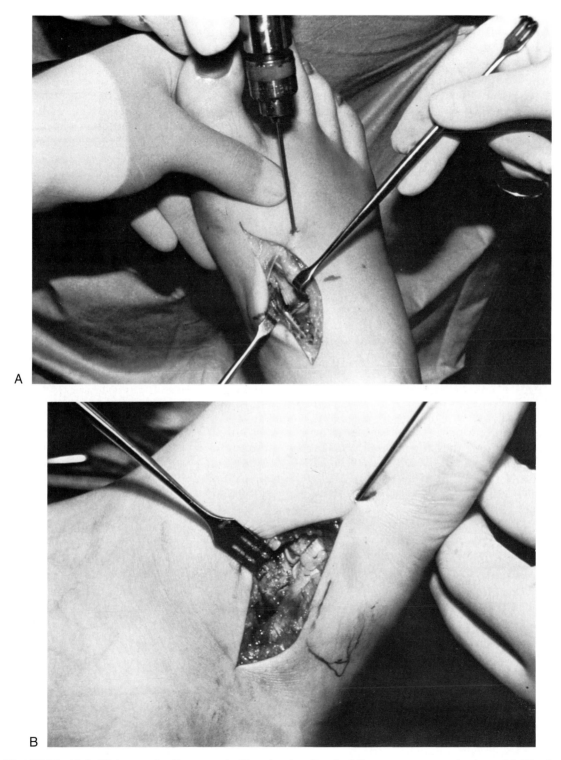

Fig. 17-16. (**A & B**) Anatomic alignment is directly visualized while percutaneous pinning with Kirschner wires is performed.

Once anatomic alignment has been accomplished, wire stabilization is used under direct visualization (Fig. 17-16). The technique for wire stabilization depends primarily on the injury pattern. Instability may exist at the intercuneiform articulations. Cuneiform instability requires wire stabilization of the cuneiforms from medial to lateral prior to stabilizing the metatarsus on the tarsus.

In type A injuries, stabilization with two wires is common but it depends on the stability of the second metatarsocuneiform joint. If severe dislocation is present at this level, the surgeon may encounter difficulty stabilizing the first metatarsocuneiform joint. Initial stabilization of the second metatarsocuneiform joint gives a significant amount of stability to the entire joint complex, permitting greater ease of medial and lateral sta-

bilization in those cases. In general, two wires are used for type A injuries, one medially across the first metatarsocuneiform joint and one laterally across the fifth metatarsal cuboid joint (Fig. 17-17).

The medial type B injuries are extremely unstable and usually require two medial fixation wires. The lateral type B injuries usually require a lateral wire through the fifth metatarsocuboid articulation. Type C injuries are extremely unstable and often require three or more wires for fixation. Cuneiform disruption seems to occur more often with this injury.

After radiographic confirmation of alignment, soft tissue repair is completed. Primary repair of the dorsomedial ligament of the first metatarsocuneiform joint and its capsule is quite possible (Fig. 17-18). Delayed closure may be necessary if

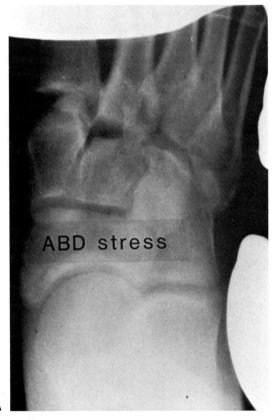

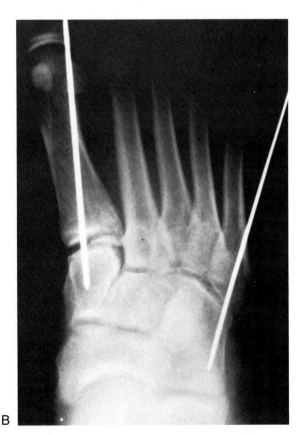

A   B

Fig. 17-17. **(A)** Abductory stress examination reveals total lateral displacement of metatarsals on lesser tarsus. **(B)** Postoperative radiograph demonstrating stabilization of first metatarsocuneiform joint and fifth metatarsocuboid joint.

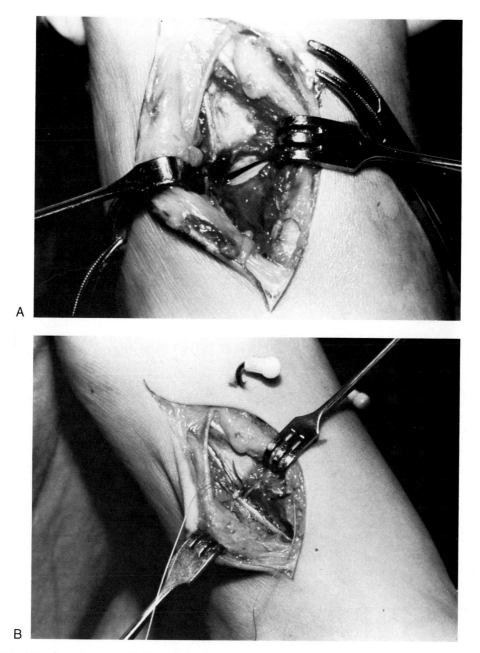

Fig. 17-18. (A) Identification of dorsomedial ligament of first metatarsocuneiform joint. (B) Primary repair of ligament and capsule. Note percutaneous wire stabilization.

severe edema or extensive trauma to the soft tissues exists.

Compressive dressings are applied following reduction until edema and the vascular status have stabilized. This depends on the extent and severity of the injury, and usually occurs in 5 to 14 days. Below-the-knee casting is then used for 6 to 12 weeks. Wires can be removed between 6 and 8 weeks. Weight bearing with supportive shoegear may begin after cast removal. Careful monitoring for redislocation is extremely important.

A number of complications have been previously mentioned. In old injuries in which there are severe destructive changes and pain or deformity, arthrodesis of the involved tarsometatarsal joints is indicated and may be performed in a variety of ways.

Fracture-dislocation of the Lisfranc's joint complex is a relatively uncommon injury. Diagnosis of the grossly edematous and painful foot with radiographic changes is not difficult. The occult disruption of this joint complex requires a high index of suspicion. Accurate anatomic reduction at initial presentation has produced the most satisfactory results. Surgical intervention in acute and chronic cases may be warranted.

FIRST METATARSOPHALANGEAL JOINT

Sporadic reports of first metatarsophalangeal joint dislocation attest to the rare occurrence of this injury. Jahss reported treating only two dislocations of this type from approximately 25,000 foot patients.[58] Giannikas et al. indicated treating only four cases in over 10,000 orthopedic patients.[59] We have recorded four such cases, two traumatic and two pathologic.[60,61] The two pathologic cases represent a type II first metatarsophalangeal joint dislocation associated with spina bifida and a previously unreported case of lateral first metatarsophalangeal joint dislocation in a patient with insulin-dependent diabetes mellitus (Fig. 17-19).

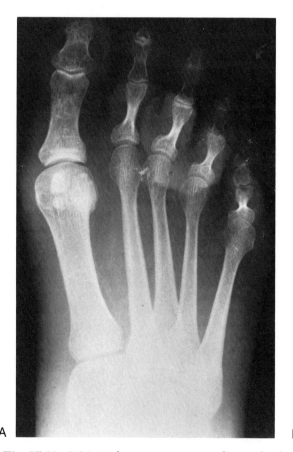
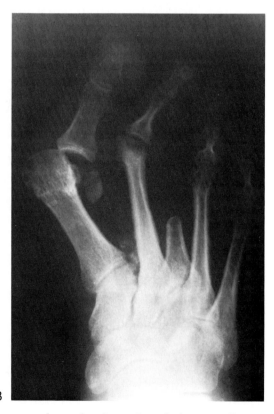

A   B

Fig. 17-19. **(A)** Initial anteroposterior radiograph of patient with insulin-dependent diabetes mellitus. **(B)** Eighteen months later following ray resection for osteomyelitis, Charcot degeneration of Lisfranc's joint, and lateral dislocation of the first metatarsophalangeal joint.

Despite the rare occurrence of this injury, dislocation of the first metatarsophalangeal joint is interesting both anatomically and pathomechanically.[22] The first metatarsophalangeal joint is extremely complex in design and function. A multitude of soft tissues including ligaments, tendons, and joint capsule bind the osseous components, including the sesamoids, metatarsal, and proximal phalanx. A thorough understanding of these anatomic relationships is needed to appreciate the injury presentation and deduce soft tissue disruptions.

Anatomy

The first metatarsophalangeal joint is formed by the articulation of the round first metatarsal head with the ovoid and concave proximal phalangeal base (Fig. 17-20). Two sesamoids exist within the flexor apparatus plantar to the metatarsal head. They can be considered as an articular extension of the proximal phalangeal cup because of their fixed position to it.[58] The entire metatarsal articular surface articulates with the phalangeal-sesamoid articular surface through dorsiflexion and plantar flexion. The sesamoids ride within grooves on the metatarsal head plantarly separated by a ridge or crista.

Five basic osseous relationships exist within this metatarsal-sesamoid-phalangeal complex of the first metatarsophalangeal joint. The soft tissues bind and support these relationships and permit the motion needed through active muscular power and the biomechanical forces of gait to permit ambulation. These five relationships include (1) metatarsal-phalanx; (2) metatarsal-sesamoid; (3) sesamoid-phalanx; (4) foot-sesamoid; (5) sesamoid-sesamoid. Each relationship is considered when assessing the soft tissue damage present in a first metatarsophalangeal joint dislocation.

The metatarsal is joined to the phalanx by the fibrous capsule surrounding the joint and by the strong medial and lateral collateral ligaments. The metatarsal is joined to the sesamoid by the

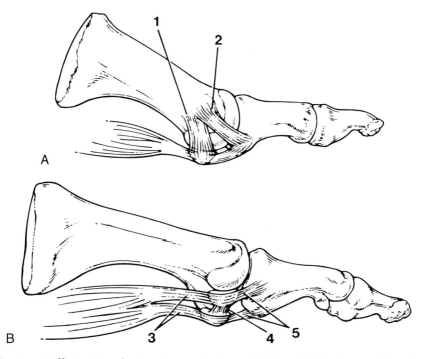

Fig. 17-20. Anatomic illustration first metatarsophalangeal joint. (**A**) Medial and (**B**) plantar-medial perspectives. 1, Sesamoidal collateral ligament; 2, collateral ligament; 3, flexor tendons, fibular and tibial; 4, intersesamoidal ligament; 5, tendinous extension flexor apparatus from sesamoid to phalanx.

sesamoidal collateral ligaments medially and laterally and by portions of the joint capsule plantarly as well. The sesamoids are firmly held to the proximal phalanx by the tendinous extensions of the flexor hallucis brevis. The tibial sesamoid is secured through the flexor hallucis brevis and abductor hallucis tendons. The sesamoids are bound to the foot proximally by the expandable and elastic muscle belly tissues of the flexor hallucis brevis, abductor hallucis, and adductor hallucis. The sesamoids are bound to each other very firmly by the intersesamoidal ligament. The deep transverse intermetatarsal ligament provides the distal interconnection from the first metatarsal to the second metatarsal.

Classification

Automobile accidents account for the vast majority of reported cases.[38,59,60,62,63] Falls from a height account for a secondary number.[64–66] Pathologic compromise of tissues would appear to account for a significant number of cases as well (Fig. 17-19).[61] A hyperextension force of the phalanx-sesamoid apparatus on the metatarsal is generally accepted as the mechanism of injury. A secondary force of direct pressure to the plantar joint may be present to complicate the hyperextension force.

During an injury episode, the proximal phalanx-sesamoid apparatus goes through a dorsiflexory range of motion on the metatarsal. The end range of motion is met and the proximal capsular attachments at the metatarsal neck level rupture plantarly. The joint then virtually turns inside-out as the sesamoids are dragged distally over the metatarsal head within the intact collateral ligaments. The phalangeal-sesamoid relationship is generally not disrupted.[59] The sesamoids remain attached to the proximal phalanx. The articular convex cuplike surface continues to be contiguous (Fig. 17-21). Giannikas et al. reported a case in which the sesamoids remained plantarly and retracted with dorsal dislocation of the phalanx on the metatarsal.[59] This is the only such case noted in the literature.

The sesamoid collateral ligaments must rupture to permit the degree of sesamoid to metatar-

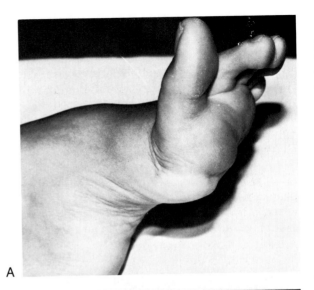

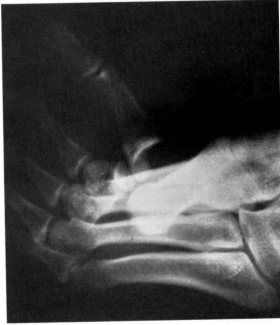

Fig. 17-21. Dislocation of first metatarsophalangeal joint. **(A)** Prereduction clinical presentation. **(B)** Prereduction radiographic presentation.

sal malalignment that exists. No such anatomic description has been found or noted in the literature. The sesamoid-foot soft tissues remain intact. The elongated and pliable muscle complex lies medially and laterally, passing from plantar to dorsal over the metatarsal head. The medial and lateral components are slung beneath the epicondyles of the first metatarsal and the insertion of the collateral ligaments. They take a right-angle turn from their plantar origins to the dorsally luxated proximal phalangeal base. The pivot point of the right-angle turn is the intact collateral ligament insertion in the metatarsal epicondyles medially and laterally. A rigid strap is created to prevent relocation. It includes the tibial and fibular foot-sesamoid-phalanx apparatus joined by the intersesamoidal ligament. Disruption of any portion of this strap will weaken it and increase the possibility of closed reduction. It must be emphasized that, to this point in the dislocation process, the only rupture of soft tissue is the plantar joint capsule from the metatarsal neck and possibly the sesamoidal collateral ligaments.

The intersesamoidal relationship is important to assess radiographically before reduction. A normal sesamoid to sesamoid relationship, although both sesamoids lie dorsal to the metatarsal, implies an intact foot-sesamoid-phalanx apparatus bound together by the intact intersesamoidal ligament. Closed reduction is virtually impossible.[59,60,64] Further traumatic hyperextension force of the proximal phalanx applies a force to pull apart the sesamoids in a medial plantar to lateral plantarward direction. This can be likened to breaking a stick over a knee. The phalanx continues to pull the sesamoids dorsally while they are still bound plantarly through the muscular origins slung around the metatarsal condyles. Thus, a medial to lateral disruptive force is applied to the intersesamoidal ligament. Two scenarios are likely to dissipate the additional force: (1) the intersesamoidal ligament ruptures, or (2) a sesamoid fractures transversely distal to the intact intersesamoidal ligament remnant.

If the intersesamoidal ligament ruptures, the sesamoid-sesamoid relationship seen radiographically is widened. This injury is much more amendable to closed reduction.[59,63–65] This is due to the slack created in the flexor appartus binding the metatarsal plantarly beneath the sesamoids. It might seem more logical that if the intersesamoidal ligament did not rupture, the sesamoid would fracture longitudinally. The strength of the sesamoid bone itself over the soft tissues is,

however, much greater. An avulsion type of transverse fracture occurs distal to the intersesamoidal ligament in the fibular sesamoid. Only the proximal fragment remains attached to the adjacent sesamoid. Closed reduction here is again more readily possible.[59,63–65] The concern here is for the distal sesamoidal fragment. It tends to act as a free fragment within the joint, not healing to the proximal major fibular sesamoidal fragment. This results in pain that may necessitate excision.[63,65] A fractured sesamoid reported by Brown healed uneventfully.[64]

Sesamoidal fracture may also occur by direct plantar force applied to the joint, as in falls from heights.[66] The tibial sesamoid is implicated more in these injuries owing to its prominence beneath the joint. The fracture pattern is potentially variable. The fibular sesamoid appears to be involved in the avulsion-type mechanism of hyperextension. The pattern of fracture is fairly regular and has a transverse orientation as described above.

Clinically, the patient will present with a prominent first metatarsal head plantarly. Some extensor tendon relaxation may be observed. The hallux interphalangeal joint may be in a plantar-flexed attitude. Attempted plantar flexory motion of the joint is restricted, resulting in pain with range of motion and palpation (Fig. 17-21). Obesity or extensive edema can mask the clinical presentation. Cases have been reported in the literature of delay in diagnosis because of the presence of multiple other injuries.[59]

Management

Jahss has described a classification scheme for first metatarsophalangeal joint dislocations.[58] The scheme is based on the position of the sesamoids and whether or not fracture of the sesamoids is present. Type I dislocations represent dorsal luxation of the sesamoid-phalanx complex upon the metatarsal head. The intersesamoidal ligaments remain intact. These dislocations are poorly reducible by closed means. Type II dislocations represent some degree of disruption of the intersesamoidal apparatus. Type IIA dislocations represent a disruption of the intersesamoidal ligament. Radiographically, the sesamoids appear well separated medially and laterally but still dorsal to the metatarsal head. Type IIB dislocations represent a fracture of the fibular sesamoid resulting in a normal tibiofibular sesamoid alignment dorsal to the metatarsal with a fracture fragment still attached to the base of the proximal phalanx. This classification scheme does not recognize the medial or lateral dislocation possibilities (Fig. 17-19) or dorsal migration of the proximal phalanx with the plantar attitude of the sesamoids.[59]

Type II dislocations are generally relocated by closed reduction methods. A distal traction force is applied to the joint, followed by plantar flexory movement. The slackening of the intersesamoidal ligament strap prevents locking of the metatarsal head, allowing plantar excursion of the proximal phalanx and relocation.

Percutaneous pinning is generally not required. Compressive dressings are applied for 3 to 4 weeks as a standard course. At approximately 3 weeks, ambulation may be started, followed by physical therapy regimens as needed. Once ambulation begins, a surgical shoe may be utilized in the recovery period as ambulatory status improves.

Type I injuries generally require open reduction. Attempts at closed reduction are notoriously unsuccessful. The first metatarsal remains trapped beneath an intact intersesamoidal ligament strap as described above. Several investigators describe a plantar transverse approach to the first metatarsophalangeal joint to permit open reduction. This approach is reported to offer the best visualization and the most direct approach to the relevant anatomic structures necessary for relocation. Other researchers prefer a dorsomedial approach utilizing an inverted L-shaped capsulotomy in the intact dorsal capsule.[60] Plantar scars are thus avoided with their potential complications.

Postoperative therapy usually does not necessitate extensive immobilization since most relocations are generally very stable. A report of recurrent dislocations has appeared in the literature.[67] A below-the-knee weight-bearing cast for approximately 4 weeks followed by hydrotherapy can be utilized. A firm compression dressing, however, is generally all that is required for 2 to 3 weeks.

First metatarsophalangeal joint dislocations when reduced early generally do not result in degenerative joint disease or prolonged disability. This appears to be the prognosis regardless of the degree of injury involved or type of injury presented. Structural or positional deformities have not been reported if prompt therapy was instituted. Pain necessitating the excision of the distal fibular sesamoidal fragment has been described. When prompt reduction is not possible, secondary adhesions and fibrosis occur, preventing relocation. A Keller arthroplasty may be necessary to achieve reduction and realignment.[59,61] Mulis and Miller presented an interesting case of first metatarsophalangeal joint soft tissue injury without gross dislocation.[68] Stress radiography demonstrated excessive varus excursion. Repair of the torn conjoined adductor tendon, collateral ligament, and joint capsule relieved symptoms and provided stability. These subtle injuries may potentially occur about any plane.[68,69]

LESSER METATARSOPHALANGEAL JOINTS

Dislocations of the lesser metatarsophalangeal joints have been rarely reported in the literature.[70,71] They have been described as involving multiple joints[70] or, although extremely rare, as isolated dislocations.[71] This injury may be associated with other lower extremity trauma. English reported on lesser metatarsophalangeal joint dislocation occurring with Lisfranc's joint trauma.[72] Chronic pathologic dislocations of the lesser metatarsophalangeal joints are common forefoot complaints, especially in patients with arthritic tendencies (Fig. 17-22).[22]

Anatomy

The anatomy of the lesser metatarsophalangeal joints is similar to that of the first metatarsophalangeal joint. Articular surfaces are present on the distal and plantar surfaces of the metatarsal

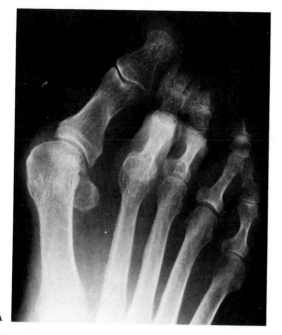 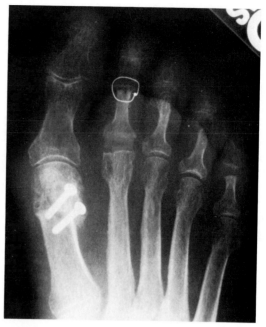

Fig. 17-22. Chronic dislocation of the second metatarsophalangeal joint. (**A**) Preoperative radiograph. (**B**) Postoperative radiograph demonstrating implant anthroplasty of the metatarsophalangeal joint with arthrodesis of the proximal interphalangeal joint.

head but do not cover it dorsally. Ligamentous structures include capsular, plantar, collateral, and deep transverse intermetatarsal ligaments.

The injury pattern is usually hyperextension, resulting from forced dorsiflexion of the proximal phalanx in relation to the metatarsal head. Accordingly, plantar ligamentous and capsular structures are ruptured from the joint.

The metatarsal head may actually buttonhole through the plantar fibrocartilaginous plate and become prominent plantarly. The metatarsal head then becomes trapped by the fibrocartilaginous plate plantarly, the deep transverse intermetatarsal ligament and dorsal capsule dorsally, the lumbrical tendons medially, and the flexor tendons laterally.[71] Open reduction is usually necessary after incarceration of the metatarsal head.[45] Strong transverse plane forces applied between the toes may result in collateral ligament disruption and medial or lateral dislocation.

Clinically, pain is elicited with joint palpation or attempted joint range of motion. Moderate to severe edema with diffuse ecchymosis may be present depending on the extent of injury. A prominent metatarsal head may be palpated where the head has extruded through the flexor plate.

Anteroposterior, oblique, and lateral radiographs without forefoot overexposure should be obtained. Classically, the anteroposterior radiograph will demonstrate an overlap of the joint margins. The lateral view will reveal an isolated proximal phalanx that is not superimposed with the other digits of the foot. Radiographic variants may exist depending on the mechanism of injury. In the anteroposterior view, foreshortening of the second toe with increased metatarsophalangeal joint space has been observed. A plantar position of the metatarsal head relative to the proximal phalanx in the lateral view has also been reported.[71]

A high index of suspicion is necessary, or subtle dislocations may be easily missed. Long-term sequelae of chronic dislocations include claw digit formation as well as painful plantar hyperkeratotic lesions and metatarsalgia. Undiagnosed or improperly treated isolated second metatarsophalangeal joint dislocation is analogous to am-

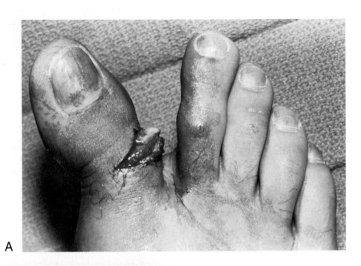

A

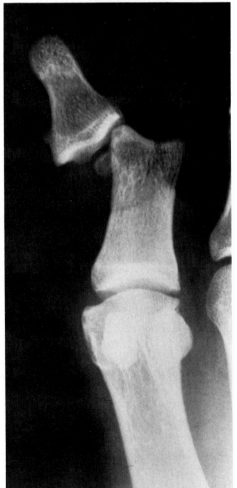

B

Fig. 17-23. Open dislocation of interphalangeal joint of hallux. (A) Prereduction clinical presentation. (B) Prereduction radiographic presentation.

putation of the second digit. Without support or buttress for the hallux, lateral drift ensues and hallux valgus is the final result. Degenerative changes of both the first and second metatarso-phalangeal joints may result, necessitating joint arthroplasty procedures.

Management

Closed reduction is usually successful in the majority of acute, dorsal dislocations.[45] A below-the-knee walking cast of a well-molded synthetic material may be utilized, or a padded metal splint may be applied.[73] Immobilization for 3 weeks is sufficient, followed by weight-bearing in a stiff-soled shoe as tolerated. Because redislocation may occur, follow-up radiographs and clinical monitoring should be performed frequently.

Unreducible dislocations occur occasionally secondary to soft tissue interpositioning resulting in trapping of the metatarsal head. Murphy reports on a case in which the fibrocartilaginous plate acted as an obstacle to closed reduction.[71] Roa et al. describe the metatarsal head incarcerated by tendon and ligamentous structures, requiring incision of the dorsal capsule, deep transverse metatarsal ligament, and fibrocartilaginous plate to achieve reduction.[70]

Rupture of a collateral ligament can result in either medial or lateral dislocation of the joint. The unstable nature of this injury may require percutaneous pinning as described by Giannestras and Sammarco.[73]

INTERPHALANGEAL JOINTS

Dislocations of the interphalangeal joints are generally rare. The most common joints involved are the hallux and the proximal interphalangeal joint of the second digit (Fig. 17-23).[45,74] The injury pattern is either isolated or multiple and may occur in association with other trauma (Fig. 17-24). Plantar or dorsal displacement of the distally located phalanx may occur. Plantar dislocations of the distal phalanx of the hallux have been described as more common than dorsally dis-

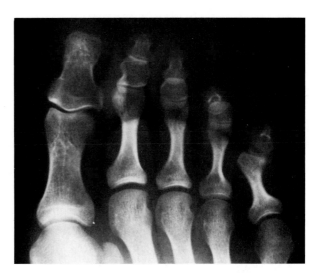

Fig. 17-24. Preoperative clinical presentation of proximal interphalangeal joint laxity following multiple traumas to fifth digit.

placed injuries. Closed reduction is usually possible, although Nelson and Uggen described an irreducible dorsal dislocation of the hallux.[74]

Anatomy

The interphalangeal joint is a hinge joint in which the trochlear surface of the phalangeal head articulates with the inversely shaped head of the phalangeal base. The joint is surrounded by an articular capsule that has two collateral ligaments arranged like those in the metatarsophalangeal joints. The plantar capsule is thickened to form a fibrous plate known as the volar plate or plantar ligament.

Injury patterns are from either forced dorsiflexion or plantar flexion of the involved joint. Transverse plane forces result in collateral ligament disruption, producing medial or lateral dislocation. Nelson and Uggen suggest that dorsal dislocations of the interphalangeal joint of the hallux are secondary to hyperextension at the interphalangeal joint with the metatarsophalangeal joint stabilized by the foot in a weight-bearing position.[74] Without stabilization of the metatarsal head, the metatarsophalangeal joint would dislocate owing to a greater lever arm and increased mobility at that joint.

Management

Interphalangeal joint dislocations almost always may be reduced by closed reduction.[75] Nelson and Uggen reported on an irreducible dorsal dislocation of the interphalangeal joint of the hallux in which exposure was obtained with a dorsal incision.[74] The collateral ligaments were intact, with the volar plate interposed into the joint and preventing relocation. The volar plate was moved plantarly and the joint was relocated.

Taping the affected digit to the adjacent digit is usually the only form of immobilization required. Cotton or felt is placed in the interdigital space, and the digits are taped together. Rarely, when the stability is questionable, a Kirschner wire may be placed percutaneously. Three weeks of immobilization is usually satisfactory whether or not wire fixation is utilized. Chronic instability of the joint may result following interphalangeal dislocation.

ACKNOWLEDGMENTS

Special thanks and appreciation are extended to Sherri Mercer for her technical assistance and dedication to this work in preparation of this manuscript.

REFERENCES

1. Leitner B: Obstacles to reduction of the talus. J Bone Joint Surg 36A:299, 1954
2. Smith H: Subastragalar dislocation. J Bone Joint Surg 19:373, 1937
3. Fahey JJ, Murphy JL: Dislocations and fractures of the talus. Surg Clin North Am 45:79, 1965
4. Christensen SB, Lorentzen JE, Krogsoe O et al: Subtalar dislocation. Acta Orthop Scand 48:707, 1977
5. Heppenstall RB, Farahvar H, Balderston R, Lotke P: Evaluation and management of subtalar dislocations. J Trauma 20:494, 1980
6. Monson ST, Ryan JR: Subtalar dislocation. J Bone Joint Surg 63A:1156, 1981
7. Shands AR, Jr: The incidence of subastraguloid dislocation of the foot with a report of one case of the inward type. J Bone Joint Surg 10:306, 1928
8. Grantham SA: Medial subtalar dislocation: five cases with a common etiology. J Trauma 4:845, 1964
9. Larsen HW: Subastragalar dislocation (luxatio pedis sub talo). Acta Chir Scand 113:380, 1957
10. Straus DC: Subtalar dislocation of the foot. J Bone Joint Surg 30:427, 1935
11. Buckingham WW: Subtalar dislocation of the foot. J Trauma 13:753, 1973
12. Leitner B: Mechanism of total dislocation of the talus. J Bone Joint Surg 37A:89, 1955
13. Main BJ, Jowett RL: Injuries of the midtarsal joint. J Bone Joint Surg 57B:89, 1975
14. Smith TF: Pedal dislocations: an overview. Clin Podiatry 2:349, 1985
15. Ganel A, Ahronson F, Heim M et al: Subtalar dislocations. J Foot Surg 20:142, 1981
16. Mulroy RD: The tibialis posterior tendon as an obstacle to reduction of a lateral anterior subtalar dislocation. J Bone Joint Surg 37A:859, 1955
17. Kenwright J, Taylor RG: Major injuries of the talus. J Bone Joint Surg 52B:36, 1970
18. Sharit FE, Cole LF: Subtalar dislocations. J Am Podiatry Assoc 74:386, 1984
19. Mindell ER, Cisek EE, Kartaliam G, Dziob M: Late results of injuries to the talus. J Bone Joint Surg 45A:221, 1963
20. Plewes IW, McKelvey KG: Subtalar dislocation. J Bone Joint Surg 26:585, 1944
21. Barber JR, Bricker JD, Haliburton RA: Peritalar dislocation of the foot. Can J Surg 4:205, 1961
22. Smith TF, Dislocation. In McGlamry ED (ed): Comprehensive Textbook of Foot Surgery. Williams & Wilkins, Baltimore, 1987
23. McKeever FM: Treatment of complications of fractures and dislocations of the talus. Clin Orthop 30:45, 1963
24. Dewar FP, Evans DC: Occult fracture-subluxation of midtarsal joint. J Bone Joint Surg 50B:386, 1968
25. Drummond DS, Hastings DE: Total dislocation of the cuboid bone. J Bone Joint Surg 51B:716, 1969
26. Sarrafian SK: Anatomy of the Foot and Ankle: Descriptive, Topographic, Functional. JB Lippincott, Philadelphia, 1983
27. Hermel MB, Gershon-Cohen J: The nutcracker

fracture of the cuboid by indirect violence. Radiology 60:850, 1953

28. Rymaszewski LA, Robb JE: Mechanism of fracture-dislocation of the navicular: brief report. J Bone Joint Surg 70B:492, 1988

29. Wiley JJ: The mechanism of tarso-metatarsal joint injuries. J Bone Joint Surg 53B:474, 1971

30. Wilson DW: Injuries of the tarso-metatarsal joints. J Bone Joint Surg 54B:677, 1972

31. Maerschalk P: Luxationsfracturen im Lisfrancschen Gelenk. Unfallchirurg 8:112, 1982

32. English TA: Dislocations of the metatarsal bone and adjacent Toe. J Bone Joint Surg 46B:700, 1964

33. Leitner B: Behandlung und Behandlungsergebnisse von 42 frischen Fallen von lusatio pedis sub talo im Unfallkrankenhaus in Wien in der Jahren 1925–1940. Ergeb Chir Orthop 37:501, 1952

34. Hesp WLEM, Van Der Werken C, Goris RJA: Lisfranc dislocations: fractures and/or dislocations through the tarso-metatarsal joints. Injury 15:261, 1984

35. Aitkin AP, Poulson D: Dislocation of the tarsometatarsal joint. J Bone Joint Surg 45A:246, 1963

36. Hardcastle PH, Reschauer R, Kutscha-Lissberg E, Schoffman W: Injuries to the tarsometatarsal joint: incidence, classification and treatment. J Bone Joint Surg 64B:349, 1982

37. Easton ER: Two rare dislocations of the metatarsal at Lisfranc's joint. J Bone Joint Surg 20:1053, 1938

38. Goossens M, DeStoop N: Lisfranc's fracture-dislocations: etiology, radiology, and results of treatment. Clin Orthop 176:154, 1983

39. Gissane W: A dangerous type of fracture of the foot. J Bone Joint Surg 33B:535, 1951

40. Romanes GJ: Cunningham's Textbook of Anatomy. 11th Ed. Oxford University Press. New York, 1972

41. Jeffreys TE: Lisfranc's fracture dislocation. J Bone Joint Surg 45B:546, 1963

42. Ashhurts APC: Divergent dislocation of the metatarsus. Ann Surg 83:132, 1926

43. Lenczner EM, Waddell JP, Graham JD: Tarsal-metatarsal (Lisfranc) dislocation. J Trauma 14:1012, 1974

44. Saft SS, Franciosi RV, Cole FL: Fracture-dislocation of the tarsometatarsal Joints. J Am Podiatry Assoc 71:162, 1981

45. Anderson ID: Injuries of the forefoot. Clin Orthop 122:18, 1977

46. Francesconi F: Sopra un caso di lussanzione di Lisfranc. Chir Organi Mov 9:589, 1925

47. Bonnel F, Barthelemy M: Traumatismes de l'artic-ulation de Lisfranc: entroses graves, luxations, fractures: etude de 39 observations. personnelle et classification biomechanique. J Chir (Paris) 111:573, 1963

48. Quenu E, Kuss G: Etude sur les luxations du metatarse du diastasis entre le 1er et le 2e metatarsien. Rev Chir 39:281, 720, 1093, 1909

49. Cook JM, Galorenzo R, Gold RH: Lisfranc's joint dislocation: a review and case report. J Am Podiatry Assoc 71:611, 1981

50. Norfray JF, Geline RA, Setinberg RI et al: Subtleties of Lisfranc fracture dislocations. AJR 137:1151, 1981

51. Foster SC, Foster RR: Lisfranc's tarsometatarsal fracture-dislocation. Radiology 120:79, 1976

52. Granberry WM, Lipscomb PR: Dislocations of the tarso-metatarsal joints. Surg Gynecol Obstet 114:467, 1962

53. Bassett FH: Dislocations of the tarsometatarsal joints. South Med J 57:1294, 1964

54. Holstein A, Joldersma RD: Dislocation of first cuneiform in tarsometatarsal fracture dislocations. J Bone Joint Surg 32:419, 1950

55. Lowe J, Yosipovitch Z: Tarsometatarsal dislocation: a mechanism blocking manipulative reduction. J Bone Joint Surg 58:1029, 1976

56. De Benedette MJ, Evanski PM, Waugh TR: The unreducible Lisfranc fracture. Clin Orthop 136:238, 1978

57. Blair WF: Irreducible tarsometatarsal fracture dislocation. J Trauma 21:988, 1981

58. Jahss MH: Traumatic dislocation of the first metatarsal phalangeal joint. Foot Ankle, 1:15, 1980

59. Giannikas AC, Papachristou G, Papavasilou N et al: Dorsal dislocation of the first metatarso-phalangeal joint. J Bone Joint Surg 57B:384, 1975

60. Daniel WL, Beck EL, Duggar GE: Traumatic dislocation of the fist metatarsophalangeal joint. J Am Podiatry Assoc 66:97, 1976

61. Schlefman BS, McGlamry ED, HIlkemann RJ: First metatarsophalangeal joint dislocation in spina bifida. J Am Podiatry Assoc 74:147, 1984

62. Salamon PB, Gelberman RH, Huffer JM: Dorsal dislocation of the metatarsophalangeal joint of the great toe. J Bone Joint Surg 56A:1073, 1974

63. DeLuca FN, Kenmore PI: Bilateral dorsal dislocations of the metatarsophalangeal joints of the great toes with a loose body in one of the metatarsophalangeal joints. J Trauma 15:737, 1975

64. Brown TIS: Avulsion fracture of the fibular sesamoid in association with dorsal dislocation of the metatarsophalangeal joint of the hallux. Clin Orthop 149:229, 1980

65. Konkel KF, Muehlstein JH: Unusual fracture-dislocation of the great toe. J Trauma 15:733, 1975

66. Mouchet A: Deux cas de luxation dorsale complete du gros orteil avel lesions des sesamoides. Rev Orthop 18:221, 1931

67. Burns JJ: Recurrent dislocation of the first metatarsophalangeal joint. J Foot Surg 15:118, 1976

68. Mullis DL, Miller WE: A disabling sports injury of the great toe. Foot Ankle, 1:22, 1980

69. Coker TP, Arnold JA, Weber DL: Traumatic lesions of the metatarsal-phalangeal joint of the great toe in athletes. Am J Sports Med 6:326, 1978

70. Roa JP, Manuel TB: Irreducible dislocations of the metatarsophalangeal joints of the foot. Clin Orthop 145:224, 1979

71. Murphy JL: Isolated dorsal dislocation of the second metatarsophalangeal joint. Foot Ankle, 1:30, 1980

72. English TA: Dislocation of the metatarsal bone and adjacent toe. J Bone Joint Surg 46B:700, 1964

73. Giannestras NJ, Sammarco GJ: Fractures and dislocations in the foot. p. 1488. In Rockwood CA, Green DP (eds): Fractures. JB Lippincott, Philadelphia, 1975

74. Nelson TL, Uggen W: Irreducible dorsal dislocation of the interphalangeal joint of the great toe. Clin Orthop 157:110, 1981

75. Schock C: Feet of clay. J Arkansas Med Soc 82:383, 1986

18

Digital Fractures and Dislocations*

David E. Marcinko, D.P.M.
Douglas H. Elleby, D.P.M.

Until recently, there was little medical literature available concerning the diagnosis and treatment of digital fractures and dislocations. This casual opinion persisted because the toes were not considered important enough to be assigned much functional significance. Fractures or dislocations were typically treated with a combination of rest, ice, compression splintage, and elevation. Closed reduction was attempted for major pathology only, and the possibility of surgical intervention was rarely entertained. The long-term prognosis for inadequately treated injuries was poor and often led to chronic deformities such as heloma formation, contracted digitis, transverse plane adductus or abductus formation, and metatarsalgia. In 1985, Elleby and Marcinko presented their review of the entire spectrum of digital fractures and dislocations.[1] They examined most known digital osseous injuries and suggested an aggressive treatment approach with an emphasis on surgical intervention. Similarly, in 1987, Downey adopted a like attitude in his discourse on digital injuries.[2] He emphasized a thorough understanding of the anatomy involved in digital fractures as a prerequisite to proper treatment. Therefore, this chapter continues to stress the need for precise clinical evaluation in the management of digital fractures and dislocations.

---

* Portions of this chapter have been adapted from Elleby DH and Marcinko DE.[1]

MEDICAL CONSIDERATIONS

The same general medical considerations of fractures and dislocations of the fingers apply equally to the management of injuries to the toes. For example, a careful history must be taken and a lower extremity physical examination performed to establish the current health status of the patient. Medications, drug allergies, and the mechanism of injury should be determined. This will allow a treatment program to be tailored to the individual needs of the patient.

Diagnosis

The diagnosis of a digital fracture or dislocation begins with the careful manipulation and palpation of the injured part. Malalignment may be first detected at this stage, and careful examination allows associated injuries to be promptly noted. Furthermore, the mechanism of injury should be elicited to determine the dominant plane of pathologic force. For example, the major plane of injury encountered in digital fracture(s) is the sagittal plane; the most common injury in this plane results from direct compaction of the involved area. Other mechanisms of injury in this plane include direct trauma from above and secondary hyperextension or hyperflexion of the joint(s) of the digit(s) involved.

In the transverse plane, the predominant injury is caused by an abduction-adduction force resulting in a spiral oblique or transverse fracture. Although the proximal phalanx is usually involved, the middle or distal phalanges may also be affected. Treatment is usually conservative.

The least frequent plane of deforming force in digital fractures is the frontal plane; injury to this area results in rotational or inversion-eversion force and is commonly associated with other pathologic conditions. Because this injury results from a high degree of torque, neurovascular damage is possible along with a potential for soft tissue injuries and an open wound. When this occurs, immediate attention must be focused on the wound to prevent contamination and possible osteomyelitis. Additionally, in open dirty wounds, tetanus prophylaxis should be administered along with appropriate antibiotics after Gram stains are done and cultures (aerobic and anaerobic) have been taken. Degloving or soft tissue loss in these injuries is of prime concern, and once the tissue defect has been appropriately addressed, the fracture itself is treated in a conventional manner.

For medicolegal justification, a complete radiographic examination is essential to the diagnostic procedure when dealing with suspected digital fractures. Radiographs are indicated if only the slightest possibility of bony injury exists. To rely solely on clinical evidence is to place important structures and function needlessly in jeopardy. Standard anteroposterior, lateral, and oblique radiographs are needed to assess possible injury in all cardinal body planes. The use of tomography, fluoroscopy, lixiscopy, xerography, or radiographic stress views also aids in the diagnosis of difficult cases.

Reduction

Sarrafian and Topouzian have demonstrated that the muscle-to-tendon insertions are relatively short in the foot, and even slight malunion can adversely affect the function of an injured digit.[3] Shortening, angulation, or rotational malalignment must therefore be prevented. Once all diagnostic factors have been gathered, reduction maneuvers may be undertaken by first exaggerating and then reversing the original injury pattern. If closed reduction cannot be achieved, open reduction and anatomic alignment are required, and osteosynthesis is performed to justify the risk of operation.

Immobilization

As a rule, most digital fractures are immobilized in the position of function. Immobilization is used for stable and undisplaced fractures, and splintage will generally consist of maintaining the injured part in a shoe with a rigid sole. Lesser digital fractures can be splinted by immobilizing them to adjacent digit(s) with felt, urethane, tape, or other materials. In the nonoperative management of digital fractures, osseous involvement is considered to be of secondary importance because successful recovery is predicated on intact or properly healed soft tissue structures. The duration of immobilization is determined by clinical and radiographic evidence. In most cases, the consolidation of bony segments will take place within 4 to 8 weeks. The physician need not wait for complete union, as evidenced by radiographs, since fracture lines often remain visible for several months.

Surveillance

The extent of fracture hematoma, or postinjury soft tissue edema, cannot be estimated in advance. Splintage must therefore be monitored for the first several days so that impaired circulation can be promptly relieved. This is especially important in small body parts such as injured toes. Crushing injuries in the sagittal plane often have associated subungual or dissecting hematoma formation that must be assessed. Pressure secondary to underlying hemorrhage can compromise the matrix cells of the nail bed if not relieved. Decompression can be performed or nail plate avulsion done if hematoma is excessive. If a nail bed laceration is discovered, the injury must

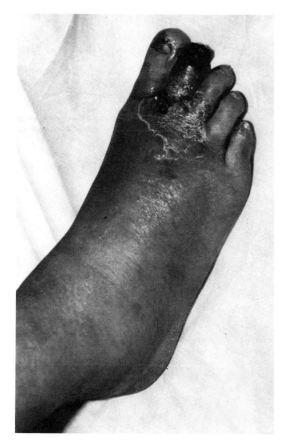

Fig. 18-1. Neurovascular compromise in crush injury of second toe.

be treated as if it were an open wound to prevent contamination of deeper structures (Fig. 18-1).

Exercise

The controlled therapeutic exercise of nonimmobilized adjacent joints and digits will promote a rapid reduction of edema and is the best treatment for disuse atrophy. In addition, it is important that the distal phalanx of the injured toe be left mobile to enable the flexor and extensor tendons to glide in the fractured region and prevent adhesion of the tendon or its sheath. Physical therapy can take the form of marble-grasping therapy, manual manipulation, or active and passive range of motion exercises.

FRACTURES OF THE HALLUX

Fractures of the hallux are among the most frequently encountered traumatic incidents to occur in the forefoot. Presenting diagnostic clinical symptoms include edema, ecchymosis, lost function, pain, and the inability to wear normal shoegear. Since a functional hallux and first metatarsophalangeal joint complex is essential for propulsive ambulation, prompt recognition and treatment of this injury is needed to prevent chronic sequelae such as growth plate arrest, hallux limitus, hallux rigidus, or other angulational deformity. Although gross fracture is usually obvious to the clinician, magnified radiography will often demonstrate underestimated bony pathology (Fig. 18-2). A typical example of this phenomenon is the exuberant callus formation and widening that may occur when the distal phalanx is comminuted in a minor crush injury (Fig. 18-3). Intra-articular metatarsophalangeal or interphalangeal joint arthrosis may also occur, along with toenail matrix pathology and subsequent onychopathology (Fig. 18-4).

Perhaps the largest review of fractures of the hallux was performed by Zrubecky in 1955.[4] His study of 122 cases revealed that one-third were subcapital in nature and involved a 10-degree dorsal tilt when associated with subluxation of the proximal phalanx. Advocated treatment was closed reduction and cast immobilization. Other researchers who reported on fracture injuries to the hallux included Taylor[5] and Zorzi and Grisostomi.[6] Jahss recently reported that one in six patients who sustained a significant interphalangeal joint stubbing injury ultimately required joint fusion for pain relief[7] (Fig. 18-5).

The most frequent mechanism of injury results from the dropping of a heavy object onto the foot. In addition, slapping injuries that occur in certain dance movements (tap, ballet, disco, clogging) may result in fractures of the hallux. In classical ballet, dancers are prone to painful hallux interphalangeal joint arthrosis owing to their repetitive "sur les pointes" posture. Therefore, interphalangeal fusion may be required for treatment upon retirement from professional

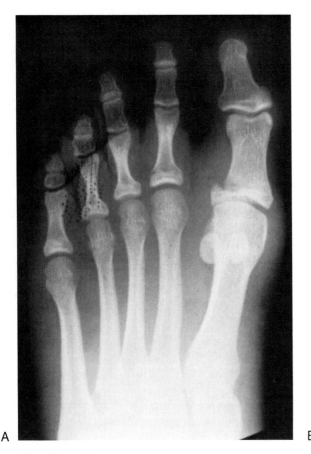 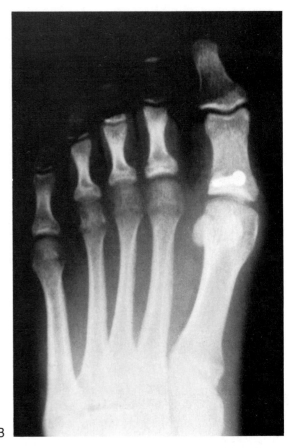

A   B

Fig. 18-2. (A) Preoperative transverse fracture of the proximal phalanx of the hallux. Note similar fracture of the base of the second proximal phalanx. **(B)** Open reduction internal fixation with 1.5-mm cortical screw. The vassal fracture of the second toe was not surgically treated.

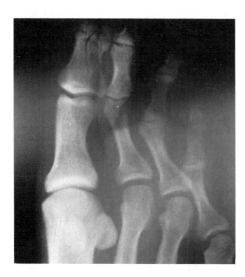

Fig. 18-3. Closed comminuted fracture of the distal phalanx.

endeavors.[8] A proximally directed shearing force may also fracture hallucal condyles, in which case fragments may be removed or fixed with miniature cortical screws according to the principles of rigid internal fixation. Tension band fixation of larger fragments is another viable alternative.

In 1981, Pinckney and associates reported on a series of six pediatric cases, each of which produced a Salter type I injury to the distal phalanx.[9] They postulated that extreme hyperflexion traumatically avulsed the distal growth plate and produced a compound fracture in all cases. An even more unusual injury was reported in 1987 by Ford and colleagues.[10] They reported a Salter type II fracture of the distal hallucal phalanx in a 14-year-old boy. The patient injured the digit while walking up a flight of steps. The so-called

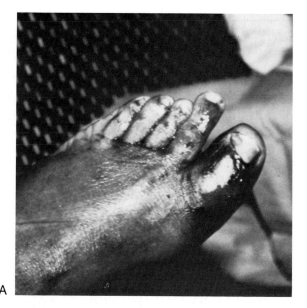

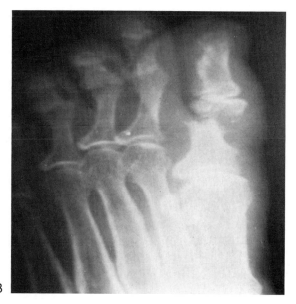

A   B

Fig. 18-4. (A) Clinical appearance of hallux following direct sagittal plane trauma. **(B)** Radiographic appearance demonstrating intra-articular fracture-dislocation.

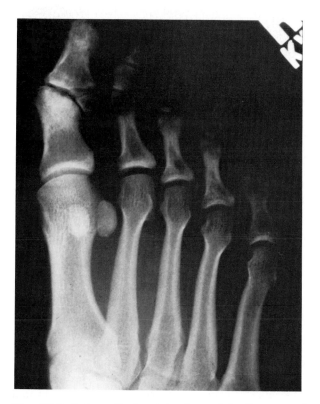

Fig. 18-5. Intra-articular lateral condyle fracture of proximal and distal phalanx of the hallux.

Thurston-Holland sign was present along with a large hematoma and partial avulsion of the nail plate. Radiographic examination further demonstrated epiphyseal widening, with a fracture along the inferior aspect of the metaphysis in the left phalanx. A slight superior displacement with mild angulation was noted, and closed reduction was initially attempted but proved unsuccessful. Surgery was needed to reduce the injury, which healed without complication.

Miscellaneous Fractures and Dislocations about the Hallux

Hallux interphalangeal joint dislocation is an unusual deformity and is rarely seen. The injury is unusual because of the intrinsic stability of the hallux, with its short lever arm, condylar joint shape, and intimacy of its collateral ligaments. The injury is usually associated with other deformities and typically occurs with medial and lateral condylar fractures of the proximal phalanx. A recent review of the literature reported the irreducible nature of this injury, presumably owing to invagination of the volar plate.[11] Noonan and Thurber documented the case report of a 26-year-old man who sustained an irreducible dorsal dislocation of the hallucal interphalangeal joint.[12] Closed reduction under general anesthesia was unsuccessful. Therefore, open reduction and external fixation was achieved using crossed Kirschner wires. A small bone fragment was also excised. Irreducibility was attributed to ligamentous joint structures, ruptured plantar capsular structures, and contracted soft tissue structures resulting from lack of immediate treatment (Fig. 18-6). Follow-up revealed a nonproblematic sequela, and interphalangeal joint arthrodesis was avoided in this case. Other injuries of this type were reported by Giannestras and Sammarco[13] in 1984 and by Nelson and Uggen in 1981.[14]

Other, miscellaneous fractures of the hallux include iatrogenic fractures of the proximal phalanx, which may occur when performing an Akin-type closing wedge osteotomy. Nonunion or painful pseudoarthrosis formation is possible when the procedure is performed blindly, without fixation, with inadequate fixation, or in the diaphyseal portion of the bone. Distally placed osteotomies may produce intra-articular fractures, with reintervention procedures such as interphalangeal joint arthrodesis or implant arthroplasty necessary for salvage.

Additionally, iatrogenic sesamoid fractures or traumatic sesamoiditis may occur with certain hallux valgus repair procedures such as the Reverdin or Peabody osteotomy. The problem is avoided by either making the osteotomy cut distal to the sesamoids or performing Green's modification of the Reverdin procedure.[15]

Fractures of the Sesamoid

The tibial and fibular sesamoid bones of the first metatarsophalangeal joint occur anatomi-

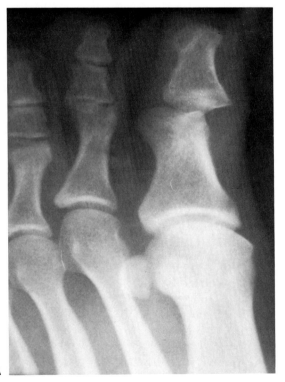 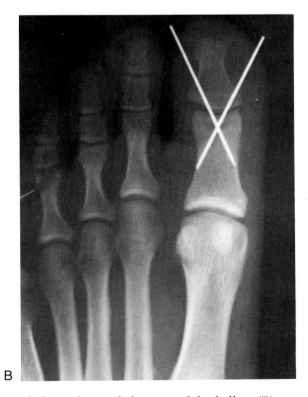

A   B

Fig. 18-6. **(A)** Preoperative oblique radiograph of interphalangeal joint dislocation of the hallux. **(B)** Postoperative dorsoplantar radiograph with crossed Kirschner wire fixation. (From Noonan and Thurber,[12] with permission.)

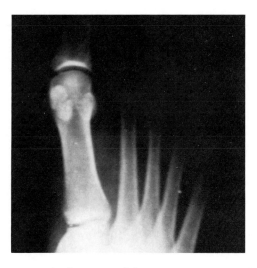

Fig. 18-7. Tibial sesamoid fracture in a young athlete.

cally within the medial and lateral tendon slips of flexor hallucis brevis muscle. Diseases of and, especially, injuries to the sesamoids have become much more common with the increasing popularity of sports such as track and field events, long distance running, or race walking, which may repetitively crush the sesamoid bones of the great toe between the first metatarsal head and supporting surface. Although the injury may be produced by such simple activity as stepping off a curb or wearing high-heeled shoes, it is usually insidious in onset with no identifiable eliciting event. Biomechanical derangements predisposed to sesamoidal injuries include the cavus foot, spasm of the peroneus longus tendon, and plantar flexed first metatarsal deformities (Fig. 18-7).

Typically, a sesamoidal fracture is transverse or comminuted, and one or both of the sesamoids may be involved. It is much more common for the tibial sesamoid to be fractured because of its increased load in closed kinetic chain gait. However, fibular sesamoidal fractures do occur. The injury must be differentiated from congenital bipartite or tripartite sesamoids that are a result from the incomplete coalition of the primordial calcification center of the ossicle. Stress radiographs, axial silhouette views, bone scans, and tomograms are helpful diagnostic aids. The clinical hallux push-up test is positive. In a true sesamoid fracture, the line of division is jagged and irregular, whereas in congenital bifurcation, the

division is smooth. Radiographic examination of the opposite foot is mandatory.

Since the fracture of a sesamoid involves the articular surface, the resulting disability may be serious and result in subsequent degenerative changes of the first metatarsophalangeal joint. Aseptic necrosis may also occur.[16] Fortunately, the condition often responds to conservative injection therapy, ultrasound therapy, or various forms of immobilization. Further conservative treatment involves the reduction of weight bearing on the sesamoids. This may be achieved by any accommodative device that allows the first metatarsophalangeal joint to "float." Stretching the heel cord may also effectively reduce first ray loading during gait. Still, it is not unusual to have to resort to surgical excision of the fractured accessory bone.

Removal of a fractured tibial sesamoid is accomplished through a medial approach, with care being taken not to violate the proper digital branch of the medial plantar nerve. The first metatarsophalangeal joint capsule is then incised, and the bone is shelled from its investment in the flexor hallucis brevis tendon. Obviously, this procedure may accentuate a present or developing hallux valgus deformity. Therefore, a medial capsulorrhaphy or musculus abductor hallucis tendon advancement may be needed to reestablish the balance of power on the first metatarsophalangeal joint. In several of our clinical cases, the distal tibial sesamoidal fragment has been excised, leaving the proximal portion intact. Results of this technique are encouraging since it presumably maintains soft tissue joint integrity. Further studies are currently in progress.

Excision of the fibular sesamoid, on the other hand, takes place through a dorsal approach located between the hallux and second toe. The bone is first skewered with a threaded Kirschner wire, and the strong intersesamoidal ligament is divided. Removal then is accomplished quickly, and a lateral capsulotomy, musculus abductor hallucis tendon transfer or tenotomy is performed as indicated. When both sesamoids have to be removed, the interphalangeal joint of the hallux must be fused to prevent a malleus deformity from occurring. Following surgery, a cutout orthosis may be worn to relieve weight bearing and limit pronation. It is often necessary for soft crepe-soled shoegear to be worn for several months.

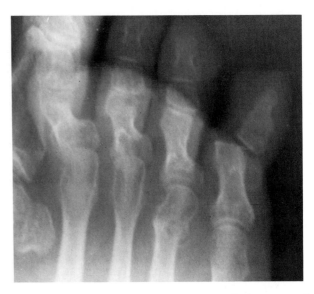

Fig. 18-8. "Nightwalker" abduction dislocation of fifth digit without fracture.

FRACTURES OF THE LESSER DIGITS

The most common type of break to occur in a lesser toe is the closed spiral-oblique fracture. This occurs while walking or running barefoot or after accidental injury. Digital stress fractures are typically reported in military personnel, who, while on maneuvers, are required to walk or run constantly, often under the burden of a 20-lb pack. Fractures of the middle three digits are uncommon because of the protective buttress effect of the hallux and fifth toe. Fractures of the fifth toe are most common and are produced by an abduction injury such as striking the toe against a piece of furniture while ambulating in the dark. Since this injury occurs at home, and the patient can still walk, medical care is seldom sought until symptoms persist. Proximal or distal interphalangeal joint dislocation can even occur without associated bony pathology, although neurovascular compromise can still result (Fig. 18-8). Fractures of the proximal phalanx usually occur through the midshaft, and dislocation is rare (Fig. 18-9). Fractures of the middle and distal phalanges are infrequent and usually result from a

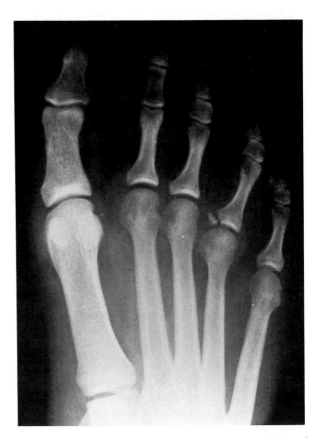

Fig. 18-9. Medial condylar fracture base of fourth proximal phalanx.

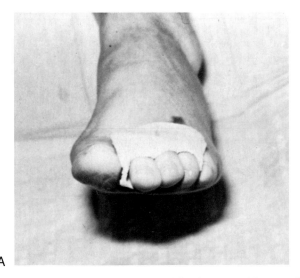
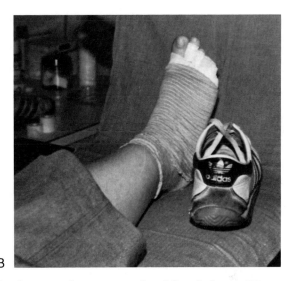

A   B

Fig. 18-10. (A) Urethane mold splintage of fractured third toe to adjacent second and fourth digits. **(B)** Immobilization of injured digit with compressive dressing to control edema.

sagittal plane crush injury. Generally, these fractures are treated conservatively with immobilization and felt splintage to adjacent un-injured toes. Urethane retainers, toe crests, moldable silicone compound, or other traditional podiatric appliances are useful modalities to reduce edema and maintain alignment. A no-salt diet is suggested, and oral diuretics are not necessary unless massive trauma has occurred. The patient may ambulate in a well-padded running shoe or reinforced surgical sandal until more normal shoegear is tolerated, usually within 4 to 6 weeks. Older patients do remarkably well (Fig. 18-10).

Phalangeal fractures may displace and become unstable consequent to the pull of anatomic structures such as the extensor tendons, flexor tendons, or interossei or lumbricale musculature. This may lead to sagittal plane, transverse plane, or frontal plane deformities. The affected toe may cease to load upon weight bearing and may "float." Hallux valgus formation may occur if the stabilizing effect of the second toe is lost in a pronated foot type. Plantar fat pad displacement with subsequent metatarsalgia may result along with metatasophalangeal joint dislocations. Closed reduction is achieved by temporary distal traction, pulp traction, skeletal traction, or the modified Quigley Chinese finger trap apparatus

(Fig. 18-11). Neurovascular status is of prime concern in these cases, and techniques of conscious sedation are useful in pediatric patients or when associated injuries have been sustained.[17] Management of these fracture-dislocations may

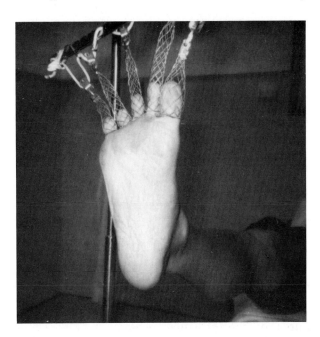

Fig. 18-11. Finger trap apparatus used for closed reduction of digital and metatarsophalangeal joint dislocations.

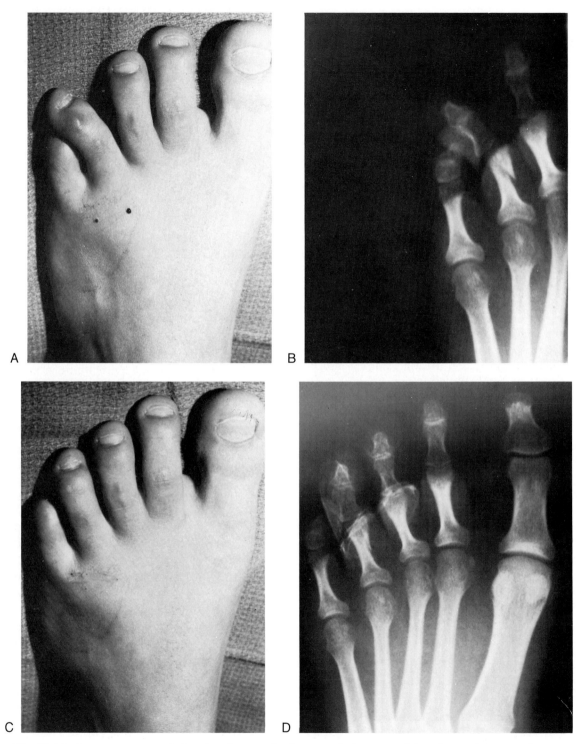

Fig. 18-12. Demonstration of closed reduction for fracture-dislocation of fourth toe: (**A**) Prereduction clinical appearance. (**B**) Prereduction radiographic appearance. (**C**) Postreduction clinical appearance. (**D**) Postreduction radiographic appearance.

require a more aggressive approach, such as blind longitudinal percutaneous Kirschner wire stabilization, to maintain alignment. Occasionally, after healing, a reduced fracture will develop exuberant callus formation and necessitate small-incision surgery to reduce painful interdigital osseous excrescences (Fig. 18-12).

Displaced irreducible fractures of any phalanx may require open reduction with internal or external fixation for adequate treatment. This may necessitate the fixation of fractured fragments with internal screws, cerclage monofilament stainless steel wire, or external smooth or threaded Kirschner wires.

Similarly, intra-articular fractures of the lesser digits are not infrequent and usually heal without complication. Occasionally, if angulational deformity develops or painful degenerative joint arthrosis persists, resection arthroplasty of the head of the proximal phalanx is required for adequate treatment (Fig. 18-13). To increase toe purchase power, Kirschner wire stabilization or flexor tendon transfer may be used in conjunction with head resection.[18] This technique is especially useful when a forefoot or ankle equinus deformity is present or the patient has a pes cavus foot type. Although digital implants have been used in the past with satisfactory results, they are currently not recommended unless all soft tissue-deforming forces on the respective toe are eliminated by either surgical or biomechanical means (Fig. 18-14).

According to Blodgett, when multiple comminuted fragments of any phalanx occur, external immobilization and longitudinal alignment are all that are needed for adequate treatment, owing to the tubular construction of the individual toe acting in splintage fashion.[19] This may or may not be a prudent treatment philosophy depending on such factors as foot type, lifestyle, shoegear, or the existence of prior foot pathology.

Pure interphalangeal dislocation, without osseous pathology, may occur at either the proximal or distal joint level. Obvious visual deformity along with palpable displacement make clinical diagnosis possible. A common presentation is lateral dislocation of the fifth proximal interphalangeal joint following an abduction injury. In a closed situation, radiographs will reveal loss of

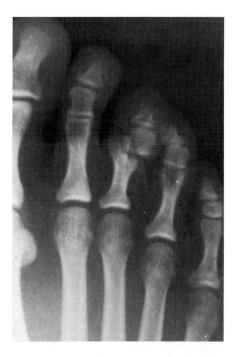

Fig. 18-13. Intra-articular fracture-dislocation of proximal third interphalangeal joint requiring head resection.

joint space congruity that may be associated with articular surface damage. Primary treatment is directed toward manual reduction followed by stabilization in the reduced attitude. If reduction cannot be achieved or maintained, a ruptured joint capsule or displaced flexor tendon has occurred. Surgical reduction is required in this case to establish normal anatomic structures. Appropriate immobilization with celastic splintage is then used to prevent redislocation. In addition to traumatic joint arthrosis, late complications of this injury include an apropulsive ray and a persistently swollen or "fat" toe (Fig. 18-15).

Finally, traumatic avulsion of any portion of the toenail following injury should arouse suspicion of possible osseous injury. The loss of a toenail and the frequently associated tearing of the nail bed may also be caused by the protrusion of crushed bone particles. Since a fracture through the distal nail bed always carries a high probability of infection and osteomyelitis, the injury should be appropriately considered a compound fracture and be treated with the protocol outlined by Malay in 1987.[20]

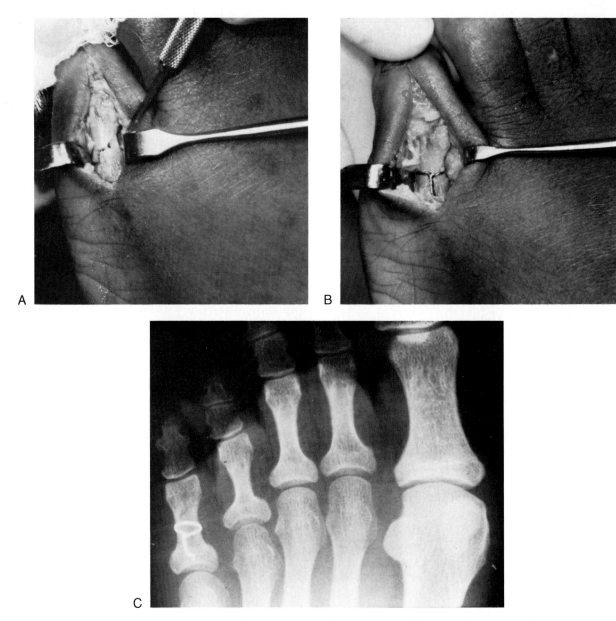

Fig. 18-14. Demonstration of open reduction internal fixation of spiral-oblique fracture of the proximal phalanx. (**A**) Intraoperative view of fracture line. (**B**) Intraoperative view of cerclage wire fixation. (**C**) Postoperative radiographic view of completed open reduction surgery.

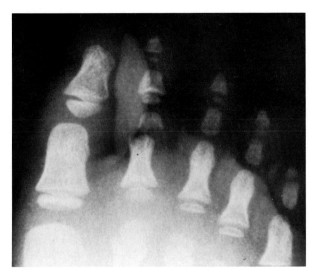

Fig. 18-15. Complex fracture-dislocation of the second proximal interphalangeal joint of a child.

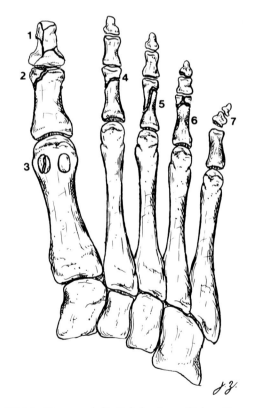

Fig. 18-16. Types of digital fracture-dislocations: (1) comminuted crush; (2) hallucal condyle; (3) sesamoid; (4) transverse; (5) spiral-oblique; (6) intra-articular; (7) abduction-dislocation. (From Elleby and Marcinko,[1] with permission.)

SUMMARY

The entire spectrum of digital fractures and dislocations has been discussed, including clinical features, diagnostic tests, mechanisms of injury, and treatment methods. Photographs accentuated important concepts and an aggressive attitude was stressed to avoid mismanagement and prolonged convalescence. Regardless of therapeutic philosophy, the goal of any treatment should be to restore lost function and maintain intrinsic stability. Emphasis was placed on surgical intervention should the need arise (Fig. 18-16).

ACKNOWLEDGMENTS

We acknowledge photographic contributions from the following clinicians: C. Fenton, R. Floros, G. Gumann, L. Harkless, S. Korn, R. Noonan, M. Rappaport, and B. Yanklowitz.

REFERENCES

1. Elleby DH, Marcinko DE: Digital fractures and dislocations—diagnosis and treatment. Clin Podiatry 2:233, 1985
2. Downey M: Digital fractures. p. 852. In McGlamry ED (ed): Comprehensive Textbook of Foot Surgery. Vol. 2. Williams & Wilkins, Baltimore, 1987
3. Sarrafian SK, Topouzian LK: Anatomy and physiology of the toes (extensor apparatus). J Bone Joint Surg 51A:699, 1969
4. Zrubecky G: Bruche der grosszeche, deren behandling and behandlungsergebnisse. Arch Orthop Trauma Surg 47:591, 1955
5. Taylor GN: Treatment of the fractured great toe. Br Med J 1:724, 1943
6. Zorzi C, Grisostomi E: Le fratture deil'alluce. Riv Infort Mal Prof 49:317, 1962
7. Jahss MH: Stubbing injuries to the hallux. Foot Ankle 1:15, 1980
8. Langford JH, Fenton CH: Hallux interphalangeal arthrodesis. J Am Podiatry Assoc 72:155, 1982

9. Pinckney LE, Currarino G, Kennedy LA: The stubbed great toe. A case of occult compound fractures and infection. Radiology 138:375, 1981

10. Ford TC, Nosacek IJ, Troisi E, Wallace JA: Salter-Harris type II fracture in the distal hallucal phalanx. Curr Podiatr Med 5:6, 1987

11. Eibel P: Dislocation of the interphalangeal joint of the big toe with inter-position of a sesamoid bone. J Bone Joint Surg 36A:880, 1954

12. Noonan R, Thurber N: Irreducible dorsal dislocation of the hallucal interphalangeal joint. J Am Podiatric Med Assoc 2:98, 1987

13. Giannestras N, Sammarco G: Fractures and dislocation in the foot. In Rockwood, Green D (ed): Fractures. Vol. 2. JB Lippincott, Philadelphia, 1984

14. Nelson T, Uggen W: Irreducible dorsal dislocation of the interphalangeal joint of the great toe. Clin Orthop 157:110, 1981

15. Beck EL: Modified Reverdin technique for hallux abducto valgus. J Am Podiatr Med Assoc 64:657, 1974

16. Mullen BR, Kashuk K: Primary avascular necrosis of halluces in a ballet dancer. J Am Podiatr Med Assoc 76:544, 1986

17. Harris WC, Alpert WJ, Gill JJ, Marcinko DE: Nitrous oxide and valium use in podiatric surgery for production of conscious-sedation. J Am Podiatry Assoc 72:305, 1982

18. Marcinko DE, Lazerson A, Dollard MD, Schwartz NH: Flexor digitorium longus tendon transfer, a simplified technique. J Am Podiatry Assoc 74:380, 1984

19. Blodgett WH: Injuries of the forefoot and toes. In Jahss MH (ed): Disorders of the Foot. WB Saunders, Philadelphia, 1982

20. Malay D: Trauma to the nail and associated structures. p. 996. In McGlamry ED (ed): Comprehensive Textbook of Foot Surgery. Vol. 2. Williams & Wilkins, Baltimore, 1987

19

Fractures of the First Metatarsal

Guido LaPorta, D.P.M.

This chapter deals exclusively with trauma to the first metatarsal, the sesamoid apparatus, and the first metatarsophalangeal joint. Emphasis is placed on the first ray because of its important function in normal ambulation. Any injury to the first ray or any of its components may drastically alter the pattern of normal gait and weight bearing. This can be very debilitating to all patients, but particularly so to the young, working, active, and athletic individual.

Forces acting across the first metatarsophalangeal joint during gait are very nearly equal to body weight.[1] During treatment of injuries to the first metatarsal, the sesamoids, or the metatarsophalangeal joint, realization of this fact, along with the knowledge of the integral function of this unit during locomotion, should lead to sound and judicious treatment of these injuries.

HISTORICAL PERSPECTIVE

Historically, treatment modalities for fractures of the first metatarsal are somewhat similar. Heppenstall notes that Hippocrates felt a fractured bone would unite if the bone ends were placed together and held in that position for an extended period.[2] Watson-Jones also thought, even as late as the 1950s, that the majority of fractures could be managed without any operative intervention. In general, most orthopedic texts and teaching advocated putting the injured part to rest with the belief that this would stimulate healing.

Orthopedic literature describes many methods and principles of treatment of skeletal fractures. However, literature on the treatment of metatarsal fractures, including the first metatarsal, is very basic and limited, primarily because these fractures have been considered to be relatively insignificant. Historically, only the most serious fractures were treated with any type of open reduction or fixation. Very little to no attention has been paid to the importance of returning the first metatarsal to a normal functional unit.

Heppenstall has cited the 1930s as the time when orthopedic advances introduced internal fixation of fractures with biologically compatible materials.[2] This began as fixation of displaced metatarsal fractures with intramedullary pins. The principle behind use of the pin was providing firm immobilization. As advances were made in types of fixation and with further application of internal fixation, it became apparent that since internal fixation applied firm immobilization across the fracture site, it could also allow for early return of surrounding soft tissues and joints to functional activity.

NORMAL FUNCTIONAL ANATOMY

The first metatarsal is considered a long bone, as are all of the metatarsals, and therefore ossifies from primary and secondary ossification centers. The primary center appears in the center of the shaft in the 10th week of intrauterine life with the secondary center appearing proximally at the base during the third year of life. Occasionally, another center is seen distally at the metatarsal head. Generally, the epiphyses fuse between the ages of 17 to 20 years.

The first metatarsal is the shortest, thickest, strongest, and most massive metatarsal. The base is reniform, concave, and covered with articular cartilage and articulates with the medial cuneiform. Laterally at its base, the metatarsal articulates with the second metatarsal. The head of the bone is covered with articular cartilage and is rounded, except on the sides, where it is flattened. The head articulates with the proximal phalanx of the hallux. The plantar aspect of the head is also covered with articular cartilage and has a median elevation, the crista, with two grooves to either side. The medial groove is larger than the lateral groove. These plantar grooves serve as articulations for the sesamoid bones plantarly. The lateral surface of the bone contains a nutrient foramina which runs distally into the bone. It is located approximately 2.7 cm proximal to the head and 0.4 cm from the dorsal aspect of the shaft.[3] The plantar surface of the first metatarsal is concave. This configuration causes the plantar surface of the bone to be the tension side when body weight is borne on it.

Located plantarly beneath the head of the first metatarsal, seated in the plantar grooves of the metatarsal head, are the tibial and fibular sesamoids. These are two constantly occurring sesamoid bones that develop within the capsule of the first metatarsophalangeal joint by intracartilaginous bone formation.[4] The tibial sesamoid is generally larger than the fibular sesamoid. They begin as islands of undifferentiated connective tissue during the eighth week of gestation and attain their adult shape by the fifth month. Ossification of these bones usually occurs between years 8 and 14 of life, usually earlier in girls than in boys.[5] The superior surface of the bones is convex and covered with articular cartilage for articulation with the plantar metatarsal head, one to either side of the median elevation. The sesamoids may have more than one ossification center, which may or may not unite. The incomplete coalition of these centers may result in bipartite or tripartite sesamoids, which could be confused with fracture.[5] Sesamoids are reported to be multipartite in 5 to 30 percent of normal asymptomatic persons,[5] with this being more commonly seen in the tibial rather than the fibular sesamoid.[5]

The medial aspect of the base of the first metatarsal is subcutaneous. Dorsally, at the base of the metatarsal, is found the first metatarsal-cuneiform ligament, and one is also present inferiorly or plantarly. No ligaments connect the base of the first metatarsal to the base of the second metatarsal. Distally, the tibial and fibular collateral ligaments course distally and plantarly from the small tubercles on either side of the metatarsal head to attach to the medial and lateral aspect of the base of the proximal phalanx of the hallux. The tibial and fibular sesamoidal ligaments pass from the same tubercles to the margins of the corresponding sesamoid. The collateral and sesamoidal ligaments are joined by an intermediate fibrous band called the plantar tibial and fibular sesamoidal ligaments. They pass from the sesamoid bones to the plantar aspect of the base of the proximal phalanx.[4] The intersesamoidal ligament is an unpaired ligament that connects the sesamoids to each other and forms part of the tunnel through which the tendon of the flexor hallucis longus passes. The deep transverse metatarsal ligament, which interconnects the lesser metatarsal plantar pads, inserts into the lateral aspect of the first metatarsophalangeal joint capsule.[4] The ligaments associated with the sesamoids collectively form a triangular mass that assists in retaining the sesamoids in their proper places beneath the metatarsal head. Also present plantarly is a fibrocartilaginous pad that thickens the inferior aspect of the joint capsule. In addition, the plantar aponeurosis sends strong fibrous slips that pass partially into the tibial and fibular sesamoids. These aponeurotic slips, together with the previously mentioned ligaments, form the tunnel through which the tendon of flexor hallucis longus travels to its insertion on the distal phalanx of the hallux.

The first ray acts as a point of insertion of several intrinsic and extrinsic muscles. Beginning proximally with extrinsic musculature, the peroneus longus tendon inserts inferiorly on the lateral aspect of the tuberosity at the base of the metatarsal. This tendon has been known to avulse a portion of the base of the metatarsal from the remainder of bone. The tibialis anterior tendon inserts at the inferior medial aspect of the base. Another extrinsic muscle crossing the first metatarsophalangeal joint is the extensor hallucis longus, which is enveloped in the extensor hood apparatus as it crosses the joint to insert dorsally on the base of the distal phalanx. Plantarly, the flexor hallucis longus tendon passes beneath the first metatarsal and travels through the fibrous tunnel and fibrocartilaginous pad of the first metatarsophalangeal joint on its way to insert on the plantar aspect of the base of the distal phalanx.

Four intrinsic foot muscles cross the first metatarsophalangeal joint and thereby act on that joint. The extensor hallucis brevis muscle approaches the joint from a lateral direction to insert lateral to the long extensor tendon onto the base of the proximal phalanx of the hallux dorsally. Plantarly, three muscles affect function of the metatarsophalangeal joint. The abductor hallucis muscle runs along the medial plantar aspect of the first metatarsal, sending an attachment into the tibial sesamoid, and inserts via a tendon into the medial plantar aspect of the base of the proximal phalanx.[4] The flexor hallucis brevis muscle runs plantarly to the shaft of the first metatarsal. Just proximal to the metatarsal head, the muscle divides into the medial and lateral heads, becomes tendinous, and envelopes the sesamoid bones. The tendons then pass distally to insert into the plantar aspect of the base of the proximal phalanx.[4] In a fashion similar to the abductor hallucis, the oblique and transverse heads of the adductor hallucis brevis form a conjoined tendon, and this tendon inserts into the fibular sesamoid and then into the base of the proximal phalanx.

A study by Jaworek[3] with cadaveric specimens revealed the constant presence of a principle nutrient artery entering the lateral aspect of the first metatarsal shaft, running in a direction from proximal to distal into the bone (Fig. 19-1). It is located approximately 2.7 cm proximal to the articular cartilage and 0.4 cm from the dorsal aspect of the lateral surface of the bone. No branches are distributed to the cortex of the shaft, but upon entering the medulla, it divides into ascending and descending branches with medial and lateral limbs. These limbs travel to the metaphyseal ar-

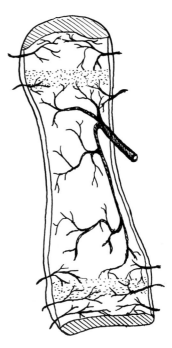

Fig. 19-1. Vascular supply to the first metatarsal. (Redrawn from Jaworek,[31] with permission.)

eas and end as a spray of vessels there. In metaphyseal bone, the vessels are arranged at right angles to the growth plate, whereas in epiphyseal bone, the pattern of vascular supply is quite random. Small branches travel toward the subchondral bone and digitate in a spray of vessels both distally and proximally to supply the subchondral bone, which in turn sustains the joint cartilage. It should be noted, however, that both metaphyseal and epiphyseal areas are well supplied with vascular elements compared with the relatively few present in diaphyseal cortical bone.

There are several vascular structures in close proximity to the first metatarsal that may be injured in closed or open fractures of the first metatarsal. First is the dorsalis pedis artery, a continuation of the anterior tibial artery. This vessel is of significant caliber, its diameter being approximately 2 to 3 mm.[6] It descends across the middle of the anterior ankle and crosses the talus, navicular, and base of the second metatarsal. At the proximal aspect of the first interspace, between the bases of the first and second metatarsals, it makes a 90 degree turn, heads plantarly in the interspace, and terminates by becoming the proximal perforating artery. This vessel then joins with the plantar metatarsal artery. Another terminal branch of the dorsalis pedis artery is the first dorsal metatarsal artery, which originates at the point where the dorsalis pedis dives plantarly at the proximal aspect of the first interspace. The artery courses distally over the first dorsal interosseous muscle and divides into the medial and lateral branches at the metatarsophalangeal joint to supply the lateral aspect of the hallux and adjacent side of the second digit. Distally, at the webspace, the first dorsal metatarsal artery plunges plantarly and divides to supply the medial and lateral plantar aspect of the hallux. Therefore, the first dorsal metatarsal artery supplies the entire hallux. It also provides muscular branches to the first dorsal interosseous muscle, articular branches to the first metatarsophalangeal joint, and cutaneous branches to the dorsum of the foot. The caliber of the first dorsal metatarsal artery is between 1 and 1.5 mm, and thus it is of significant size.[6]

Another vascular structure plantarly that needs be considered when evaluating damage to soft tissue structures near the first metatarsal is the first plantar metatarsal artery. This artery is considered to be a terminal branch of the dorsalis pedis artery or of the lateral plantar artery. It arises at the inferior aspect of the base of the second metatarsal and runs distally, separated from the dorsal metatarsal artery by the first dorsal interossoeus muscle. It runs along the lateral surface of the first metatarsal and, proximal to the metatarsophalangeal joint, divides into medial and lateral branches. The lateral branch courses next to the fibular sesamoid and joins the first dorsal metatarsal artery where it bifurcates in the first webspace. The medial branch passes next to the tibial sesamoid and anastomoses with the tibial plantar hallucal artery, a branch of the first dorsal metatarsal artery. Finally, the medial plantar artery sends a branch at the level of the medial aspect of the base of the first metatarsal to supply the medial aspect of the hallux.[6]

Nerve structures that could be involved in injuries to the first metatarsal or joint include the superficial and deep peroneal nerve as well as the medial plantar nerve. The medial dorsal cutaneous nerve is the largest branch of the superficial peroneal nerve, and it has medial, middle, and lateral branches.[6] The middle branch runs in the first interspace and supplies the lateral dorsal aspect of the hallux but receives reinforcement from the deep peroneal nerve here in the interspace. The medial branch runs medially, crosses over the extensor hallucis longus tendon, then runs parallel to it to supply the dorsomedial portion of the hallux. This nerve is quite superficial and, at the level of the metatarsophalangeal joint, anastomoses with the saphenous nerve.

The medial terminal branch of the deep peroneal nerve accompanies the dorsalis pedis artery in the foot, lying directly on the bone lateral to the artery. In the first intermetatarsal space, it is located between the extensor hallucis brevis tendon and the long extensor tendon to the second digit. Here it divides into two branches to supply the dorsolateral aspect of the great toe and the medial second toe. The medial plantar nerve has cutaneous branches that supply the skin of the inner aspect of the sole of the foot and plantar and dorsal hallux. Muscular branches supply the abductor hallucis, flexor digitorum brevis, flexor hallucis brevis, and first lumbrical. Articular branches supply the joints of the tarsus and metatarsus including the first metatarsophalangeal joint.

KINEMATICS OF THE FIRST RAY AND FIRST METATARSOPHALANGEAL JOINT

The first ray is a functional unit consisting of the first metatarsal and medial cuneiform. Both the first metatarsal cuneiform joint and the cuneiform navicular joint move together around a common axis of motion.[7] The axis is oriented from anterior, lateral, and plantar through the foot and is angled 45 degrees from the frontal and sagittal planes and only slightly from the transverse plane. The first ray exhibits triplane motion, nearly all of which occurs equally in the frontal and saggital planes. Because the axis of motion goes from anterior, lateral, plantar to posterior, medial, dorsal, the ray inverts as it dorsiflexes and everts as it plantar flexes.

The minimum amount of dorsiflexion and plantar flexion of the first ray needed for locomotion is unknown. Plantar flexion of the first ray is needed for propulsion because as the foot inverts during propulsion, the medial aspect of the forefoot elevates from the ground. The first ray must have a range of plantar flexion that will allow the first metatarsal head to maintain ground contact while the foot inverts.

The first metatarsophalangeal joint has two axes of motion.[8] The verticle axis provides the transverse plane motion of abduction and adduction of the hallux. This motion occurs in a hinge-like fashion, and the joint behaves as a ginglymus joint. Transverse plane motion at this joint is thought to be insignificant during locomotion.

Normally, no motion is available at the first metatarsophalangeal joint in the frontal plane. The transverse axis, however, provides sagittal plane motion of dorsiflexion and plantar flexion at the metatarsophalangeal joint, which is extremely important for normal locomotion. The transverse axis lies in the first metatarsal near the surgical neck. During motion in the sagittal plane, the metatarsophalangeal joint acts both as a ginglymus and as an arthrodial joint.[8] Throughout all of plantar flexion and the initial 20 to 30 degrees of dorsiflexion, the hallux rotates upon the head of the first metatarsal. Within this range of motion, the joint acts as a ginglymus joint. However, dorsiflexion greater than 20 to 30 degrees requires an arthrodial motion at the metatarsophalangeal joint as well as plantar flexion of the first metatarsal.

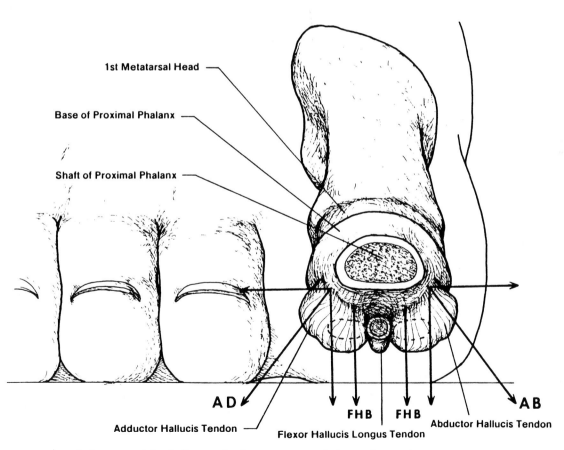

Fig. 19-2. Stabilization of the hallux at the first metatarsophalangeal joint during the propulsive phase of gait. (From Root et al.,[8] with permission.)

Root et al. describe a sequence of events that occur at the first metatarsophalangeal joint during the propulsive phase of locomotion.[8] During the first 20 to 30 degrees of dorsiflexion, the first metatarsal begins to move around a stable, fixed hallux; however, 60 to 75 degrees of dorsiflexion is necessary for propulsion. After the initial 20 to 30 degrees, the first metatarsal head must move plantarly relative to the base of the proximal phalanx. This motion results in a shift of the axis of motion to a more dorsal and posterior direction. The dorsal articular surface of the first metatarsal articulates with the proximal phalanx at this point to provide the 60 to 75 degrees of dorsiflexion. As heel lift develops during propulsion, the first ray must plantar flex to maintain the first metatarsal head against the ground. As propulsion continues, the first ray plantar flexes, and the first metatarsal head moves posteriorly and glides on top of the sesamoid until the distal plantar aspect of the first metatarsal comes to rest on the sesamoids. There, the sesamoids serve a pulley function for muscles that stabilize the hallux against the ground during propulsion. The hallux remains firmly on the ground during propulsion, stabilized by the plantar extrinsic and intrinsic muscles as depicted in Figure 19-2. It is important to note that the hallux does not move as first metatarsophalangeal joint motion occurs. Full dorsiflexion cannot be achieved unless the first ray has its necessary range of plantar flexion.

As stated by Root et al., certain conditions exist that interfere with normal mechanics of the first metatarsal phalangeal joint.[8] These conditions are (1) a congenital or acquired dorsiflexed first ray deformity; (2) ankylosis of the first ray so it cannot plantar flex; (3) a first metatarsal that is too long; (4) ankylosis of the sesamoid-metatarsal joint; (5) ankylosis of the first metatarsophalangeal joint; and (6) eversion of the foot in propulsion caused by increased subtalar joint pronation. Ground forces in this last instance will restrict plantar flexion of the first ray. Any condition that interferes with dorsiflexion of the first metatarsophalangeal joint will lead to subluxation of the first metatarsophalangeal joint, which will result in pain, formation of a dorsal exostosis, articular erosion, marginal proliferation, and eventual ankylosis of the joint. Therefore, anatomic reduction of fractures of the first metatarsal is extremely important to prevent these conditions from occurring, thereby preventing their sequelae of deformity and disability.

TRAUMATIC DISLOCATIONS OF THE FIRST METATARSOPHALANGEAL JOINTS

Traumatic dislocations of the first metatarsophalangeal joints are rare, there being only 12 reported in recent literature by Jahss.[9] Mouchet, however, cited 50 cases prior to 1913. The mechanism for this type of injury is usually forceful hyperextension of the joint, usually caused by a vehicular accident or a fall from a height.

During normal dorsiflexion and plantar flexion of the first metatarsophalangeal joint, the sesamoids go through an excursion of approximately 1 cm. In plantar flexion, they lie under the proximal portion of the first metatarsal head plantarly. In dorsiflexion, they move distally and slightly dorsally near the distal end of the metatarsal head.[9]

Jahss' classification (Fig. 19-3) of these dislocations shows that there are two basic types.[9] Type I occurs when there is dorsal dislocation in which, as the hallux is dorsiflexed, the plantar capsule ruptures at its attachment at the plantar aspect of the metatarsal neck. The hallux then rides over the metatarsal head with the sesamoids still attached to each other and the base of the proximal phalanx. The medial and lateral conjoined tendons lie very tautly to either side. This makes closed reduction of the dislocation nearly impossible, and open reduction is necessary.

Type II can occur as two types. Type IIA occurs as further dislocation occurs at the joint, causing rupture of the intersesamoidal ligament and wide separation of the sesamoids. This is usually reducible by closed reduction. Type IIB occurs when the dorsiflexion causes the intersesamoidal ligament to remain intact, but causes a transverse fracture of one or both sesamoids. The distal fragment(s) moves in normal relationship

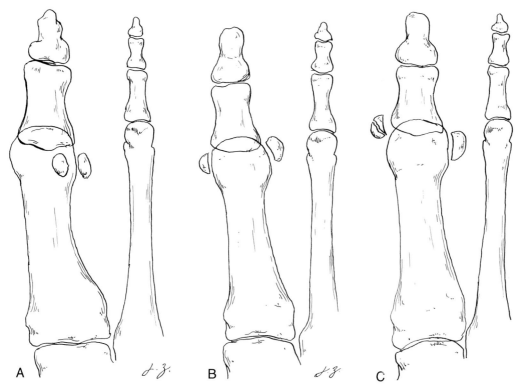

Fig. 19-3. First metatarsophalangeal joint dislocations. **(A)** Type I dislocation. The intersesamoidal ligament remains intact. **(B)** Type IIA dislocation. The intersesamoidal ligament sustains further injury and ruptures, resulting in wide separation of the sesamoids. **(C)** Type IIB dislocation, with intersesamoidal ligament rupture and sesamoidal fracture.

with the other sesamoid. This is also usually reducible by closed manipulation.

FORCES ACTING ON THE FIRST METATARSAL

In 1983, Hutton and Dhanendran devised a method of quantitatively measuring the forces acting across a section of metatarsal.[1] Figure 19-4 shows the forces acting across a section (X-X) of a metatarsal. F_T in the diagram is the ground force to the toe. F_M is the ground force applied to the metatarsal, and L is the combined force exerted by the long and short toe flexors and the tension of the plantar aponeurosis. F_T and L combine to form F_J, the resultant joint force acting across the metatarsophalangeal joint:

$$F_J = F_T{}^2 + L^2$$

Hutton and Dhanedran found that F_J, or the resultant force acting across the first metatarsophalangeal joint, is very nearly equal to body weight, with the maximum forces and movements acting on the metatarsals decreasing from the first to the fifth metatarsal. These findings reaffirm the need to maintain the normal weight-bearing capacity of the first metatarsal in the event of fracture or dislocation.

MECHANISMS OF INJURY TO THE FIRST METATARSAL

The most common mechanisms for injury to the first metatarsal are listed.

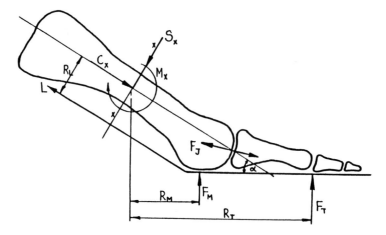

Fig. 19-4. Forces acting on the first ray. (From Hutton and Dhanendran,[1] with permission.)

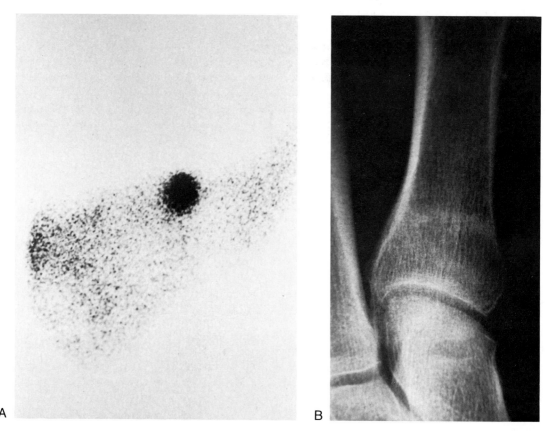

Fig. 19-5. First metatarsal stress fracture. **(A)** Technetium 99 m bone scan identifying a stress fracture at the base of the first metatarsal. **(B)** Radiograph taken 9 months later showing evidence of fracture healing. (Courtesy of Barry L. Scurran, D.P.M.)

Blunt Trauma

Blunt trauma includes a direct crushing type of injury in which a heavy weight falls on the dorsum of the foot.[2,10–12] The metatarsal shaft and neck absorb the energy from the blow, resulting in fracture. This type of force may also cause damage to the sesamoids.

Twisting Injury

A fracture of the metatarsal may result from a twisting type of injury in which the forefoot is fixed as a heavy object falls on it and the patient turns, causing a medial or lateral torque.[10]

Hyperextension Injury

Severe hyperextension injury at the metatarsophalangeal joint causes the metatarsal head to be driven through the flexor plate and fractured.[13]

Impaction Injury

Impaction injury is an injury in which the patient lands on the ball of a plantar flexed foot (i.e., from a height). In this injury, the plantar aspect of the base becomes impacted against the medial cuneiform, causing fracture of the bone.[14]

Avulsion Injury

Avulsion injury is seen in a plantar flexion and inversion type of injury in which the base of the first metatarsal is avulsed by the peroneus longus at its attachment.

Microtrauma or Stress Fracture

Many investigators suggest that metatarsal stress fractures are the result of an overuse of the bone.[15,16] Frankel has proposed a theory that there are four causes for stress fractures of metatarsals.[17] (1) Stress fractures are caused by an overload brought on the bone by excess muscle contraction; (2) stress distribution in the bone is altered by continued activity in the presence of muscle fatigue; (3) stress fractures may be caused by an abrupt change in walking or running surface; and (4) high repetition of stress may cause fracture. Slowick similarly believes that they are caused by the inability of a bone to remodel at a fast enough pace to meet the demands placed on it.[18] Stress fractures of the first metatarsal, although not common, do occur and are reported in the literature (Fig. 19-5). Therefore, they should be included in the differential diagnosis when assessing a patient with pain in the arch or first metatarsal area following forefoot trauma or exercise.

Other

Other mechanisms of injury resulting in fracture of the first metatarsal are various types of major forefoot trauma, including motor vehicle accidents, lawn mower accidents, bullet wounds (Fig. 19-6) or shell fragments, and industrial accidents. Injuries of this magnitude many times result in serious injury to surrounding soft tissue, vessels, and nerves. Immediate attention must be paid to these injuries to avoid loss of the limb, and only after the patient is stable are the fractures themselves addressed.

TREATMENT

My approach to the patient who sustains forefoot trauma includes a thorough examination of the injured part, with particular attention paid to surrounding soft tissue structures. It cannot be overemphasized that in a traumatic injury, especially those involving blunt trauma or motor vehicle, lawn mower, or bullet wound accidents, soft tissue damage can be devastating and should be addressed as a first priority. A thorough vascular and neurologic examination, therefore, is performed first. Radiographic examination of the first metatarsal should reveal the fracture on at least two, but preferably three, views. Sesamoid

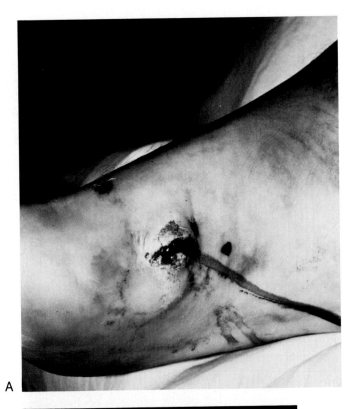

A

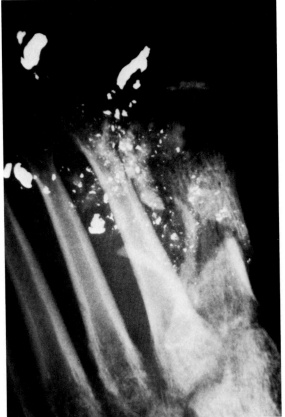

B

Fig. 19-6. Gunshot wound. (A) Clinical example of a gunshot wound resulting in extensive soft tissue and osseous involvement. (B) Radiograph of first metatarsal fracture with missile fragments. (Courtesy of Barry L. Scurran, D.P.M.)

axial views are also suggested to evaluate damage to these structures and also to rule out first metatarsophalangeal joint disruption or dislocation.

After the neurovascular status of the foot has been evaluated and found to be intact, attention can then be directed to the stabilization of the fracture. Although several different methods of treatment will be discussed as options for treatment, my preferred treatment for these farctures will be covered first.

Goals of treatment for any fracture are to heal the fracture and prevent deformity with an early return to function. However, this is especially important in the first metatarsal fracture because of the important biomechanics of the first metatarsal and first metatarsophalangeal joint in locomotion. For this reason, fractures of the first metatarsal are treated more aggressively than fractures of the lesser metatarsals.

I find that simple fractures of the shaft of the first metatarsal that are in good alignment respond well to 6 weeks of non-weight-bearing casting (Fig. 19-7). This is usually followed by several weeks in a rigid-shank shoe with firm support. In situations in which, for some reason, casting is contraindicated, the patient may be placed in a heeled surgical shoe that allows the forefoot to be elevated from the weight-bearing surface. Again, this should be done for 6 weeks, followed by ambulation in a shoe with firm support.

Displaced fractures of the first metatarsal, or any fracture that alters the weight-bearing surface of the first metatarsal as seen on a sesamoid axial view, should be reduced and fixed. Short oblique fractures of the shaft respond well to fixation with a single cortical screw (Fig. 19-8). Long oblique or spiral fractures are excellent indications for interfragmentary compression by a lag screw technique. However, as the fracture approaches a more transverse orientation, a combination of interfragmentary compression with screw fixation and a neutralization plate is recommended. These procedures are followed by non-weight-bearing casting for 6 weeks and then progression into a firm shoe. Because of its importance in locomotion, any fracture of the first metatarsal that interferes with motion at the

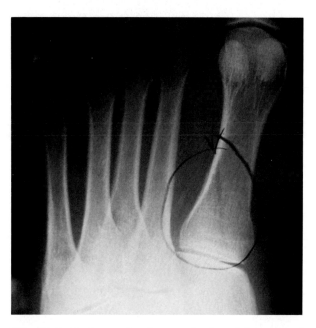

Fig. 19-7. Radiograph of a nondisplaced fracture of the base and shaft of the first metatarsal. Despite the intra-articular nature of this fracture, anatomically aligned fractures respond well to conservative care.

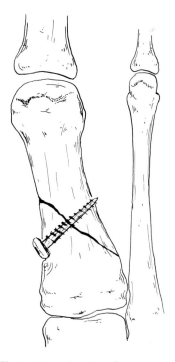

Fig. 19-8. Illustration showing lag screw technique for intrafragmentary compression of oblique first metatarsal fracture.

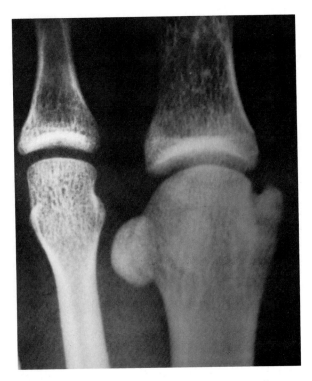

Fig. 19-9. Radiograph of displaced intra-articular medial collateral ligament avulsion fracture. An asymptomatic functional result followed conservative care.

metatarsophalangeal joint, plantar flexion of the first metatarsal, or motion of the first ray must be treated very aggressively. These types of fractures usually require open reduction with internal fixation. Concerning intra-articular fractures (Fig. 19-7 and 19-9), I recommend fixation of any fragment larger than one-fifth to one-fourth of the articular surface. This applies especially to fractures of the first metatarsal head and base. However, the decision of whether to reduce these fractures by the open technique largely depends on the activity level of the patient. A very active, athletic individual who needs to be aggressively rehabilitated is the best candidate for open reduction and internal fixation in these types of injuries. A patient with a more sedentary lifestyle whose ambulation is limited or one who may not be a good surgical candidate may best be treated by closed reduction and casting.

Finally, if the injury is an avulsion fracture in which the intra-articular fragment has the anterior tibial or peroneus longus tendon attached to (Fig. 19-10), open reduction is indicated. These fractures, seen at the metatarsal base, are best fixed with a single cancellous screw or the tension band wiring technique, followed by nonweight-bearing casting (Fig. 19-11). The exception to this is if only a small fleck of bone is avulsed, which could be managed by casting alone. If the patient is symptomatic following casting, excision of the small fragment is indicated.

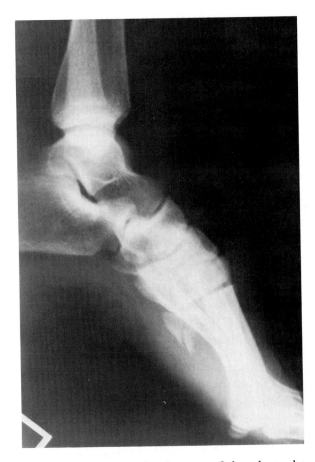

Fig. 19-10. Intra-articular fracture of the plantar-lateral aspect of the first metatarsal base caused by peroneus longus avulsion. (Courtesy of William W. Kirchwehm, D.P.M.)

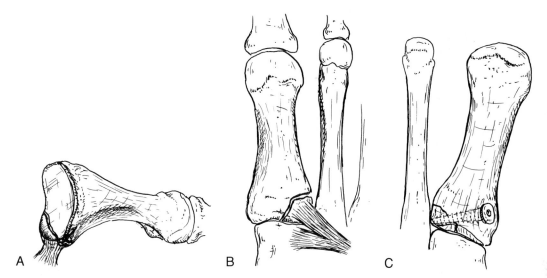

Fig. 19-11. (**A**) Lateral view and (**B**) Plantar view of the first metatarsal base identifying the insertion of the peroneus longus and a plantar lateral avulsion fracture fragment. (**C**) Open reduction and internal fixation is accomplished by the lag screw technique (dorsal view).

OPTIONS FOR TREATMENT

There are many options for treatment of open and closed fractures of the first metatarsal. In open fractures of the metatarsal or of any part of the foot, the initial step is copious irrigation of the wound and debridement of necrotic tissue with appropriate antibiotic coverage and tetanus prophylaxis. Debridement, according to Omer and Pomerantz,[19] has two objectives: to excise contaminated necrotic tissue and to incise fascial sheets choking edematous muscle. They also suggest that bone fragments attached to soft tissue not be removed. However, larger detached bony fragments should be removed, cleansed, and placed back into debrided, healthy tissue to act as bone grafts. If nerves are encountered during debridement, they should be placed in the best available bed of healthy debrided tissue. Particular attention must also be paid to the neurovascular status in open fractures of the foot. This is especially true in blunt trauma or crush injuries of the foot, which may cause devastating edema. Ischemic contracture of the intrinsic foot muscles will occur unless decompressive fascial

incisions are performed. Omer and Pomerantz state that the importance of fasciotomy cannot be overemphasized in these cases, and it should be performed whenever circulation appears to be threatened.[19] Also important during debridement of an open would is hemostasis. If a tourniquet is used during debridement, it should be released and bleeding completely controlled before a dressing is applied.

Wound closure is a topic that should be mentioned when discussing open fractures. Primary wound closure is not indicated in this type of injury.[19] Delayed primary closure, however, can be performed in 3 to 5 days on the dorsum of the foot. Undermining skin edges for delayed primary closure in these instances should be avoided. Adhering to these principles can lead to excellent cosmetic and functional results.[19] Delayed primary closure of the plantar aspect of the foot should not be performed in a severe injury before 5 to 10 days. The safest and most successful procedure for the plantar aspect of the foot is the application of a split- or full-thickness skin graft.[19]

In severe traumatic injuries of the foot, extensive soft tissue disruption as well as multiple fractures result in gross instability of the entire foot or portions of it. Many researchers recommend axial Kirschner wire fixation to stabilize the fracture fragments and to provide soft tissue stability so that healing can occur.[5,19] Omer and Pomerantz suggest delaying this procedure until the time of safe wound closure.[19] Such severe trauma is usually accompanied by gross edema, and compression of the wound and entire extremity is, therefore, very important. This should be attained with a fluff dressing and minimal circular dressings. Importantly, compression should be provided by the number of bandages, not the force of circular constriction.[19] Elevation should be continuous at this time, and may be better accomplished with a sling instead of resting on pillows. Also, the foot should be suspended in neutral position with minimal varus or valgus. Occasionally, external fixation devices are necessary for comminuted fractures to maintain length and position.

It is generally accepted that closed, nondisplaced fractures of the first metatarsal are treated by casting alone (Fig. 19-7 and 19-12). However, this type of casting and length of time of immobilization varies in orthopedic literature. Giannestras and Sammarco[20] and Garcia and Parkes[21] all recommend that nondisplaced fractures of the first metatarsal should be treated with a short leg, non-weight-bearing cast for 2 or 3 weeks, followed by a short leg walking cast for 3 additional weeks. Similarly, DiPalma advocates a short leg cast with no weight bearing on the extremity for 2 weeks, followed by a walking cast for an additional 4 weeks.[12] He then suggests avoiding early callus formation and also a stiff-soled shoe with support of the longitudinal and transverse arches. Heppenstall, however, believes that these nondisplaced fractures can be successfully managed with a below-the-knee, partial weight-bearing cast for 6 weeks.[2] Mann recommends a short leg walking cast well molded beneath the first metatarsal, with weight bearing beginning in 7 to 10 days.[5] The cast is removed when there is radiographic evidence of healing. The foot is then placed in a still-soled shoe with good support in the arch.

A few researchers have actually not recommended casting for these fractures. Johnson rec-

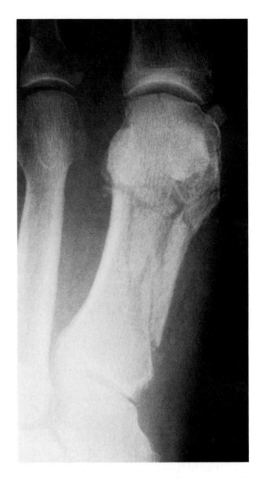

Fig. 19-12. Radiograph of a closed, minimally displaced, comminuted, intra-articular fracture of the first metatarsal.

ommends a simple treatment with compression dressings applied to the foot, several pairs of socks, and a snug-fitting work boot with return to ambulation immediately.[22] He believes that immediate ambulation and weight bearing is the key to rapid return to work with minimal disability. Likewise, Morrissey recommends application of a simple molded leather arch support that is applied to the foot with tape.[23] This taping is changed weekly for four weeks, and physical therapy such as whirlpool soaking is performed at the dressing changes. He also found that this method deceased the average period of disability compared with cast immobilization.

Closed reduced and casting are performed for first metatarsal fractures that are displaced and are attempted before open reduction is performed unless it is very obvious to the physician that closed reduction is virtually impossible. Generally speaking, most metatarsal fractures cannot be anatomically reduced by a closed technique if displacement is significant.[13] This is especially true in fractures of the head or neck area of the metatarsal since these fragments usually displace plantarly and posteriorly. Contracture of soft tissue around the displaced fragment makes closed reduction and maintenance of reduction virtually impossible, even with the use of a well-molded cast and traction.[13] Painful plantar keratoses are common because of an angularly displaced metatarsal head and metatarsalgia resulting from malalignment of the healed neck fracture.[13] Maxwell outlines steps for closed reduction that include (1) prereduction films to evaluate the type of fracture and displacement; (2) anesthesia, either local or general, to provide adequate muscle relaxation, so closed reduction can be attempted; (3) steady traction-countertrac-

tion provided while manipulation is attempted; and (4) postreduction films taken to confirm alignment.

Giannestras,[11] Mann,[5] and Heppenstall[2] believe that closed reduction is best achieved by using a finger trap applied to the toe. Patients are placed in a supine position with the knee flexed and the foot hanging, with weight applied to the distal tibia (Fig. 19-13). This will allow gentle reduction and is best performed shortly after injury. After adequate reduction is achieved on radiographs, a plaster cast is applied from the toes to the midfoot, and the cast is continued to the tibial tubercle. The patient then does not bear weight for 6 weeks, especially if the fracture is comminuted (Fig. 19-14). Weight bearing is then allowed as tolerated.[5,21]

Once reduction is attained, Chapman prefers percutaneous Kirschner wire fixation to maintain the reduction.[24] Mann suggests a transfixing pin from the first metatarsal into the second metatarsal percutaneously to maintain length (Fig.

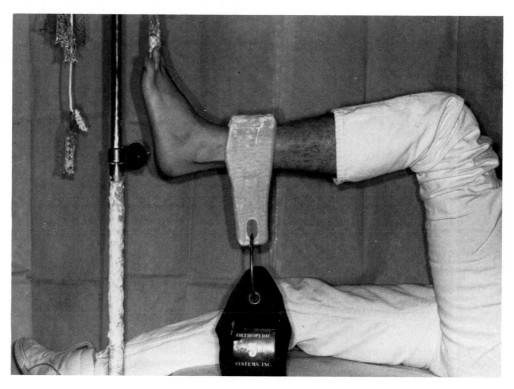

Fig. 19-13. Finger traps used for closed reduction. Note: the patient is lying supine and a 5-pound counterweight is applied for distraction prior to fragment manipulation.

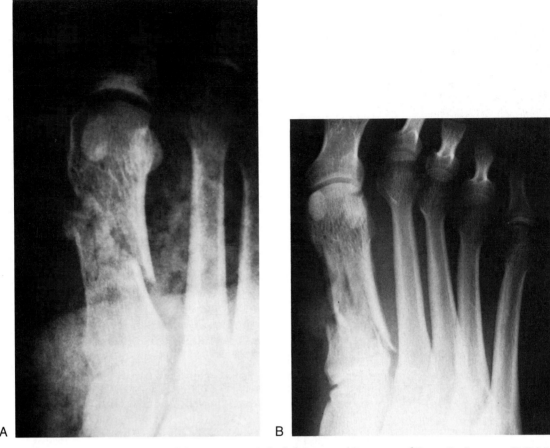

Fig. 19-14. **(A & B)** Comminuted first metatarsal shaft fractures. (Courtesy of Barry L. Scurran, D.P.M.)

19-15).[5] Garcia and Parkes, however, believe that as long as alignment is maintained, either by closed or open means, one should accept axial shortening rather than subjecting the foot to fixed traction.[21] They believe that this leads to stiffness in the forefoot that is more disabling than the metatarsal fracture itself. They believe that surgery can always be performed at a later date if a bony prominence occurs. For fractures located specifically at the base of the first metatarsal (Fig. 19-16), Mann suggests first attempting closed reduction.[5] He stresses, however, that attention must be paid to the integrity and congruency of the metatarsal cuneiform joint. He suggests applying traction until the articular surfaces are reduced and then running Kirschner wires transarticularly or into the shaft of the second

metatarsal. If the joint continues to dislocate or if the fracture fragments continue to displace, then open reduction is performed. For fractures at the base where comminution is too severe to permit open reduction and internal fixation, Mann suggests closed reduction with application of a short leg cast, well molded into the arch to support the metatarsal base.[5] The foot then does not bear weight for 2 to 4 weeks, and eventually the patient begins wearing a steel-soled shoe. Arthrodesis of this joint may be required if pain persists after healing.

If closed reduction attempts fail to reduce the fracture fragments, or if the acquired reduction is lost after casting, open reduction is necessary. Medullary wire fixation is a method of open reduction used and advocated throughout much of

the base of the first metatarsal. The wire is left
out of the skin by some clinicians and buried by
others. This method is used for treatment of shaft
as well as neck fractures. The Kirschner wire remains in place for 3 to 4 weeks only, and the
patients are kept non-weight bearing in a cast
until the wire is removed. The patient is then
recast in a weight-bearing case for an additional
3 weeks.

Giannestras and Sammarco advocate crossed
Kirschner wire fixation for a displaced fracture of
the first metatarsal shaft.[20] This is done through a
medial incision and is followed by application of
a non-weight-bearing short leg cast until healing
is complete, or approximately 6 to 8 weeks. Mann
suggests using a dorsal incision and keeping the
foot in a non-weight-bearing short leg cast for 4
weeks, following by a walking cast for an additional 2 weeks.[5] Fixation is removed between
weeks 4 and 6.

Figura suggests the use of cerclage wire in fixation of oblique fractures of the metatarsal.[26] This
type of wire fixation has been a source of debate
in the past. However, Rheinlander performed
studies on the effects of cerclage wiring on the
microcirculation of bone and found that, since
the periosteal blood supply does not run longitudinally in bone, the blood supply is not compromised.[27] Smith and Green describe the use of intramedullary Krischner wire to restore and
maintain alignment of an impacted metatarsal
neck fracture, followed by cerclage wiring at the
fracture site.[28] Figura has also suggested through
and through monofilament wire fixation for transverse fractures of the metatarsal.[28] The use of this
type of fixation provides good passive compression, minimal stabilization, and no active compression.

Rigid internal fixation of fractures of the first
metatarsal, owing to its important weight bearing
and biomechanical function, may be more effective than traditional methods discussed previously. The goal of rigid fixation is exact anatomic
reconstruction of the plantar arch with a rigid
type of fixation and early motion of the part, but
without early weight bearing.[29] However, use of
internal fixation of this type in the foot is more
difficult than in the hand because the implants
must be applied to the dorsum of the bone, which

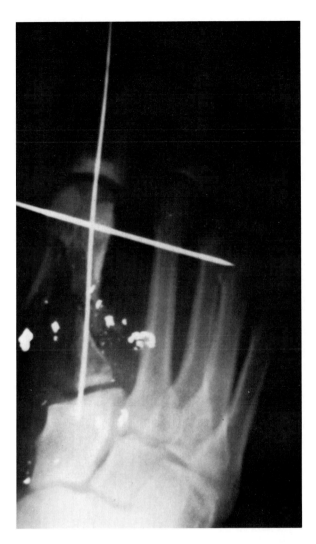

Fig. 19-15. Radiograph of a first metatarsal fracture
with bone loss. Stability and length are maintained by
transmetatarsal Kirschner wire fixation. (Courtesy of
Barry L. Scurran, D.P.M.)

orthopedic literature.[2,5,12,21,25] It involves making
a dorsal incision and driving a Kirschner wire
into the proximal portion of the distal fragment,
then dorsiflexing the metatarsophalangeal joint
and allowing the wire to puncture through the
skin at the plantar area of the metatarsophalangeal joint. The fracture is then anatomically reduced and the wire is driven proximally through
the medullary canal, across the fracture site, into

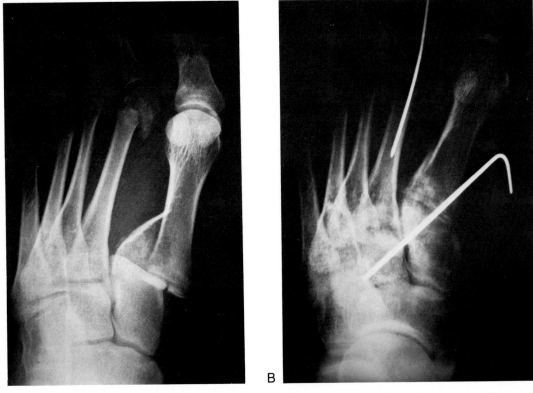

Fig. 19-16. (A) Radiograph of a closed, displaced, intra-articular fracture of the first metatarsal base. (B) Radiograph following open reduction and internal fixation utilizing Kirschner wire fixation. (Courtesy of William W. Kirchwehm, D.P.M.)

is not the tension side. Plates should be placed, therefore, on the lateral side of the metatarsal, which improves the stabilizing effect but cannot achieve a real tension-band effect. Heim and Pfeiffer suggest for fractures of the shaft of the first metatarsal use of a one-third tubular plate or a small T-plate.[29] This should be placed as far as possible on the plantar aspect where it will act as a tension-band plate, (Fig. 19-17). Small plantar wedge-shaped fragments must be addressed, as they can lead to delayed healing, as do comminuted areas. Cancellous grafting may be indicated in these instances to fill in the gaps. Muller et al. suggest that for a displaced T or Y fracture through the base of the first metatarsal, a lag screw or screws and a small T-plate is effective[30] (Fig. 19-18).

COMPLICATIONS OF FIRST METATARSAL FRACTURES

A major complication that could be encountered in fractures of the first metatarsal is delayed union or nonunion. Different opinions exist as to the definition of these terms, however. Muller et al. describe a delayed union as any fracture that has not healed in 4 months and a nonunion as one that has failed to heal in 8 months.[30] Heppenstall more generally describes a delayed union as being present when an adequate interval of time has occurred between initial injury and the average time to union for a particular bone without any radiographic or clinical evidence of union.[2] He states that a nonunion occurs when all repara-

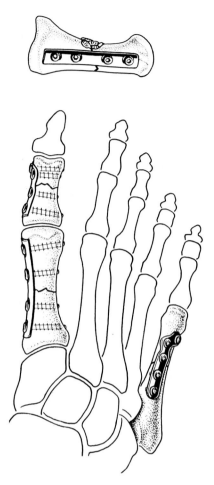

Fig. 19-17. Tubular plate fixation of the first metatarsal. (From Heim and Pfeiffer,[29] with permission.)

tive processes of healing have stopped, yet bony continuity has not been restored.

Heppenstall cites several factors that are implicated in the production of a delayed union or nonunion of a first metatarsal fracture.[2] Inade-

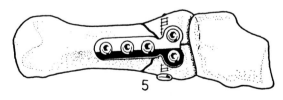

Fig. 19-18. Placement of T-plate and screws. (From Muller et al.,[30] with permission.)

quate reduction of the fracture can result in this problem. Fractures that are inadequately reduced or those that are reduced with soft tissue interposition have a greater chance of resulting in delayed union or nonunion than do properly and adequately reduced fractures. Excessive soft tissue disruption causes an increased healing time owing to the disruption of blood supply to the fracture site. Although most blood supply to the fracture is via endosteal vessels, some blood is supplied by periosteal and soft tissue structures around the fracture site. Also, surrounding musculature attachments applying forces to bone are thought to supply electrical forces across the fracture site that may stimulate healing. Inadequate immobilization in the form of loose casts allows excessive motion around a fracture site and thereby delays healing. Osseous distraction will increase healing time. Compression stimulates bone healing, but tension or distraction prevents it. If there is an increased distance between bone ends, it requires more callus to fill the gap and an increased distance over which the vascular supply must be reestablished. Good bone-to-bone apposition is therefore extremely important for normal healing to occur. Inadequate apposition occurs when adequate or rigid immobilization necessary for fracture healing is not provided. Excessive sacrifice of osseous stock will also impair union. An attempt must be made to preserve all bone present at the fracture site during operative management. Free fragments will act as a free bone graft, and this is much better than leaving a gap or defect. Finally, unnecessary surgical intervention will delay healing time. Surgery performed to treat a fracture that would normally heal with conservative treatment adds the risk of infection and the adverse effect of periosteal stripping to the adverse effect of anesthesia required for the operative procedure.

Heppenstall notes several radiographic signs suggestive of nonunion that should be monitored when treating these fractures.[2] Sclerosis of bone ends at the fracture site suggests nonunion, although a nonunion can be seen with the absence of sclerosis (see Chap. 32). Failure to show progressive radiographic changes or bony remodeling over 3 months suggests delayed union or nonunion. Bowing or deformity at the fracture site, an increase in bony atrophy above and below the fracture, or excess callus around the fracture site with lucency within the callus are all ominous signs. These radiographic signs, combined with clinical signs of persistent edema and pain with ambulation or pain on palpation of the fracture site, are highly suggestive of a delayed union or nonunion, and this problem must be addressed.

Another serious complication of first metatarsal fractures is malunion. As previously mentioned, the first ray, including the first metatarsophalangeal joint, plays an integral role in the function of the foot in the normal gait cycle. For this reason, any fracture of the first metatarsal that interferes with the weight-bearing ability of the first metatarsal can greatly and seriously alter the biomechanical function of this unit. Of particular importance is the saggital plane deviation of fracture fragments. Plantar displacement of a fragment causing excessive plantar flexion of the metatarsal will lead to a rigid plantar-flexed metatarsal, causing painful debilitating lesions beneath the metatarsal head. This may lead to a life-long antalgic gait and an inability of the patient to resume preinjury activity levels.

REFERENCES

1. Hutton W, Dhanendran M: Load distribution under the foot. p. 897. In Harris N (ed): Postgraduate Textbook of Clinical Orthopedics. John Wright & Sons, Boston, 1983
2. Heppenstall R (ed): Fracture Treatment and Healing. WB Saunders, Philadelphia, 1980
3. Jaworek T: The intrinsic vascular supply to the first metatarsal: surgical considerations. J Am Podiatry Assoc 63:555, 1973
4. McCarthy D, Grode S: The anatomical relationships of the first metatarsophalangeal joint: a cryomicrotomy study. J Am Podiatry Assoc 70:493, 1980
5. Mann R (ed): Surgery of the Foot. 5th Ed. CV Mosby, St. Louis, 1986
6. Sarrafian S: Anatomy of the Foot and Ankle: Descriptive Topographic, Functional. JB Lippincott, Philadelphia, 1983
7. Ebisui J: The first ray axis and the first metatarsophalangeal joint. J Am Podiatry Assoc 58:160, 1968
8. Root M, Orion W, Weed J: Normal and Abnormal Function of the Foot. Vol. 2. 1st Ed. Clinical Biomechanics, Los Angeles, 1977
9. Jahss M: Traumatic dislocations of the first metatarsophalangeal joint. Foot Ankle. 1:15, 1980
10. Rockwood C, Green D (eds): Fractures. Vol. 1. JB Lippincott, Philadelphia, 1975
11. Giannestras N (ed): Foot Disorders: Medical and Surgical Management. 2nd Ed. Lea & Febiger, Philadelphia, 1973
12. DePalma A: The Management of Fractures and Dislocations. 2nd Ed. Vol. 2. WB Saunders, Philadelphia, 1970
13. Maxwell J: Open or closed treatment of metatarsal fractures. J Am Podiatry Assoc 73:100, 1983
14. Guman G, Engle A, Snowden H: Comminuted intra-articular fractures of the first metatarsal base. J Am Podiatry Assoc 72:521, 1982
15. Jesse J: Hidden Causes of Injury, Prevention and Correction, for Running Athletes and Joggers. p. 581. Athletic Press, Pasadena, 1977
16. Salter R: Disorders and Injuries of the Musculoskeletal System. Williams & Wilkins, Baltimore, 1970
17. Frankel V: Editorial comment. Am J Sports Med 6:396, 1978
18. Slowick A: Stress fractures of the first metatarsal. J Am Podiatry Assoc 50:333, 1969
19. Omer G, Pomerantz G: Initial management of severe open injuries and traumatic amputations of the foot. Arch Surg 105:696, 1972
20. Giannestras N, Sammarco G: Fractures and dislocations in the foot. p. 1400. In Rockwood C, Green D (eds): Fractures. Vol. 1. JB Lippincott, Philadelphia, 1975
21. Garcia A, Parkes J: Fractures of the foot. p. 517. In Giannestras N (ed): Foot Disorders: Medical and Surgical Management. 2nd Ed. Lea & Febiger, Philadelphia, 1973
22. Johnson V: Treatment of fractures of the forefoot in industry. In Bateman J (ed): Foot Science. WB Saunders, Philadelphia, 1976
23. Morrissey E: Metatarsal fractures. J Bone Joint Surg 28:594, 1946
24. Chapman M: Fractures and fracture-dislocation of the ankle and foot. In Mann R (ed); Du Vrie's Surgery of the Foot. 4th Ed. CV Mosby, St. Louis, 1978

25. Sisk T: Fractures of the lower extremity. p. 1607. In Edmonson A, Crenshaw A (eds): Campbell's Operative Orthopedics. 6th Ed. Vol. 1. CV Mosby, St. Louis, 1980

26. Figura M: Metatarsal fractures. p. 247. In Scurran B (ed): Clinics in Podiatry: Symposium on Osseous Trauma of the Foot. Vol. 2. WB Saunders, Philadelphia, 1985

27. Rheinlander R: Normal microcirculation of the cortex. J Bone Joint Surg 50A:784, 1968

28. Smith G, Green A: Cerclage wiring of metatarsal fractures, a case report. J Am Podiatry Assoc 73:25, 1983

29. Heim U, Pfeiffer K: Small Fragment Set Manual. 2nd Ed. Springer-Verlag, New York, 1982

30. Muller M, Allgower M, Schneider R, Willenegger H: Manual of Internal Fixation. 2nd Ed. Springer-Verlag, New York, 1979

31. Jaworek T: The intrinsic vascular supply to first and lesser metatarsals: surgical considerations. Sixth Annual Northlake Surgical Seminar, Chicago, 1976

20

Fractures of Internal Metatarsals

William W. Kirchwehm, D.P.M.
Michael A. Figura, D.P.M.
Timothy A. Binning, D.P.M.
Stanley B. Leis, D.P.M.

Metatarsal fractures are among the most common fractures of the foot. Spector et al. reviewed 29,668 emergency department admissions at Kaiser Permanente Medical Center in Hayward, California, from December 1, 1981, through May 31, 1982.[1] Foot trauma was diagnosed 868 times. Of those foot injuries, 153 pedal fractures were diagnosed, 53 of which involved one or more metatarsal bones. In this time period, 1,005 fractures of one or more skeletal bones were noted. Therefore, metatarsal fractures comprised 35 percent of of foot fractures, 6 percent of foot injuries, 5 percent of total skeletal fractures and 0.2 percent of emergency department admissions. (Fig. 20-1).

Although these fractures are seen by almost every health care professional, their real significance is often not appreciated. This chapter describes the anatomy of the internal metatarsals, gives a workable classification of metatarsal fractures, and provides an insight into their proper diagnosis and treatment and a guideline for evaluation and therapy of any sequelae that may develop after treatment.

ANATOMY

A detailed knowledge of the local anatomy of the forefoot and especially the lesser metatarsals is crucial for understanding osseous injuries to these structures. The internal metatarsals—the second, third, and fourth metatarsals—are relatively more stable than the first and fifth metatarsals as a result of their more confined location and relative lack of extrinsic muscular insertions.[2–4] This anatomic difference that separates the internal metatarsals from the first and fifth metatarsals justifies their exclusive treatment in this discussion.

Metatarsal bones are long bones in structure and function. Their anatomic adaptations provide solutions for local mechanical problems.[4] Biologic evolution has arrived as the most economic solution to the local functional needs of the host. The foot is no less well adapted than other anatomic regions. Long bones throughout the body are composed of an elongated, tubular, diaphyseal shaft with thickened compact cortical bone and a central medullary cavity. Epiphyses are the

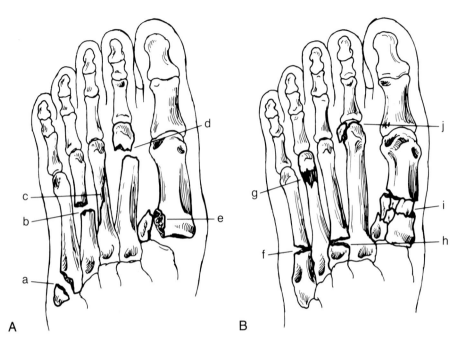

Fig. 20-1. (A & B) Types of metatarsal fractures. (a) Avulsion fracture of the fifth metatarsal base. (b) Transverse metatarsal shaft fracture. (c) Spiral metatarsal shaft fracture. (d) Transverse metatarsal neck fracture. (e) Fracture-dislocation of the first metatarsal base. (f) Jone's fracture of the fifth metatarsal. (g) Compression fracture of the metatarsal neck. (h) Transverse fracture of the metatarsal base. (i) Comminuted fracture of the first metatarsal base. (j) Intra-articular metatarsal head fracture.

enlarged ends and are primarily composed of spongy cancellous bone with a thin cortical shell adapted as the articular constituent. The physis is the site of bone-lengthening growth. The trabecular lattice network of these bones provides the strongest and lightest possible arrangement. The metaphysis is the highly vascular cancellocortical bridge between the diaphyseal shaft and the articular epiphyses.

The bases of the internal metatarsals are the proximal epiphyses. The bases articulate with the lesser tarsus as well as with the adjacent metatarsals via their articular cartilage covering. Distally the heads of the metatarsals articulate with the bases of the proximal phalanges of each corresponding digit. The bases of the second and third metatarsals are triangular, while that of the fourth is rectangular. The heads of these lesser metatarsals form condylar joints with the bases of the proximal phalanges of their respective digits.

The bases of the internal metatarsals have a variable pattern of articulating facets. The second metatarsal base is the most stable and is recessed in a fashion similar to a dado-type joint used in woodworking. It articulates on all three sides with the three cuneiforms and the first and third metatarsal bases. In addition, the second metatarsal base is stabilized by the constantly present first interosseous tarsometatarsal ligament or Lisfranc's ligament. All of the metatarsal bases are further stabilized by plantar, dorsal, and interosseous ligaments that form the tarsometatarsal joint or Lisfranc's joint. Gliding motions of flexion, extension, abduction, and adduction are permitted at Lisfranc's joint.

Adjacent soft tissues and soft tissue attachments are important anatomic features in light of the substantial soft tissue destruction that occurs during fracture trauma. Some investigators implicate soft tissue as an etiology in overuse syndromes and stress fractures.[5] As previously emphasized, there is a relative lack of insertion of extrinsic musculature on the internal metatarsals. However, the intrinsic musculature originates from these metatarsals, forming the majority of local soft tissue support. Metatarsal bases two, three, and four, along the plantar medial aspect, provide the origin for the oblique head of the adductor hallucis muscle. Both dorsal and plantar interosseous muscles originate from the internal metatarsal shafts and bases. The plantar interosseous muscles originate from the medial base and shaft of the third, fourth, and fifth metatarsals. The dorsal medial and dorsal lateral shafts of metatarsals two through four form the origin of the dorsal interosseous muscles. Draves states that both tibialis posterior and peroneus longus may send tendinous slips to the bases of the second, third, and fourth metatarsals on their way to their respective sites of primary insertion.[2] Thus, we describe these internal metatarsals as having a relative lack of extrinsic muscular insertions.

Jaworek investigated the intrinsic vascular supply to the first metatarsal and to the lesser metatarsals using cadaveric specimens.[6] The principle nutrient artery of the lesser metatarsal enters the lateral diaphyseal cortex approximately 3.1 cm from the distal articular cartilage and approximately 0.2 cm from the dorsal aspect of the metatarsal. Ascending and descending subcortical branches reach each end of the metatarsal. The terminal branches form a plexus of small vessels that anastomose with metaphyseal nutrient arteries. These highly vascular metaphyseal and epiphyseal regions are well supplied and thus less likely to suffer nonunion in fracture healing. External metatarsal blood supply derives from the periosteal circulation. Care should always be exercised with the periosteum during fracture surgery or any elective metatarsal osteotomy.

ETIOLOGY

Metatarsal fractures can be caused by either direct or indirect trauma. Direct trauma, such as crush injuries or sudden impact forces, can cause fractures to the internal metatarsals. Indirect trauma includes torque or twisting forces, abnormal biomechanical stress, and avulsion fractures.[7–12]

Direct trauma is self-explanatory and will not be included in this discussion. However, the mechanism of indirect traumatic fractures is more complicated. The most common fracture of the lesser internal metatarsal bones is the fatigue or stress fracture caused by indirect repetitive microtrauma. Metatarsal stress fractures are also known as march fractures and are frequently seen in athletes and military recruits, individuals who are exposed to a rapid increase in rate of activity. Bone is continually adapting to new loading patterns. When this adaptive response is overwhelmed by increasing loads, failure points develop. Increased workload coupled with biomechanical imbalance contributes to the mechanism of stress fracture formation. Bakers et al. concluded that muscle fatigue leads to altered gait patterns and, therefore, abnormal stress distribution.[5] New or different activity alters the delicate relationship between growth and repair of osseous tissues. Bone remodeling that predominates over repair will result in bone injury. Continual fatigue of the periosteum, periosteal inflammation, and subperiosteal new bone formation eventually precipitate fracture of the metatarsals.

Although rare, pathologic fractures can occur in the lesser metatarsal bones. A pathologic fracture is found in abnormal bone where the osseous structure and trabecular pattern are not able to withstand forces that may otherwise be harmless to normal bone. These fractures may also occur with major traumatic stress. Numerous underlying conditions can weaken osseous tissue. Salter presents an exhaustive list of disorders that predispose bone to pathologic fractures.[12] The categories include the following:

1. Congenital abnormalities
    Localized
    Disseminated
    Generalized
2. Metabolic bone disease

3. Disseminated bone disorders of unknown etiology
4. Inflammatory disorders
5. Neuromuscular disorders
6. Avascular necrosis of bone
7. Neoplasms of bone
    Primary neoplasmlike lesions
    True primary neoplasms
    Metastatic neoplasms in bone

In addition, Harkess cites osteoporosis as a cause of pathologic fracture, especially in the elderly.[9]

CLASSIFICATION

Salter devised a working classification to allow accurate description of long bone fractures.[12] Since long bone fractures present in an infinite variety, an organized system is necessary to describe them. A clear description will aid in the establishment of an appropriate treatment regimen. Salter's classification consists of five categories including the site of fracture, extent of fracture within the bone, configuration of fracture, relative position of fracture fragments, and the relationship of the fracture to the external environment. Gudas added a sixth category specific to metatarsal fractures.[13] The internal metatarsals have minimal extrinsic muscular attachments, whereas the external metatarsals are major insertion points. Therefore, these muscles must be properly neutralized to maintain proper apposition and alignment of the fracture. In addition, the first metatarsal is larger and bears more weight, thus requiring a more precise reduction and stable immobilization.

The site of a fracture specifies the area of bony involvement. With regard to metatarsal fractures, these areas include the diaphysis, metaphysis, and epiphysis or intra-articular area. The physis in the skeletally immature individual has a separate classification of fractures and will be included elsewhere.

A fracture may extend completely or incompletely through the bone. Greenstick or buckle fractures are common types of incomplete fractures seen in children secondary to the increased bony pliability of skeletal immaturity.

The configuration of the fracture may be spiral, transverse, or oblique, to name a few of the possible shapes. A comminuted fracture results from two or more fracture lines with three or more osseous fragments.

The fourth descriptive category is the relationship of the fragments to each other. If the fragments are displaced, they can be shifted in any plane. They may be rotated, shifted laterally, distracted, overriding, angulated, impacted, and compressed. They also may occur in combinations. Fractures in good anatomic alignment are designated as nondisplaced.

The relationship of the fragments to the external environment will determine whether the fracture is open or closed. Previous terminology respectively referred to these fractures as compound or simple. Open fractures communicate with the outside environment, whereas closed fractures do not. Open fractures may communicate from without as a result of penetration by a sharp object.

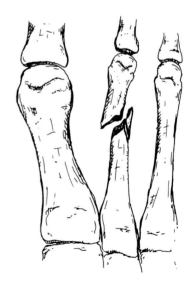

Fig. 20-2. An example of a common long bone fracture. Fracture, second metatarsal shaft, complete, displaced, comminuted, internal metatarsal.

An example of a fracture description using this classification system is given in Figure 20-2. This type of description would provide a good mental picture of the fracture if described over the telephone. If an emergency room physician provided this description, one could make a medically sound assessment and treatment until able to examine the patient and radiographs personally.

DIAGNOSIS

A thorough history and physical examination is required to evaluate the degree of injury and to determine proper treatment of metatarsal fractures. The uniqueness of each case makes it essential to assess the injury carefully prior to initiation of treatment. The general medical health of the patient is a major consideration. The patient's age, occupation, and ambulatory status prior to injury are vital factors in formulating a treatment plan.

Pertinent information elicited in the history should include the mechanism of injury, if possible. Often metatarsal fractures are a result of blunt, crushing trauma. The patient may relate a twisting injury resulting from a fall. The patient may suspect a fracture if a popping or cracking sound was heard. Patients often complain of swelling, bruising, and the inability to bear weight.

Physical examination of potential fractures begins with observation, followed by palpation and assessment of functional capability. Inspection of the patient should include a thorough evaluation for evidence of multiple traumatic injuries. Pedal fractures, including metatarsal fractures, may coexist with other fractures. Calcaneal fractures, for example, often are observed with concomitant compression fractures of the lumbar vertebrae.[14,15] Visible signs of metatarsal fractures include edema, subcutaneous ecchymosis, and obvious deformity. Open fractures may be obvious with inspection of the injury site. Digital vascular status can be assessed by observation of the color, temperature, tone, and turgor of the skin as well as by assessment of the subpapillary venous plexus filling time.

Palpation should include evaluation of the point of maximum tenderness. Isolation of the individual metatarsal, however, may be difficult because of their close proximity. Palpation may elicit crepitus and sharp pain. Careful neurovascular testing should always accompany the evaluation of any suspected fractures.

Compartment syndrome, although rare in the foot, has been reported secondary to trauma.[16,17] Pain resistant to analgesics, pallor, paresthesias, and intrinsic muscle paralysis are the findings present in compartment syndrome of the foot. A high index of suspicion requires further evaluation by compartment pressure measurements. This syndrome should be included in the differential diagnosis whenever multiple pedal fractures are present.

Gentle passive range of motion examination is useful in intra-articular metatarsophalangeal joint injury. Active range of motion testing is used to assess major tendon integrity. Finally, clinical evaluation for metatarsal fractures may be aided by the c-128 tuning fork. This method is often helpful in determining the site of maximum tenderness. Any findings suggestive of fracture should be followed by radiographic evaluation.

Radiographic examination of metatarsal fractures is normally a simple procedure but should include at least two views at 90 degrees to one another. The standard three view foot series of anteroposterior, medial-oblique and lateral views are usually sufficient. The anteroposterior view assesses the amount of coronal plane displacement, metatarsal shortening, and parabolic curve of the metatarsals. The medial-oblique view decreases the overlap of the lateral metatarsals and assists in determining the fracture fragment relationships in the dorsal and plantar directions. The lateral view assesses sagittal plane displacement, but can be misleading owing to the overlap inherent in this view.

If proper anatomic position is in question, a plantar axial or sesamoidal view must be considered. The axial radiograph is important because it may reveal the relative position of the metatarsal heads in the sagittal plane.[18]

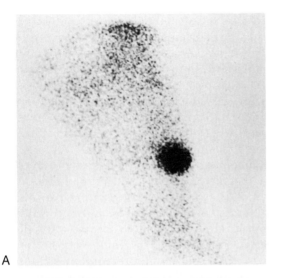

A

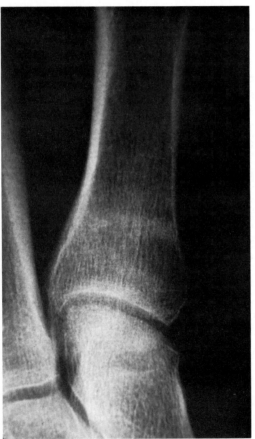

B

Fig. 20-3. (A) Technetium 99 bone scan identifying a stress fracture of the base of the first metatarsal. **(B)** Radiograph taken 9 months later showing evidence of fracture. (Courtesy of Barry L. Scurran, D.P.M.)

Bone scanning with radionuclide imaging is a useful technique in the diagnosis of stress fractures throughout the body. Many articles have been published documenting the usefulness of this technique in diagnosis of fatigue fractures in the foot.[19–24] Standard radiography identifies the healing process in stress fractures; medullary sclerosis, periosteal new bone growth and callus formation become apparent 2 to 4 weeks after injury.[19] Greaney et al. showed that 75 percent of metatarsal stress fractures could not be diagnosed without a scintigram.[20] This profound difficulty in diagnosis by standard techniques makes technetium 99 bone imaging a logical indication (Fig. 20-3).

PATHOMECHANICS

During the normal gait cycle, at heel lift during the propulsive phase, vertical ground reactive force approaches 125 percent of body weight.[25] A large percentage of this force is isolated to the forefoot, primarily the metatarsophalangeal joints. Normally, the soft tissues of the forefoot are adapted to withstand this force. During propulsion, these tissues also resist injury by the routine linear and transverse shearing force and torque associated with leg rotation. Clearly, the margin of error in the skin and subcutaneous tissues is minimal. Minimal increases in these forces combined with plantar-flexed metatarsals, metatarsus primus elevatus, hypermobile first ray, increased age, or a displaced or decreased subcutaneous fat pad may lead to pathologic lesions. Ambulation and its associated repetitive microtrauma may initiate inflammatory hyperplasia and hyperkeratotic sequelae. Constant or increased forces with subsequent nucleated lesions may eventually be infiltrated by neurovascular elements to become heloma neurovasculare. The metatarsalgia secondary to these neurovascular lesions may be intractable to the degree that an antalgic gait pattern develops and disability ensues.

This consideration of the pathomechanics of hyperkeratoses may also be applied to post-traumatic malunion of metatarsal fractures. Consider, for example, the malalignment of a metatarsal fracture in the sagittal plane leading to a plantar flexion deformity. The unfortunate individual in this example would be obliged to bear weight on this plantar-flexed metatarsal. Single or multiple fractures of the internal metatarsals, if inappropriately treated, may ultimately result in plantar hyperkeratotic lesions. Metatarsal fractures that heal either dorsiflexed or plantar flexed may cause plantar lesions. Sagittal plane malalignment in an individual with peripheral neuropathy is poorly tolerated, with potential for tissue breakdown and neurotrophic ulceration. The practitioner with an awareness of these problems must strive to achieve good anatomic alignment of displaced internal metatarsal fractures to avoid future debilitating sequelae.

TREATMENT

Treatment of internal metatarsal fractures takes many factors into consideration.[26] Accurate anatomic alignment of the fracture fragments is recommended in the ideal situation. However, this treatment is not always possible. The physical condition and biomechanical needs of the patient should always be considered. In a debilitated patient who does not have a normal gait cycle, a closed manipulation and casting may be all that is necessary to reduce the fragments to an appropriate alignment for satisfactory healing.[1,11,27] However, in a young, athletic individual or an active adult, an accurate anatomic open reduction with rigid internal fixation and early mobilization might be indicated.[28] Furthermore, the correct choice of treatment for metatarsal fractures requires the intangible quality of the practitioner's clinical experience and time-proven expertise to determine whether the fracture should be treated by open or closed methods. Open reduction is the treatment of choice only when the advantages are clearly superior to the disadvantages. Anderson outlines three considerations when treating any fracture.[29] (1) To obtain union is the primary objective of treatment since function of the adjacent soft tissue parts and joints depends on it. (2) Functional results are proportional to the position of bones after healing. Some variation from the normal anatomy is compatible with good or even normal function. However, the limit of error is small in fractures that involve joint surfaces or are near joints. (3) Early mobilization of soft tissues and adjacent joints is the key to early return of function.

There is a tremendous variation of opinions regarding criteria for open versus closed reduction of metatarsal fractures. The following criteria are guidelines intended to assist the trauma physician in determining whether an internal metatarsal fracture is best treated open or closed. In addition, the common methods and techniques of treatment are discussed. Basic fracture management principles and the tenets of fixation should always be kept in mind.[7,8,10–12,20,30–32] Fixation of the internal metatarsal bones should include techniques affording active compression, passive compression, stabilization, and neutralization. Table 20-1 shows a comparison of the advantages and disadvantages of Kirschner wire, monofilament wire, and ASIF technique.[30]

Residual displacement of the second, third, and fourth metatarsal shafts or heads in the frontal plane does not usually leave the patient with significant complicating sequelae.[29] These fractures heal by conservative management despite significant fragment separation. Transverse plane

Table 20-1. Methods of Fracture Fixation

	Active Compression	Passive Compression	Stabilization
Monofilament wire	None	Good	Minimal
Kirschner wire	None	Minimal	Very good
ASIF technique	Excellent	Excellent	Excellent

displacement, again, does not result in significant late complications because the metatarsals lie deep within the foot musculature and are protected medially and laterally by the first and fifth metatarsals, respectively. However, Mann notes several uncommon complications secondary to residual transverse plane malunion.[33]

As described in the pathomechanics section, sagittal plane displacement, either dorsal or plantar, or significant metatarsal shortening from fracture fragment overlap will result in painful irritation or hyperkeratotic lesions. Careful radiographic evaluation of subtle displacements of any easily identifiable fracture is imperative. Proper management depends upon it if restoration of acceptable anatomic alignment and an asymptomatic result are the goals. Both open and closed reduction techniques have been successful with internal metatarsal fractures. The principles of fracture management must be strictly observed to achieve an early return to full functional capacity without complications.

Early evaluation and treatment is very important as reactive edema can complicate both open and closed techniques. Optimally, a fracture should be treated within hours of the initial injury. Significant edema obliterates palpable landmarks and renders osseous manipulation impossible. Open surgical reduction is usually contraindicated in the presence of severe edema; wound closure may be impossible and postoperative wound complications such as dehiscence may occur. In these situations, reduction, whether open or closed, should be postponed several days until local management of edema is completed. Bed rest, ice, elevation, use of nonsteroidal anti-inflammatory agents, and compression (Jones-type splinting) will resolve edema and allow further treatment.

Return of the osseous components to acceptable alignment should be first attempted by closed methods. Maxwell emphasizes the guidelines for closed reduction as (1) radiographic evaluation both before and after reduction, (2) anesthesia as required, and (3) reduction technique.[11] Radiographic evaluation has been discussed in detail previously. Anesthesia choices are many and varied. Our choice is local anesthetic ankle block combined with a hematoma block technique,[34] similar to that described by Dinley and Michelinski[35] used in Colles' fracture of the wrist. Closed reduction can also be attempted with intravenous narcotic analgesia combined with intravenous sedation with a short acting benzodiazapine. Demerol (meperidine hydrochloride) and Valium (diazepam), respectively, are often used. Care must be taken to avoid central respiratory depression and apnea when using narcotics. A narcotic antidote such as naloxone must be immediately available for narcotic reversal in an emergency situation. Local anesthetic agents administered as intravenous regional anesthesia are also useful for both open and closed treatment.[36,37] Failure of these methods may require spinal, epidural, or general anesthesia.

Manipulation is attempted to align the fracture fragments. Distal traction, generally the first manipulative force applied, can be executed by manual maneuvers, by applying force via surgical tape, or by "hanging" the extremity or digit in finger traps.[38] Once the fragments are separated, manual manipulation of individual fragments reduces the malalignment. Plaster cast application of a well-molded, below-the-knee cast follows manipulation. Again, successful reduction is evaluated by radiography or image intensification devices.

Failure of closed reduction methods requires open reduction and rigid internal fixation. Proper evaluation and appropriate treatment of foot trauma must only be initiated and performed by a well-qualified practitioner. This becomes more important when open reduction and internal fixation are required to treat foot and ankle fractures. A good understanding of the rules of surgical fixation is a minimal requirement for operative management. Several texts will provide the foot surgeon with the fundamentals of open techniques.[8,10,11,29–32,37,39,40] As emphasized previously, fixation techniques utilized in conjunction with open reduction include Kirschner wires, monofilament wire, and AO technique. AO techniques used in the foot include tension band wiring, interfragmentary compression with screws, neutralization plating, buttress plating and mini-Hoffman-type external compression devices.[30,31] A classic method of open reduction and internal

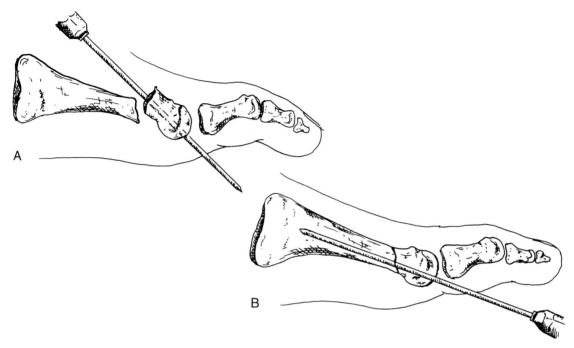

Fig. 20-4. (A & B) Diagram outlining a classic technique for Kirschner wire fixation of a metatarsal fracture.

fixation is illustrated in Figure 20-4.

Although regaining anatomic alignment is the goal of trauma surgery, certain situations prohibit open surgical reduction. Clearly, the general contraindications of open reduction can be applied to metatarsal fractures. We recommend the following: (1) In the presence of active infection, open reduction should be temporarily postponed. The surgeon should immobilize the patient in a cast or splint and proceed to treat the infection until resolved. Open reduction may be performed upon resolution. (2) When fracture fragments are of insufficient size to allow use of fixation devices, open treatment should be avoided. (3) Inadequate bone stock secondary to osteoporosis or other conditions may technically limit the surgeon. Care should be exercised in treatment. (4) Nondisplaced or impacted fractures are usually successfully treated by closed methods. (5) Patients with traumatic skin conditions, fracture blisters, or abrasions along the proposed surgical site should be assessed according to the potential risks versus the benefits of surgi-

cal treatment. Resolution of these conditions by local wound care is suggested prior to surgical intervention.

Fractures of the Metatarsal Head

If a significant intra-articular fracture of the metatarsal head is sustained, open reduction is recommended to restore anatomic alignment of the articular surface. If the fragments are too small, the best treatment is nonsurgical. Utilization of a rigid-bottomed shoe or an accommodative orthosis as well as early range of motion exercises is essential for management of these fractures.[28]

Fractures of the Metatarsal Neck

Fractures of the distal metaphyseal area are common because the traumatic force is often per-

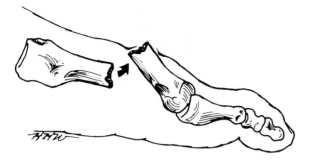

Fig. 20-5. Diagram showing dorsal displacement of a metatarsal neck fracture with concomitant metatarsophalangeal joint subluxation.

pendicular to the long axis of the metatarsal. These fractures are usually transverse. The distal fragment may be displaced plantarly and laterally owing to the pull of the strong flexor tendons. Fracture at this level with metatarsophalangeal joint dislocation may occur (Fig. 20-5). In this case, it is important to achieve reduction of the dislocation and the fracture. Given the likelihood of sagittal malalignment, closed reduction should be attempted with traction and manipulation. Finger traps, used in conjunction with a local anesthetic block, are an excellent method of applying distal traction while attempting manipulation in the sagittal plane (see Fig. 19-13). Edema, tendinous interposition, and muscular contracture surrounding the metatarsal head are factors that increase the level of difficulty associated with closed reduction of the metatarsal neck. Often closed reduction fails, and then open reduction with internal fixation should be performed. Residual sagittal plane displacement or angulation is an important contribution to late sequelae as described above in the discussion of pathomechanics of metatarsal fractures.

Case One

A 44-year-old man fell from a ladder while trimming branches from a tree. His left foot contacted the ground in a plantar flexed and inverted position. Experiencing pain and inability to bear weight on the foot, he went to the emergency room and was subsequently referred to our service.

The clinical findings revealed forefoot edema, ecchymosis, and tenderness to palpation at the second, third, and fourth metatarsalphalangeal joints and Lisfranc's joint. Neurovascular compromise was not present. In all other respects the patient was in good health.

The anteroposterior and medial-oblique radiographic views demonstrated displaced comminuted fractures of the second and third metatarsal necks and a displaced intra-articular fracture of the fourth metatarsal head. Furthermore, fractures of the third and fourth metatarsal bases were noted, as well as a displaced comminuted intra-articular fracture of the second metatarsal base (Fig. 20-6A and B).

Our criteria for open reduction and internal fixation was the presence of metatarsal neck fractures with significant residual plantar angulation after attempted closed reduction and unstable intra-articular fractures of the fourth metatarsal head and second metatarsal base.

Considering the small fracture fragment size, Kirschner wire fixation was the preferred method of fixation. Crossed Kirschner wires were used to stabilize the comminuted, intra-articular fracture involving the second metatarsal base. Intraoperative radiographs revealed satisfactory reduction and stabilization of all components of the injury (Fig. 20-6).

Postoperatively, the patient remained casted and non-weight bearing for 6 weeks, at which time all Kirschner wires were removed. Six weeks of modified footgear consisting of a wooden surgical shoe and a stiff soled shoe allowed protected weight bearing. At 6 months postsurgery, the patient was asymptomatic and radiographs revealed good joint congruity and fracture healing (Fig. 20-6).

Diaphyseal Fractures

Fracture of the diaphysis of the internal metatarsal is usually caused by direct trauma or a twisting torque of the foot. The fracture configuration is usually oblique, although transverse, spiral, and comminuted injuries occur as well. If the fracture is nondisplaced, a well-molded, non-weight-bearing cast for 4 to 6 weeks nearly guar-

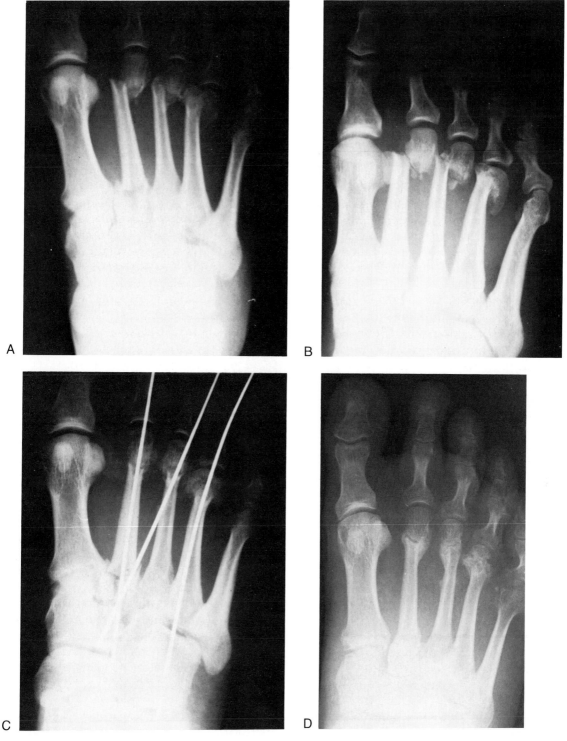

Fig. 20-6. (A) Anteroposterior view and (B) oblique view showing metatarsal neck fractures of the second and third metatarsals, and intra-articular fractures of the fourth metatarsal head and second metatarsal base. (C) Intraoperative radiograph shows satisfactory reduction and stabilization using crossed Kirschner wires. (D) Joint congruity is reestablished and fracture healing has occurred as visualized in radiographs taken 6 months postsurgery.

antees success. More conservative management includes weight-bearing casts (with heel walker), soft casting, orthoses and arch supports have been recommended. Displaced metatarsal shaft fractures with separation of fragments have been treated conservatively with acceptable results.[27]

Oblique diaphyseal fractures can present further difficulty if displaced in the sagittal plane. Similarly, if significant shortening occurs from proximal displacement of the distal fragment, then the metatarsal parabola is lost and weight-bearing biomechanical complications result. Closed reduction should be attempted under anesthesia followed by cast immobilization and re-evaluation with post-reduction radiographs. Failures require open reduction with rigid internal fixation. Oblique fractures are amenable to fixation by several techniques including cerclage wire[41,42] (Fig. 20-7), intramedullary pinning with Kirschner wire,[30,43] and interfragmentary compression by the lag screw technique.[11,30,31,39,44]

Transverse fractures of the diaphysis with angulation in the sagittal plane may also require open reduction and internal fixation. Kirschner wire, through-and-through monofilament wire, a tension band fixation for axial compression or a semitubular plate are options for fixation techniques. The more difficult comminuted fracture of the internal metatarsal is successfully treated with circlage wire, Kirschner wire, lag screw technique, and buttress plating. In a severely comminuted fracture, a mini-Hoffman compression device with bone grafting may be necessary.[45] Initial non-weight-bearing casting or splinting is recommended. Once evidence of fracture healing is present, vigorous physical therapy is initiated to facilitate the return to normal functional capacity.

Case Two

A 22-year-old man injured his right foot while working with heavy construction equipment. The patient was seen immediately after the injury in the emergency room following his severe forefoot injury.

Clinically, there was an open fracture involving the second, third, fourth, and fifth metatarsals of the left foot. There was considerable soft tissue damage with contamination. Additionally, there was neurovascular compromise to the forefoot.

Radiographically, there were open, displaced fractures of the second, third, fourth, and fifth metatarsal shafts. Obvious disruption of the lesser transverse metatarsal arch was noted (Fig. 20-8A and B).

Criteria for open reduction and internal fixation included open fracture, neurovascular compromise, and severely displaced fractures with total disruption of the metatarsal parabola. Therefore, the goals of surgical treatment were debridement and cleaning of the wound, restoration of neurovascular status, and reduction and immobilization of the fractures in a normal weight-bearing position. These goals were met, and neutralization plates were used for fixation (Fig. 20-8C and D).

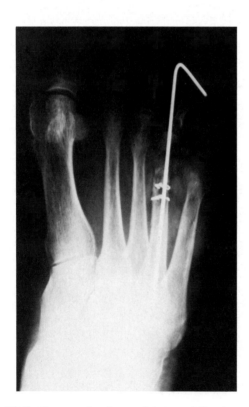

Fig. 20-7. Open reduction and internal fixation of an oblique fracture of the fourth metatarsal shaft utilizing both cerclage wire and intramedullary Kirschner wire.

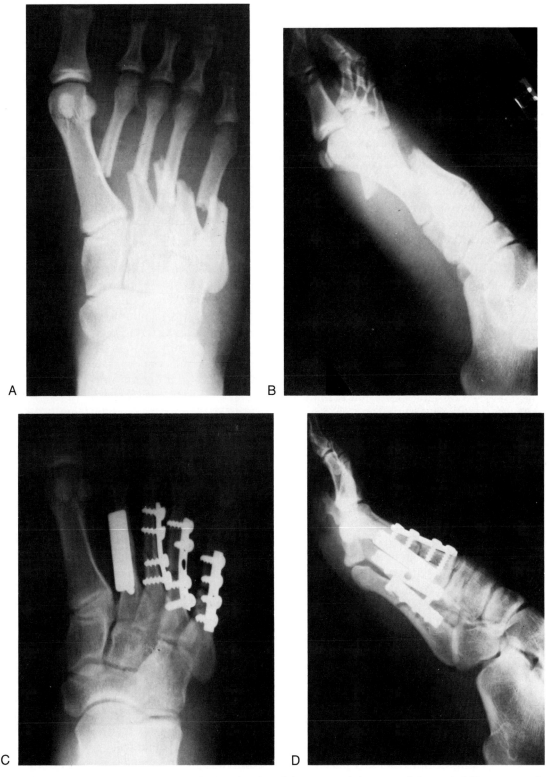

Fig. 20-8. (A) Anteroposterior view of open displaced fractures of the second through fifth metatarsals. (B) Lateral view of the same injury. (C) Anteroposterior view and (D) lateral view after open reduction and internal fixation utilizing neutralization plates for fixation.

Metatarsal Base Fractures

Fractures of the metatarsal base are usually nondisplaced transverse fractures that often occur approximately 1 cm distal to the articular surface. When evaluating these fractures, emphasis should be placed on the assessment of Lisfranc's joint integrity and intra-articular continuity. Extensive ligamentous attachment confers stability to these fracture fragments. Thus, if the fracture is extra-articular and does not involve disruption of Lisfranc's ligament or the tarsometatarsal joint, conservative treatment will often yield a good result. Cast immobilization with a well-molded below-the-knee cast until the appearance of radiographic evidence of healing is appropriate.

Displaced internal metatarsal fractures are included in Chapter 17 on dislocations (Fig. 20-6). Occasionally, a significantly displaced metatarsal base fracture will occur without articular dislocation. This fracture should be treated in the same manner as a Lisfranc's fracture with accurate reduction by either external or internal immobilization depending on postreduction stability. If more than one internal metatarsal is fractured and unstable, the most unstable displaced fracture should be reduced. Spontaneous reduction of the other fractures will normally occur. This phenomenon has been described as the vassal effect.[30]

Percutaneous Kirschner wire fixation and plaster immobilization may be necessary to manage unstable metatarsal base fractures. Rarely is open reduction with extra-articular internal fixation necessary for closed internal metatarsal base fractures not involving Lisfranc's joint.

Open fracture management and metatarsal fractures in children are addressed in detail in Chapters 3 and 25, respectively.

COMPLICATIONS

Numerous complications to metatarsal fracture healing and treatment have been reported, and nearly all are complications observed in general fracture healing. These complications are only briefly discussed here.

Delayed unions and nonunions are uncommon complications observed in internal metatarsal fractures. However, this complication has often been observed in Jones-type fractures of the fifth metatarsal shaft. The internal metatarsals are located within the depth of the foot, with extensive soft tissue coverage providing an excellent environment for bone healing. Delayed union or slow healing is a multifactorial phenomenon and is identified when clinical and radiographic evidence of healing goes beyond what is statistically average for a particular bone.[10] Nonunion is diagnosed when sufficient time has elapsed for expected union without evidence of healing or, conversely, with radiographic or clinical evidence of nonunion. Several elapsed time period estimates are found in the literature for both delayed union and nonunion. We agree with the rule of thumb reported by Oloff and Jacobs,[46] that failure to demonstrate any progressive radiographic changes over a 3-month period is highly suggestive of a nonunion.

Disability from delayed union or nonunion of a metatarsal fracture may be significant. The delayed union or nonunion should be accurately diagnosed and aggressively treated to avoid the possibility of disability. Nonunion requires surgical treatment for resolution. Debridement of necrotic soft tissue and bone, rigid internal fixation, and bone grafting are some of the techniques used in these situations. Delayed union may respond to improved and prolonged external cast immobilization, but the potential for cast disease and its consequences must also be recognized. Bioelectrical stimulation has been utilized to stimulate osteogenesis and bone union in delayed union and nonunion.[47]

Malunion is a more common but less serious complication of internal metatarsal fractures. Malunion in any cardinal body plane may lead to debilitating sequelae, however. Sagittal plane malunion is of highest concern regarding the internal metatarsals. Residual plantar displacement in metatarsal neck fractures will lead to a rigid plantar-flexed metatarsal. This will result in painful debilitating plantar lesions under the metatarsal phalangeal joint as described in the pathomechanics section of this chapter. Figure 20-9 shows radiographic evidence of a malunion re-

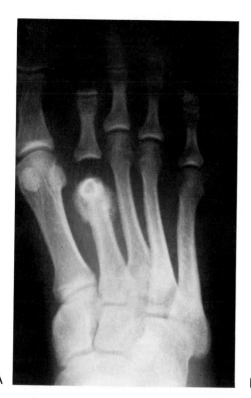
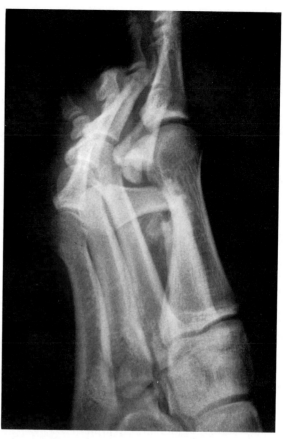

A   B

Fig. 20-9. (**A**) Gun-barrel appearance and large fracture callus at the site of a second metatarsal neck malunion. (**B**) Lateral view showing the verticle orientation of the second metatarsal head with complete metatarsophalangeal joint dislocation. (Courtesy of Jeffrey M. Karlin, D.P.M.)

sulting from inadequate treatment of a fourth metatarsal neck fracture. This unfortunate patient sought surgical correction of his prominent plantar-flexed metatarsal head. Figure 20-10 shows the results of open reduction, bone grafting, and external fixation with an outrigger device to establish a more normal weight-bearing surface.

Post-traumatic degenerative joint disease occurs as a late complication of intra-articular fracture of joint surfaces with residual incongruity. This complication is especially common in the lower extremity weight-bearing joints.[12] Although rare, intra-articular fractures of the lesser metatarsals do occur. Harrison states that a common sequela of this type of fracture is Freiberg's infraction or aseptic necrosis of the metatarsal

head.[48] Gauthier and Elbaz agree that Freiberg's infraction is osteonecrosis of a lesser metatarsal head secondary to osteochondral fracture.[49] They further describe five stages of anatomic evolution of Freiberg's lesions; "stage 0: subchondral bone march fracture, x-ray normal; stage 1: osteonecrosis without deformation; stage 2: deformation of the metatarsal head by crushing of osteonecrosis; stage 3: gradual cartilaginous tearing; stage 4: arthrosis" (Fig. 20-11). They describe successful treatment by deflexion osteotomy to realign viable cartilage to necrosed areas in stage 2 and 3 lesions. Total joint arthroplasty with or without prosthesis has been useful for this lesion.

Mann reveals two less common complications of treatment of metatarsal fractures.[33] The first is a painful pressure lesion induced by shoe irrita-

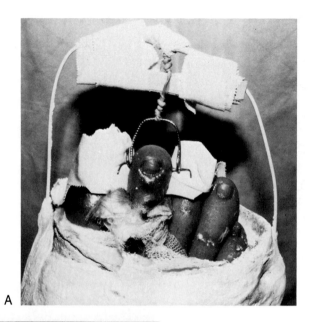

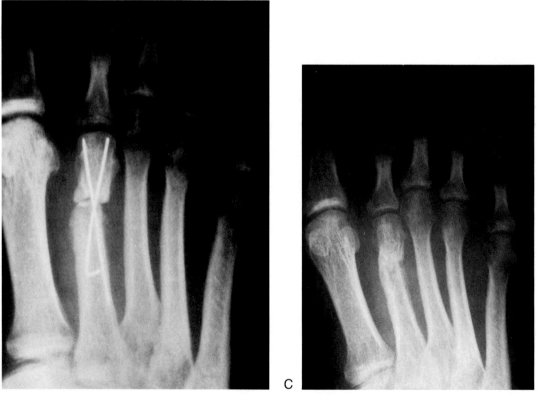

Fig. 20-10. (**A**) Outrigger used to maintain second metatarsal length after bone grafting and internal fixation of malunion. (**B**) Realignment, bone grafting, and crossed Kirschner wire fixation utilized for malunion repair. (**C**) Bone graft incorporation and complete union. (Courtesy of Jeffrey M. Karlin, D.P.M.)

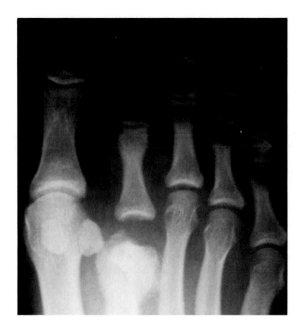

Fig. 20-11. Freiberg's infraction, stage 4. Arthrosis, a late complication of intra-articular metatarsal head fracture.

tion on an overabundant healing bone callus. The slow resorption of bone callus during the consolidation phase of bone healing usually will decrease excess external callus and relieve the localized symptoms. If symptoms persist, surgical excision of excess callus may be clinically indicated.

Although transverse plane malunion is thought to be a benign outcome of internal metatarsal fractures, painful sequelae do occur. Mann cites two painful lesions that are complications secondary to medial-to-lateral deviation of the metatarsal head.[33] Formation of an interdigital neuroma and head impingement against an adjacent metatarsal may occur, both resulting in painful symptoms.

Almost any forefoot trauma is capable of resulting in compartment syndrome of the foot[16,17] as well as reflex sympathetic dystrophy.[12] Although both are considered rare in forefoot trauma, their course can be catastrophic. However, early diagnosis and appropriate treatment result in full recovery.

The other general complications of fracture treatment are discussed in Chapter 32. All surgeons are aware that open fracture care has its potential complications. Surgical management can lead to wound dehiscence, superficial infection, osteomyelitis, anaesthesia reactions, deep venous thrombosis, hematoma, skin slough, nerve trauma, and pulmonary embolus. Similarly, conservative management has potential complications. Closed fracture treatment with cast immobilization can lead to pressure sores, cast disease, loss of reduction, common peroneal nerve damage, and hidden infection, among others.

REFERENCES

1. Spector F, Karlin J, Scurran B et al: Lesser metatarsal fractures: incidence management and review. J Am Podiatry Assoc 74:259, 1984
2. Draves D: Anatomy of the Lower Extremity. Williams & Wilkins, Baltimore, 1986
3. Sarrafian S: Anatomy of the Foot and Ankle: Descriptive, Topographic, Functional. JB Lippincott, Philadelphia, 1983
4. Williams P, Warwick R: Gray's Anatomy. 36th Ed. WB Saunders, Philadelphia, 1980
5. Bakers J, Frankel V, Burstein A: Proceedings. J Bone Joint Surg 54A:1345, 1972
6. Jaworek TE: The intrinsic vascular supply to the first and lesser metatarsals: surgical considerations. Sixth Annual Northlake Surgical Seminar, Chicago, 1976
7. DePalma A: The Management of Fractures and Dislocations. 2nd Ed. Vol. 2. p. 2058. WB Saunders, Philadelphia, 1970
8. Giannestras N: Foot Disorders: Medical and Surgical Management. 2nd Ed. Lea & Febiger, Philadelphia, 1973
9. Harkess J: Principles of Fractures and Dislocations. p. 1. In Rockwood C, Green D (eds): Fractures. Vol. 1. JB Lippincott, Philadelphia, 1975
10. Heppenstall R (ed): Fracture Treatment and Healing. WB Saunders, Philadelphia, 1980
11. Maxwell JR: Open or closed treatment of metatarsal fractures. J Am Podiatry Assoc 2:100, 1983
12. Salter RB: Disorders and Injuries of the Musculoskeletal System. WB Saunders, Philadelphia, 1970
13. Gudas CJ: Traumatic fractures and dislocations of the foot and ankle. p. 100. Seventh Annual Northlake Seminar, Chicago, 1977

14. Edwards C: Fractured os calcis and lumbar vertebrae. Trauma Rounds 103:177, 1970

15. Wilson D: Functional capacity following fractures of the os calcis. Can Med Assoc J 95:908, 1966

16. Bonatti P, Bell G: Compartment syndrome of the foot. J Bone Joint Surg 68A:9, 1986

17. Whitesides T: Compartment syndromes. p. 1201. In Jahss M (ed): Disorders of the Foot. WB Saunders, Philadelphia, 1982

18. Pritsch M, Heim M, Horoszowski H et al: The significance of axial foot projection in the diagnosis of metatarsal pathology. Arch Orthop Trauma Surg 98:139, 1981

19. Altman M: Stress fractures: revisited. JRSH 4:139, 1985

20. Greaney R et al: Distribution and natural history of stress fractures in U.S. Marine recruits. Radiology 146:339, 1983

21. Markey K: Stress fractures. Clin Podiatr Med Surg 4:969, 1987

22. Milgrom C: Stress fractures in military recruits. J Bone Joint Surg 67B:732, 1985

23. Orava S: Stress fractures. Br J Sports Med 14:40, 1980

24. Phillips G, Matthews P: Consecutive stress fractures in a metatarsal. J Foot Surg 3:186, 1982

25. Root M, Orion W, Weed J: Normal and Abnormal Functions of the Foot. Clinical Biomechanics. Vol. 2. 1st Ed. Clinical Biomechanics, Los Angeles, 1977

26. Dorfman G: Determinations of treatment in fractures of the fifth metatarsal. J Foot Surg 1:16, 1978

27. Maxwell J: Open or closed treatment of metatarsal fractures. J Am Podiatry Assoc 2:100, 1983

28. Figura M: Metatarsal fractures. Clin Podiatry 2:247, 1985

29. Anderson L: Fractures. p. 477. In Edmonson A, Crenshaw A (eds): Campbell's Operative Orthopedics. 5th Ed. Vol. 1. CV Mosby, St. Louis, 1963

30. Heim U, Pfeiffer KM: Small Fragment Set Manual. 1st and 2nd Ed. Springer-Verlag, New York, 1974

31. Muller M, Allgower M, Schneider R, Willenegger H: Manual of Internal Fixation. 2nd Ed. Springer-Verlag, New York, 1979

32. Rockwood C, Green D (eds): Fractures. Vol. 1. JB Lippincott, Philadelphia, 1975

33. Mann R: Complications of treatment of fractures and dislocations of the foot. p. 604. In Epps C (ed): Complications of Orthopedic Surgery. JB Lippincott, Philadelphia, 1978

34. Raggi R: Balanced regional anesthesia for hand surgery. Orthop Clin North Am 17:473, 1986

35. Dinley R, Michelinski E: Local anaesthesia in the reduction of Colles' fracture. Injury 4:435, 1973

36. Sorbie C, Chacha P: Regional anaesthesia by the intravenous route. Br Med J 1:957, 1965

37. Cavaliere R, Bergman R: Anesthesia. p. 315. In McGlamry ED (ed): Fundamentals of Foot Surgery. Williams & Wilkins, Baltimore, 1987

38. Inman VT: DuVries' Surgery of the Foot. 3rd Ed. CV Mosby, St. Louis, 1973

39. Mann R (ed): Surgery of the Foot. 5th Ed. CV Mosby, St. Louis, 1986

40. Wu KK: Surgery of the Foot. Lea & Febiger, Philadelphia, 1986

41. Smith G, Green A: Cerclage wiring of metatarsal fractures: a case report. J Am Podiatry Assoc 1:25, 1983

42. Subotnick SI: Open reduction of spiral fracture of the second metatarsal: a case report. J Foot Surg 3:110, 1977

43. Arango G: Proximal diaphyseal fractures of the fifth metatarsal (Jones fracture). Two cases treated by cross pinning with review of 106 cases. Foot Ankle 3:293, 1983

44. Levy I: Stress fractures of the first metatarsal. Am J Roentgenol 130:679, 1978

45. Walter J, Pressman M: External fixation in the treatment of metatarsal nonunion. J Am Podiatry Assoc 6:197, 1981

46. Oloff L, Jacobs A: Fracture nonunion. Clin Podiatry 2:379, 1985

47. Friedenberg Z, Andrews E, Smolenski B et al: Bone reaction to varying amounts of direct current. Surg Gynecol Obstet 131:894, 1970

48. Harrison M: Fractures of the metatarsal head. Can J Surg 11:511, 1968

49. Gauthier G, Elbaz R: Freiberg's infraction: a subchondral bone fatigue fracture. Clin Orthop 142:93, 1979

21

Fractures of the Fifth Metatarsal

William W. Kirchwehm, D.P.M.

This chapter deals with trauma to the fifth metatarsal. Unique fractures of the fifth metatarsal include the proximal diaphyseal fracture or the Jones fracture as well as the more common avulsion-type fractures involving the tuberosity of the fifth metatarsal.

In addition, this chapter describes the anatomy of the fifth metatarsal, classifies fractures of the fifth metatarsal, and provides a rationale for diagnosis and treatment.

ANATOMY

A review of the anatomy is essential to best understand osseous injuries to the fifth metatarsal. The proximal portion of the fifth metatarsal has a tuberosity referred to as the styloid process on the lateral side of its base. This base articulates proximally with the cuboid and medially with the fourth metatarsal. The tuberosity can be seen grossly as well as palpated midway on the lateral border of the foot. The tendon of the peroneus tertius attaches to the medial portion of the dorsal surface and the medial border of the fifth metatarsal shaft. The peroneus brevis tendon attaches to the dorsal surface of the tuberosity. The lateral portion of the plantar aponeurosis attaches to the fifth metatarsal tuberosity as well as the lateral process of the calcaneal tuberosity. The plantar surface of the metatarsal base is grooved by the tendon of the abductor digiti minimi. The flexor digitorum brevis originates from the plantar surface of the fifth metatarsal base. The me-

dial border of the shaft serves as the origin of the lateral head of the fourth dorsal and the third plantar interosseous muscles.[1,2] Distally, the head of the fifth metatarsal articulates with the base of the proximal phalanx of the fifth toe.

The intrinsic vascular supply of the fifth metatarsal has been investigated by Jaworek using cadaveric specimens.[3] The principal nutrient artery of the fifth metatarsal enters the lateral diaphyseal cortex. Ascending and descending subcortical branches reach the end of the metatarsal. The terminal branches form a plexus of small vessels that anastomose with the metaphyseal nutrient arteries. The metaphyseal and epiphyseal portions of the metatarsal are well vascularized. The vascular supply to the diaphyseal cortical bone is less abundant. This is one factor that might explain the high incidence of delayed union and nonunion in proximal diaphyseal fractures of the fifth metatarsal.

The sural nerve must be considered in injuries about the fifth metatarsal. This nerve runs anteriorly and inferiorly to the lateral malleolus and continues along the lateral aspect of the foot to the fifth digit.

BIOMECHANICS OF THE FIFTH RAY

Root et al. describe the fifth ray as consisting of the fifth metatarsal only.[4] They further describe the fifth metatarsal as moving in the directions of supination and pronation about a triplane axis of motion. The axis of motion lies at an angle of approximately 20 degrees from the transverse plane and 35 degrees from the sagittal plane. They further state that the amounts of inversion-eversion and plantar flexion-dorsiflexion are great and that the amount of adduction-abduction is small as the fifth metatarsal is supinated and pronated. These three components of motion are great enough to be clinically significant.

The function of the fifth ray during locomotion is not fully understood.[4] The osseous mechanisms that move the fifth ray about its independent axis of motion during locomotion have not been adequately studied. In addition, the function of the muscles that are responsible for its stability while bearing weight are not clearly known.

Clinically, the normal fifth ray exhibits approximately equal ranges of plantar flexion and dorsiflexion as it supinates and pronates. In other words, the fifth metatarsal should normally move the same distance below and above the transverse plane position of the three central metatarsal heads when a weight-bearing load is applied.

Congenital anomalies of fifth ray motion include an abnormal direction of motion in the presence of a full range of motion.[4] These are one-plane sagittal deformities, and the range of motion is usually symmetrical in the two feet.

Acquired fifth ray deformities include triplane deformities that are characterized by a measurable decrease in or absent range of motion. The range of fifth ray motion is usually asymmetrical in the two feet.

The required range of fifth ray motion necessary for locomotion is unknown.

MECHANISM OF INJURY

Kavanaugh et al. reviewed 22 patients with 23 fractures involving the proximal part of the diaphysis of the fifth metatarsal (Fig. 21-1).[5] Each patient described the ankle and foot position, which was elevation of the heel, "breaking" at the metatarsophalangeal joints, and maximum loading over the lateral aspect of the foot. In this type of fracture, at no time was the foot in the

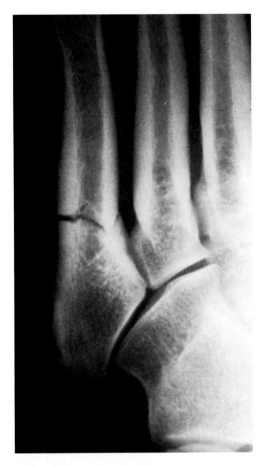

Fig. 21-1. Proximal diaphyseal fifth metatarsal "Jones" fractures induced by vertical or mediolateral forces without inversion of the foot.

inverted position. Eleven of these patients underwent high-speed cinematography and force-platform analysis to reproduce the exact foot position at the time of injury. The results indicated that in the Jones-type fracture, a vertical force or a mediolateral force, or a combination of the two, acts on the base of the fifth metatarsal in conjunction with a posterior ground (braking) force, bringing the patient up on the metatarsal heads and concentrating the vertical and mediolateral forces on the lateral metatarsal. Body positions of these patients fell into two distinct categories.[5] In five patients, the positions of the body's center of gravity and the position of the foot at the time of injury precluded the capacity of inversion. In the remaining patients, the body's center of gravity was in a position to allow inversion of the foot, but this did not occur. It was concluded that the inability or failure of the foot to go into inversion produces the large vertical and mediolateral ground forces responsible for the Jones-type fracture.

I suggest that if vertical and mediolateral forces are applied more distal, fractures of the distal shaft, neck, and head may also result.

The mechanism of injury for avulsion-type fractures of the tuberosity, aside from a direct blow, is inversion of the foot. Giannestras and Sammarco[6] as well as Joplin[7] describe in some detail the avulsion-type fractures of the tuberosity. The inverted stress applied to the foot causes pull on the peroneus brevis tendon, resulting in fractures of the tuberosity (Fig. 21-2).

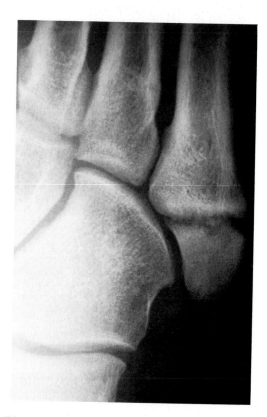

Fig. 21-2. Avulsion fracture of the fifth metatarsal base induced by inversion stress against the pull of the peroneus brevis tendon.

CLASSIFICATION

Salter has devised a working classification that allows accurate description of long bone fracture.[8] An organized system describing such fractures will be beneficial in determining specific treatment regimens. This classification consists of five categories, including the site of fracture, extent of fracture within the bone, configuration of fracture, relative position of fracture fragments, and relationship of fracture to the external environment. In addition, Gudas further added a sixth category specific to metatarsal fractures.[9] For details in regard to the working classification of metatarsal fractures, please refer to Chapter 20.

DIAGNOSIS

The history and physical examination are essential in determining an accurate diagnosis. The history should be taken in such a manner so as to reconstruct the mechanism of injury. Questions pertinent to fractures of the fifth metatarsal may include the following: Did the patient fall with the foot inverted, as in a lateral ankle sprain? Did the patient have a vertical force and mediolateral force applied to the lateral column of the foot without true inversion? The patient may describe a heavy weight dropped on the dorsum of the metatarsal or a forceful blow to the lateral aspect of the foot. The patient may describe falling from a height, and if so, one must inquire as to the foot position upon landing. If the fifth metatarsophalangeal joint has been injured, was this due to lateral displacement of the fifth digit, as noted in the "bedpost fracture," or was the digit hyperextended? The patient may describe an audible popping or cracking sound that occurred at the time of injury.

A detailed inquiry may be beneficial in further assessing the extent of neurovascular and soft tissue damage in such injuries as those occurring from motor vehicle accidents, lawn mower accidents, gunshot wounds, and industrial accidents.

The physical examination at the time of acute injury to the foot must immediately address the neurovascular status. The capillary filling time to the fifth toe is the initial test to assess the vascular status following injuries to the fifth metatarsal. Presence or absence of pedal pulses must be noted. I also confirm the status of the sural nerve by soft touch and pinprick testing. Clinical findings of the fractured metatarsal include edema, ecchymosis, instability, and deformity.

The radiographic examination of the fifth metatarsal fracture should include at least two views, but preferably three standard positions. Comparative radiographs of the opposite foot may also be beneficial. The anteroposterior, medial-oblique, and lateral views are usually sufficient to make an accurate diagnosis. A plantar axial or sesamoidal view may be beneficial in evaluating displaced fractures of the fifth metatarsal head in the sagittal plane. Radionuclide imaging is valuable in assessing the extent of healing in proximal diaphyseal fractures, or in the diagnosis of subtle fractures (e.g., stress fractures).

TREATMENT

The goals of treatment are well summarized by Anderson.[10] Below are noted the three primary considerations when treating any fracture.

1. Obtaining union is the primary objective, as function of the adjacent joints and soft tissue depends on it.
2. Functional results are proportionate to the position of bones after healing. Some variation from the normal anatomy is compatible with satisfactory or even normal function. However, the limit of error is small in fractures that involve joint surfaces.
3. Early mobilization of soft tissues and adjacent joints is paramount to early return of function.

Simple fractures of the metatarsal shaft, neck, and head that are not displaced respond well to 5 to 6 weeks of immobilization. I prefer non-weight bearing for 3 weeks, with a weight-bearing bivalved fiberglass cast for the final 3 weeks. This is done to encourage early mobilization of the soft tissues and adjacent joints. Many clinicians believe 5 to 6 weeks in a short leg walking cast will suffice. Other modalities include immobilization with tape, Unna's paste boot, or a postoperative shoe.

If the fracture involving the metatarsal shaft, neck, or head is displaced, an attempt should be made to manipulate and align the fracture fragments by closed methods. Distal traction applied to the fifth toe may reduce the displaced fracture fragments. I have used surgical tape anchored to the base of the fifth toe to distract it distally with leverage. This is similar to the use of a finger trap apparatus, as described by Giannestras[11] (Fig. 21-3).

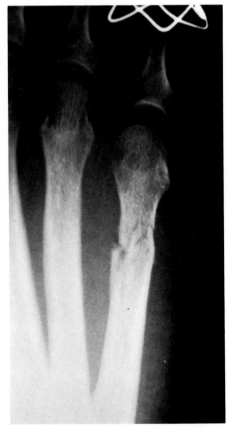

Fig. 21-3. Distal diaphyseal fracture reduced with distal traction using a simulated finger trap apparatus. Counter pressure using elevation (gravity) or small 2.5- to 5-lb weights may be necessary.

Before the indications for open reduction are discussed, contraindications must be noted. Contraindications include fracture fragments of insufficient size, inadequate bone stock, nondisplaced fractures, impacted fractures, and those fractures posing a high risk of infection or in which significant vascular compromise exists. In addition, certain medical conditions may contradict open reduction such as uncontrolled diabetes mellitus, advanced arteriosclerotic occlusive peripheral vascular disease, and extensive osteoporosis. Further, the patient's ambulatory status must be considered in choosing open versus closed reduction. The active and athletic individual is certainly a better candidate for open reduction and internal fixation, as compared with the older, more sedentary individual, for whom one would attempt a more conservative course of management.

Closed Reduction

Restoration of the osseous components to "normal" anatomic alignment should be first attempted by closed reduction. Maxwell outlines the steps for appropriate closed reduction,[12] which include (1) prereduction films to evaluate the type of fracture and degree of displacement; (2) anesthesia, either local or general, to provide adequate muscle relaxation for attempted closed reduction; (3) steady traction and countertraction provided while manipulation is attempted (for a more detailed description of closed reduction techniques, see Ch. 5); (4) postreduction films to confirm acceptable alignment.

SPECIFIC FRACTURES

Fractures of the Fifth Metatarsal Head

The majority of intra-articular fractures of the fifth metatarsal head should be reduced to restore normal function of the joint and minimize the development of degenerative arthritis. If the fragments are quite small, they should be excised if symptomatic. However, small Kirschner wires can be used to fixate larger fragments. The foot should be immobilized for 6 weeks. Depending on the placement of the pins, the patient may be required to remain non-weight bearing until radiographic evidence of healing is noted. Early, gentle, passive range of motion exercise of adjacent joints and soft tissues should be encouraged. A bivalved cast in the fourth week of healing may prove useful toward that end. Impaction fractures, intra-articular fractures, and isolated fifth metatarsal head fracture are relatively uncommon (Fig. 21-4).

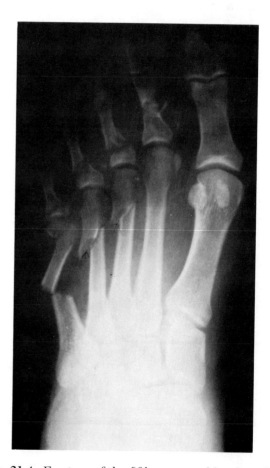

Fig. 21-4. Fracture of the fifth metatarsal head rarely occurs as an isolated phenomenon. Here associated, displaced diaphyseal fractures of the lateral three metatarsals are noted. Reduction is required.

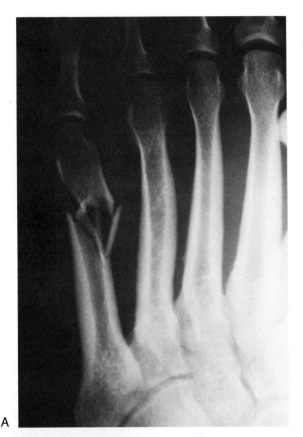

A

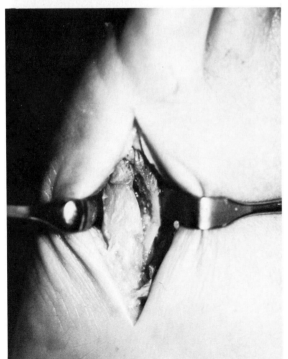

B

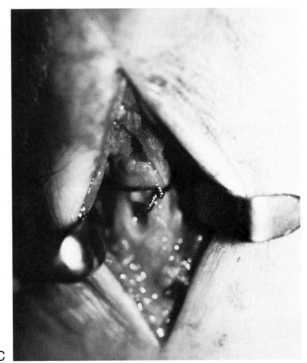

C

Fig. 21-5. (**A**) Distal diaphyseal-metaphyseal fracture which is comminuted and displaced. (**B**) Exposure of the fracture fragments. (**C**) Reduction and fixation with cerclage monofilament wire. (Courtesy of Barry L. Scurran, D.P.M.)

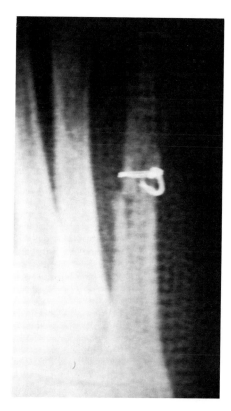

Fig. 21-6. Radiograph showing reduction of the larger segments of a spiral fracture with single cerclage wire fixation.

Fractures of the Metatarsal Neck

Fractures of the distal metaphysis region of the fifth metatarsal are more common than the previously described type of fracture. Fractures in the transverse plane should be reduced only if there is abnormal angulation or displacement. Malaligned fractures in the sagittal plane are particularly critical since alignment directly affects the weight-bearing load on the fifth metatarsal head.

The method most often described in the orthopedic literature for open reduction of this type of fracture is medullary wire fixation.[13–20] This method of fixation is particularly advantageous in the short transverse fracture. Figura has recommended monofilament wire for this type of fracture[20] (Fig. 21-5). A small L- or T-plate with axial compression is another preferred choice in reducing the shorter transverse type of fracture.[18,19]

Oblique or spiral fractures of the metatarsal neck can be reduced by using medullary wire fixation or cerclage wire (Fig. 21-6). I have used cerclage wire with or without medullary wire fixation with much success. If cerclage wire is used alone, two separate sites of fixation may be utilized whenever possible to prevent rotation or displacement (Fig. 21-7). Interfragmentary compression with lag screw fixation and a neutralization plate has been an excellent means of internal fixation. Comminuted fractures may also be reduced by using the small L- or T-plate.[18,19]

Proximal Diaphyseal Fractures (Jones Fracture)

The Jones fracture is a transverse proximal diaphyseal fracture approximately 1.5 to 3.0 cm distal from the tuberosity of the fifth metatarsal

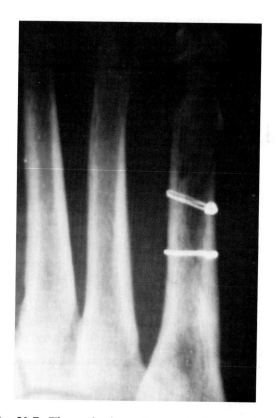

Fig. 21-7. The author's preference is the use of two sites of cerclage wire fixation to prevent rotation or displacement.

(Fig. 21-1). This type of fracture is less commonly seen than the avulsion fracture. The injury is produced by a large vertical or mediolateral ground force with failure of the foot go into inversion.[5] In 1896 at New Brighton, England, Robert Jones himself suffered this type of fracture. The injury occurred while he was dancing around a tent pole at a military garden party. In his original article, published in 1902,[21] he clearly describes the fracture and stresses the role of the constraining ligaments between the fourth and fifth metatarsals and the cuboid.

Jones initially noted that this fracture was an incomplete fracture and was wider on the lateral cortex.[21] Irwin commented that on the day of injury, the fracture often could not be visualized radiographically, but with continued weight bearing the fracture "widened" and became more apparent radiographically.[22] The first direct reference to this type of fracture as a stress-related injury was made by Devas.[23] Kavanaugh and co-workers, in their study, also thought that this was more a stress fracture since callus formation was noted on the lateral cortical margin.[5] Kavanaugh further described this type of lesion as being comparable to stress fractures seen in the superior femoral neck, femoral shaft, and tibial shaft.[5] All of these fractures involve only one cortex, can slowly transverse the bone, and are typically difficult to heal.

A review of the literature documents the increased incidence of nonunion or delayed union involving this type of fracture. Wharton[24] and Young[25] in 1908 and Christopher[26] in 1923 all described fractures of the proximal portion of the fifth metatarsal. All cases were treated with partial weight-bearing immobilization, and the results of the studies were unknown. Carp, in 1927, reviewed 20 cases of fifth metatarsal base fractures in adults, with delayed union occurring in five patients.[27] Poor vascular supply was also discussed as the cause of this delay in healing. Key and Conwell, in 1934, also described the increased frequency of nonunion of fifth metatarsal fractures and recommended excision of the loose fragment if symptoms persisted.[28] In 1937, Morrison described the possible necessity of bone grafting to repair a fracture of the proximal end of the fifth metatarsal.[29] Bohler, in 1958, described a

delayed union of a Jones fracture, stating that this was the natural course following such an injury.[30] Stuart, in 1960, stated that during World War II members of his military unit required bone grafting to secure union of some fractures involving the fifth metatarsal.[31]

In more recent literature, Dameron describes 20 acute fractures all treated with partial weight-bearing immobilization.[32] Fifteen healed uneventfully, but five patients developed nonunions. All five patients were treated with bone grafting and went on to heal uneventfully. Kavanaugh et al. presented 22 patients with 23 fractures of the proximal diaphysis of the fifth metatarsal.[5] Of 18 patients treated conservatively, delayed union occurred in 12 patients or 66.7 percent. In their series, four athletes with acute fractures were treated with primary open reduction utilizing intramedullary screw fixation. All four patients healed uneventfully and returned to sports in 2 months. Further, their study describes nine patients with delayed unions who also had open intramedullary screw fixation. All nine healed both clinically and radiographically. Zelko and colleagues described a series of proximal diaphyseal fractures in athletes.[33] They presented 21 patients, of whom 19 were treated with partial weight-bearing immobilization. The remaining two patients were treated by primary bone grafting. In this series, three patients progressed to union, seven demonstrated symptoms of symptomatic delayed union, and eight had asymptomatic delayed union. Of the two cases involving primary bone grafting, both progressed to union. Torg has presented two significant papers on fractures of the base of the fifth metatarsal distal to the tuberosity.[34,35] His initial paper, in 1980, described classification and guidelines for nonsurgical and surgical management.[34] In acute fractures, Torg's methods resulted in 100 percent clinical and radiographic union utilizing casting and non-weight bearing as compared with 48 percent achieving clinical and radiographic union with partial weight-bearing immobilization. He further describes the dynamic muscles attaching to the fifth metatarsal proximal diaphysis that predisposed this area to motion. In 1983, Arangio described two cases of successful percutaneous cross pinning of one acute and one delayed union of Jones fracture.[36] Torg et al. describe 46 fractures presented between 1973 and 1982.[35] In this study, of the 25 acute fractures treated with non-weight-bearing immobilization, 14 healed in a mean of 7 weeks. Of the other 10 fractures treated by various weight-bearing methods, only four progressed to union. Of the 12 patients with delayed union, 10 were treated by immobilization in a plaster cast with weight bearing. Of these 10, 7 healed in a mean time of 15.1 months and 3 eventually required bone grafting for nonunion. Nine nonunions in this series were treated by medullary curettage and bone grafting, with eight healing uneventfully in approximately 3 months. Of the 20 fractures treated surgically with autogenous corticocancellous graft, 19 progressed to complete healing and 1 remained an asymptomatic nonunion. Torg and associates concluded that the treatment of choice for acute fractures would be immobilization of the limb with a non-weight-bearing cast.[35] Further, fractures with delayed union or nonunion, particularly in active or athletic individuals, should benefit from medullary curettage and bone grafting.

The decision to treat these fractures by open reduction seems to depend significantly on the activity level of the patient. A very active and athletic individual may be a more appropriate candidate for open reduction than a more sedentary individual, whose treatment would be conservative. If conservative measures are attempted initially, immobilization techniques with partial weight-bearing are not adequate. The patient must be treated with a non-weight-bearing cast for approximately 6 to 8 weeks. If open reduction is performed, there are several alternatives that have proved successful. These include percutaneous cross pinning,[35] medullary curettage and bone grafting,[29,32,33,35] and intramedullary screw fixation.[5]

Fractures Involving the Base of the Fifth Metatarsal (Tuberosity)

The *Small Fragment Set Manual*[18] describes two ways to injure the tuberosity of the fifth metatarsal. The first is an avulsion fracture that is produced by the sudden pull of the peroneus brevis muscle that inserts into the base of the metatarsal. This occurs in supination trauma and results in a small displaced fragment. This type of avulsion is quite common with lateral ankle sprain injuries (Fig. 21-8). The second fracture is produced by excessive weight bearing on the lateral aspect of the foot, which is supinated. Further, fracture may be caused by a direct blow. In these incidences, the fracture is larger and may be comminuted (Fig. 21-9).

The mechanism of injury to the tuberosity is primarily that of inversion of the foot. Further, it was the opinion of the Swiss Association for the Study of Internal Fixation that the treatment of choice should be either a small tension-band wire or screw fixation, depending on the size of the fragment.[18,19] It was their opinion that cast immobilization resulted in a high incidence of pseudoarthrosis.

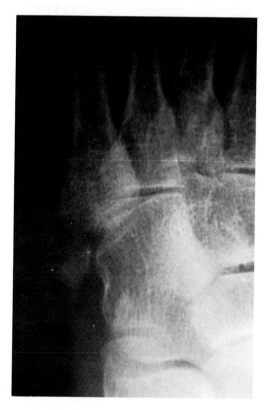

Fig. 21-8. Small avulsion fracture produced by a sudden pull of the peroneus brevis tendon against a supinated foot.

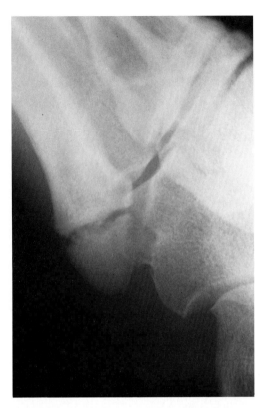

Fig. 21-9. Large avulsion fracture produced by an excessive loading force applied directly to the supinated foot.

Giannestras and Sammarco[6] and Joplin[7] each described in some detail the avulsion fracture of the tuberosity. The most common description in the orthopedic literature is "a fracture caused by inversion of the foot resulting in pulling of the peroneus brevis where it inserts into the base of the fifth metatarsal." Further, the treatment for the majority of these fractures was with a weight-bearing below-the-knee cast for approximately 6 weeks. In cases of severe avulsion in which closed reduction is unsuccessful, open reduction may be required.[6,7,11,13,17,28,29]

Criteria for open reduction include significant displacement or rotation of the fracture fragments or fragment. If the bone is completely avulsed, closed reduction is extremely difficult owing to the pull of the peroneus brevis tendon.

If smaller fragments are present, the use of multiple small, crossed Kirschner wires or tension-band wiring is preferred (Fig. 21-10). If the fragment is larger and avulsed, intramedullary screw fixation may be used (Fig. 21-11).

Multiple Fractures

If the fourth and fifth metatarsals are simultaneously fractured, a mechanical interdependence between the two fractures is noted (Fig. 21-12). The dominant fracture is that of the fifth metatarsal, and if this is reduced initially, the fourth metatarsal or vassal fracture will reduce spontaneously.[18,19] If the fifth metatarsal is reduced by one of multiple appropriate techniques (e.g., a lag screw with L-plate), then the fourth metatarsal will spontaneously reduce. Once passively reduced, the fourth metatarsal fracture may be either left alone or fixed with an axial Kirschner wire or single screw.

Comminuted Fractures

In comminuted fractures of the fifth metatarsal in which displacement is noted, open reduction and internal fixation with a buttress-type plate is preferred.[18,19] If the comminuted fractures are severe and involve bone defects, a cancellous or corticocancellous bone grafting is obligatory.

Open Fractures

It is critical to assess initially the neurovascular status of the fifth toe, as previously discussed. In addition, careful assessment of the soft tissue injury and damage as well as contamination of the wound must be made. The use of intermedullary Kirschner wire or an external fixator are the preferred methods of reduction for unstable fractures. With these methods, a significant decrease in the rate of infection has been reported.[18,19]

Additional information on fractures of the fifth metatarsal may be found in Chapters 25 and 28.

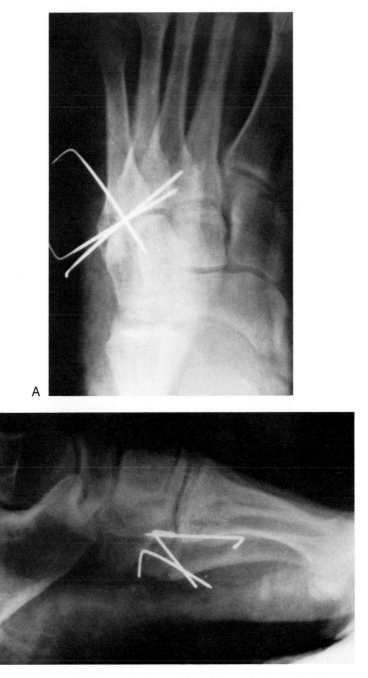

Fig. 21-10. (A) Anteroposterior and (B) lateral radiographs of the reduction of a displaced fifth metatarsal base avulsion fracture. Anatomic reduction has been stabilized using triplane Kirschner wires. Tension banding may also be utilized.

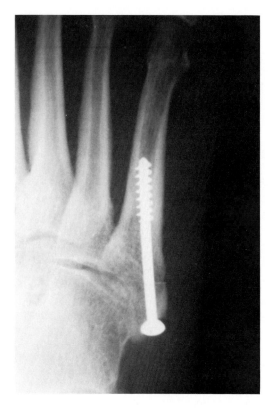

Fig. 21-11. Intramedullary screw fixation of a large fifth metatarsal base tuberosity fracture.

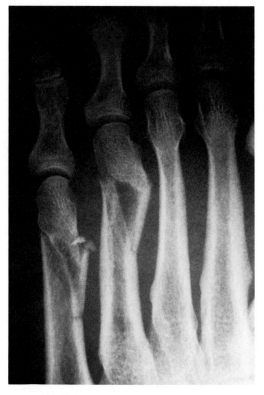

Fig. 21-12. Simultaneous distal diaphyseal fractures of the fourth and fifth metatarsals. Since these fractures are mechanically interdependent, reduction of the fifth metatarsal will generally allow spontaneous reduction of the "vassal" fourth metatarsal fracture.

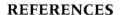

REFERENCES

1. Draves D: Anatomy of the Lower Extremity. Williams & Wilkins, Baltimore, 1986
2. Williams P, Warwick R: Gray's Anatomy. 36th Ed WB Saunders, Philadelphia, 1980
3. Jaworek T: The Intrinsic Vascular Supply to the First and Lesser Metatarsals; Surgical Considerations. Sixth Annual Northlake Surgical Seminar, Chicago, 1976
4. Root M, Orion W, Weed J: Normal and abnormal functions of the foot. p. 53. In Clinical Biomechanics. Vol. 2. 1st Ed. Clinical Biomechanics Corp., Los Angeles, 1977
5. Kavanaugh J, Brower T, Mann R: The Jones fracture revisited. J Bone Joint Surg 60A:6, 1978
6. Giannestras N, Sammarco G: Fractures and dislocations in the foot. p. 1482. In Rockwood C, Green D (eds): Fractures. Vol. 2. JB Lippincott, Philadelphia, 1975
7. Joplin R: Injuries of the foot. p. 851. In Cave E, Burke J, Boyd R (eds): Trauma Management. Year Book Medical Publishers, Chicago, 1974
8. Salter R: Disorders and Injuries of the Musculoskeletal System. WB Saunders, Philadelphia, 1970
9. Gudas C: Traumatic Fractures and Dislocations of the Foot and Ankle. Seventh Annual Northlake Surgical Seminar, Chicago, 1977
10. Anderson L: Fractures. p. 477. In Edmonson A, Crenshaw A (eds): Campbell's Operative Orthopedics. 5th Ed. Vol. 1. CV Mosby, St. Louis, 1963
11. Giannestras N: Foot Disorders: Medical and Surgical Management. 2nd Ed. Lea & Febiger, Philadelphia, 1973
12. Maxwell J: Open or closed treatment of metatarsal fractures. J Am Podiatry Assoc 2:100, 1983

13. Mann R (ed): Surgery of the Foot. 5th Ed. CV Mosby, St. Louis, 1986
14. Heppenstall R (ed): Fracture Treatment and Healing. WB Saunders, Philadelphia, 1980
15. DiPalma A: The Management of Fractures and Dislocations. 2nd Ed. Vol 2. WB Saunders, Philadelphia, 1970
16. Sisk T: Fractures of the lower extremity. p. 539. In Edmonson A, Crenshaw A (eds): Campbell's Operative Orthopedics. 6th Ed. Vol. 1. CV Mosby, St. Louis, 1980
17. Garcia A, Parkes J: Fractures of the foot. p. 517. In Giannestras N (ed): Foot Disorders: Medical and Surgical Management. 2nd Ed. Lea & Febiger, Philadelphia, 1973
18. Heim U, Pfeiffer K: Small Fragment Set Manual. 1st and 2nd Ed. Springer-Verlag, New York, 1974
19. Muller M, Allgower M, Schneider R, Willenegger H: Manuel of Internal Fixation. 2nd Ed. Springer-Verlag, New York, 1979
20. Figura M: Metatarsal fractures. Clin Podiatry 2:247, 1985
21. Jones R: Fracture of the base of the fifth metatarsal bone by indirect violence. Ann Surg 35:697, 1902
22. Irwin C: Fractures of the metatarsals. Proc Soc Med 31:789, 1938
23. Devas M: Stress Fractures, pp. 1, 163, and 230. Churchill Livingstone, Edinburgh, 1975
24. Wharton H: Fractures of the proximal end of the fifth metatarsal bone. Ann Surg 47:824, 1908
25. Young J: Fractures of the proximal end of the fifth metatarsal. Ann Surg 47:824, 1908
26. Christopher F: Fractures of the fifth metatarsal. Surg Gynecol Obstet 37:190, 1923
27. Carp L: Fractures of the fifth metatarsal bone, with special reference to delayed union. Ann Surg 86:308, 1927
28. Key J, Conwell H: The Management of Fractures, Dislocations and Sprains. p. 1116. CV Mosby, St. Louis, 1934
29. Morrison G: Fractures of the bones of the feet. Am J Surg 38:721, 1937
30. Bohler L: The Treatment of Fractures. English Ed. 5th Ed. Vol. 3. p. 2147. Grune & Stratton, Orlando, FL, 1958
31. Stewart I: Jone's fracture: fracture of the base of fifth metatarsal. Clin Orthop 16:190, 1960
32. Dameron T: Fractures and anatomical variations of the proximal portion of the fifth metatarsal. J Bone Joint Surg 57A:788, 1975
33. Zelko R, Torg J, Ruchun A: Proximal diaphyseal fractures of the fifth metatarsal. Treatment of the fractures and their complications in athletes. Am J Sports Med 7:95, 1979
34. Torg J: Fracture of the Base of the Fifth Metatarsal Distal to the Tuberosity Classification and Guidelines for Non-Surgical and Surgical Management. Presented at the American Academy of Orthopedic Surgeons' Meeting, Feb. 6, Atlanta, GA, 1980
35. Torg J, Baldini F, Zelko et al: Fractures of the base of the fifth metatarsal distal to the tuberosity. J Bone Joint Surg 66A:2, 1984
36. Arangio G: Proximal diaphyseal fractures of the fifth metatarsal (Jones' fracture). Two cases treated by cross-pinning with review of 106 cases. Foot Ankle 3:293, 1983

22

Midfoot Fractures

Flair Goldman, D.P.M.

In the past, fractures of the midfoot, which include the navicular, cuneiform, and cuboid bones (Fig. 22-1), were considered rare and generally insignificant. Reviewing older literature, one finds a reported frequency of 2.6 percent of all fractures involving the tarsus in general, with only 0.5 percent of all fractures involving the midfoot.[1] A total of 0.6 percent of all tarsal injuries were reported as compound. As recently as 1969, in a review of 260 stress fractures, there were no midfoot fractures identified.[2] The reasons for underdiagnosis, missed diagnosis, or delay in diagnosis of midfoot fractures vary and are numerous. Generally speaking, the identification of midfoot fractures requires a high index of suspicion on the part of the clinician. Often midfoot fractures are complicated by other fractures of the foot and other serious body trauma, sometimes associated with loss of consciousness. In such cases, more subtle midfoot fractures may be overlooked initially and become discovered only later as patients begin ambulating. Many midfoot fractures are missed if they are not considered in the differential diagnosis of midfoot pain. This is especially true for stress fractures in athletes and nonathletes and in osteochondral fractures of the midfoot, which have only recently been described.[3] Finally, radiographs of the midfoot may be difficult to evaluate because of multiple overlapping irregular bones giving rise to double densities and because of the possibility of misinterpreting accessory ossicles, ligamentous and vascular calcifications, and epiphyseal variations as chip or avulsion fractures (Fig. 22-2).

Some simple measures that can help diagnose midfoot fractures include comparison views of the opposite foot, magnification views, spot views, and use of high-resolution radiographic film. Recently, many investigators have suggested that with a high index of suspicion, thorough history, and careful physical examination and the use of newer diagnostic studies including bone scans, tomograms and CT and MRI scans, many previously missed midfoot fractures will be recognized.[4–10] The general approach to the use of such studies is to first obtain a technetium 99 bone scan to identify and localize the bony source and then obtain further information with tomograms or CT scans directed to that area.[11]

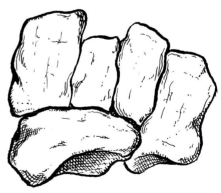

Fig. 22-1. Midfoot bones: Navicular, cuneiforms, and cuboid.

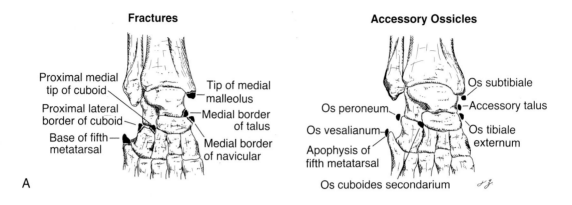

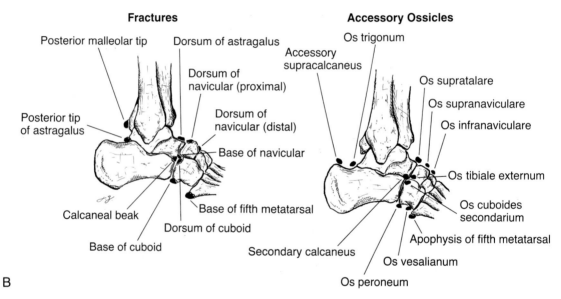

Fig. 22-2. Accessory ossicles of the foot and fractures in similar places. (**A**) Anteroposterior view, (**B**) lateral view. (From Zatzkin,[42] with permission.)

SPECIFIC INJURIES

Tarsonavicular fractures are the most common midfoot fracture, making up 62 percent of all fractures of the midfoot and 0.37 percent of all fractures. They occur most often between 10 and 20 years of age.[1] Ten of every 12 navicular fractures occur in this age group. Of navicular fractures, dorsal avulsion fractures, sometimes referred to as cortical avulsion fractures, are the most common, representing 47 percent of all navicular fractures.[12]

CLASSIFICATION

Five categories of navicular fractures are discussed in this chapter: (1) dorsal avulsion fractures; (2) tuberosity fractures; (3) body fractures, further subdivided as vertical, horizontal, crush, or stress; (4) displaced fractures; and (5) osteochondral fractures. Other classifications have been used. Wilson classified navicular fractures as chip, comminuted, and crush[1]; Watson-Jones as dorsal, lip, tuberosity, and transverse; De-Palma as dorsal, lip, avulsion, tuberosity, and fracture-dislocation.[13] Rockwood and Green described fracture of the body with and without dislocation, chip fracture, and tuberosity fracture.[14]

Dorsal Avulsion Fracture

Dorsal avulsion fractures are best visualized on lateral radiographs. The mechanism of injury is plantar displacement of the foot followed by either eversion or inversion. During plantar flexion and eversion, the dorsal tibionavicular ligament, part of the deltoid ligament, becomes taut and avulses the dorsal cortex of the navicular bone at its insertion. During plantar flexion and inversion, the talonavicular ligament becomes stressed and acts in a similar manner. The avulsed fragment usually contains a small portion of articular surface as well as dorsal (Fig. 22-3). Examination of the patient shows tenderness and edema at the fracture site. Usually, open reduction and internal fixation are not necessary. When there is a large fragment with displacement, it may be helpful to manipulate the fragment. Prior to manipulation, a field block of local anesthesia is achieved. Then, using the thumbs to place downward pressure over the fragment, the fragment may be manipulated into better position. Since the region is edematous and the fracture does not have any interdigitating fragments or an opposing surface for instability, an incomplete reduction with modest improvement is typical. Kent recommends open reduction with internal fixation if the fragment involves more than 20

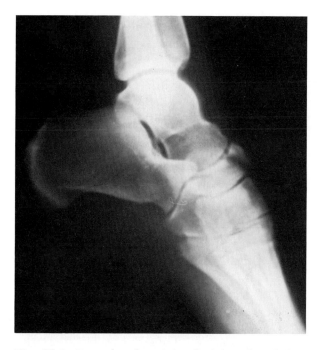

Fig. 22-3. Lateral radiograph of plantar-flexed foot showing dorsal avulsion fracture of navicular. (From Goldman,[39] with permission.)

percent of the articular surface.[15] Observation of the natural history of such fractures without open reduction and internal fixation demonstrates less distraction as edema subsides and as healing progresses, although when bone healing is complete it is common to have an irregular dorsal bump, which is apparent on a lateral radiograph. Subsequent painful arthrosis is generally not the rule. Such fractures are treated with a short leg walking cast for 4 to 6 weeks with the foot in a neutral position relative to inversion and eversion and in a slight calcaneus position if possible. Some patients may not be candidates for casting. These include older patients with balance problems, pre-existing knee, hip, and low back problems, and hygiene problems. Symptomatic treatment with an Ace bandage and wooden-soled shoe may be appropriate. Rarely, if the dorsal exostosis forms a painful impingement or fails to join, excision of the fragment may be indicated.

Fractures of the Navicular Tuberosity

Fractures of the navicular tuberosity are relatively common, representing 24 percent of all navicular fractures in one series.[12] The navicular tuberosity can be palpated about 2.5 cm anterior and inferior to the medial malleolus as the medial surface roughens and enlarges to form a tuberosity. The size and shape of the tuberosity vary greatly. Between 2 and 12 percent of the time, an accessory navicular in this location is present. It is commonly referred to as an os tibial externum or a navicular secondarium. This accessory ossicle can articulate with the true navicular by either fibrous union or a true synovial joint.[16,17] The accessory navicular has been classified into two types[18]: type I is small, round, and discrete from the main body; type II is closely related to the body but separated by dense fibrocartilage. Type II is more common and further confuses the diagnosis of fracture. The os tibial externum when observed in 14 children totally fused to the main body in 5, partially fused in 3, and remained independent in 6 children.[17] Such tuberosity fractures generally occur as an avulsion (Fig. 22-4A). The tendon of the posterior tibial muscle is the only tendon inserting on the navicular and exerts force when the foot is forcibly everted. The fracture shows up well on oblique and anteroposterior radiographs. At least one researcher has implied that stress on the calcaneonavicular ligament and deltoid ligament may also produce tuberosity avulsion fractures.[12] Rarely, a direct blow will cause such a fracture.

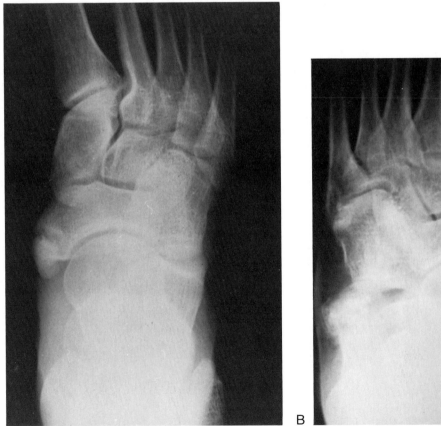

Fig. 22-4. (A) Avulsion fracture of navicular. **(B)** Anteroposterior view showing avulsion fracture of navicular with severe abduction injury. Note displaced calcaneal fracture. (Part A from Goldman,[39] with permission.)

Characteristically, these fractures are nondisplaced by virtue of the multiple ligamentous attachments to the navicular and the broad insertion of the posterior tibial tendon. The anterior component of the posterior tibial tendon is the largest and inserts onto the navicular tuberosity. It also sends fibers to the inferior surface of the first cuneiform. The middle component sends fibers to the second and third cuneiforms and cuboid, subsequently forming metatarsal slips to the second, third, fourth, and sometimes fifth metatarsal as well as the origin of the flexor hallucis brevis. The posterior component is recurrent and inserts into the sustentaculum tali. Many investigators have pointed out the need to distinguish fractures of the tuberosity from those of the accessory navicular.[13,19–21] As pointed out above, type II accessory navicular fractures may be very difficult to distinguish from fractures of the tuberosity of the navicular. Radiographically, the classical differentiation is based on three criteria: (1) the os tibial externum is "usually bilateral"; (2) fractures are "usually" sharp with jagged edges; (3) the os tibiale externum usually has smooth, round edges. To further complicate such a distinction, cases involving traumatic disruption of a fibrous union or synovial joint can be as symptomatic and disabling as true avulsion fractures; often these cases are more troublesome in subsequent management because bony healing will never occur in such cases. Treatment is similar in either case.

Treatment

Generally, significant edema is not a problem, but if it is, a compression dressing with posterior splint holding the foot in mild talipes equinovarus is indicated. The foot should not bear weight for 24 to 72 hours. During this time, it should be kept elevated as much as possible. Crutches should be used for ambulation. If swelling is not a problem or swelling has been controlled by compression dressings, a short leg walking cast with a well-molded arch is applied for 6 to 8 weeks. Although some clinicians may prefer a more cavalier approach such as an Ace wrap and postoperative shoe or a multitude of other noncasting techniques, these often prove unsatisfactory. For most active patients, greater comfort and greater mobility are achieved in a snug below-the-knee walking cast with a well-molded arch. Even with early diagnosis and immobilization in plaster, a significant number of these injuries will remain bothersome and may require surgical treatment. Casting for longer than 2 months is not generally indicated even if radiographs do not show bony healing. Many of these cases may represent disrupted fibrous unions and not true fractures. Additionally, cases that do not go on to bony healing may develop asymptomatic nonunions. Conversely, many cases even with prolonged casting will not show bony unions. For these reasons, periods of immobilization in plaster for greater than 2 months do not seem indicated. When mild or occasional activity-related pain persists, orthotics may be helpful in reducing symptoms. When there is more significant pain and when function is compromised, surgical excision of the fragment is indicated. Surgery is performed through a medial longitudinal incision centered over the tuberosity. The capsule is incised and the posterior tibial tendon reflected. The fragment is identified and removed completely, being sure to smooth any rough edges. At times the fragment will appear clinically united and difficult to identify. In such cases, simply use an appropriate-sized osteotome and proceed as if you were excising an enlarged navicular tuberosity, and invariably this force will separate the nonunited fragment from the body of the navicular. When remodeling the remainder of the navicular, take care not to remove so much bone that the head of the talus will be significantly uncovered when the foot is in a maximally pronated attitude. For closure, reapproximate the capsule-tendinous flap and secure it to the undersurface of the navicular or spring ligament. Following wound closure, a short leg cast is applied for approximately 4 to 6 weeks. Follow-up with orthotics may be indicated.

Fractures of the Body of the Navicular

Fractures of the body of the navicular represent 29 percent of all fractures of the navicular.[12] Navicular body fractures may be either vertical,

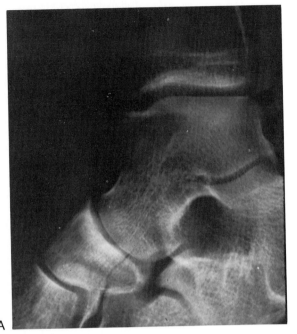

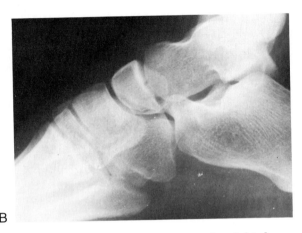

A   B

Fig. 22-5. **(A)** Nondisplaced body fracture of the navicular starting at interval between second and third cuneiforms. **(B)** Nondisplaced horizontal fracture of navicular. (Part A from Goldman,[39] with permission.)

horizontal, crush, stress, or displaced fractures. The simplest and most common fracture of the body of the navicular is the nondisplaced vertical or horizontal fracture (Fig. 22-5). Usually these fractures remain nondisplaced as the result of the multiple tendinous ligamentous investments and buttressing of surrounding bones.

Such fractures occur by a variety of mechanisms, including falling with the foot striking the ground in plantar flexion,[1,22] or plantar flexion and abduction at the midtarsal joint,[23,24] Hect describes force-dorsiflexion[25] and Eichenholtz and Levine state that a twisting injury may produce such a fracture from "stress applied from the bone by opposite rotatory forces from the short dorsal and plantar talonavicular and navicular cuneiform ligaments."[12] In such injuries, the navicular may become compressed between the talar head and the cuneiforms. Generally, these fractures appear on oblique and lateral radiographs. Often vertical fractures will show the fracture line passing through the interval between the second and third cuneiforms, suggesting that their alignment on the navicular and the interval

between the three facets on the anterior surface of the navicular act as a stress riser. There are conditions that must be considered in the differential diagnosis of navicular body fractures, including bipartite tarsonavicular fractures[26] (Fig. 22-6) or lithiasis of the navicular.[27]

Treatment

Nondisplaced vertical or horizontal fractures of the navicular are treated with a short leg walking cast for 6 to 8 weeks. Such fractures will generally heal without any sequelae. Following removal from plaster immobilization, treatment should be symptomatic and vigorous activities such as running and jumping may need to be curtailed. The foot can be protected with an orthosis to eliminate excessive subtalar and talonavicular motion.

Fractures of the Body of the Navicular with Displacement

Fractures of the body of the navicular with displacement occur when the foot strikes the ground

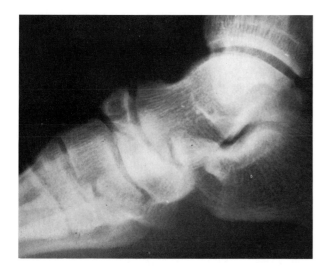

Fig. 22-6. Lateral radiograph showing bipartite navicular that is asymptomatic. (From Goldman,[39] with permission.)

plantar flexed, causing a buckling of the midfoot. Stress is placed in the region of the dorsal capsular and ligamentous structures of the midfoot by the long bones of the forefoot and rearfoot acting as lever arms against the midfoot bones, thus wedging the navicular between the cuneiforms

distally and the talus proximally. This results in a dorsal extrusion of the navicular once the soft tissue has given way. This mechanism is similar to dislocations of the cuneiforms and cuboid and has been likened to the splitting of a pod and the resulted ejection of a pea[14] (Fig. 22-7). Acute inversion and adduction of the foot have been said to produce fracture-dislocations in a similar manner.[24] Again, plantar extrusion of fracture fragments is most unlikely since the dorsal capsular ligamentous structures are much weaker than the plantar structures, the plantar structures being reinforced with strong ligaments, muscular origins, and tendinous insertions. However, isolated plantar dislocation of the navicular has been reported[28] (Fig. 22-8) and a proposed mechanism has been described. The displaced dorsal fragment has been found to be prone to developing aseptic necrosis.[13]

Treatment

In body fractures of the navicular with displacement, closed reduction has been described as improbable, and open reduction has been advocated.[22] There are however, some reports advocating closed reduction. Bohler in 1958 recommended skeletal traction through the calca-

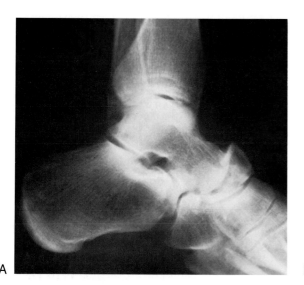
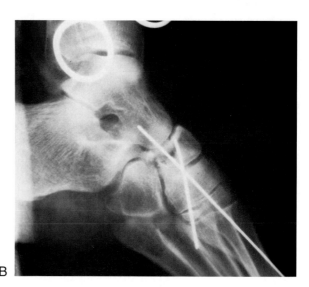

A   B

Fig. 22-7. **(A)** Lateral view showing horizontal fracture of the navicular with dorsal displacement of dorsal fragment. **(B)** Lateral view showing relocation with pin fixation. (From Goldman,[39] with permission.)

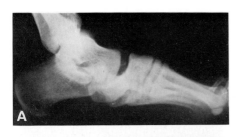

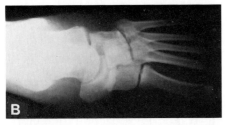

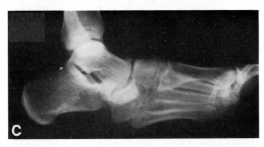

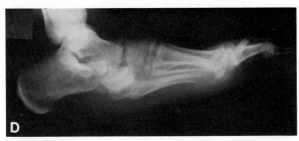

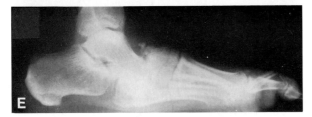

Fig. 22-8. Isolated plantar tarsonavicular dislocation, neuropathic foot. (**A**) Lateral view. (**B**) Anteroposterior view. (**C**) Lateral view after immobilization, early. (**D**) Lateral view after immobilization, intermediate. (**E**) Lateral view after several years of weight bearing. (From Goldman,[28] with permission.)

neus. Wilson recommended forced plantar flexion of the forefoot with pressure on the dorsal surface of the fracture to achieve closed reduction.[1] In fractures older than 8 days or if complete reduction was not accomplished, he recommended talonavicular arthrodesis. Day suggested manipulation[24] and pointed out that Hendison noted that considerable force would be necessary. Day also reviewed cases by Penhalo and Lehman, who claimed good results with manipulation, but Day cautioned that good results may only be early results and suggested that later results may show degenerative changes. Day also thought that isolated talonavicular fusion would be inadequate and suggested triple arthrodesis combined with naviculocuneiform arthrodesis in selected cases.[24] Eichenholtz and Levine concluded that the treatment of such fracture-dislocations is controversial.[12] They suggested that closed reduction should be attempted; however, they cautioned that redislocation or partial redislocation occurs frequently enough to make this method uncertain. DePalma advocated manipulation followed by the application of a short leg cast and the use of crutches for 3 weeks, after which a short leg walking cast is used for 9 weeks.[13] Eftekhar et al. believed that anatomic reduction was important by either open or closed measures.[23] Duvries noted that there was no consensus of opinion in the treatment of such fracture-dislocations.[19] He recommended open reduction with internal fixation with pins or screws. Giannestras suggested that closed reduction be attempted but admitted that open reduction with internal fixation would usually be necessary.[20] Rockwood and Green noted that closed reductions are usually ineffective and thought that open reduction with internal fixation is necessary to maintain reduction.[14] Open reduction is usually effected by a dorsomedial longitudinal incision placed lateral to the anterior tibial tendon and extending from the talus to the cuneiform.[13,14,23,29] Following open reduction and internal fixation, patients are immobilized in a nonweight-bearing short leg cast until union occurs in approximately 8 weeks. Ashurst and Crossan reported several cases in which open reduction was "impossible" in old cases of navicular fractures that were missed and recommended

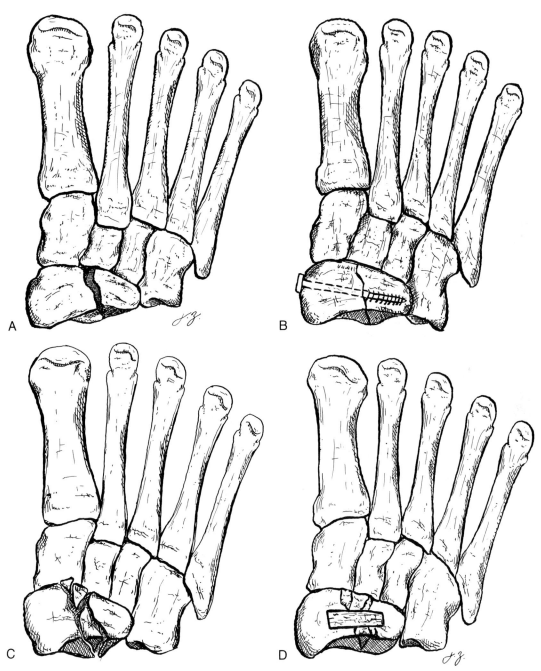

Fig. 22-9. (**A**) Diagram of displaced navicular fracture, vertical. (**B**) Reduction with screw fixation. (**C**) Comminuted navicular fracture. (**D**) Elevation of displaced fracture and packing with bone graft.

removal of the navicular as the only means of relieving symptoms.[22] Mann recommended in selected cases of severe comminution the use of internal fixation with Kirschner wires through the fracture fragments and into the surrounding bones to preserve the architecture of the arch.[30] Mann also recommended in cases of collapse that reconstruction with elevation of depressed fragments and bone graft be considered (Fig. 22-9). He cautioned that later degenerative changes may require fusion. In cases that show severe comminution of the navicula, talus, or cuneiform, primary arthrodesis has been indicated.[20,23] In less active elderly patients, aggressive surgical treatment may not be indicated.[14]

Stress Fractures of the Tarsonavicular

Bateman first described navicular fractures in greyhounds.[31] The dogs run counterclockwise on the tracks, stressing their outer limbs and fracturing their right hind limb. The condition is referred to as broken hock. In humans, this fracture typically involves the middle third of the body of the navicular. Stress fractures of the navicular have been described as complete or incomplete. Complete fractures may result in dislocation if care is not sought.[9,18] This fracture has been described as being underdiagnosed and requires a high index of suspicion for diagnosis. These fractures mostly occur in young male athletes who present with symptoms ranging from weeks to years, showing an average delay in diagnosis of 7.2 months.[9] The pain is poorly localized to the dorsum of the foot and to the medial long arch. It is described as having an insidious onset. Physical examination shows pain to direct palpation of the tarsonavicular area. Characteristically, there is little swelling. As with all stress fractures, the symptoms are made worse during activity and are relieved with rest. This is just the opposite of what one would expect to find with a soft tissue strain or tendinitis in which, typically symptoms will improve during activity once past "warm-up" but then will become more painful once the activity has ceased. Routine radiographs will generally demonstrate underpenetration of the central one-third of the navicular, and for that

reason routine radiographs may fail to show the fracture. In one study,[8] anteroposterior radiographs visualized the fracture in only 9 of 23 cases, and the fracture was never evident on oblique or lateral views. In suspected cases, technetium 99 bone scan should be ordered. Once a positive bone scan is obtained a tomogram or CT scan directed by the bone scan should be ordered. When ordering tomograms, it is important to specify an "anatomic tomogram" of the navicular since normal tomograms may fail to show the lesion. Anatomic tomograms in one study showed the lesion 17 of 23 times, while standard tomograms only showed a yield of 1 of 23. The difference between the standard tomogram and the anatomic tomogram is the position of the foot (Fig. 22-10).

Treatment
Failure to treat such fractures with non-weight-bearing short leg casts may precipitate delayed union or nonunion. In one report,[9] all uncomplicated fractures treated with non-weight-bearing casting for 4 to 6 weeks healed. In these cases, it was 3 to 6 months before full activity was resumed, with an average of 3.8 months.

Osteochondritis Dissecans of the Navicular

Only one case of navicular osteochondral fracture has been reported.[3] The diagnosis was by tomogram guided by a bone scan and plane radiographs. Treatment consisted of excision of the fragment and drilling of the cavity. Limited follow-up revealed a good course. The authors recommended a trial of conservative treatment.

Fractures of the Cuneiforms and Cuboid

Taken together, fractures of the cuneiforms and cuboid constitute 8.4 percent of all tarsal fractures and 0.24 percent of all fractures. A statement made regarding the navicular fractures also applies to cuboid and cuneiform fractures and that is that the diagnosis is sometimes obvious,

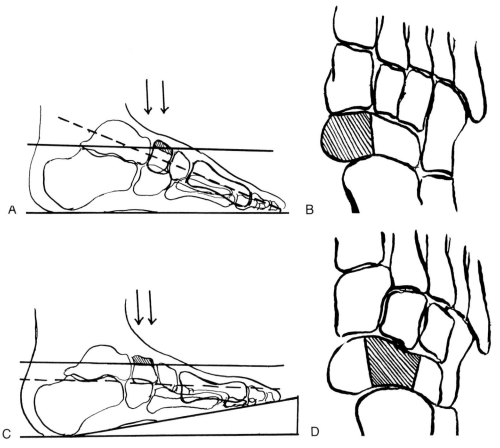

Fig. 22-10. **(A)** Standard anteroposterior tomogram position. **(B)** Shaded area is the central third of the navicular as seen obliquely. **(C)** Anatomic anteroposterior tomogram. **(D)** Shaded area is the central third of the navicular as seen en face. (Modified from Pavlov et al.,[8] with permission.)

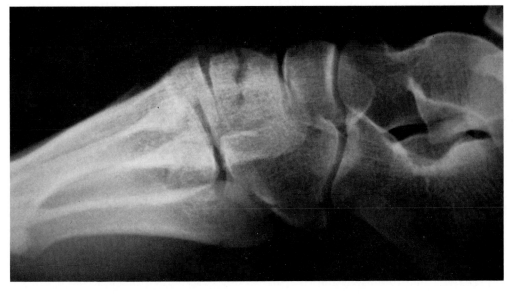

Fig. 22-11. Lateral view of nondisplaced cuneiform fracture.

frequently difficult, occasionally elusive, and surprisingly not rare. Furthermore, these fractures are often neglected, usually unsuspected, frequently undiagnosed, and occasionally mismanaged.[12]

Fractures of the Cuneiforms

Incidence. Cuneiform fractures represent 4.2 percent of tarsal fractures, and 1.7 percent are isolated and 0.5 percent are associated with other foot and ankle injuries.[1]

Classification. Fractures of the cuneiforms are classified as avulsion or body fractures. Body fractures are further classified as simple, comminuted and crush, fracture-dislocation, and osteochondral. Avulsion fractures may occur on the medial side of the first cuneiform and may represent avulsion of the anterior tibial tendon. Fractures of the body may be caused by direct trauma or by axial and rotational force transmitted through the foot. Isolated fractures rarely show displacement since they are strongly bound by intertarsal ligaments and surrounding bone (Fig. 22-11). Generally these fractures will heal readily if immobilized for 6 to 8 weeks in a short leg walking cast. After removal of the cast, patients may benefit from supportive shoes or orthotics to help limit medial motion. Injuries caused by a direct blow should be observed for edema, and compression dressings may be necessary before casts are applied. In addition, the condition of the skin must be assessed.[20] Stress fractures of the cuneiforms have been described[5,6] (Fig. 22-12). As with other midfoot stress fractures, a high index of suspicion is necessary, and in suspect cases bone scans should be performed and results of the bone scan should direct tomographic or CT scan studies. Not infrequently, cuneiform fractures are associated with midtarsal and tarsometatarsal dislocations.[13,20,32–34] With such fracture-dislocations, the force is axial and the foot generally strikes the ground in a plantar-flexed attitude. Thus, the long bones of the forefoot and rear foot act as levers, wedging the midfoot bones and causing fracture and dislocation (Fig. 22-13). Generally these bones dislocate dorsally and laterally. Dislocation occurs dorsally because the dorsal capsular ligamentous structures are weaker than the plantar structures and because the anatomy of the medial longitudinal arch buckles the foot in a dorsal direction. Dislocation occurs laterally because the tarsometatarsal joint is angulated from distal to proximal as it progresses from the second to fifth metatarsals. The second metatarsal is recessed between the first and third cuneiforms. It is the most stable, and generally either fracture or dislocation of the second metatarsal base must occur before the other metatarsals can dislocate. A variation of this has been described in which the second cuneiform dislocated and the second metatarsal remained intact.[35] The second metatarsal's stability depends on Lisfranc's ligament, a ligament between the first cuneiform and the base of the second metatarsal. Once this ligament is ruptured, not only are the metatarsals at risk for dislocation but so is the first cuneiform.

Treatment. In reducing such fracture-dislocations, there are two fundamentals. (1) The foot needs to be brought out to length. Usually this is accomplished by using finger traps and hanging the foot from an intravenous-bottle pole. Additional traction is obtained by draping a cervical collar over the lower leg and applying weights as necessary (Figs. 22-14 and 22-15). At times the toes are so swollen that finger traps will not fit. In such instances, it may be necessary to use a heavy percutaneous pin through the involved metatarsals to apply traction (Fig. 22-16). Visualization by C-arm fluoroscopy is helpful for pin placement. To obtain adequate reduction, complete muscular relaxation and cessation of pain is necessary, usually requiring general or spinal anesthesia. (2) The keystone effect of the second metatarsal is only as good as the mortise that the cuneiforms create for it; therefore, anatomic reduction of the cuneiforms with secure fixation is necessary.[35,36]

Fractures of the Cuboid

Cuboid fractures can occur in isolation but very often they are associated with other fractures, most commonly fractures in the lateral column including the calcaneus and the fifth metatarsal or fractures of the navicular (Fig. 22-17). As with other fractures in the midfoot, displacement of cuboid fractures is rare because of the strong capsular ligamentous attachments and adjacent artic-

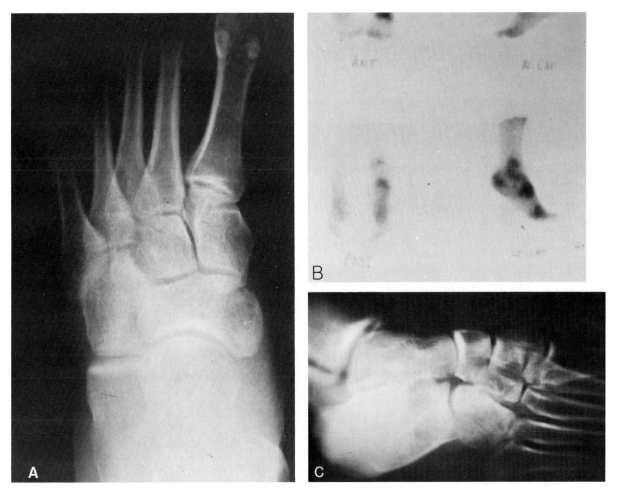

Fig. 22-12. (**A**) Anteroposterior radiograph showing second cuneiform stress fracture. (**B**) Bone scan showing uptake in cuneiform region. (**C**) Tomogram confirming stress fracture of the cuneiform. (From Goldman,[39] with permission.)

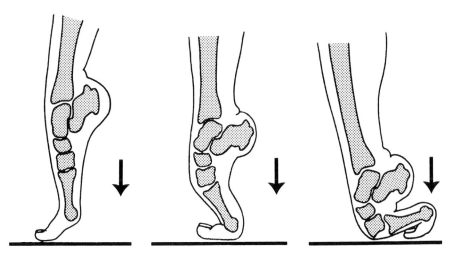

Fig. 22-13. Diagrammatic representation of plantar-flexed position of foot striking ground and axially loading the foot, causing midfoot to buckle with subsequent fractures and dorsal dislocations. (From Wargon and Goldman,[35] with permission.)

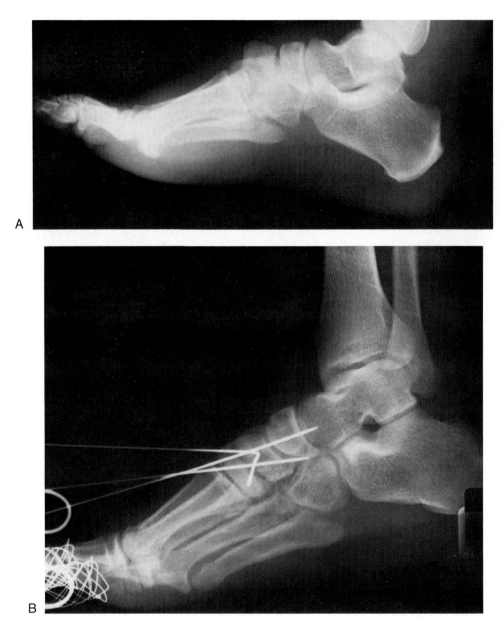

Fig. 22-14. (**A**) Lateral view showing dorsal displacement of the medial cuneiform. (**B**) Reduction with pin fixation. Finger traps are attached to toes distally.

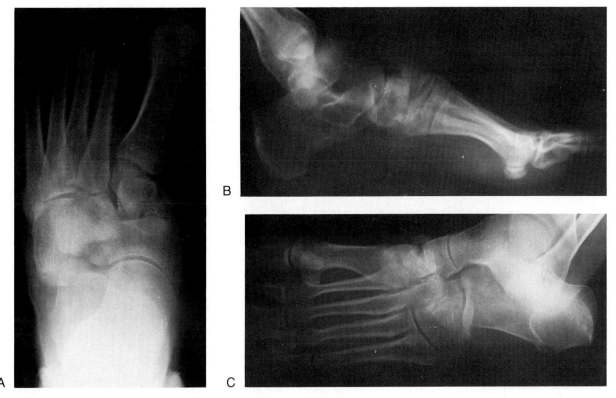

Fig. 22-15. (**A**) Fracture dislocation of medial cuneiform, anteroposterior view. (**B**) Lateral view. (**C**) Oblique view. (*Figure continues.*)

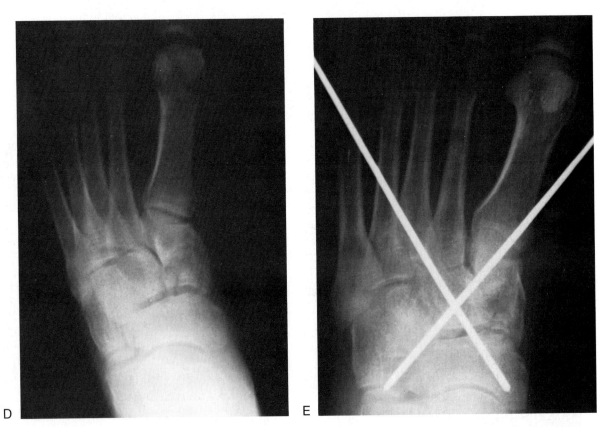

Fig. 22-15 (*Continued*). (**D**) Anteroposterior view showing reduction in finger traps. (**E**) Percutaneous pin fixation, anteroposterior view.

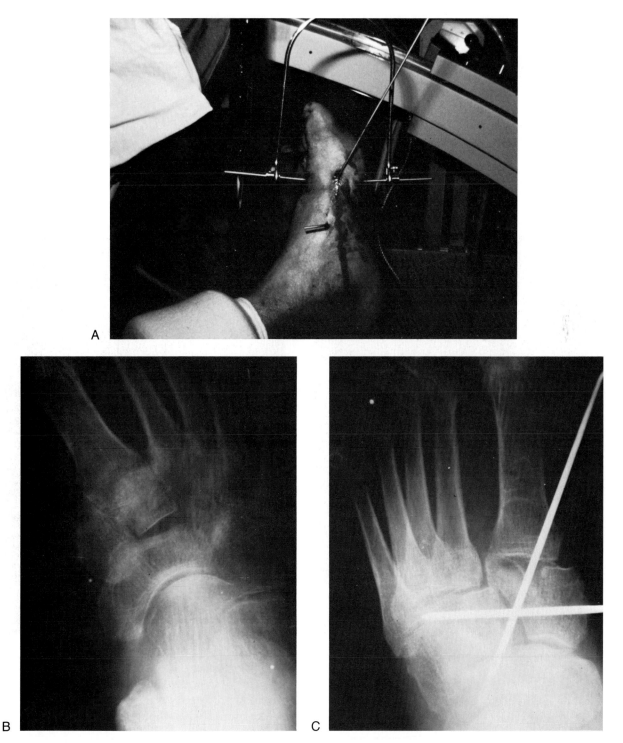

Fig. 22-16. **(A)** Use of percutaneous pins to achieve traction on metatartsals when the toes are too swollen to accept finger traps. Note use or C-arm fluoroscopy to confirm pin placement and fracture reduction. This was a missed injury and therefore edema had developed prior to reduction. Also, this patient was quite elderly and had other serious injuries making open reduction undesirable. **(B)** Prereduction view. Note fractured and displaced first cuneiform with cuneiform being dorsally displaced on top of navicular and first metatsal. **(C)** Postreduction view.

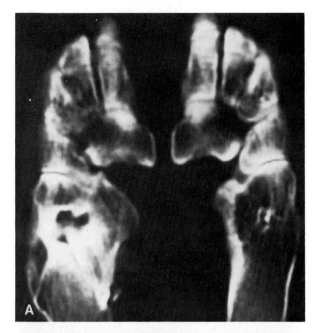

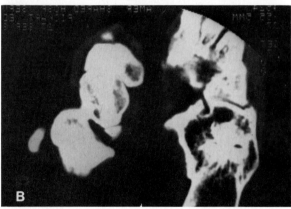

Fig. 22-17. (A & B) CT scan of calcaneal fractures with involvement of calcaneocuboid joint. (From Goldman,[39] with permission.)

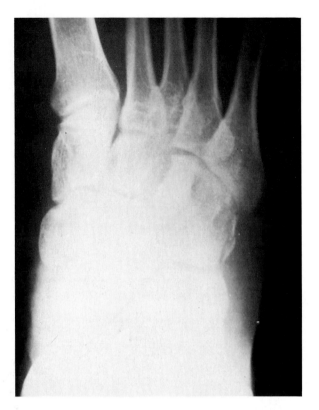

Fig. 22-18. Lateral avulsion fracture of cuboid.

ulations. Fractures of the cuboid can be classified as either avulsion fractures or body fractures, which are further classified as simple, stress, comminuted or crush, or fracture-dislocation. Avulsion fractures of the cuboid most often occur on the lateral surface.[24] Benassi described an avulsion fracture of the cuboid tuberosity and attributed it to the pull of the inferior calcaneal

cuboid ligament (Figs. 22-18 and 22-19). The lateral calcaneal cuboid ligament may also cause an avulsion fracture as the cuboid is adducted on the calcaneus. Simple body fractures of the cuboid usually occur when the foot hits the ground in a plantar-flexed position when axial and rotatory forces are directed up the rigid lateral column of the foot. The force transmitted from the fifth metatarsal then produces a crescent-shaped fracture (Figs. 22-20 and 22-21). Such fractures are interarticular and less than anatomic reduction can lead to degenerative changes (Fig. 22-21). Direct trauma is another common cause of simple body fractures. In such cases, soft tissue and skin condition should be monitored initially. Avulsion fractures and nondisplaced body fractures generally heal well when placed in short leg walking casts for 6 to 8 weeks. Crush fractures of the cuboid generally occur from the above mech-

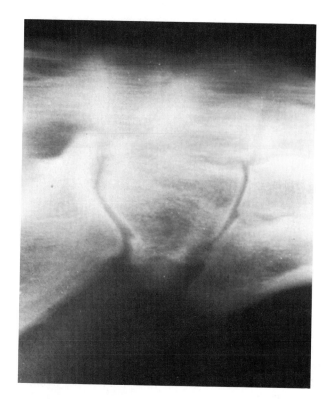

Fig. 22-19. Tomogram of old missed avulsion fracture with articular offset of cuboid at calcaneocuboid joint.

recommended for depressed fractures with bone graft as necessary (Figs. 22-23 and 22-24). Positive bone scans suggesting stress fractures of the cuboid have been reported[39] (Fig. 22-25); however, confirmation with a tomogram was lacking. Other causes for pain in the cuboid region are (1) dropped cuboid, (2) peroneus longus tendinitis, (3) os peroneum degenerative changes, (4) calcaneo cuboid joint arthritis, (5) capsuloligamentous strain associated with cavus foot type, (6) extensor digitorum brevis myositis, and (7) stress fracture.

anism but require more force. Hermel and Gershon-Cohen describe a nutcracker fracture of the cuboid in which the cuboid is "caught like a nut in a nutcracker between the base of the fourth and fifth metatarsal in the calcaneus."[37] Such fractures occur with severe abduction of the forefoot and are often associated with an avulsion fracture of the navicular. Figure 22-4B shows a variation in which the navicular has an avulsion fracture and, rather than the cuboid fracture, the anterior calcaneus collapsed at the calcaneo cuboid joint. In cases of severe comminution and articular damage, primary arthrodesis of the involved joint surfaces may be indicated. Total dislocation of the cuboid is rare but has been reported.[38] Fracture-dislocation is also rare and requires open reduction with internal fixation (Fig. 22-22) if closed reduction is not successful. Open reduction with internal fixation has been

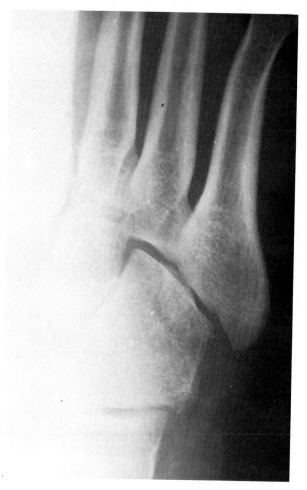

Fig. 22-20. Nondisplaced crescent-shaped fracture of the distal lateral cuboid, fifth metatarsal joint.

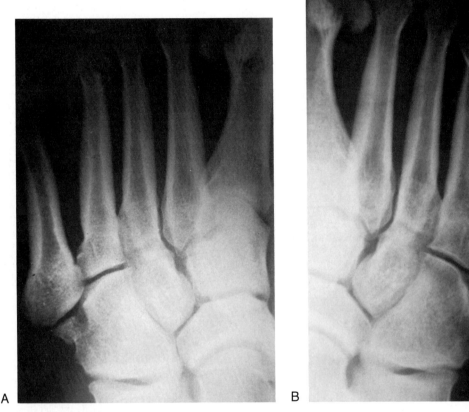

Fig. 22-21. **(A)** Small crescent-shaped distal lateral cuboid fracture, displaced, again probably resulting from axial loading force on the fifth metatarsal. **(B)** Healed fracture. Fragment was not reduced anatomically. Note the degenerative changes at the cuboid, fifth metatarsal, and at the base of the fourth and fifth metatarsals; the fifth metatarsal has now assumed the more proximal position. (*Figure continues.*)

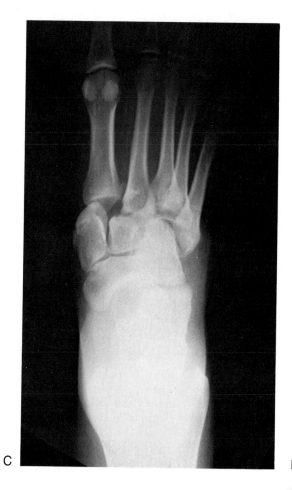

C

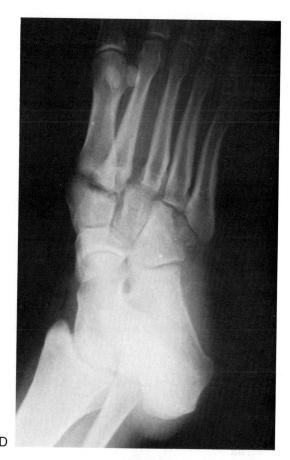

D

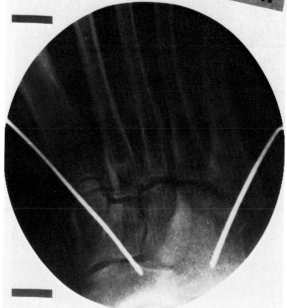

E

Fig. 22-21 (*Continued*). (**C**) Crescent-shaped distal lateral cuboid fracture associated with Lisfranc's fracture-dislocation, anteroposterior view. (**D**) Medial-oblique view. (**E**) Anteroposterior view of reduced fracture dislocation. Note the restoration of the fifth metatarsal cuboid joint.

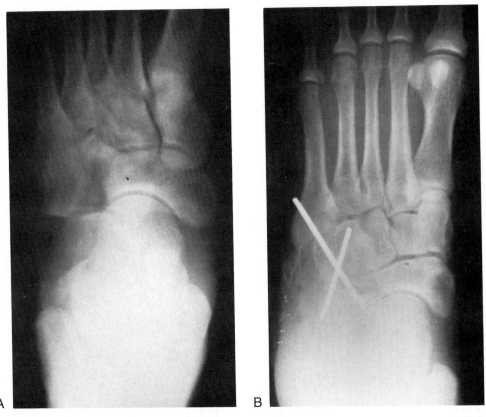

Fig. 22-22. **(A)** Anteroposterior view of displaced cuboid fracture. **(B)** Anteroposterior view following open reduction with internal fixation of cuboid. (From Goldman,[39] with permission.)

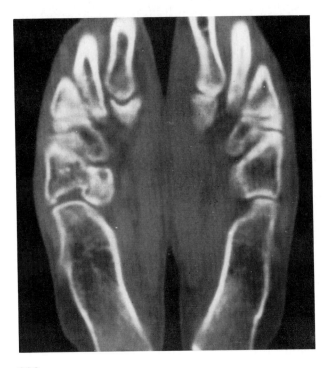

Fig. 22-23. Tomogram revealing central depression of cuboid at calcaneocuboid joint. Standard radiographs failed to reveal this fracture.

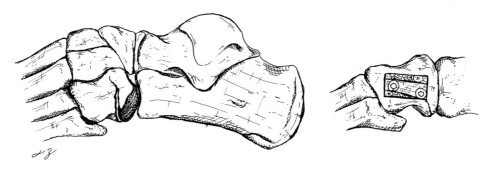

Fig. 22-24. Diagram showing open reduction and internal fixation with elevation of depressed cuboid fracture and bone grafting. (Modified from Mann,[30] with permission.)

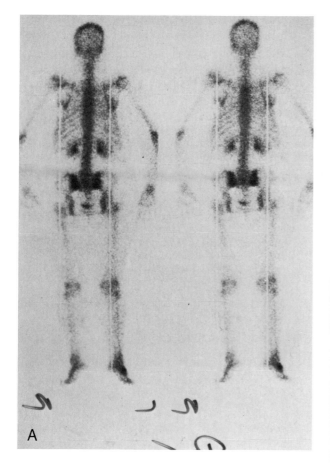

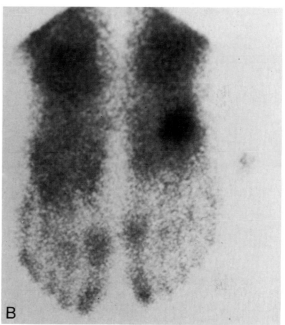

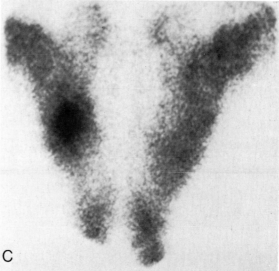

Fig. 22-25. (A) Full body bone scan showing localization to the left foot. (B) Anteroposterior view showing localization to the cuboid region. (C) Lateral view showing localization to the cuboid region. (From Goldman,[39] with permission.)

NEUROPATHIC JOINT DISEASE

As with other midfoot fracture-dislocations, neuropathic joint disease requires a high index of suspicion. Asymptomatic swelling in the insensate patient should be suspect for neuropathic joint disease.[28] Often such patients are diagnosed as having idiopathic edema, phlebitis, or cellulitis. Radiographs should be ordered. The midfoot is a favorite site for such fracture-dislocations. Diabetes is currently the most common cause for Charcot's joints of the foot. Generally, such patients are asymptomatic, although pain may be present at times. On examination, the foot is usually warm with bounding pulses since patients with such neuropathy may have an autosympathectomy. Radiographs often show complete destruction of normal bony architecture and bony disintegration in later stages (Fig. 22-26). Early stages may show more subtle fracture-dislocations and periarticular bony fragmentation dorsally in the midfoot (Fig. 22-27). Later changes may be confused with osteomyelitis radiographically.

Treatment

Treatment consists of keeping weight off the foot and elevating the affected extremity until the edema subsides. Once edema has diminished,

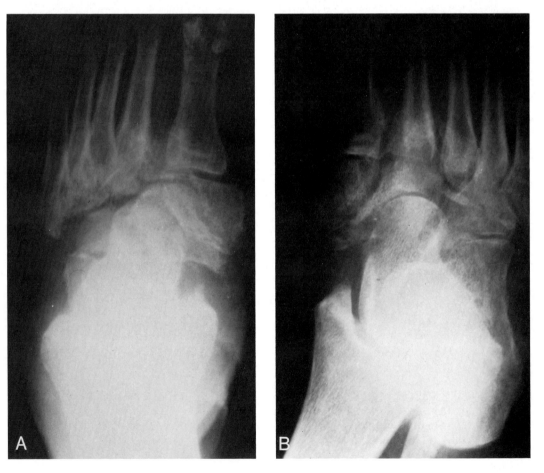

Fig. 22-26. (A) Anteroposterior view of Charcot changes of the midfoot with complete loss of bony architecture and disintegration of midfoot bones. **(B)** Oblique view of same. (From Goldman,[39] with permission.)

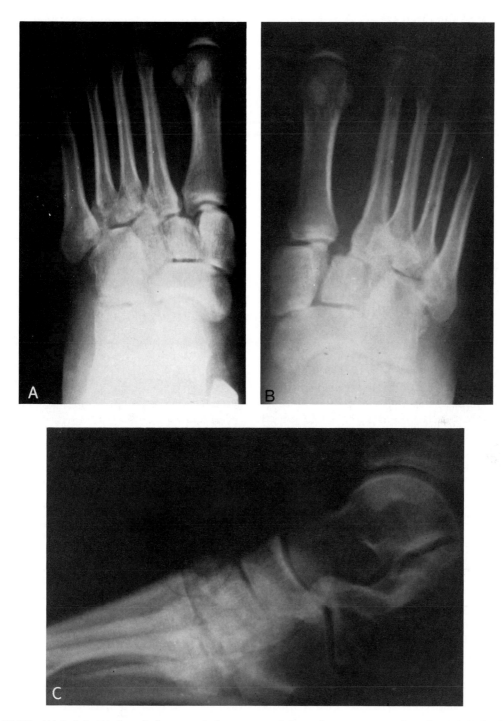

Fig. 22-27. (A) Subtle Lisfranc's fracture-dislocation with loss of intermetatarsal angle and slight diastasis between first and second metatarsals in neuropathic foot. (B) More advanced stage of same. Anteroposterior view with increased diastasis between the first and second cuneiforms and the first and second metatarsals. (C) Lateral view showing dorsal midfoot Charcot changes. (From Goldman,[39] with permission.)

the extremity is immobilized in a short leg bivalved walking cast or patellar tender bearing cast until remaining edema and warmth resolve and, if possible, until signs of bony consolidation are present on radiographs. Patients may then be treated with supportive and accommodative foot gear including ankle-foot orthoses. Attempts at fusion may fail and result in infection and amputation. If fusion is to be attempted, it is best performed after the hyperemic stage has passed and the consolidation stage has started. In general, conservative approach in the management of these patients will allow continued ambulation. Palliative surgery in selected cases may be indicated, including excision of sinus tracts and exostosectomy.

matic arthritis. Since each midfoot bone articulates with at least four other bones, and since these joints are weight bearing, even small articular incongruities can lead to degenerative changes and pain. For this reason and since newer imaging techniques allow more precise diagnosis, I anticipate a greater interest in anatomic reduction of such injuries in the future. Hillegass has suggested such for cuboid fractures.[41] Symptoms can result from nonunions of small avulsion fractures, which are unusual, or from bony prominences associated with avulsion fractures causing irritation in shoegear. In either case, simple excision will generally resolve the problem. Midfoot fractures and fracture-dislocations may heal with residual stiffness and edema of the foot.

SUMMARY

Most injuries to the midfoot involve small avulsion, stress, or nondisplaced body fractures. Treatment is generally nonoperative and consists of rest, elevation, and immobilization. When there is significant displacement of fractures or fracture and dislocation when closed reduction fails, open reduction with internal fixation is necessary. In cases involving joint depression, reduction with internal fixation and bone grafting may be indicated at the discretion of the treating surgeon. Naturally, such cases are rare and the experience of any one surgeon in treating such cases is equally rare. In cases of severe comminution and destruction of articular surface, primary fusion may be indicated. As in all cases of trauma, the neurovascular status of the foot and toes must be assessed, the overlying skin should be evaluated, and the patient should be evaluated for any other associated injuries. In cases involving compound injury, tetanus prophylaxis status should be ascertained. Finally, the patient's medical status and ultimate functional needs will influence the treatment plan.

Most simple midfoot injuries heal without serious complications. Nonunion of the body of a midfoot bone is rare because of the basic arrangement of numerous radially penetrating vessels.[40] The most common long-term problem is trau-

REFERENCES

1. Wilson PD: Fractures and dislocations of the tarsal bones. South Med J 26:833, 1933
2. Wilson ES, Katz FN: Stress fractures and analysis of 250 consecutive cases. Radiology 92:481, 1969
3. Lehman R, Gregg JR: Osteochondritis dissecans of the mid foot. Foot Ankle 7:171, 1986
4. Hunter LY: Stress fracture of the tarsal navicular, more frequent then we realize. Am J Sports Med 9:217, 1981
5. Marymont JH, Mills GQ, Merritt WD: Fracture of the lateral cuneiform bone in the absence of severe direct trauma: diagnosis by radionucleotide bone scan. Am J Sports Med 8:135, 1980
6. Meurman, Koa, Elfvings: Stress fracture of the cuneiform bones. Br J Radiol 53:157, 1980
7. Meurman, Koa: Less common stress fractures in the foot. Br J Radiol 54:1, 1981
8. Pavlov H, Torg J, Freiberger RH: Tarsal navicular stress fractures: radiographic evaluation. Radiology 148:641, 1983
9. Torg JS, Pavlov H, Cooley LH et al: Stress fracture of the tarsal navicular. J Bone Joint Surg 64A:700, 1982
10. Towne LC, Blazina ME, Cozen LN: Fatigue fracture of tarsal navicular. J Bone Joint Surg 52A:376, 1970
11. Maurice HD, Newman JH, Watt I: Bone scanning of the foot for unexplained pain. J Bone Joint Surg 16B(3):448, 1987

12. Eichenholtz SN, Levine DB: Fractures of the tarsal navicular. Clin Orthop 34:142, 1964

13. DePalma AF: The Management of Fractures and Dislocations. An Atlas. 2nd Ed. Vol. 2. WB Saunders, Philadelphia, 1970

14. Rockwood CA, Green DP: Fractures. JB Lippincott, Philadelphia, 1975

15. Kent K: Surgery of the Foot. Lea & Febiger, Philadelphia, 1986

16. Lemont H, Eravisano V, Lyman J: Accessory navicular: appearance of a synovial joint. J Am Podiatry Assoc 71:423, 1981

17. Sarrafian SK: Anatomy of the Foot and Ankle. 1st Ed. JB Lippincott, Philadelphia, 1983

18. Voutsinas S, MacNicol MF: Surgical treatment of the symptomatic accessory navicula. J Bone Joint Surg 66B:218, 1984

19. Duvries: In Mann RA (ed): Surgery of the Foot. 4th Ed. CV Mosby, St. Louis, 1978

20. Giannestras NJ: Foot Disorders, Medical and Surgical Management. 2nd Ed. Lea & Febiger, Philadelphia, 1976

21. Rogers L, Campbell R: Fractures and dislocations of the foot. Semin Roentgenol 131:157, 1978

22. Ashurst APC, Crossan ET: Fractures of the tarsal scaphoid and the os calcis. Surg Clin North 10:1477, 1930

23. Eftekhar NM, Lyddon DW, Stevens J: An unusual fracture dislocation of the tarsal navicular. J Bone Joint Surg 51A:577, 1969

24. Day MA: Treatment of injuries to the tarsal navicular. J Bone Joint Surg 29:359, 1947

25. Hect CV: Fractures of the bones of the foot except the talus.

26. Wiley JJ, Brown DE: The bipartite tarsal scaphoid. J Bone Joint Surg 63B:583, 1981

27. Wiley JJ, Brown D: Lithiasis of tarsal scaphoid. J Bone Joint Surg 56B:586, 1974

28. Goldman FD: Identification, treatment and prognosis of Charcot joint in diabetes mellitus. J Am Podiatry Assoc 72:485, 1982

29. Nadeau P, Templeton J: Vertical fracture dislocation of the tarsal navicular. J Trauma 16:669, 1976

30. Mann RA: Surgery of the Foot. 5th Ed. CV Mosby, St. Louis, 1986

31. Bateman J: Broken hock in the greyhound: repair methods and plastic scaphoid. Vet Rec 70:621, 1958

32. Cain PR, Seligson D: Lisfranc's fracture dislocation with inter-cuneiform dislocation; presentation of two cases and a plan for treatment. Foot Ankle 2:156, 1981

33. Gopal-Krishnan S: Dislocation of the medial cuneiform and injuries of the tarsometatarsal joints. Int Surg 58:805, 1973

34. Schiller MG, Ray RD: Isolated dislocation of the medial cuneiform bone: a rare injury of the tarsus. J Bone Joint Surg 52A:1632, 1970

35. Wargon C, Goldman FD: Lisfranc's fracture dislocation: a variation. J Am Podiatr Med Assoc 76:466, 1986

36. Brown DC, McFarland GB: Dislocation of the medial cuneiform bone in the tarsometatarsal fracture dislocation. J Bone Joint Surg 57A:858, 1975

37. Hermel MB, Gershon-Cohen J: The nutcracker fracture of the cuboid by indirect violence. Radiology 60:850, 1953

38. Drummond DS, Hastings DE: Total dislocation of the cuboid bone. J Bone Joint Surg 51B:716, 1969

39. Goldman FD: Fractures of the midfoot. Podiatry 2:259, 1985

40. Waugh W: Deossification and vascularization of the tarsal navicular and their relation to Köhler's disease. J Bone Joint Surg 40B:765, 1958

41. Hillegass RC: Injuries to the mid foot. A major case of industrial morbidity. p. 266. In Bateman J (ed): Foot Science. WB Saunders, Philadelphia, 1976

42. Zatzkin HR: Evaluation of post-traumatic x-rays of the foot. Mod Med Mar 6:107, 1972

23

Fractures of the Talus

Stephen H. Silvani, D.P.M.

Owing to their fascinating complexity, injuries of the talus have challenged the expertise and ingenuity of surgeons throughout history. The first account of a dislocated talus was by Fabricius of Hilden in 1608. The term *aviator's astragalus* was used by Anderson in 1919 to describe a common talar fracture incurred in airplane accidents.[1] Coltart reported on 228 talar fractures treated by surgeons of the Royal Air Force during World War II.[2] Postreduction complications are common and management is difficult because of the unique anatomic, functional, and vascular aspects of the talus.

This chapter describes the proposed mechanisms of injury, the clinical features of the fractures, and the treatment alternatives for injuries of the talus.

ANATOMY

The talus, the most distal bone of the ankle, consists of the body, dome, head, and neck. The body of the talus is cuboidal, and its superior surface, the dome, is covered by a trochlear articular surface that articulates with the tibial plafond to form the ankle joint. The dome is convex from anterior to posterior, and slightly concave from side to side. It is widest anteriorly. The lateral surface is triangular and articulates with the lateral malleolus, and inferiorly its apex forms the lateral process. The medial surface is comma shaped, articulates with the medial malleolus, and is pitted inferiorly by numerous vascular foramina. The posterior surface contains an oblique groove for the flexor hallucis longus tendon. This is located between the larger lateral tubercle and the less prominent medial tubercle. The plantar surface of the body is covered with an oval, concave facet that articulates with the posterior facet of the calcaneus.

The neck of the talus is a constricted part that is set obliquely on the body and inclines medially. Its roughened surface provides attachment for ligaments and plantarly contains a deep groove, the sulcus tali. This forms the roof of the sinus tarsi, which contains the interosseous talocalcaneal and cervical ligaments.

The head of the talus contains an oval and convex articular surface distally that articulates with the navicular. Its plantar surface contains three articular facets, which sometimes are indistinct. These rest on the sustentaculum tali of the calcaneus, the anterior calcaneal articular surface, and the plantar calcaneonavicular ligament, respectively.

Numerous important ligaments attach to the talus, but no muscles insert on this bone. The talus is subjected to tremendous stress forces during normal walking, running, and jumping. Its composition of dense cancellous bone prevents injury despite its anatomic vulnerability. Since most of the surface is articular, post-traumatic deformity or incongruity is poorly tolerated. Healing with fibrocartilage can predispose to arthritic changes. The talus is integrally involved in the ankle, subtalar, and talonavicular joints. Together these joints translate rotational motion of the leg into pronation and supination of the foot.

405

A normally functioning talus is necessary for the foot to alternate between a mobile adaptor for ground contact and a rigid lever for propulsion. Coltart referred to the talus as the "universal joint of the foot."[2]

The unique blood supply of the talus also predisposes it to severe post-traumatic complications, including delayed union and avascular necrosis. Because three-fifths of this bone is covered by cartilage, only two-fifths of the surface can contain vascular foramina. Many researchers have attempted to describe this blood supply[3–6]; however, Mulfinger and Trueta published the most complete description of the intraosseous and extraosseous arterial circulation.[3]

Arteriographic studies demonstrate that the blood supply is retrograde from three main sources: through the neck of the talus, through the foramina in the sinus tarsi and tarsal canal, and through the foramina on the medial side of the body. Additional contributions are supplied by the continuation of the peroneal artery to the lateral talar tubercule and by the posterior tibial artery and its calcaneal branch to the medial tubercle and posterior process. Peterson et al. in 1974 reported another artery within the joint capsule that enters the neck region.[4] One can readily understand why fractures of the talar neck with any posterior displacement of the body result in a high incidence of avascular necrosis. This precarious blood supply must also be taken into account during open reduction, and soft tissue dissection must be kept to a minimum.

CHIPS AND AVULSIONS

Chips and avulsions occur at ligamentous or capsular attachments on the superior surface of the neck, or on the medial, lateral, or posterior aspects of the body. A plantar flexion or dorsiflexion force at the ankle plus an appropriate rotational stress of the leg or foot are the speculated causes of the these talar fractures.

The most common chip is from the anterosuperior surface of the neck on the lateral aspect (Fig. 23-1). This probably results from a longitudinal compressive force combined with a plantar flexion stress that avulses this flake. If small, this piece of bone usually reattaches or reabsorbs when the patient is placed in a below-the-knee weight-bearing cast for 4 to 6 weeks. When large or greatly displaced, the flakes should be excised.

Fractures of the lateral aspect of the talar body are also common, but may be missed in the initial diagnosis of ankle trauma. This fracture usually involves the posterior articular facet where it projects laterally beneath the tip of the fibular malle-

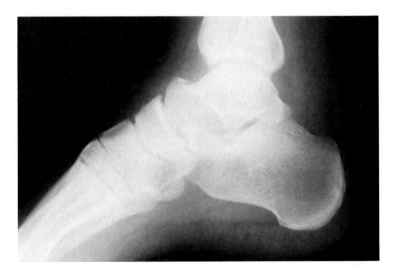

Fig. 23-1. Chip fracture on the superior aspect of the talar neck.

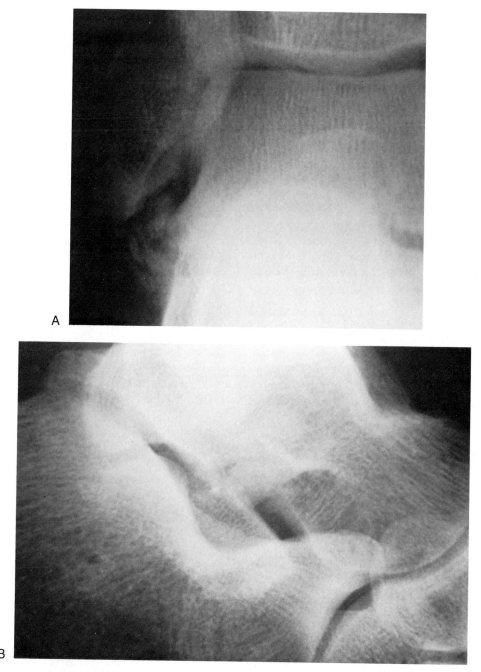

Fig. 23-2. Lateral process fracture as seen on the (**A**) anteroposterior and (**B**) lateral views (stage III).

olus (Fig. 23-2). Therefore, it may be an intra-articular fracture involving one or both of the subtalar and talofibular joints. The mechanism is forced dorsiflexion and inversion of the foot with possible rotational stress. Hawkins reported 13 lateral process fractures among 50 talar fractures.[7] Fjeldborg described three stages of this fracture consisting of fissure (stage I), fracture with displacement (stage II), and fracture with subtalar dislocation (stage III).[8]

Initial treatment is a below-the-knee walking cast for 6 weeks if the lateral process fracture is small or nondisplaced. If the fragment is large or significantly displaced, rigid internal fixation or early excision is appropriate. Late symptomatic displacement or delayed union or malunion is best treated by excision. Post-traumatic arthritis may be a disabling complication caused by misdiagnosis or improper treatment.

Avulsion fractures may occur where the deep fibers of the deltoid ligament attach to the medial surface of the talus. The fracture line may extend posteriorly to involve the medial portion of the groove of the flexor hallucis longus tendon. The mechanism for medial process fractures is dorsiflexion with external rotation or pronation of the foot. Treatment is a below-the-knee weight-bearing cast for 6 weeks. When displacement is evident on the anteroposterior or oblique ankle radiograph (Fig. 23-3), excision of small fragments or attempted fixation of larger fragments is warranted. A surgical approach involves plantar retraction of the posterior tibial neurovascular bundle and tendon. Care must be taken to avoid the arteries supplying the medial body of the talus as they penetrate beneath the deltoid ligament.

The posterior process of the talus (Stieda's process) is located on the lateral side of the groove for the tendon of the flexor hallucis longus. This injury is also referred to as a fracture of a fused os trigonum as described by Lapidus[9] and Ihle and Cochran.[10] During severe plantar flexion injuries, this fracture occurs as the process is jammed between the tibia and calcaneus (Fig. 23-4). This fracture is distinguished from the accessory bone at this location, the os trigonum, by its irregular outline, tilting, or rotation. Immobilization in a slight equinus with a short leg non-weight-bearing cast for 4 to 6 weeks usually results in an osseous union. When displacement with disability persists, excision through a posterolateral approach is indicated. Care should be exercised to avoid damaging the flexor hallucis longus tendon. Postoperatively, the patient is casted for 4 weeks in a weight-bearing below-the-knee cast.

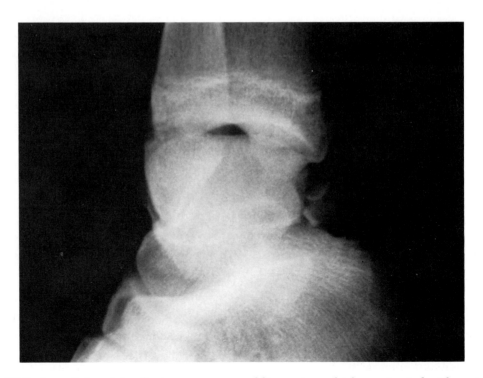

Fig. 23-3. A medial avulsion fracture seen on an oblique view which was treated with excision.

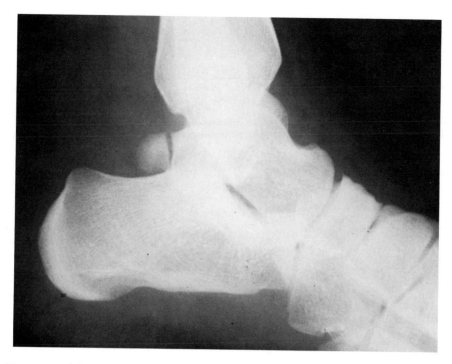

Fig. 23-4. Fractures of the posterior process of the talus are distinguished from an os trigonum by their tilting and irregularity.

FRACTURES OF THE TALAR HEAD

The rare fractures of the talar head result from a longitudinal force while the foot is plantar flexed. Coltart reported these fractures to occur when a fully plantar-flexed foot is violently dorsiflexed, as in an airplane crash with the foot on the rudder pedal.[2] Also, an impact to a completely dorsiflexed foot compresses the talar head against the anterior tibial lip, fracturing the head. Usually the medial portion of the talar head is fractured without displacement. Immobilization for 4 to 6 weeks in a short leg weight-bearing cast is usually adequate. Open reduction with internal fixation is necessary in the rare instances of displacement, larger fragments with slight comminution, or symptomatic nonunions (Fig. 23-5). Persistent symptomatic small fragments of bone in the talonavicular joint may be excised. Posttraumatic arthritis of the joint may occur, and an isolated talonavicular joint arthrodesis is warranted if symptoms are severe.

FRACTURES OF THE BODY OF THE TALUS

Fractures of the body of the talus account for approximately 10 to 20 percent of talar fractures.[11–13] These are classified as nondisplaced, displaced, and comminuted. The mechanism of these injuries is severe dorsiflexion with or without a compressive force. This usually occurs with a fall from a height or the force that is produced as the foot strikes the floorboard of an automobile during a motor vehicle accident. Vigilance must be exercised in ruling out other lower extremity, hip, or thoracolumbar injuries in these patients.

Nondisplaced Body Fractures

Radiographs may not reveal the full extent of nondisplaced talar body fractures. CT is extremely helpful in determining the extent of the tibiotalar and talocalcaneal joint involvement

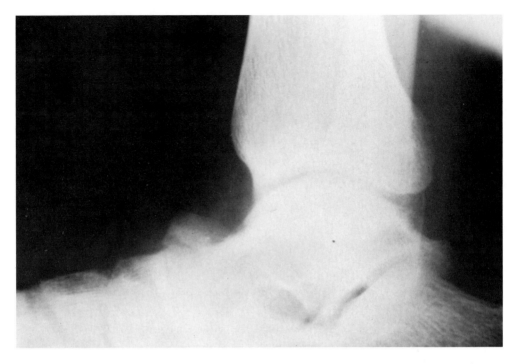

Fig. 23-5. A displaced talar head fracture that extends into the talonavicular joint. Open reduction with internal fixation is required in this injury.

(Fig. 23-6). Nondisplaced fractures through the body of the talus should be immobilized for 6 to 8 weeks in a short-leg non-weight-bearing cast (Fig. 23-7). The consensus of reports from the literature is that the incidence of avascular necrosis in nondisplaced body fractures is low.[13,14] Figure 23-8A reveals another vertical, nondisplaced talar body fracture that healed without incident. The rationale for the percutaneous pinning is discussed in the next section.

Displaced Body Fractures

Displaced fractures of the body of the talus usually require open reduction with rigid internal fixation. However, acceptable results have been achieved with manipulation and closed reduction in some cases. If post-traumatic swelling is significant, a Jones compression dressing should be utilized initially. Immobilization consists of a well-molded short leg non-weight-bearing cast with the foot held in neutral or slight equinus for 6 to 8 weeks. At this time, if radiographs show evidence of early osseous union, weight bearing is permitted in a short leg cast for 6 to 8 additional weeks. If no healing is seen radiographically, the non-weight-bearing immobilization should be continued for 6 to 8 weeks.

The two factors most affecting the ultimate results are the amount of initial displacement and the anatomic accuracy of reduction. Long-term results are less favorable with severe injury. If closed reduction of the fracture fails, an anatomic reduction must be achieved through surgical intervention. The approach is best accomplished through an anteromedial incision. An osteotomy of the medial malleolus is potentially necessary to visualize and manipulate the fragments. The talar body fracture is fixed with large pins or cancellous lag screws. The malleolar osteotomy is fixated with malleolar screws, as dictated by the size and angle of the osteotomy. Initial postoperative swelling is reduced with a Jones compression dressing. The foot is immobilized in a short leg non-weight-bearing cast for 6 to 8 weeks with

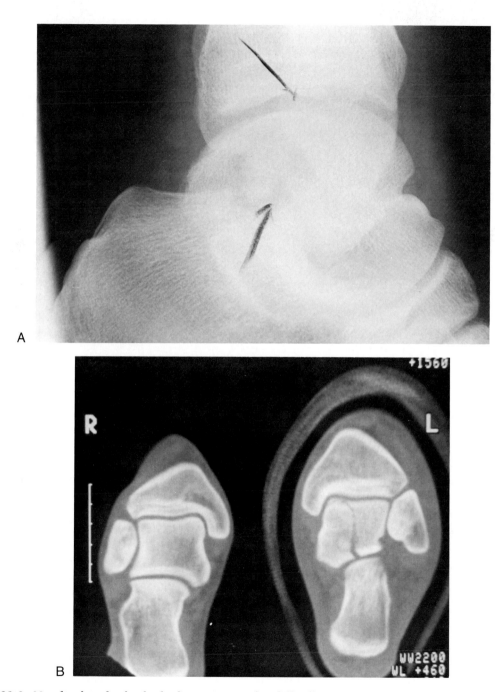

Fig. 23-6. Nondisplaced talar body fractures may be difficult to visualize on plain radiographs. CT scanning is useful to determine the articular involvement. (**A**) Lateral plain radiograph. (**B**) CT scan.

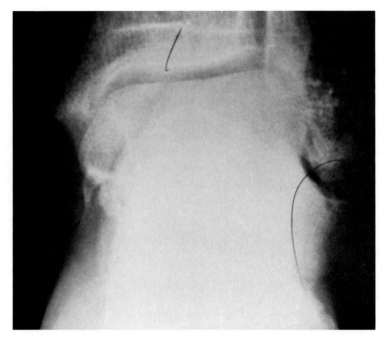

Fig. 23-7. Eight weeks of short leg non-weight-bearing immobilization healed this nondisplaced body fracture that extended into the tibiotalar joint. A lateral process fracture (stage I, nondisplaced) is also present.

the foot in slight equinus. At this time, if radiographs reveal early osseous union, weight bearing is permitted in a short leg cast for an additional 4 to 6 weeks. However, if healing is not evident, non-weight bearing is continued for 6 to 8 additional weeks or until the union is radiographically demonstrated.

Complications of displaced talar body fractures include avascular necrosis and post-traumatic arthritis of the tibiotalar and the subtalar joints. Avascular necrosis of the talus occurs in fewer than 50 percent of the patients whose talar body remains in the ankle mortise. This is contrast with almost 100 percent occurrence of avascular necrosis with posterior talar body dislocation.[15,16] Treatment of avascular necrosis is discussed under the section on complications of talar neck fractures. Treatment of post-traumatic arthritis may include nonsteroidal anti-inflammatory drugs, orthoses to limit subtalar joint motion, cortisone injections, and possible arthrodesis of the affected joint.

An illustrative case is demonstrated in Figure 23-8. This 19-year-old woman fell from a second story window, landing on both heels and suffering bilateral talar fractures. Since difficulty was expected in compliance with the bilateral non-weight-bearing status necessary for 3 months, the left nondisplaced fracture was percutaneously pinned to allow partial weight-bearing. This permitted the severely displaced comminuted right talar body fracture to remain totally non-weight bearing. The intraoperative radiograph (Fig. 23-8B) reveals the position of the percutaneously placed trial pins. Only two pins remained for the final fixation. The right talus (Fig. 23-8C), resisted attempts at closed reduction. A large osteochondral fragment, approximately one-fourth of the talar dome (Fig. 23-8D) had been driven into the body of the talus, thus preventing reduction. Once this was removed, the body fracture was easily reduced with two 4.0-mm cancellous lag screws (Fig. 23-8E). The large osteochondritic fragment, a vital portion of the articular surface,

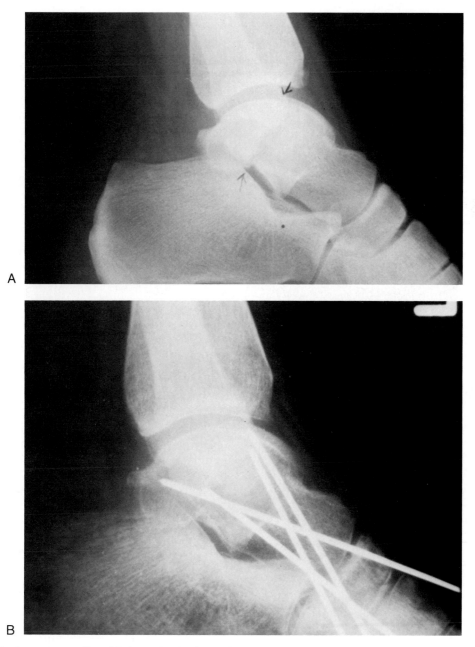

Fig. 23-8. A patient suffered bilateral talar body fractures. (**A**) The nondisplaced body fracture of the left talus. (**B**) Intraoperative radiography of the percutaneously placed pins. (*Figure continues.*)

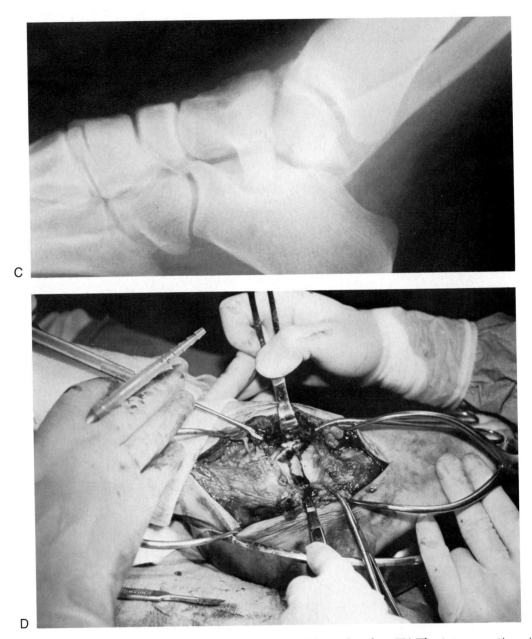

Fig. 23-8 (*Continued*). (**C**) The displaced body fracture of the right talus. (**D**) The interoperative view shows the impaction of the large dome osteochondral fracture into the displaced body fracture. This prevented closed reduction (lateral view of the right foot with the digits to the right). (*Figure continues.*)

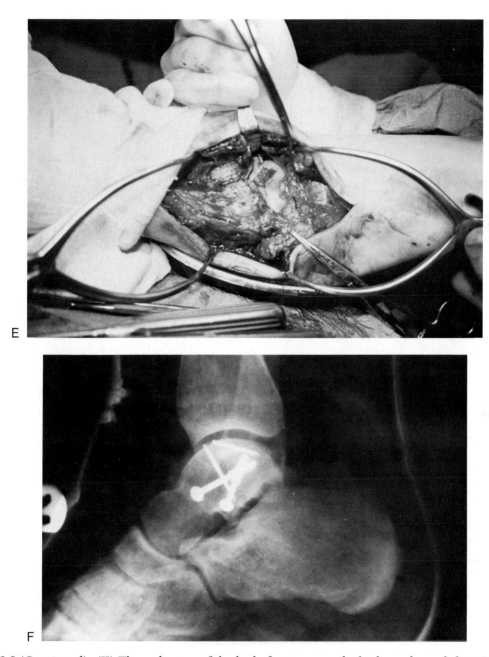

Fig. 23-8 (*Continued*). (**E**) The reduction of the body fracture reveals the large dome defect. (**F**) The postreduction radiograph shows the restoration of talar anatomy with rigid internal fixation. (*Figure continues.*)

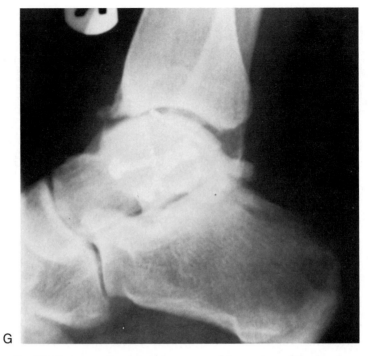

G

Fig. 23-8 (*Continued*). (**G**) Degenerative joint changes and loosening of the hardware are seen 2 years after reduction.

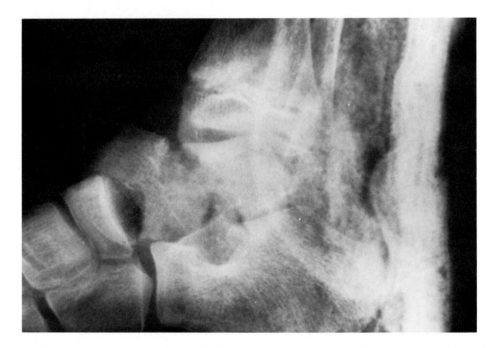

Fig. 23-9. A severely comminuted talar body fracture destroys the general morphology of the talus. The body height is diminished and all of the surrounding articulations are disrupted. This also exemplifies a type IV neck fracture.

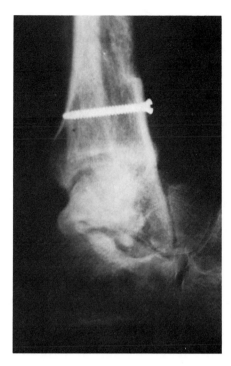 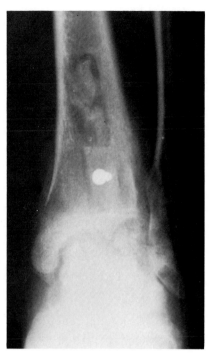

Fig. 23-10. A modified Blair fusion is utilized for a comminuted talar body fracture with avascular necrosis.

was replaced, using Smillie nails (Richards Manufacturing Co., Inc., Memphis, TN) (Fig. 23-8F). The right side was kept non-weight bearing for 3 months. Early passive and active range of motion exercises were initiated at 4 weeks to aid in fibrocartilaginous remodeling of the talar dome. The osteochondritic chip survived and avascular necrosis did not occur. Radiographs 2 years postoperatively revealed early degenerative changes of the ankle joint, as well as loosening of the hardware (Fig. 23-8G). The joint was surgically debrided and the hardware was removed at that time. The patient remains asymptomatic 7 years following the trauma.

Comminuted Fractures

A severely comminuted talar body fracture is accompanied by a poor prognosis for a normally functioning ankle joint mortise (Fig. 23-9). The cartilaginous surface of the talar dome is irre-pairably shattered, and poor long-term results are reported by many clinicians.[12,14,16–18] Initial management should include a compression dressing, ice, elevation, and non-weight bearing for 3 to 4 weeks. At that time, operative intervention is indicated, but controversy exists in the literature as to what surgical procedure should be performed. The results of a talectomy alone are disappointing and include persistent pain, edema, instability, and powerless propulsion.[13,19] A tibiocalcaneal fusion is recommended by most investigators to obtain a stable functioning unit.[12,16–18] Blair described excising the comminuted body fragments and fusing the tibia to the remaining head and neck of the talus, with an anterior sliding bone graft[17] (Fig. 23-10). Fusion of the ankle joint is recommended because the foot remains plantigrade and the major limb shortening encountered in direct tibiocalcaneal fusion is avoided. This fusion allows some flexion and extension of the foot on the leg. Dennis and Tyllos found that most patients after Blair arthrodeisis had approximately 20 degrees of apparent ankle joint motion, originating in the anterior and middle facets of the subtalar joint.[20] Additional motion occurred at the midtarsal joint, facilitating a functional gait pattern. However, this procedure cannot be performed if there is significant loss or total collapse of the talar body. The ankle joint fusion is performed by denuding the cartilaginous surfaces and fixating the joint with rigid internal hardware or external compression devices. The postoperative care for either procedure is 12 to 16 weeks of non-weight-bearing immobilization, until osseous union is achieved as assessed radiographically.

NECK FRACTURES

Talar neck fractures are common, second only to chip and avulsion fractures. In 1919, Anderson reported on 18 cases of fracture dislocations of the talus, and coined the term aviator's astragalus.[1] Fractures of the talar neck are usually caused by tremendous force, such as that involved in motor vehicle accidents, aircraft accidents, and falls from heights. The commonly accepted mechanism of marked ankle joint dorsiflexion with talar neck impingment across the anterior margin of the tibia may be erroneous. The demonstrated lack of damage to this region and the concave column tali lend credence to experiments in which ankle joint motion was blocked.[19,21] With the talus fixed between the tibia and calcaneus, typical neck fractures were produced with a forceful blow to the sole of the foot.[22] Whatever the mechanism, talar neck fractures are associated with disabling long-term effects, notably avascular necrosis of the talar body secondary to severe disruption of the blood supply.

Various schemes for classification of talar neck fractures have been proposed in the literature. The most functional seems to be that of Hawkins,[15] who modified that of Coltart,[2] with an addition by Canale and Kelly[23] (Fig. 23-11).

Type I: A vertical fracture through the talar neck without displacement. Possibly only the blood supply of the neck is disrupted.

Type II: A vertical fracture through the neck with subtalar joint subluxation or dislocation, but no dislocation from the tibial talar joint. At least two of the three sources of blood (talar neck and tarsal canal) are disrupted.

Type III: A vertical fracture of the talar neck with displacement of the talar body from both the subtalar and tibiotalar joints. All three sources of blood supply are disrupted.

Type IV: A vertical fracture of the neck with talar body displacement from subtalar and tibiotalar joints and subluxation or dislocation of the talar head from the talonavicular joint. All three sources of blood supply again are disrupted.

This classification can be criticized for its failure to differentiate slight subluxation from frank dislocation of the subtalar and tibiotalar joints or to recognize a transient subluxation that reduces itself prior to radiographic assessment. However, this classification scheme is useful in order to predict the possibility of future avascular necrosis. Type 1 fractures occur in approximately 20 percent of the cases, type II in approximately 42 percent, type III in 34 percent, and type IV in 4 percent in most of the reported series.[12,15,23,24] To some extent, all types of talar neck fracture-dislocations threaten the vulnerable blood supply. The greater the displacement, the greater the destruction of the vascular supply and the higher the incidence of avascular necrosis.

Type I fractures require simple immobilization in a short leg, non-weight-bearing cast until osseous union occurs, usually in 6 to 8 weeks (Fig. 23-12). Nonunion has not been reported, and avascular necrosis is rare. Such cases may represent type II fractures that have spontaneously reduced after disrupting talar blood supply.

With type II, III, and IV neck fractures, closed reduction is routinely attempted initially. A reduction that shows less than 5 mm of displacement or less than 5 degrees of malalignment is deemed adequate. However, surgical reduction is generally necessary to obtain accurate anatomic alignment. The commonly encountered compound talar neck fracture demands special treatment, including debridement and meticulous wound care.

The type II fractures involving subtalar joint

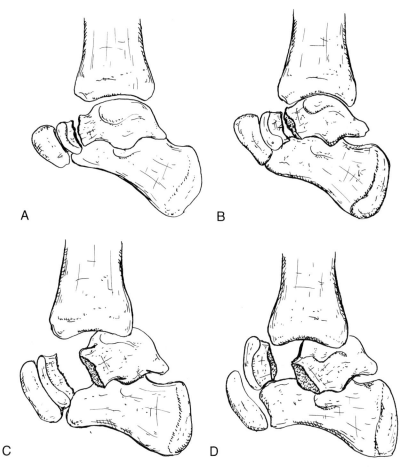

Fig. 23-11. Classification of talar neck fractures. **(A)** Type I. **(B)** Type II. **(C)** Type III. **(D)** Type IV.

dislocation should be reduced immediately under general or spinal anesthesia to ensure muscle relaxation. In anterior subtalar joint dislocation, the talar body is in equinus (Fig. 23-13). Manipulation is performed with traction in equinus with posterior displacement of the foot. In lateral subtalar joint dislocation, the foot is displaced laterally and the head and neck of the talus appear to be prominent medially. The calcaneus will slip under the talus if the foot is brought into adduction. A long leg well-padded cast is applied, and immediate radiographs are obtained. A special anteroposterior projection of the foot in pronation, as described by Canale and Kelly,[23] detects varus angulation of the talar head, or offset in the neck. Repeat radiographs are recommended at 2, 7, and 14 days after reduction, as the potential for redisplacement of the fracture exists.

When the above-described treatment fails to reduce a type II fracture, open reduction is indicated. A medial approach with osteotomy of the malleolus is preferred to disruption of the deltoid ligament. Meticulous care must be taken during soft tissue dissection to avoid disrupting the deltoid vascular supply to the medial talar body. The subtalar joint dislocation is first stabilized with Kirschner wires, and the neck fracture should be anatomically reduced with cancellous compression screws (Fig. 23-14). Avascular necrosis is seen more commonly in fractures in which surgical reduction has been performed, owing to the soft tissue dissection, but less commonly when secure fixation is achieved[24] (Fig. 23-15). A short leg non-weight-bearing cast is applied for 8 to 12 weeks, or until the fracture healing is successfully demonstrated radiographically.

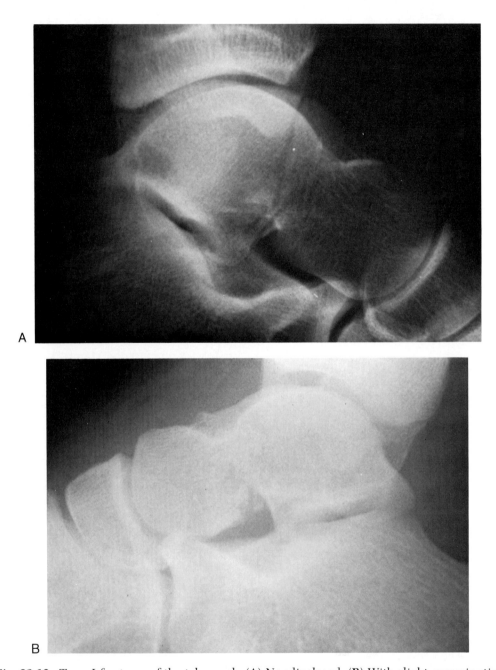

Fig. 23-12. Type I fractures of the talar neck. (**A**) Nondisplaced. (**B**) With slight comminution.

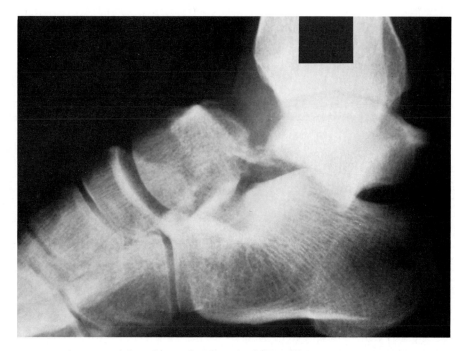

Fig. 23-13. Type II fracture of the talar neck. The talar body is in equinus with an anterior subtalar joint dislocation.

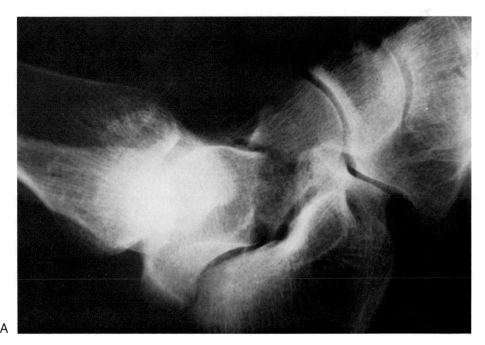

A

Fig. 23-14. (**A**) An adequate anatomic reduction of a type II talar neck fracture with suboptimal fixation. (*Figure continues*).

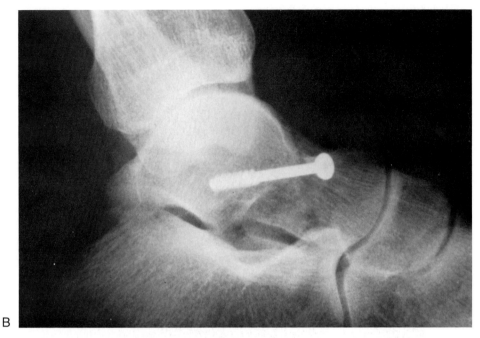

B

Fig. 23-14 (*Continued*). **(B)** An additional cancellous screw or Kirschner wire would provide more stability.

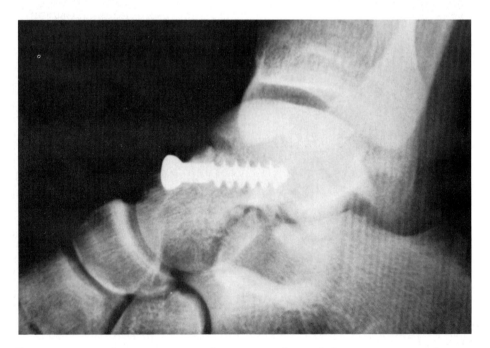

Fig. 23-15. Inappropriate fixation is seen in this type II talar neck fracture. Proper technique requires two lag screws with threads not crossing the fracture site. However, this talus healed without avascular necrosis.

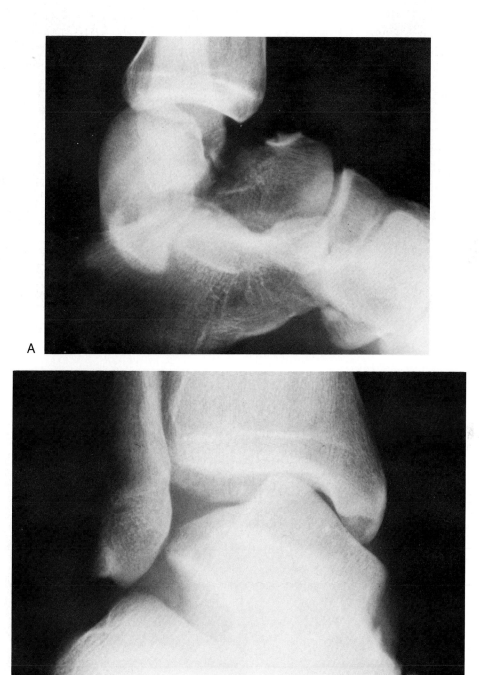

Fig. 23-16. A type III talar neck fracture occurring with a posterior rotation of the talar body from the ankle mortise. **(A)** Lateral view. **(B)** Anteroposterior view. (*Figure continues.*)

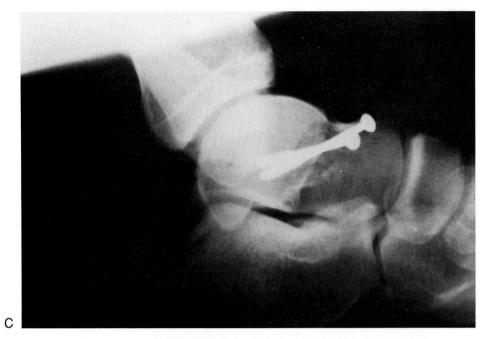

C

Fig. 23-16 (*Continued*). (**C**) Lateral view after open reduction with internal fixation.

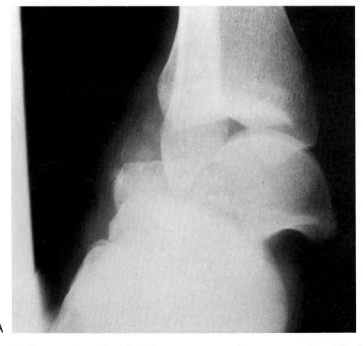

A

Fig. 23-17. A type III fracture associated with a neurovascular compromise. The body has rotated medially, and produced an impingement on the posterior tibial artery and nerve, which was relieved by fracture reduction. (**A**) Anteroposterior view. (*Figure continues.*)

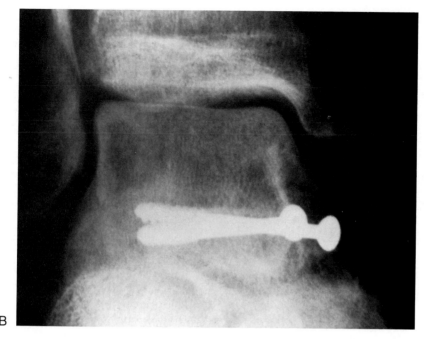

B

Fig. 23-17 (*Continued*). (**B**) Postreduction (8 weeks) anteroposterior view without signs of avascular necrosis.

Type III fractures are associated with massive disruption of the blood supply in the branches of the deltoid ligament, as well as the neck. The talar body is usually dislocated posteriorly and medially, with intact medial soft tissue. The lateral soft tissues are usually torn or stretched. The body of the talus may rotate and be located between the posterior surface of the tibia and Achilles tendon (Fig. 23-16). The posterior tibial neurovascular bundle usually escapes direct injury, but can be contused and occasionally may thrombose, resulting in gangrene distally. Persistent nerve injury can also occur with this dislocation (Fig. 23-17). Immediate closed reduction is usually attempted, but most often open reduction is necessary. A transverse heavy Kirschner wire through the calcaneus is used for distal traction to allow reduction of the talar body into the ankle mortise. The medial subtalar joint dislocation should be reduced by applying distal traction to the forefoot and a lateral force to the calcaneus with the foot in equinus. The talar neck fracture is aligned, temporarily stabilized with pins, and fixed with cancellous lag screws. The foot is then

immobilized in equinus with a long leg non-weight-bearing cast for 10 to 12 weeks.

Type IV talar neck fractures were first described by Canale and Kelly in 1978.[23] In this category, the talar neck fracture is associated not only with the dislocation of the body from the ankle and subtalar joints, but with an additional dislocation of the head of the talus from the talonavicular joint as well (Fig. 23-9). In their series, the incidence of this type of fracture was found to be 4.2 percent. Type IV fractures require reduction and temporary fixation of the talonavicular joint, in addition to the maneuvers described for type III fractures.

COMPLICATIONS

Talar fractures may be complicated by postreduction avascular necrosis, malunion, traumatic arthritis, and deep infections. In most series, type I fractures had an incidence of avascular necrosis of less than 15 percent. The occurrence of avascular necrosis in type II fractures ranges from 15 percent in Peterson and colleagues' study[24] to 50 percent in the study by Canale and Kelly.[23] Most patients have subsequent problems related to talocalcaneal and tibiotalar joint arthritis, rather than to the collapse of the body of the talus. Degenerative arthritis of the subtalar joint was reported in 80 percent of patients with type II talar neck fractures.

Type III and type IV fractures had the poorest long-term results, primarily because of a 90 to 100 percent incidence of avascular necrosis. Hawkins' sign, a subchondral radiolucency, is apparent on the anteroposterior view of the ankle (out of plaster 6 to 8 weeks after reduction) when no avascular necrosis is present (Fig. 23-18). Hawkins postulated that this was caused by disuse osteopenia or vascular congestion, which suggested maintenance of blood supply to the talar body. This can be a reliable indicator, but absence of the sign does not necessarily suggest that avascular necrosis will occur. A more timely method of predicting avascular necrosis is provided by the technetium 99 bone scan. Utilizing a pinhole collimator, a bone scan performed at 48 hours post-trauma will provide a reliable assess-

ment of blood supply to the talar body. If no uptake is seen in the posterior body of the talus, one may assume that avascular necrosis may occur and precautions should be taken to prevent talar body collapse. When a repeat bone scan at 5 to 6 weeks post-trauma shows no evidence of avascular necrosis, some investigators recommend allowing weight-bearing without fear of further talar injury. Magnetic resonance imaging is currently utilized in assessing the potential for avascular necrosis of the femoral head. This technique assesses the viable fat content within the bone. In the future, this technique may also be utilized in analyzing the talus. Avascular necrosis of the talar body appears as increased density on plain radiographs 6 to 8 weeks following talar trauma (Fig. 23-19). Regardless of method, once the diagnosis of avascular necrosis is made, the patient must be kept totally non-weight bearing for an average of 8 months to prevent catastrophic talar body collapse. A patellar tendon brace with partial weight bearing is considered superior to unprotected weight bearing.

Many researchers recommend definitive initial procedures for treatment of type III and type IV fractures in attempt to prevent avascular necro-

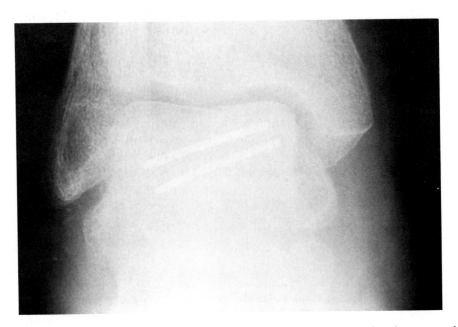

Fig. 23-18. Hawkins' sign occurs when *no* avascular necrosis is present. Hawkins' sign is only present in the lateral dome; the medial fragment has avascular necrosis.

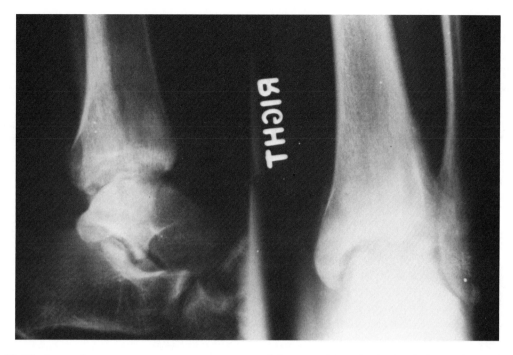

Fig. 23-19. Avascular necrosis appears as an increased density of the talar body of plain radiographs 6 to 8 weeks after talar trauma.

sis. These range from primary subtalar fusion or ankle fusion to pantalar arthrodesis in an attempt to revascularize the talar body. However, recent studies have shown these procedures to be less than satisfactory.[16,23] With protection against talar collapse by prolonged non-weight bearing, revascularization develops slowly. Even in the presence of avascular necrosis, a satisfactory result is therefore achievable.

Malunion of these fractures with dorsal or varus angulation of the talar neck was noted in 25 percent of the patients in Canale and Kelly's study.[23] This occurred most often with closed reduction. If malunions are symptomatic, dorsal talar neck exostectomies or triple arthrodesis are performed. The most common cause of degenerative arthritis of the ankle following talar neck fractures appears to be avascular necrosis. Degenerative arthritis of the subtalar joint was also a common finding. Arthrodesis of the tibiotalar joint for treatment of arthritis is acceptable, except when subtalar joint arthritis is evident. A triple arthrodesis is satisfactory for localized talocalcaneal joint arthritis without ankle joint in-

volvement. When both the tibiotalar and subtalar joints are symptomatic, a tibiocalcaneal fusion is recommended. Compound fractures of the talus and surgically reduced fractures may occasionally become infected. Meticulous surgical technique and appropriate debridement can lessen the incidence of infection. However, chronic osteomyelitis is best treated by resecting all infected bone and performing an ankle, subtalar, or tibiocalcaneal arthrodesis. Occasionally, an amputation may be necessary as a salvage procedure for this serious sequela.

OSTEOCHONDRAL FRACTURES OF THE TALAR DOME

Transchondral fractures of the dome of the talus are produced by jamming it against the tibial plafond. These injuries are commonly overlooked since they are often associated with other gross disruptions of the malleoli or soft tissue injuries. These fractures were first described in

1932 by Rendu.[25] Berndt and Harty described the mechanism of injury and classified the fractures according to the degree of displacement.[26] In their series, 43 percent of the fractures were located on the lateral portion of the dome, usually on the middle one-third. Fifty-seven percent occurred on the medial dome, usually in the posterior area. In their cadaver limb experiments, they demonstrated that the lateral lesions were caused by inversion and strong dorsiflexion. The medial lesion was caused by inversion, plantar flexion, and external rotation of the leg on the talus.

These fractures are classified as follows[26]: (Fig. 23-20) Stage I is a small area of subchondral bone compression. Stage II is a partially detached osteochondral fragment (Fig. 23-21). Stage III is a completely detached osteochondral fragment remaining in its crater (Figs. 23-22 and 23-23). Stage IV is a displaced osteochondral fragment, or one that is inverted in its crater (Fig. 23-24).

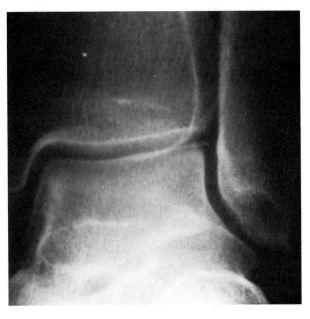

Fig. 23-21. A lateral stage II fracture of the talar dome.

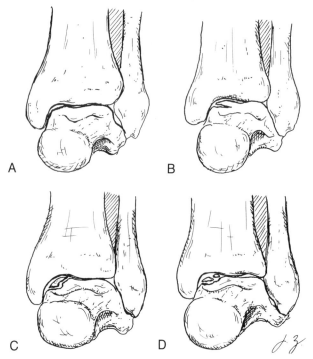

Fig. 23-20. Classification of osteochondral fractures of the talar dome. **(A)** Stage I. **(B)** Stage II. **(C)** Stage III. **(D)** Stage IV.

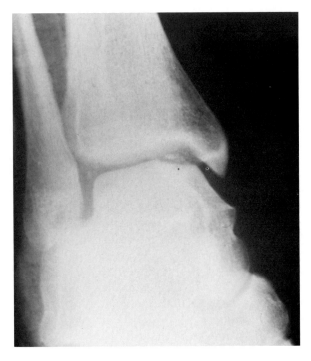

Fig. 23-22. A medial stage III fracture of the talar dome.

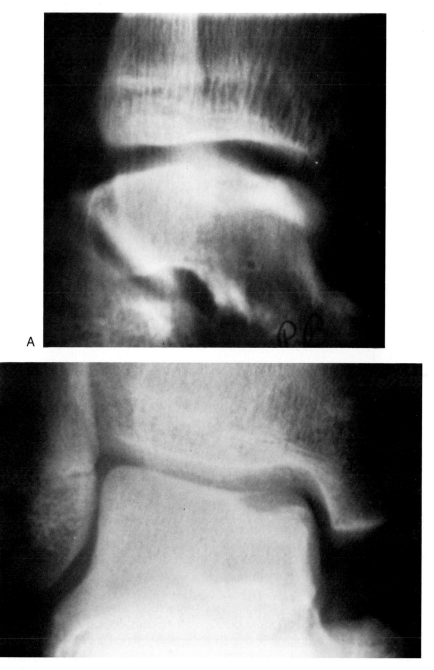

Fig. 23-23. A medial stage III lesion whose exact location is determined by tomography. (**A**) Anteroposterior and (**B**) lateral views.

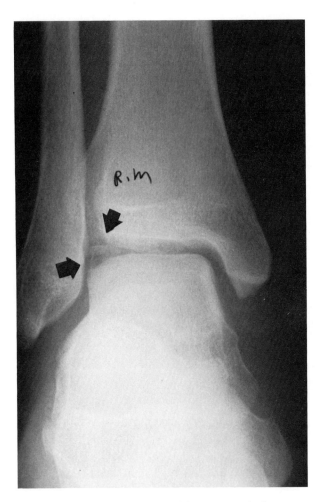

Fig. 23-24. A lateral stage IV fracture with fragment dislocation. (From Silvani,[36] with permission.)

If initially missed, these lesions may progress to a chronic, more symptomatic stage. Since the fracture may be initially difficult to visualize, meticulous radiography must be employed in those suspect injuries. Additionally, stress views, arthrograms, air-contrast tomography, CT, and MRI will help delineate the dome defect, extent, and exact location. Arthroscopic examination will help in staging the lesion, as well as offering the potential for excision or debridement. There is a noted lack of correlation between the radiographic appearance of the lesions and the quality of the articular cartilage overlying them as visualized by arthroscopy.[27]

Correct staging and early definitive treatment will prevent most future complications. Inosculation is inhibited by motion at the fracture site. If immobilization is inadequate, the fracture may proceed to delayed union or an established nonunion. Osteoarthritic changes may develop, and a painful ankle joint ensues.

Following the recommendations of Berndt and Harty[26] and Canale and Belding[28] stage I and II and medial stage III lesions should be initially treated by conservative means. A short leg non-weight-bearing cast is applied until radiographic evidence of osseous union is seen, usually after 8 to 12 weeks. Lateral stage III and medial and lateral stage IV lesions should be treated through surgical intervention.

Lateral lesions can usually be reached by anterolateral arthrotomy (Fig. 23-25). A fibular osteotomy may be necessary to obtain adequate visualization. Predrilling and insertion and then retraction of a self-tapping screw into the fibula will aid in later fixation of this osteotomy. Some medial lesions can be resected by arthrotomy alone with the foot in extreme plantar flexion, but most require a similar osteotomy in the medial malleolus. Joint inspection should be meticulous. A probe is used to palpate the talar dome for softness, depression, or color variations that indicate the location of the fracture. Large fractures may be reduced utilizing subchondral fixation (Smillie nails). Small lesions are treated by excision of the fragment, curettage of the subchondral bed, and drilling of holes into the cancellous bone to stimulate revascularization.

For those patients treated by simple arthrotomy, curettage, and drilling, it is advisable to begin early range of motion and partial weight bearing at 2 weeks. Full weight bearing is allowed at 6 to 8 weeks. Patients with malleolar osteotomy require bony union (approximately 6 weeks) until weight bearing, but passive and active range of motion is allowed at 2 weeks. Patients with internal fixation of the dome fracture require total non-weight bearing until osseous union is demonstrated radiographically (8 to 12 weeks).

An arthroscopic examination provides treatment for these lesions with much less morbidity than the traditional arthrotomy and considerably less disability than utilizing a malleolar osteot-

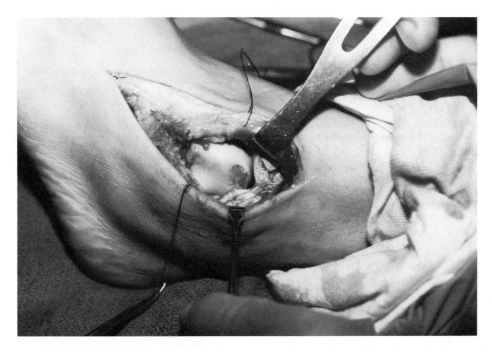

Fig. 23-25. A lateral ankle arthrotomy visualizes a stage III fracture (postdebridement). (From Silvani,[36] with permission.)

omy. The arthroscopic examination is done under local or general anesthesia, utilizing a pneumatic tourniquet. The technical details of arthroscopy of the ankle are described elsewhere in this text. The arthroscopic and not the radiographic appearance of the lesions should determine treatment. If the overlying cartilage is firm and of normal appearance, the lesion can be treated simply by restriction of the patient's activity until symptoms disappear. If the cartilage is frayed, the lesion should be treated by curettage and drilling. Arthroscopy also provides an excellent method for removal of loose bodies such as displaced stage IV osteochondral fractures. Postoperatively, the limb is elevated for 24 hours, after which full weight bearing is allowed and range of motion exercises are begun. The immediate relief of symptoms as reported by some patients after arthroscopic surgery may be falsely optimistic. It is probably due to lavage of the joint. Although some patients experienced continued relief of symptoms, other patients reported recurrence of minimal symptoms. Alexander and Lichtman reported that gradual improvement can be expected for as long as 18 months postoperatively.[29] However, the ultimate efficacy of this procedure in preventing late arthritic conditions has not yet been documented.

Unfortunately, since this lesion is often missed initially, there is much clinical evidence that if it is left untreated, degenerative arthritis will develop. The degree of degenerative changes varies according to the size and location of the lesion, body weight, activity level, and associated ligamentous laxity.

DISLOCATION OF SUBTALAR AND MIDTARSAL JOINTS

Peritalar dislocation occurs when there is combined dislocation of the talonavicular and talocalcaneal joints, usually with preservation of the tibiotalar relationship. The causative factor is usually torsional forces incurred with falls from a height or automobile and motorcycle accidents.

These injuries are classified by the direction taken by the foot in relation to the talus.

Medial Dislocations

Medial dislocation is the most commonly reported peritalar dislocation in the literature.[2,30–33] A severe inversion force causes disruption of the talonavicular joint and rotatory subluxation of the talocalcaneal joint. The talar head now faces laterally and the calcaneus is displaced medially. Concomitant fractures of the malleoli, talar body margins, fifth metatarsal, and navicular must be excluded.

An example of this type of medial peritalar dislocation is seen in Figure 23-26. This patient's inverted foot was rammed against a car's firewall during a rear-end auto collision. The talus was dislocated to the lateral side from the talonavicular and talocalcaneal joints.

Reduction is done immediately under total muscle relaxation provided by general or spinal anesthesia. With the leg stabilized proximally, the foot is distracted, then pronated, abducted, and dorsiflexed. If this fails to relocate the talus, open reduction must be performed. Impaction of the talar head onto the lateral side of the navicular, buttonholing of the talar head through the extensor retinaculum, or entrapment by the peroneal tendons may prevent reduction. Through the lateral approach, the talus is gently levered into its normal anatomic relationship with the navicular with concomitant reduction of the talocalcaneal joint. Internal fixation is rarely necessary because the reduction is usually anatomically stable. Traditionally, the foot is immobilized in a short leg non-weight-bearing cast for 6 weeks. Current trends in treatment confirm McKeever's findings that early, limited ambulation prevents subtalar joint stiffness.[16] Therefore, 2 weeks of nonweight-bearing immobilization are followed by 4 weeks of weight bearing in a cast.

Lateral Dislocation

In lateral dislocations, the foot is everted and the head of the talus is forced through the ta-

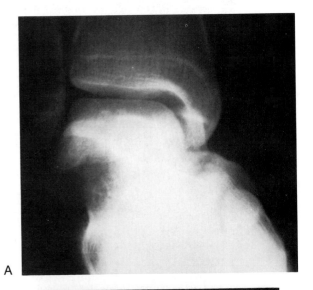

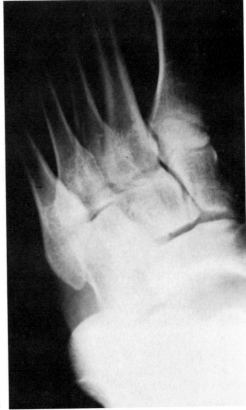

Fig. 23-26. A compound medial peritalar dislocation that occurred in a motor vehicle accident. **(A)** Anteroposterior ankle radiograph demonstrating the maintenance of the tibiotalar joint with the foot dislocated medially. **(B)** Anteroposterior foot radiograph shows the talar head protruding laterally (through the skin laceration). (*Figure continues.*)

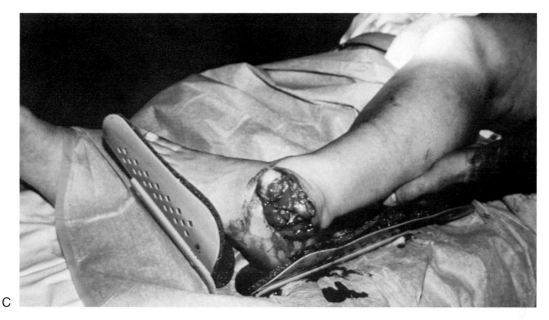

C

Fig. 23-26 (*Continued*). (**C**) Clinical photograph showing the peroneal tendons wrapped medially around the talar head, thus preventing reduction. (Courtesy of Barry L. Scurran, D.P.M.)

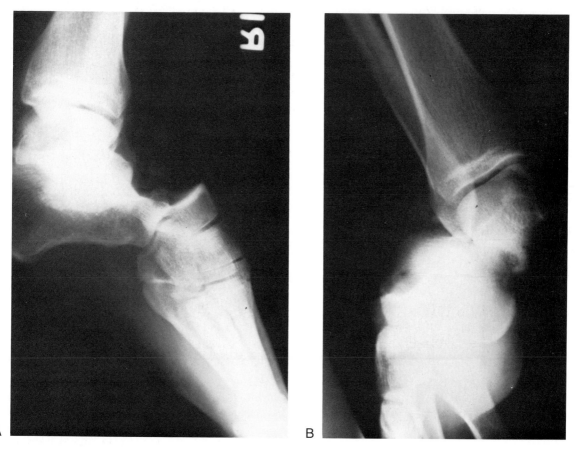

A

B

Fig. 23-27. A lateral peritalar dislocation with the talar head protruding medially through the talonavicular joint capsule. (**A**) Lateral and (**B**) anterior views.

lonavicular joint capsule medially. The calcaneus dislocates laterally (Fig. 23-27).

General or spinal anesthesia is again induced for total muscle relaxation. Distal traction and gentle manipulation of the talus with the foot in pronation should allow reduction. If reduction fails, soft tissue interposition must be suspected.

Usually, the posterior tibial muscle or the flexor digitorum longus is wrapped laterally around the talar neck. Bohler's reported method of maximally dorsiflexing and plantar flexing the foot may free the tendon from the talar neck.[23] If this fails, open reduction is performed through an anterolateral incision. The subtalar and midtarsal

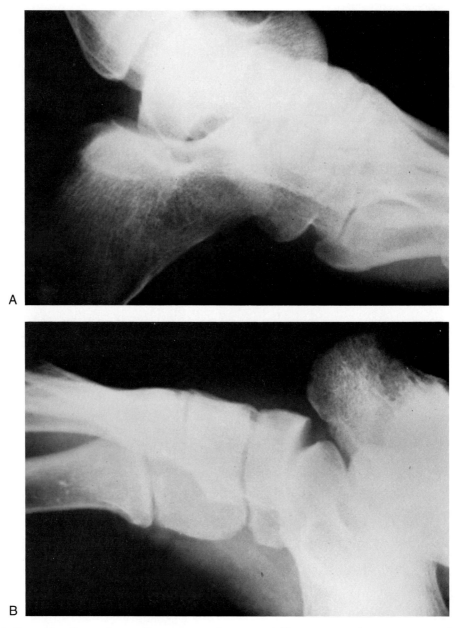

A

B

Fig. 23-28. Lateral radiographs are diagnostic in these two different cases of posterior peritalar dislocations. **(A)** Closed reduction. **(B)** Needed open reduction owing to extensive soft tissue interposition.

joints are easily exposed, all interposed soft tissue is removed, and the talus is repositioned. The foot is immobilized for 2 weeks in a non-weight-bearing short-leg cast, followed by 4 weeks of weight bearing in a cast.

Posterior Dislocation

Posterior dislocation is rare and may occur as the result of a fall from a height onto an outstretched foot in the plantar-flexed position. Dislocation is best visualized on a lateral radiograph, and the posterior tubercule of the talus should be closely examined for fractures (Fig. 23-28).

Closed reduction under general or spinal anesthesia is initiated by plantar flexion of the foot to release the talar neck from the dorsal margin of the navicular. The calcaneus is pulled distally and the foot is moved dorsally. If this fails, open reduction is performed through a lateral incision to restore the talar relationships. Again, the foot is immobilized in a short leg non-weight-bearing cast for 2 weeks, followed by 4 weeks of weight bearing in a cast.

Anterior Dislocation

Anterior dislocation also occurs with falls from heights. Lateral radiographs are usually diagnostic and closed reduction is attempted under general or spinal anesthesia. Distal traction frees the posterior aspect of the calcaneus from the talar sulcus. The foot is manipulated posteriorly to obtain the reduction. As with all such reductions, a radiograph should be obtained in the operating room to assess the accuracy of the reduction. A short leg cast should be applied for 6 weeks, with weight bearing allowed for the last 4 weeks. Satisfactory results are usually achieved with definitive early care. Delaying reduction can lead to skin necrosis and neurovascular compromise of the foot. Avascular necrosis is rare, secondary only to the loss of the blood supply in the tarsal canal. Peritalar arthritis with pain, stiffness, and prolonged edema are common. This is best treated initially with conservative methods, and if no relief is obtained, a triple arthrodesis is indicated.

TOTAL DISLOCATION OF THE TALUS

Total talar dislocation is complete extrusion of the talus from the surrounding joints. This rare injury is serious and difficult to manage owing to the extensive skin pressure from the massive edema, direct skin slough from displaced bone, and impending neurovascular compromise.[34,35] Infection and almost certain avascular necrosis are frequent complications.

This injury demands immediate reduction for relief of pressure on the deep neurovascular structures and soft tissues. Closed manipulation should be attempted in those total dislocations that are closed initially. Additional aid for distraction of the area can be provided by placing large Steinmann pins transversely through the calcaneus and distal tibia to allow distraction in an attempt to relocate the talus.

Extension of the compounding wound in open dislocations will afford access to the talus. Skeletal traction distally and proximally aids in replacing the bone. Thorough debridement and meticulous wound toilet are mandatory. The scarcity of soft tissue that can be debrided and still provide adequate coverage for deep structures adds to the difficulty of treating these problems. If possible, capsular repair to provide coverage will aid in preventing subsequent infection. If the joint capsule can be closed, delayed primary closure of the skin wound may minimize necrosis and slough. If the skin can be closed primarily, deep drainage with outflow suction will prevent formation of a hematoma. This will aid in reduction of postoperative edema and the likelihood of infection.

An example of a total talar dislocation can be seen in Figure 23-29. This injury was suffered by a young gymnast while working on a trampoline. He broke through the cloth and hit the underlying floor with sufficient force to completely extrude the talus through the anterior ankle joint. When he was seen in the emergency room, the talus was lying in a bursting-type anterior laceration with wound edges that appeared to be ischemic. Open reduction was performed, and the talus was repositioned with pins. Continuous el-

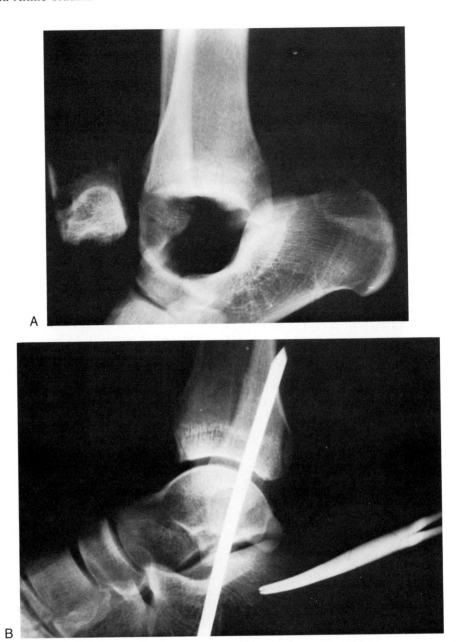

Fig. 23-29. Total talar dislocation. **(A)** Lateral radiograph showing the talus lying on the anterior ankle region. **(B)** Postreduction radiograph. Definitive treatment for avascular necrosis was a modified Blair tibiocalcaneal arthrodesis. (Courtesy of Hardin Jones, M.D.)

evation of the leg with overhead traction was necessary to reduce the massive swelling characteristic of this injury. The leg was immobilized in a Jones compressive dressing with a posterior splint holding the foot in the neutral position for 4 weeks.

Owing to the severing of all talar blood supplies, a total dislocated talus is rendered avascular. In this patient, avascular necrosis was noticed radiographically 4 weeks after reduction. A modified Blair tibial calcaneal arthrodesis was performed with no subsequent complications.

SUMMARY

The diversity of fractures and injuries suffered by the talus have been described. The practitioner may follow these guidelines in dealing with these complex and somewhat frustrating injuries.

REFERENCES

1. Anderson HG: The Medical and Surgical Aspects of Aviation. Oxford University Press, London, 1919
2. Coltart WD: Aviator's astragalus. J Bone Joint Surg 34B:535, 1952
3. Mulfinger GL, Trueta J: The blood supply of the talus. J Bone Joint Surg 52B:160, 1979
4. Peterson L, Goldie I, Lindell D: The arterial supply of the talus. Acta Orthop Scand 45:260, 1974
5. Sneed WL: The astragalus: a case of dislocation, excision and replacement: an attempt to demonstrate circulation in this bone. J Bone Joint Surg 7A:384, 1925
6. Haliburton R, Sullivan R, Kelly P, Peterson L: The extra-osseous and intra-osseous blood supply of the talus. J Bone Joint Surg 40A:1115, 1958
7. Hawkins LG: Fracture of the lateral process of the talus. A review of thirteen cases. J Bone Joint Surg 47A:1170, 1965
8. Fjeldborg O: Fracture of the lateral process of the talus. Supination-dorsal flexion fracture. Acta Orthop Scand 39:407, 1968
9. Lapidus PW: A note on the fracture of the os trigonum. Report of a case. Bull Hosp Joint Dis 33:150, 1975
10. Ihle CL, Cochran RM: Fracture of the fused os trigonum. Am J Sports Med 10:47, 1982
11. Garcia A, Parker JC: Fractures of the foot. p. 89. In Giannestras NJ (ed): Foot Disorders, Medical and Surgical Management. 2nd Ed. Lea & Febiger, Philadelphia, 1973
12. Kenwright J, Taylor RG: Major injuries of the talus. J Bone Joint Surg 52B:36, 1970
13. Pennal GF: Fractures of the talus. Clin Orthop 30:53, 1963
14. Mindell ER, Cisek EE, Kartalion G, Dziob JM: Late results of injuries to the talus: analysis of forty cases. J Bone Joint Surg 45A:221, 1963
15. Hawkins LG: Fractures of the neck of the talus. J Bone Joint Surg 52A:991, 1970
16. McKeever FM: Treatment and complications of fractures and dislocations of the talus. Clin Orthop 30:45, 1963
17. Blair HC: Comminuted fractures and fracture dislocations of the body of the astragalus. Am J Surg 59:37, 1943
18. Morris HD, Hand W, Dunn AW: The modified Blair fusion of fractures of the talus. J Bone Joint Surg 53A:1289, 1971
19. Schrock RD: Fractures and dislocation of the astragalus. p. 361. In American Academy of Orthopedic Surgeons. Instructional Course Lectures. Vol. 9. Edwards, Ann Arbor, 1982
20. Dennis MD, Tyllos HS: Blair tibiotalar arthrodesis of the talus. J Bone Joint Surg 62A:103, 1980
21. Rockwood CA, Green DP (eds): Fractures. JB Lippincott, Philadelphia, 1975
22. Peterson L, Romanus B, Oahlberg E: Fractures of the collum tali—an experimental study. J Biomech 9:277, 1976
23. Canale ST, Kelly FB: Fractures of the neck of the talus. J Bone Joint Surg 60A:143, 1978
24. Peterson L, Goldie IF, Irstam C: Fracture of the neck of the talus. Acta Orthop Scand 48:696, 1977
25. Rendu A: Fractures intra-articulaire parcellaire de la poulie astraglienne. Lyon Med 150:220, 1932
26. Berndt AL, Harty M: Transchondral fractures (osteochondritis dissecans) of the talus. J Bone Joint Surg 59:37, 1943
27. Pritsch M, Horoshovski H, Farine I: Arthroscopic treatment of osteochondral lesions of the talus. J Bone Joint Surg 68A:862, 1986
28. Canale ST, Belding RH: Osteochondral lesions of the talus. J Bone Joint Surg 62A:97, 1980
29. Alexander AH, Lichtman DM: Surgical treatment of transchondral talar dome fractures (osteochondritis dissecans). Long term follow-up. J Bone Joint Surg 62A:646, 1980
30. Barber JR, Brucker JD, Haliburton RA: Peritalar dislocation of the foot. Can J Surg 4:205, 1961
31. Buckingham WW: Subtalar dislocation of the foot. J Trauma 13:753, 1973
32. Grantham SA: Medial subtalar dislocations; five cases with a common etiology. J Trauma 4:845, 1964
33. Leitner B: Obstacles to reduction in subtalar dislocations. J Bone Joint Surg 36A:299, 1954
34. Leitner, B: The mechanism of total dislocation of the talus. J Bone Joint Surg 37:89, 1955
35. Detenbeck LC, Kelly PJ: Total dislocation of the talus. J Bone Joint Surg 51A:283, 1969
36. Silvani S: Injuries to the talus. Clin Podiatry 2:287, 1985

24

Fractures of the Calcaneus

John M. Schuberth, D.P.M.
Jeffrey M. Karlin, D.P.M.
Nicholas Daly, D.P.M., M.S.

The os calcis is the largest bone of the foot and is the major weight-bearing osseous structure of the foot. It is one of the components of the tritarsal articulation and has important functional tasks with regard to normal ambulation. With a bone so vital to the normal mechanics of locomotion it is easy to see why a fracture of the calcaneus is attended by considerable morbidity. The mere mention of the word fracture as applied to the calcaneus brings to mind the image of a bone with its structure and shape grossly disrupted and its articular relationship seriously disorganized. What follows then are arduous and complicated efforts to attain a satisfactory reduction, prolonged disability, and the tedious stages of functional restoration.

Calcaneal fractures make up about 2 percent of all fractures. They account for 60 percent of major tarsal injuries. According to Rockwood and Green, the os calcis is fractured more than any other tarsal bone.[1] Seventy-five percent of all calcaneal fractures result from a vertical fall from 3 to 50 feet with an average height of 14 feet.[2] Twisting type injuries are second in frequency with 15 percent of the cases.[3] The remaining 10 percent of the cases result from blunt trauma or ballistic injury. Calcaneal fractures usually occur between the ages of 30 and 50 years, with men affected five times as often as women.[4,5]

Calcaneal fractures can be classified into two major groups: extra-articular and intra-articular fractures. Intra-articular fractures account for 75 percent of all injuries to the calcaneus.[6,7] Intra-articular fractures have a high morbidity with loss of time from work, persistent pain, and possible permanent disability.[8] The Industrial Commission has rated the average disability of a calcaneal fracture as a 22 percent loss of the limb in some cases.

CALCANEAL FRACTURES IN CHILDREN

Calcaneal fractures in children are rare. Matteri and Frymoyer reported a 6 percent incidence of calcaneal fractures in children.[9] Extra-articular fractures are more common than intra-articular fractures in children. Schmidt and Weiner found a 63 percent incidence of extra-articular fractures in this age group.[10] There are fewer intra-articular fractures in children because of the resiliency of cartilage and because the soft tissues tend to absorb impact from vertical compression load. When they do occur, intra-articular fractures in children are less severe than in adults because of these factors.

The joint involvement in childhood injuries is usually very subtle, and the fracture may be overlooked on initial radiographic examination. Minor involvement of the posterior subtalar joint is usually identified by a bursting of the lateral wall of the calcaneus, producing a longitudinal sliver of bone. This is only seen on the calcaneal axial view.

In children, the treatment of choice is conservative, particularly in the age group under 10 years of age. Satisfactory results are related to the growth potential and remodeling of the osteocartilaginous bone in young children.[11] Treatment usually is a short leg cast for 3 to 4 weeks or until bony union occurs.[12]

ANATOMY

The calcaneus is the largest bone of the foot. It is shaped like an irregular rectangular solid and presents six surfaces: superior, inferior, lateral, medial, posterior, and anterior.

Superior

On the superior surface lies the posterior, middle, and anterior facets that articulate with the talus (Fig. 24-1). The posterior facet is the largest and is the major weight-bearing facet of the three. It spans almost the entire width of the body. The surface is convex along the longitudinal axis. Manter[13] and Inman[14] both studied the shape of the posterior articular facet. Manter[24] concluded that the articular surface was screw shaped.[13] Inman found screwlike behavior in only 58 percent of his specimens and noted a high degree of variability in the articular geometry.[14]

The anterior and middle facets are supported by the beak of the calcaneus and the sustentaculum tali, respectively. They may be separate, confluent, or united into a single surface. The middle facet is contained on the superior surface of the sustentaculum. These facets form a concavity that articulates with the head of the talus. The three articular facets all lie at different angles to one another, with none of the facets being parallel or perpendicular to one another. This complex and variable arrangement can be difficult to reconstitute with injury to any or all of the facets.

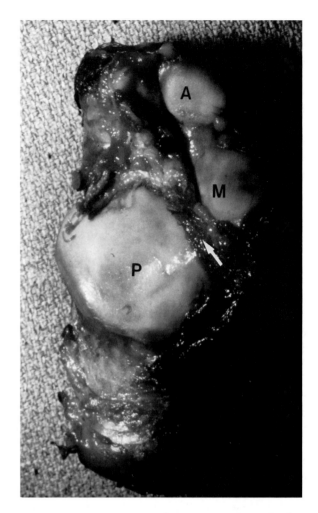

Fig. 24-1. Superior view of superior surface of calcaneus. In this specimen there are three distinct facets. The posterior facet (P) is the largest and is separated from the middle (M) and anterior (A) facets by the tarsal canal (arrow).

Between the middle and posterior facets lies the tarsal canal. The interosseous talocalcaneal ligament and the medial root of the inferior extensor retinaculum insert into the floor of the canal.

The tarsal canal opens laterally into the sinus tarsi. The sinus tarsi provides attachment for the extensor digitorum brevis, the intermediate and inferior roots of the extensor retinaculum, the cervical ligament, the bifurcate ligament, and the dorsal calcaneocuboid ligament.

There is a strong cortical strut extending along the superolateral aspect of the calcaneus from the calcaneocuboid joint to the anterior margin of the posterior facet that forms the crucial angle of Gissane. The talocalcaneonavicular joint is formed by the anterior and middle calcaneal facets, the navicular facet that articulates with the head of the talus, and the inferior and superomedial calcaneonavicular ligaments. These structures form the acetabulum pedis.[15]

Inferior Surface

The inferior surface of the calcaneus is triangular with the base posterior and the apex anterior. The larger medial and smaller lateral tuberosities occupy the base of the triangle while the anterior tuberosity occupies the apex. The medial and lateral tuberosities are structures that have intimate contact with the ground, thereby transmitting the forces of body weight to the supporting surface. The medial tuberosity also is the origin of the abductor hallucis muscle, while the lateral tuberosity is the primary origin for the abductor digiti minimi. The triangular surface between the medial and lateral tuberosities gives rise to the long plantar ligament. The anterior tuberosity serves as the origin for the short plantar ligament and provides insertion for the deep fibers of the long plantar ligament. The calcaneal pitch is maintained by these ligamentous structures attaching to the inferior surface. The plantar aponeurosis and flexor digitorum brevis insert on both tuberosities.

Lateral Surface

The lateral surface is flat and almost subcutaneous with an elevated ridge, the peroneal tubercle, located in the middle third (Fig. 24-2). The peroneus longus rides in a groove inferior to the tubercle, while the peroneus brevis passes superiorly. This surface is primarily composed of very thin cortical bone that has a strong tendency to comminute when placed under a compressive load. The inferior peroneal retinaculum lies directly over the peroneal tubercle. Its deeper fibers attach to the tubercle, dividing the peroneal sheath into two distinct components at this level.

Medial Surface

The medial surface is concave and includes the sustentaculum tali. The sustentaculum is triangular in shape, projects anteromedially, and is inclined downward at an average of 45 degrees. The middle facet lies on its superior surface, while the inferior surface forms a groove for the flexor hallucis longus and its tendon sheath. The medial surface of the sustentaculum tali serves as the insertion for the tibial calcaneal component of the deltoid ligament, the superior medial calcaneal navicular ligament, and the recurrent band of the posterior tibial tendon. The posterior border of the sustentaculum tali serves as the insertion of the medial portion of the talocalcaneal ligament and forms the medial entrance of the tarsal canal. The quadratus plantae partly originates from the inferior two-thirds of the medial surface of the calcaneus.

Posterior Surface

The posterior surface is shaped like an inferiorly based triangle. The middle third of this surface is the site of the Achilles tendon attachment. The superior third is generally smooth owing to its variable contact with the Achilles tendon. As the foot is dorsiflexed at the ankle or the knee is fully extended, the anterior aspect of the Achilles tendon gains more purchase of the superior one-third of the surface. The inferior one-third is broad and marks the point of confluence of the plantar fascia and the Achilles tendon.

Anterior Surface

The anterior surface essentially comprises the calcaneal articulation for the cuboid. The lateral surface meets the anterior surface to form the lateral corner of the joint. The anterior aspect of the sustentaculum tali courses anterolateral to blend into the medial aspect of the cuboidal

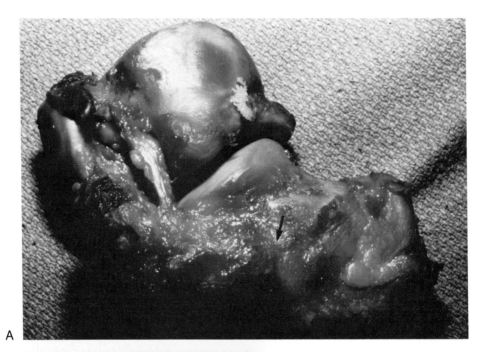

A

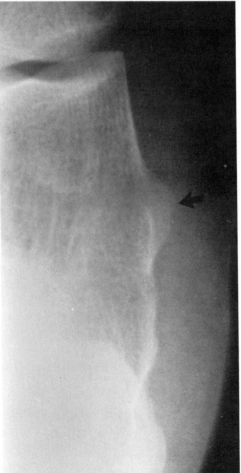

Fig. 24-2. (A) Lateral view of articulated talus and calcaneus. The arrow indicates the peroneal tubercle. (B) Anteroposterior radiograph indicating the large peroneal tubercle (arrow).

B

facet. The articular surface itself is a complex saddle shape.

PHYSICAL EXAMINATION

When evaluating a patient with a calcaneal fracture, a thorough musculoskeletal examination must be performed owing to the high incidence of concomitant injuries. Spinal fractures occur approximately 10 to 20 percent[16–18] of the time, with L1 the most frequently involved vertebra. Other related injuries are to other tarsal bones, ankle, femur, and wrist, as well as soft tissue injuries to the heel. Concomitant injuries occur about 40 percent of the time. Obvious deformities of the foot usually represent either concomitant ankle fracture or dislocation of the midfoot or hindfoot joints. Violations of skin integrity should be searched for in any patient.

Although neurovascular compromise is rare with calcaneal fractures, careful assessment of the pulses is mandatory. Severe swelling may develop rapidly after the injury and make pulses difficult to locate. Doppler assistance should be used if they are not easily palpable. In severe crush-type injuries, there may be both subjective and objective loss of sensation on the plantar aspect of the foot. This can be related to the excessive buildup of pressure in the deep compartments of the foot. Usually sensation will return to normal with several days of elevation. However, progression into a full-blown compartment syndrome is exceedingly rare. It is diagnosed only when there is pain on passive stretch and documented elevation of pressures in the deep central compartment. If these criteria exist, then immediate release should be performed.

Ecchymosis will often develop several days after the injury. It usually parallels the amount of intra-articular disruption and typically is bimalleolar. Fracture blisters also develop within 48 hours and are more common laterally where the skin adheres less to the deep fascia (Fig. 24-3).

Most patients with severe intra-articular fractures will be quite uncomfortable with any attempts at examination of the skeletal components of the foot. However, at a minimum, the practi-

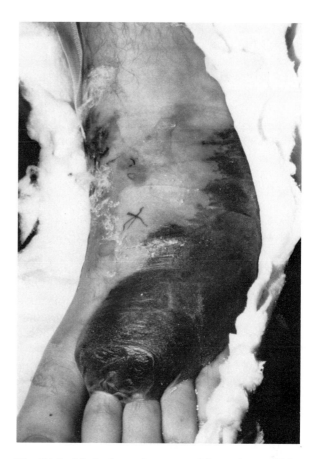

Fig. 24-3. Marked eccyhmosis and large fracture blisters in patient with grossly comminuted calcaneal fracture.

tioner should palpate the entire foot systematically to include the appropriate radiographic views in the work-up. If there is no significant ankle injury, most patients will be able to move the ankle with coaxing.

CLASSIFICATION

Calcaneal fractures has been classified in various ways by different investigators.[7,9–21] The multitude of classification schemes is testimony to the lack of suitability of any single scheme. The simplest method of classification is to differentiate calcaneal fractures into extra-articular and intra-articular fractures. The classification of Rowe et al. best describes extra-articular fractures and is predicated on the injury to specific anatomic structures (see Extra-articular Fractures).[20] Essex-LoPresti identified two distinct intra-articular fracture subtypes: the tongue fracture and the joint depression fracture.[7] This system is mechanistically based and founded on the sequential appearance of various fracture lines and ultimate radiographic appearance. Since the tongue fracture mechanism is so infrequent, essentially most intra-articular fractures are in the class of joint depression.

We favor the combined classification scheme of Rowe et al.[20] for extra-articular injuries and that of Essex-Lopresti[7] for intra-articular fractures. It is important not to place too much emphasis on the classification of intra-articular fractures as it applies to treatment. This is because each calcaneal fracture has its own unique characteristics that must be addressed. However, it is critical to identify each primary fracture fragment. There can be anywhere from two to four main fracture fragments (see Intra-articular Fractures). Generally, the more main fragments there are, the more severe the injury. There is a concomitant increase in the complexity of open repair and a worsening of the prognosis as the number of fracture fragments increases.

RADIOGRAPHIC EVALUATION

Radiographs are essential in making the correct diagnosis of a calcaneal fracture. Because clinical examination capabilities are limited by patient guarding, specific views should be ordered liberally to assess the entire calcaneus and surrounding structures. Radiographs may not show all of the involvement in these severe injuries, but they do demonstrate parameters that are most important in making a diagnosis and formulating a treatment plan.

The essential imaging views and techniques may include the following:

1. The lateral view gives one the overall appearance of the body of the calcaneus. The position of the posterior facet can be judged from this view. It enables the tuber-joint angle to be measured.[22] The angle normally measures 25 to 45 degrees, but should be compared with the opposite side when determining the significance of the measurement. A difference of 5 degrees or more is said to be significant, with the injured side measuring less than the noninjured side. A discrepancy indicates depression of the posterior facet (Fig. 24-4).

2. The axial view of the calcaneus demonstrates the tuberosity, the body, the sustentacular joint, and the posterior facet. This view will show the presence or absence of medial displacement and overriding of the superomedial fragment and the degree of heel widening. It is often helpful in assessing the congruity of reduction of the posterior facet. The degree of comminution of the lateral wall is also shown on this view.

3. The dorsal plantar view allows visualization of the calcaneocuboid joint and the amount of bursting of the lateral calcaneal wall.

4. The medial oblique view is ideal for assessment of the anterior process as well as the calcaneocuboid joint.

5. Broden views were described by Broden to evaluate the posterior facet and the associated articulation.[23] The foot is positioned with heel on the cassette and the foot internally rotated 45 degrees. The radiograph is taken with the central ray aimed at the sinus tarsi and at 10, 20, 30, and 40 degrees cephalad. They are quite useful in evaluating the degree of congruity of the postoperative reduction of the posterior facet (Fig. 24-5).

6. The availability of computed axial tomography (CT) has enabled surgeons to evaluate completely the degree of pathology, and the extent of comminution and therefore administer the optimal form of treatment (Fig. 24-6).

7. A limited or complete ankle series should be obtained to rule out concomitant fracture of the malleoli, talus, or distal tibia.

8. Lumbar spine films are indicated with any history of back pain as a result of the injury or if there is any tenderness along the posterior spinous processes. They are also indicated if there is any neurologic deficit that cannot be explained as a result of the pedal injury.

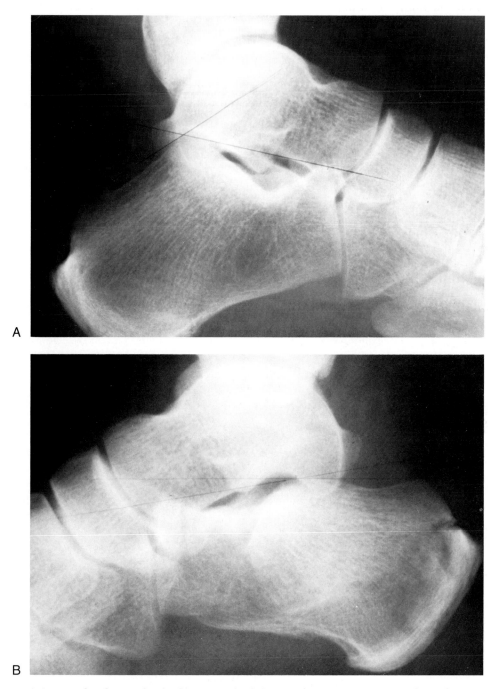

Fig. 24-4. (**A**) Lateral radiograph of calcaneus which has not been injured. Böhler's angle measures 40 degrees. (**B**) Lateral radiograph with obvious reduction of Böhler's angle (degrees) indicating depression of posterior facet.

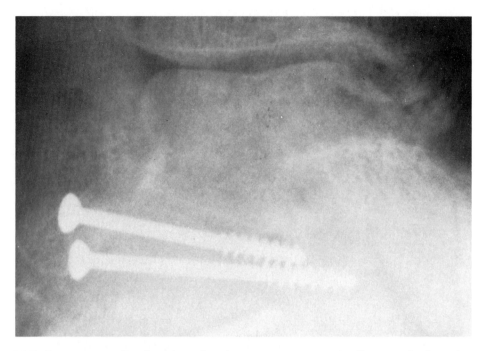

Fig. 24-5. Postoperative Broden view showing congruous posterior facet on the lateral aspect.

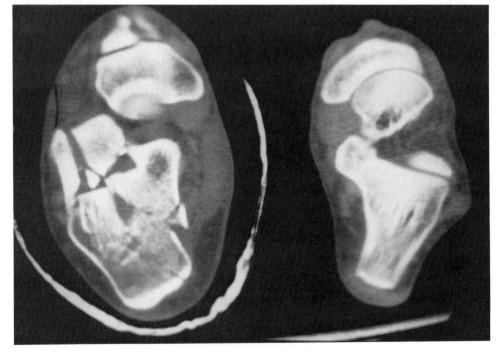

Fig. 24-6. CT scan showing extensive comminution of fracture.

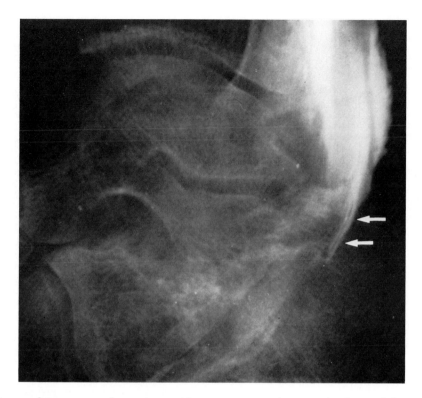

Fig. 24-7. Peroneal tenogram of a patient with a conservatively treated calcaneal fracture. Note the point of constriction from expansion of the lateral wall (arrow). Also note the relative congruency of the posterior facet.

9. Peroneal tenography can be a valuable adjunct in the assessment of calcaneal fracture pathology. It can be used during the treatment of the acute injury in isolated cases but is more applicable in the later phases of treatment when peroneal tendon dysfunction is evaluated. Here the constriction or irritation of the tendon sheath is visualized at the lateral aspect of the calcaneus. It is often a consequence of the explosion and expansion of the lateral calcaneal wall (Fig. 24-7).

EXTRA-ARTICULAR FRACTURES

Fracture of the Calcaneal Tuberosities

Fracture of the calcaneal tuberosities is a Rowe type Ia fracture usually resulting from a fall with the heel inverted or everted. With the heel everted, the medial tuberosity is fractured, and with the foot inverted, the lateral tuberosity is fractured. These are shear-type fractures and appear more commonly on the medial side. They are best viewed with an axial calcaneal view. Nondisplaced or moderately displaced fractures should be treated with a cast for 4 to 6 weeks (Fig. 24-8). Severely displaced fractures should be treated by closed manipulation and casted for 4 to 6 weeks. Rarely, open or closed pinning is indicated. The major complication of these fractures is widening of the heel.

Fracture of the Sustentaculum Tali

Fracture of the sustentaculum tali is a Rowe type Ib fracture resulting from a fall with the foot in marked supination. There is usually pain and

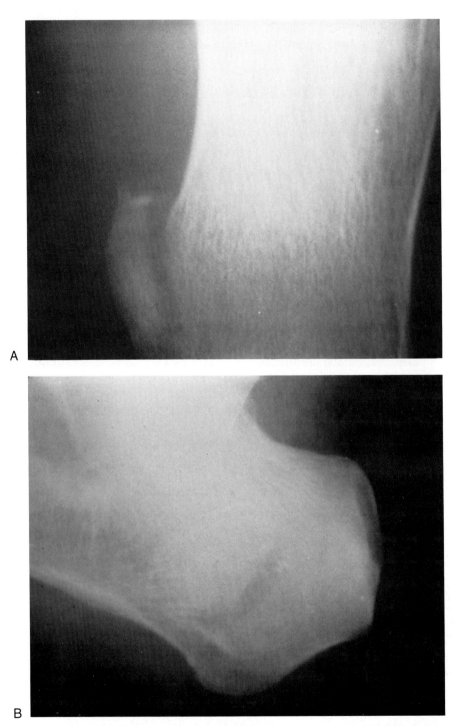

Fig. 24-8. (**A**) Axial view of type Ia calcaneal fracture. The heel is slightly widened but preservation of the weight-bearing cortex is evident. (**B**) Lateral view of same patient. The loss of the normal contour of the tubercles is evident. Compression accounts for the relative increase in bony density.

swelling below the medial malleolus and associated pain with flexion of the hallux. This is best viewed by the calcaneal axial radiograph. There is almost always less displacement of the fracture than actually occurred owing to the recoil of the sustentaculum. This is because of the strong ligamentous attachments from the talus and the sling effect of the flexor hallucis longus tendon. This may represent instability in a seemingly harmless nondisplaced fracture. Treatment for undisplaced fractures consists of a short leg walking cast for 4 to 6 weeks with the foot slightly inverted. Severely displaced fractures should be treated with open manipulation and internal fixation. Cancellous screw fixation or staple fixation in the manner of McReynolds[24] (see Indications for Open Reduction) are the preferred methods of choice. The prognosis is usually good. If painful nonunion occurs, surgical excision of the fragment is the treatment of choice.

Fracture of the Anterior Process

There are two fracture patterns involving the anterior portion of the calcaneus: avulsion fractures of the anterior process and compression fractures of the anterior calcaneus. Both mechanisms may involve a variable portion of the calcaneocuboid joint. This is referred to as a Rowe type Ic fracture (Fig. 24-9).

Avulsion fractures of the calcaneus are the most common type of extra-articular calcaneal fracture. Carey et al. reported a 15 percent occurrence in one large series of calcaneal fractures.[25] The mechanism of this fracture is supination-plantar flexion with tension placed on the bifurcate ligament avulsing the anterior process.[20] Norfray et al. reported a 10 percent incidence of a dorsolateral avulsion fracture at the origin of the extensor digitorum brevis muscle.[26] Many times the patient is misdiagnosed as having an ankle sprain.[27–29] The typical history in these injuries is a twisting injury with pain over the sinus tarsi. The point of maximal tenderness on examination is anterior and inferior to the anterior talofibular ligament. This fracture is best visualized on the medial oblique radiograph. The diagnosis may be missed unless this view is requested. If seen in a usual emergency room setting with the chief complaint of a twisted ankle, this view is seldom ordered in a routine ankle series.

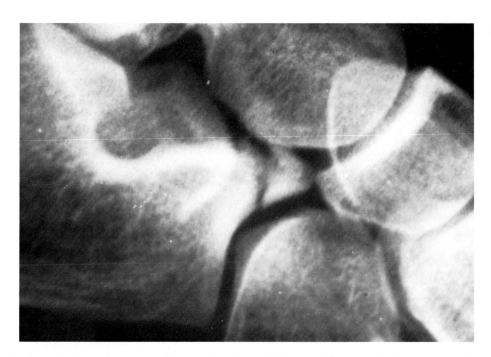

Fig. 24-9. Lateral view of patient with type Ic calcaneal fracture. There is clearly some involvement of the articular surface of the calcaneal cuboid joint.

Another mechanism for this fracture is a compression of the calcaneal articular surface.[28,30] It involves a forced forefoot abduction with compression of the calcaneocuboid joint. This fracture is usually displaced superiorly and posteriorly, resulting in joint incongruity.

Regardless of the mechanism of injury, there is controversy as to what represents the best treatment. The significance of this fracture is related to the size of the fragment and the amount of the calcaneocuboid joint that it comprises. Degan et al. have classified this fracture into three different types.[27] Type I is a nondisplaced fracture involving the tip of the anterior process. Type II is a displaced fracture that does not involve the calcaneocuboid joint. Type III is a fracture that involves a variable portion of the calcaneocuboid joint. This type is usually seen with the compressive mechanism of injury.

Various treatment schemes for this injury exist ranging from an Ace bandage to a short leg walking cast to non-weight bearing for 2 to 8 weeks.[28,30,31] It is our opinion that all type I and II injuries can be treated with weight-bearing immobilization for 4 to 6 weeks. Bony union is more common in type I injuries and less common in type II fractures. However, prognosis does not seem related to the occurrence of fracture union. Type III injuries should be carefully evaluated for the degree of articular involvement (Fig. 24-10). If there is a significant amount of articular disruption, then open reduction and internal fixation should be considered. There is more of an indication for open reduction and internal fixation in the patient with a compressive type of injury because subsequent loading of the calcaneocuboid joint in normal gait is likely to cause symptoms. On the contrary, if there is an avulsion type of injury, weight bearing and loading of the calcaneocuboid joint may reduce the fracture into a more anatomic position.

The fracture fragment is often a source of significant discomfort in those cases in which there is no bony union. However, the practitioner should be aware that often a prolonged recovery period is required before more aggressive treatment is indicated. Many of these patients will become asymptomatic after 6 to 9 months of conservative treatment. If, however, the patient wishes intervention, then excision of the nonunited fragment is the procedure of choice. Degan et al. recommend injection of local anesthetic into the fracture area to ascertain whether the source of pain is emanating from the fracture site.[27] They also emphasize the prolonged postoperative recovery period often necessary to become asymptomatic.[27]

Fracture of the Tuberosity

Fractures of the calcaneal tuberosity can be classified as beak or avulsion fractures. These fractures are usually broken down into Rowe's classification of type II extra-articular fractures. Rowe et al.[20] and Essex-LoPresti[7] believed that beak fractures were caused by direct trauma and avulsion fractures were caused by direct pull on the Achilles tendon (Fig. 24-11). However, Lowry[32] and Lungstaades[33] have shown that the Achilles tendon may insert into the superior portion of the tuberosity. Thus, avulsion can be the mechanism of fracture of all or any part of the tuberosity. Rarely is direct trauma the cause of avulsion fractures. Another possible mechanism for beak fractures is a push-off injury of the anterior aspect of the Achilles tendon as the tendon becomes taut. A combined position of dorsiflexion of the ankle and extension of the knee will increase the articulation of the Achilles tendon with the posterior aspect of the calcaneus. A shearing mechanism can result in a fracture of the superior aspect of the body, although this rarely extends into the subtalar joint.

These fractures occur in individuals 50 to 70 years old. These injuries occur in this age group presumably because of the more osteoporotic bone; younger patients suffer Achilles tendon ruptures with a similar mechanism. The patient has tenderness over the posterior process of the calcaneus at the Achilles tendon insertion. They may have weakness, an antalgic gait, and difficulty standing on tiptoes and climbing stairs. A displaced avulsion fracture may tear the skin and could cause skin necrosis to the relatively avascular posterior skin. Diagnosis can be made with a lateral radiograph, which will demonstrate the size of the fragment and degree of displacement.

The most important factor in treatment of any calcaneal avulsion fracture is the degree of dis-

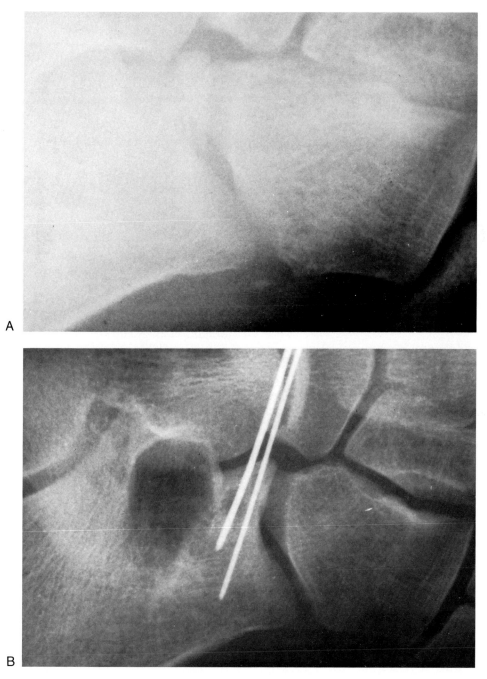

Fig. 24-10. (**A**) Oblique view of same patient in Figure 24-9 showing that the extent of articular involvement (arrows) is greater than seen on the lateral view. (**B**) Intraoperative view indicating anatomic reduction and internal fixation.

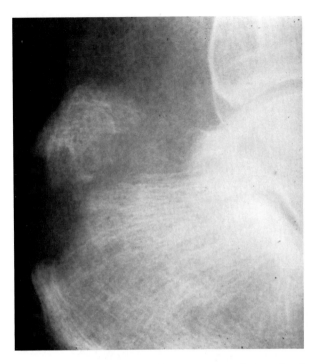

Fig. 24-11. Lateral view demonstrating the avulsed fragment of the calcaneal tuberosity. Note that the fracture line is at the middle third of the posterior surface.

placement. Undisplaced fractures can be treated with closed reduction with a long leg non-weight-bearing cast with the foot in gravity equinus for approximately 6 weeks. Careful and frequent follow-up is necessary because of the tendency for the fracture to displace. Displaced fractures should be treated with open reduction and internal fixation with the patient in the prone position. Fixation devices are the choice of the surgeon but the fracture can best be handled with cancellous screws. The foot is then placed in a gravity equinus non-weight-bearing cast for 6 to 8 weeks or until bony union occurs. In some cases, modification of the tension-band principle can be used to facilitate early postoperative range of motion (Fig. 24-12).

Fracture of the Body Without Involvement of the Subtalar Joint

Fracture of the body without involvement of the subtalar joint is a Rowe type III fracture and composes about 20 percent of all calcaneal fractures. The injury usually results from a fall, forcing the edge of the talus into the calcaneus. The diagnosis is made with lateral calcaneal axial and anteroposterior views of the foot. Broden views or a CT scan should be obtained to be certain that there is no involvement of the subtalar joint. A lateral radiograph of the opposite foot should be taken to compare Bohler's tuber-joint angle.[22]

The symptoms in these fractures may be similar to those of intra-articular fractures. There may be extreme swelling pain and inability to bear weight. The swelling and ecchymosis may become apparent within 1 to 2 hours after the injury. Fracture blisters may appear within 24 hours.

Treatment of fractures of the body of the calcaneus should initially consist of bed rest, elevation, compression, and ice for 48 hours to minimize swelling and the presence of fracture blisters. For nondisplaced and most displaced fractures, treatment should include active range of motion exercises to prevent ankle and subtalar stiffness. If there is significant widening of the calcaneus, then closed reduction with manual compression should be performed to reduce the chance of peroneal tendon irritation. When there is significant displacement and flattening of Bohler's angle,[22] traction or open reduction of the fracture should be considered to restore calcaneal height. These fractures also require careful and frequent follow-up to ensure no interim displacement occurs owing to the pull of the gastro-soleus complex. The prognosis is good in these fractures because they spare the subtalar joint.

INTRA-ARTICULAR FRACTURES

Mechanism of Injury

The mechanism of injury of intra-articular fractures is poorly understood and has inconsistent descriptions in the literature. Clinical experience with large numbers of these injuries has shown us that no two calcaneal fractures are alike but that there are some similarities that may be relied on during the interpretation of radiographic stud-

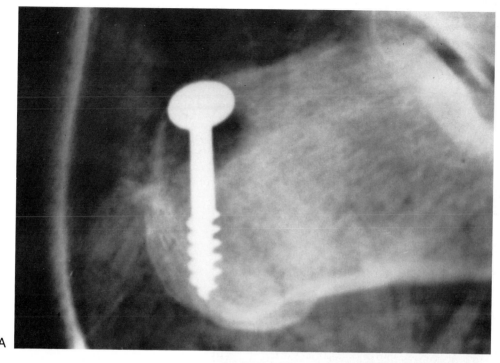

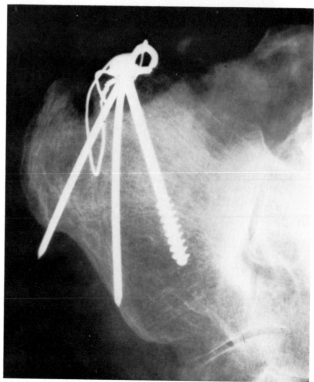

Fig. 24-12. **(A)** Avulsion fracture fixated with a cancellous screw. **(B)** Avulsion fracture fixated with intraosseous wiring technique.

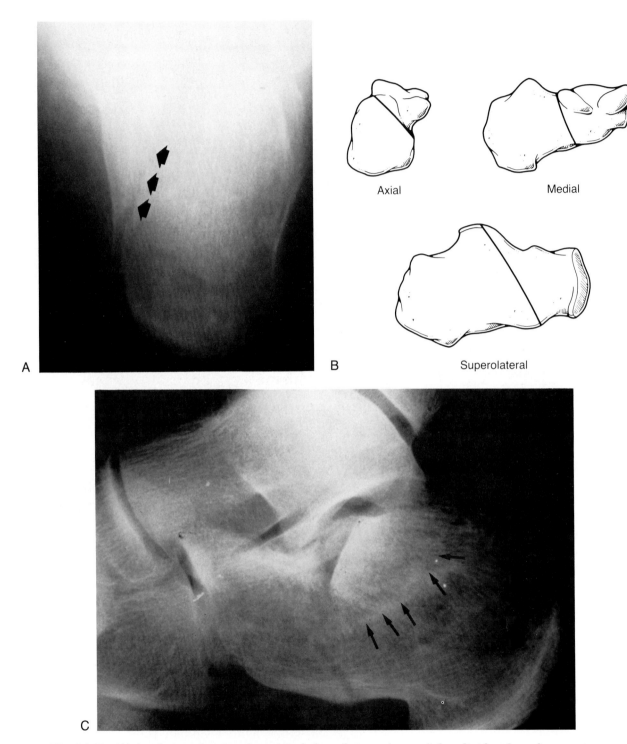

Fig. 24-13. (A) Axial view showing the vertical shear fracture (arrows) that divides the calcaneus into two major fragments. **(B)** Diagram depicting the two major fragments from the initial fracture line. **(C)** Lateral view showing the fracture line that isolates the lateral portion of the posterior facet. (*Figure continues.*)

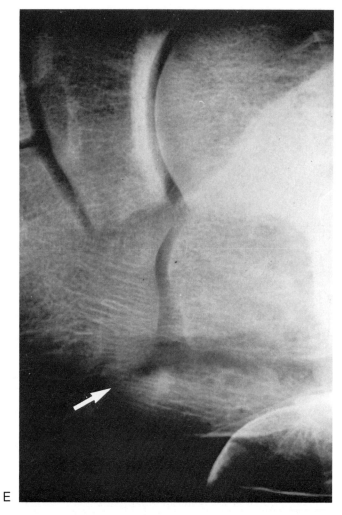

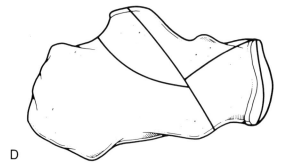

Fig. 24-13 (*Continued*). (**D**) Diagram showing that there are now three large fragments which result from the isolation of this facet. (**E**) Oblique view showing the lateral cortical fracture extending into the calcaneal cuboid joint (arrows).

ies. Likewise, understanding of the mechanism of injury will aid in determining the most appropriate treatment.

There are three constant components to most intra-articular calcaneal fractures.[34,35] They are the vertical shearing fracture resulting in the sustentacular fragment, the lateral portion of the posterior facet, and the lateral cortical fracture (Fig. 24-13). The sequence of events leading to this final fracture pattern varies among investigators.

Once initial impaction occurs, there is some controversy over what happens next. Essex-Lopresti thought that the primary fracture line results from the lateral process of the talus impacting into the lateral cortical strut of the calcaneus or the angle of Gissane (also known as the critical angle).[7] Continued force from the moment of body weight then shears off the superior medial fragment of the sustentaculum. This essentially cuts the calcaneus into anterior and posterior portions. Further forces then comminute

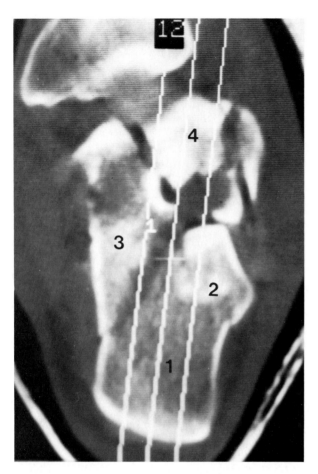

Fig. 24-14. CT scan showing the four major fragments. (1) The main body; (2) the sustentaculum; (3) the posterior facet; and (4) the anterior body fragment.

the lateral wall as the lateral portion of the posterior facet is driven down into the body of the calcaneus.

However, as Cavaliere points out,[16] this mechanism is not sufficient when considering the work of Burdeaux[36] and Palmer.[34] These two clinicians described the primary fracture line as that occurring through the posterior facet. This fracture line is attributed to the shearing fracture of the sustentaculum tali. This leaves two major fragments—the superiomedial one and the remainder of the os calcis. It is unusual to observe a fracture with only two major fragments. Continued downward loading then causes the lateral portion of the posterior facet to be driven into the softer cancellous bone of the body. This is then

the third large fragment. The so-called four-part fracture results when the comminution of the lateral wall extends into the calcaneocuboid joint and leaves the anterior portion of the body as the fourth large fragment (Fig. 24-14).

TREATMENT

Indications for Open Reduction

The indications for open reduction of an intra-articular calcaneal fracture depend on many factors. These include age of the patient, occupation, general health status, activity level, ability of the surgeon, and the degree and type of fracture. None of these factors can be considered absolute determinants with regard to the type of treatment rendered. However, the totality of the situation must be prudently considered. The single most important question to answer is: Can the patient definitely be helped with an open reduction procedure? Careful consideration and honest assessment of the entire situation will enable the most efficacious treatment to be applied. Therefore, open reduction is indicated when the articular surfaces can be reconstructed and the normal height and width of the calcaneus can be reestablished with some degree of predictability.

Although advancing age is not an absolute contraindication to surgical intervention, one must be aware of the physiologic barriers that might adversely affect the result. Bone stock is likely to be compromised, especially in women. Rigid fixation may be impossible. There is also a loss of resilience in all soft tissue structures with advancing age.[7] If either of these conditions prevails, then the patient is usually best treated by some alternative method.

The patient's occupation and activity level are also important in determining the ultimate treatment plan. The goal with any treatment of these fractures is return to previous occupation and activity level without pain. Certainly, those with more physically demanding occupations and active athletic individuals would require more exacting results if one expects the patient to return to the previous occupation. Although stiffness of the subtalar joint is often observed postfracture, it is seldom a deterrent to the attainment of the stated goal.

Technique of Open Reduction

The optimal time to perform open reduction and internal fixation is immediately after the injury.[37] The relatively scant edema present at this time makes dissection and subsequent wound closure much easier without additional risk of wound complications. If surgery must be delayed for any length of time, then firm compression dressings should be applied until surgery. Strict elevation also aids in reducing the amount of edema. We prefer to admit the patient to the hospital prior to the day of surgery so the leg can be placed in an overhead sling to reduce edema. If fracture blisters ensue, we believe it is more advantageous to proceed with the surgery and cut through any offending blister. If one waits for the blisters to dissipate, it usually takes at least 2 weeks for the skin to return to an acceptable condition. The fracture margins are beginning to become obscured by this time and anatomic reduction is more difficult. It is also more difficult to discern the tissue layers at a later date. There is no better time to disrupt the fracture blisters than on the operating table in a sterile environment.

When surgical intervention has been chosen for the treatment of an intra-articular calcaneal fracture, several preparatory maneuvers must be performed. First, arrangements for an autogenous bone graft must be made. In almost all cases, the quantity of bone that will be necessary is not obtainable from the tibia without severe compromise to the tibia and a significant risk of fracture. Therefore, the bone graft must be obtained from the iliac crest. The posterior iliac crest has a more abundant supply of cancellous bone and is easily obtainable while the patient is in the prone position.

The use of allogenic bone graft is not recommended in most cases of calcaneal fractures because of its slower rate of incorporation. It is also generally stronger than autogenous cancellous bone and can act like a wedge, thereby compressing the softer autogenous bone when subjected to weight bearing. The only acceptable use of allogenic bone is the absolute inability to procure autogenous bone. If this is the case, the patient must be maintained in the non-weight-bearing position for a longer period. This is necessitated by a longer incorporation time of the graft.

Our recommended approach to the comminuted intra-articular fracture is the lateral one, followed by the medial approach if necessary.[38,39] In our experience, the medial approach is seldom necessary. However, in situations in which there is no lateral comminution and only a large posteromedial sustentacular fragment is present (the two-part fracture), the isolated medial approach is indicated. It is logical to approach the fracture from the side where most of the damage is identified by the preoperative radiographs and diagnostic studies. We have been unable to reproduce the level of results touted by those who favor only the medial approach. It clearly makes more sense to individualize the approach to the individual fracture pattern.

Unless only the medial approach is going to be utilized, we position the patient prone on the operating table. The hips are well padded and chest rolls are usually placed. The ipsilateral hip is externally rotated and the knee is flexed about 90 degrees (Fig. 24-15). This usually allows the medial side of the foot to be placed flat on the operating table. If it does not, then appropriate bolstering under the ipsilateral hip is indicated. A large bolster is then placed under the medial ankle, well proximal to the subtalar joint. This allows for easy manual inversion of the subtalar joint, facilitating exposure. It is also helpful if a medial approach is needed by raising the leg off the table. If the medial approach becomes necessary, then the knee is straightened and the hip is internally rotated. Bolstering of the contralateral hip may be necessary. A thigh tourniquet is placed, and the leg and iliac crest are then prepared and draped. Tourniquet control is not mandatory but is highly recommended.

The incision must be fashioned to allow access to the subtalar joint, the calcaneocuboid joint, and the lateral wall of the calcaneus. This is best accomplished by an incision paralleling the peroneal tendons with the foot dorsiflexed 90 degrees. This accentuates the angle of curvature at the apex. The advantage is better exposure by the elevation of an L-shaped flap. The disadvantage is increased risk of wound slough at the apex.

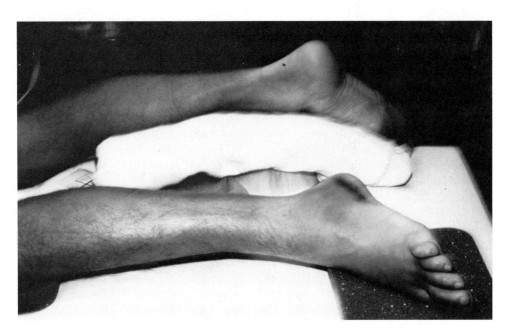

Fig. 24-15. Patient positioned for open reduction and internal fixation. All bony prominences are well padded.

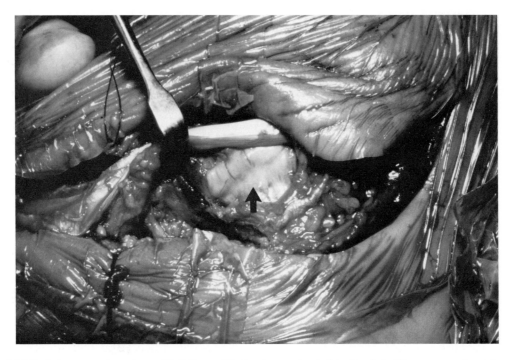

Fig. 24-16. Intraoperative view of left foot with the toes oriented to the left. The peroneal tendons are retracted superiorly. The arrow marks the portion of the sheath that overlies the peroneal tubercle.

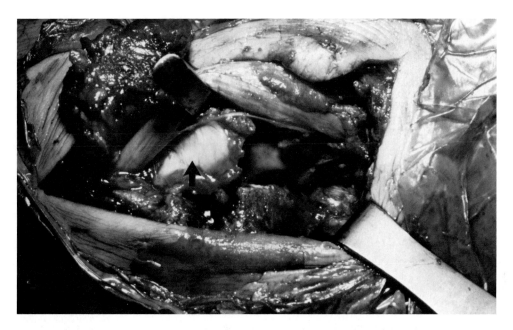

Fig. 24-17. A second intraoperative view of the same patient in Figure 24-16. With further dissection the entire lateral wall is exposed. Note that the peroneal tubercle is contained in a portion of the free-floating lateral wall.

The skin is incised to the level of the subcutaneous tissue. Here the sural nerve must be identified, examined, and mobilized either inferiorly or superiorly. Usually it is preferable to leave it intact in the inferior skin margin, but it is not always possible to preserve its anatomicity owing to its branches or its course across the corner of the incision line. If it is necessary to mobilize the nerve, it should be handled with care. Rarely, it is necessary to sacrifice the entire nerve owing to its interference with the procedure. This should be avoided unless absolutely necessary or undue manipulation of the nerve has occurred during the procedure. However, it is acceptable to sacrifice smaller branches of the nerve with impunity. The peroneal tendon sheath is encountered and fully exposed by elevating the entire subcutaneous layer and skin as a unit off this deep fascial component. It is of the utmost importance to handle the skin flap with skin hooks only and avoid the use of pick-ups. Self-retaining retractors are also not utilized in this area.

An attempt is then made to displace the peroneal tendons superiorly over the lateral malleolus. Both of the peroneal retinacula must be incised to facilitate mobilization. This is done by incising the sheath over the tendons and tagging each retinaculum for later repair. The medial wall of the sheath, which is well adhered to the lateral calcaneal wall, should be left in place over the peroneal tubercle, which is often contained in the free-floating lateral wall (Fig. 24-16). The incision of the sheath is carried anteriorly to the inferior margin of the extensor digitorum brevis muscle belly. The muscle belly and the contents of the sinus tarsi are reflected subperiostally in a superior direction. After the incision of the calcaneofibular ligament, the entire lateral wall of the calcaneus should be exposed (Fig. 24-17).

The extent of the comminution and articular damage should then be assessed. First, the foot is forcibly inverted over the bolster to directly visualize the subtalar joint. The lateral fragment of the posterior facet should then be identified. It is usually found to be depressed below the medial fragment. Often the lateral wall of the calcaneus will need to be retracted to fully assess the size of the fragment. An elevator is then inserted to elevate the lateral fragment. It is best to insert the elevator anteriorly just at the critical angle. Reduction is best accomplished with a combination of elevation and anterior translation to optimally

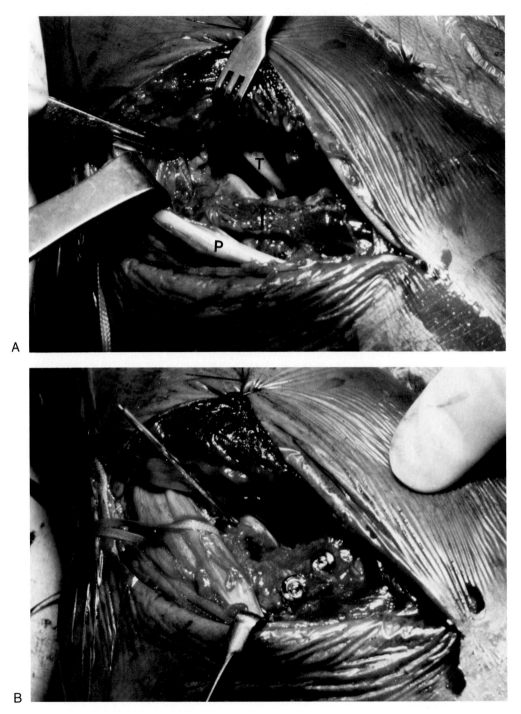

Fig. 24-18. (A) Intraoperative view of right calcaneal fracture. Note the stepoff of the posterior facet (arrow). (T) talus; (P) peroneal tendons. The toes are to the right. **(B)** Reduced posterior facet with Kirschner wire placed across the fracture site. The cancellous screws will be placed after the temporary fixation. In this case the calcaneal cuboid joint was repaired first.

disimpact the fragment. Reduction is done under direct vision, using the visible posterior facet articular surface as a template. Temporary fixation to the sustentacular fragment is maintained with a Kirschner wire, and then a 4.0-, 6.5-, or 7.0-mm cannulated screw is introduced. It is desirable to place the screw near or in the subchondral cortex to ensure good compression, especially in patients with soft bone (Fig. 24-18).

If the patient sustained a three-part fracture, then the inferior void created by the compression of the posterior facet is filled with cancellous autograft. We believe that the vast majority of these injuries should be bone grafted. It is common to underestimate the amount of graft necessary to firmly pack the void. Therefore, the donor site should not be closed until the primary foot surgeon is absolutely sure that sufficient graft has been harvested. Once the graft is inserted, the lateral wall is replaced and fixated if it is large enough. If fixation is impractical, then small loose pieces should be discarded as they will most likely necrose and be resorbed.

The calcaneocuboid joint is attended to next if the fracture pattern has extended into this articulation. Typically, there is a vertical or saggital split of the distal calcaneal articular surface. This is also reduced under direct vision, and again the sequence of temporary Kirschner wire and screw fixation is followed. This is an ideal application for the small cannulated screw system. Again, the subchondral cortex affords better fixation in patients with softer bone, but care must be taken to avoid intra-articular penetration in this irregular, saddle-shaped joint.

In a four-part fracture, the relationship of the anterior and posterior portions of the calcaneus may be uncertain owing to cleavage of one from the other. In this instance more fixation is necessary. We prefer the use of either the Arbeitgemeinshaft für Osteosynthesisfragen (AO) multifragment plate or a small customized AO reconstruction plate (Fig. 24-19). The most difficult part is the reestablishment of the anatomic relationship between the two free-floating fragments. The best landmark is the cortical aspect of the critical angle as this area seldom comminutes owing to its cortical nature. If appropriate landmarks are obtained, temporary fixation is best accomplished with obliquely placed Kirschner wires from the anterolateral corner of the calcaneus to the sustentaculum tali or the area just posterior. Radiographs are taken to ensure normal restoration of Böhler's angle and anatomic restoration of the anterior and posterior aspects of the calcaneus. Customized or premade AO plates are then used to secure the reduction. Ideally, the plate is placed to avoid the peroneal tendons, but this is practically impossible. Surprisingly, it is seldom a problem postoperatively.

Occasionally, we have used intraoperative traction to assist in the establishment of the proper osseous relationships.[40] The AO external fixator or a standard femoral distractor works equally well. The inferior pin is placed in the tuber and the superior pin is placed in the tibia. Caution should be used not to place the inferior pin through any areas suspicious of fracture so additional fracture patterns won't be propagated. Experience will enable one to distract the proper amount as judged by the tension of the Achilles tendon and radiographically.

Final intraoperative radiographs are taken to ensure satisfactory reduction and placement of the fixation. These must include axial calcaneal views to assess the restoration of the proper calcaneal width and lateral decompression of the peroneal tendons. Judicious positioning of the foot will allow for adequate visualization of the middle and posterior facets. Axial views are best taken with the knee extended. The plate is placed flat against the sole of the foot and the sterilely covered x-ray tube is aimed almost parallel to the leg.

When satisfactory reduction has been achieved, the wound is closed in layers, with care taken to anchor the peroneal sheath back to its original location. It is usually only possible to secure it at the anterior and posterior retinacula with a heavy suture of choice. The retinacula are repaired after the tendons are placed into the sheath. A small closed suction drain is usually used. The skin is closed with care taken to reduce any tension on the edges.

Medial Approach

Although the medial approach is used sparingly by us, there are some distinct indications

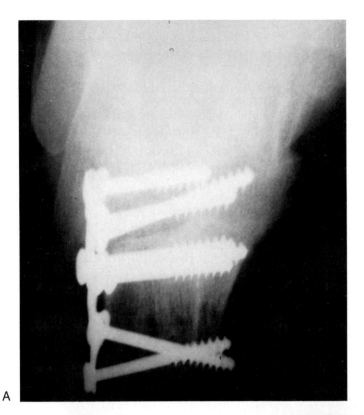

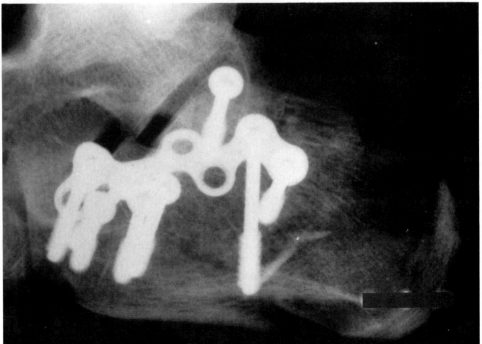

Fig. 24-19. (**A**) Axial and (**B**) lateral views of fracture fixated with AO multi-fragment plate. Care should be taken to ensure that the talus does not impinge on the hardware during pronatory movements.

for this method.[38,39] The first is the situation in which there is a two-part fracture consisting of the sustentacular fragment and the main tuber fragments only. Here, the medial fragment can be anatomically reduced and fixated to the tuber with staples or screws (Fig. 24-20).

The second indication is in the presence of a four-part fracture with disruption of the lateral anatomic landmarks. Here, the medial approach can be used to align the anterior and posterior portions of the calcaneus. Often the only remaining reliable landmark is the fractured medial cortex. The posterior facet should be rigidly fixed to the superomedial fragment prior to the medial exposure. Once this is done, the alignment of the medial cortex will place the intact posterior facet into proper arrangement relative to the anteromedial aspect of the calcaneus and the rest of the tuber. The fourth fragment of the lateral anterior calcaneus can then be fixated to the remaining three fragments with the proper anatomic relationship of the anterior and posterior calcaneus ensured.

The approach is patterned after that of McReynolds.[24] The incision is made roughly in line with the inclination of the calcaneus in the midportion of the bone. Care should be taken to find, preserve, and retract the neurovascular bundle posteriorly after incising the deep fascia. By dissecting the intrinsic muscle bellies and extrinsic tendon away from the medial cortex, the fracture line is visualized. It is helpful to place a large stout retractor such as an Army-Navy retractor along the muscle belly and retract anteriorly and medially. Although one will be looking into a cavity, access to the fracture is improved in this difficult approach.

A narrow elevator is then used to manipulate and rotate the fragment. The posterior aspect of the fragment must be rotated inferiorly, and the anterior end superiorly. One is often able to interdigitate the edges anatomically when the proper derotation has been attained. We find it easiest to use two-point staples of medium caliber. It is preferable to predrill to avoid iatrogenic comminution of the fragile medial wall. If the approach is for a two-part fracture, then the wound is closed in layers. If a four-part fracture is being reduced, temporary staple fixation is done

and attention to the lateral side is given. Here the final fixation of the fragments is done as outlined above. The medial staples are usually left in place regardless of the application.

Closed Reduction and Percutaneous Pinning

The combined technique of closed reduction and percutaneous pinning is useful in those patients in whom anatomic reduction may be difficult owing to the amount of comminution or the fragility of bone secondary to age or disease. It may also be the procedure of choice when the primary goals are narrowing of the heel and decompression of the peroneal tendons when the above limitations are present.

Although the method of Essex-LoPresti[7] has been classically employed with the tongue fracture, we have had success with the use of the maneuver with the joint depression injury. Its main purpose is again decompression of the peroneal tendons. This is made possible by the use of a heavy Steinmann pin placed percutaneously and used to lever the posterior facet up to disimpact the wedge and permit manual reduction.

The technique for reduction requires the use of a C-arm fluoroscope. The patient is positioned prone on the table with the foot hanging free off of the table. A fluoroscopy table is not necessary. A small 2-cm incision is made between the peroneal and Achilles tendons commencing approximately 5 to 7 cm proximal to the Achilles tendon insertion and proceeding distally. A large Steinmann pin (9/64th inches) is then inserted at the superior aspect of the incision and directed under fluoroscopic control to the lateral fragment of the posterior facet. Whether one is dealing with a smaller joint depression fragment or the larger tongue fragment, the pin is advanced and manipulated to engage the fragment so the pin is oriented parallel to the posterior articular surface. The pin is then advanced to the anterior margin of the free fragment (Fig. 24-21).

The surgeon then takes the pin and pulls on the free end in a plantar direction, levering the skewered fragment up. The skin incision may

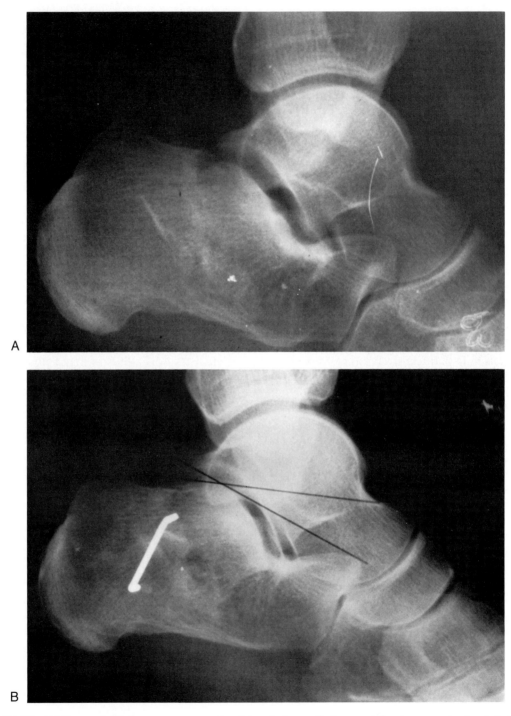

Fig. 24-20. **(A)** Pre- and **(B)** 1-year postoperative lateral views of a two part fracture repaired solely from the medial side. (*Figure continues.*)

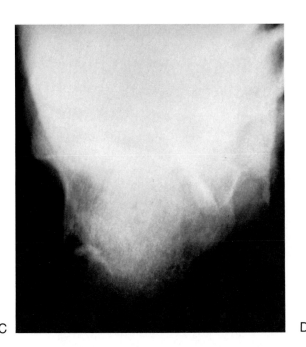
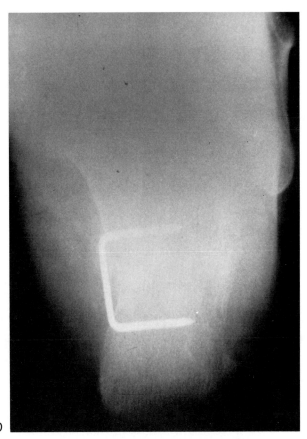

Fig. 24-20 (*Continued*). (**C & D**) Pre- and 1-year postoperative axial views of the same fracture.

need to be extended as more force is applied. The maneuver is extended as far as necessary to pry the fragment against the inferior aspect of the talus. When this is accomplished the pin is advanced. We find it most helpful to keep the power source attached to the pin so that speedy pin advancement may occur. The pin is advanced to the tarsus while ensuring that it is engaging bony structures. Fluoroscopic control is essential throughout.

The lateral wall can then be reduced by placing the palms on either side of the heel and compressing together the sides of the calcaneus.[41] One should feel actual narrowing of the breadth of the calcaneus during this procedure. Axial fluoroscopic or radiographic images should confirm the decompression of the peroneal tendons and

narrowing of the heel. If there are other large fragments that are amenable to closed pinning, then they are secured, again under fluoroscopic control.

The large posterior pin is incorporated into the plaster cast. We prefer to wrap the pin in cast padding to facilitate removal of the cast. The foot is casted with the ankle at 10 to 15 degrees of plantar flexion. A long leg cast is seldom necessary.

Postoperative Care

Following open reduction and internal fixation, the patient is placed at bed rest for 24 to 48 hours with the leg elevated. Suction drains are

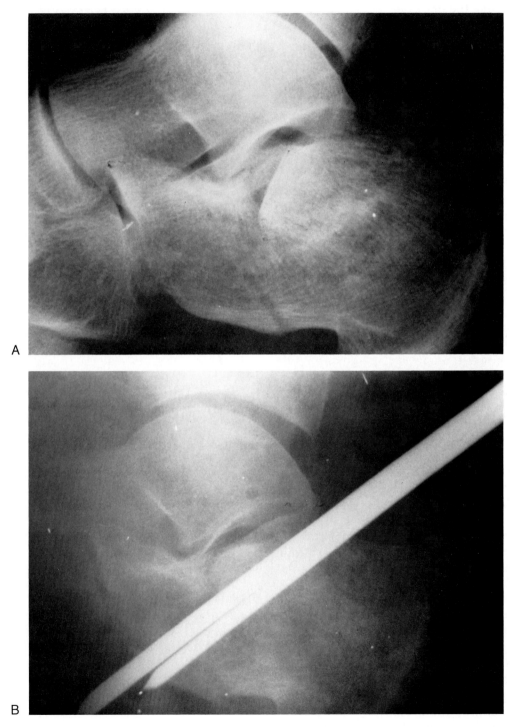

A

B

Fig. 24-21. **(A)** Pre- and **(B)** postoperative lateral views of joint depression fracture treated by closed pinning. Here two pins were used for stabilization of the posterior facet after the initial pin was used to elevate the facet. Note the reduction of the posterior facet.

removed when the drainage slows to less than 10 ml/8 hours. This is often on the second postoperative day.

If the surgeon has achieved rigid internal fixation, then active and passive range of motion exercises are begun on the second or third postoperative day. It is critical to impress upon the patient the importance of early motion for the attainment of a good functional result. It is often necessary to use oral or parenteral narcotics prior to each therapy session. Patient-controlled analgesic technology may be instituted in cases in which a prolonged hospital stay is anticipated. The patients are taught to make the figure of eight with the toes as well as active ankle dorsiflexion.

If available, a partner is taught to perform passive range of motion exercises of the subtalar and midtarsal joints with vigor. Again, narcotic assistance may be necessary. When therapy is not being performed, the leg is immobilized in a removable short leg splint or cast.

If fixation was tenuous, then only gentle active range of motion exercises are permitted early. Weight bearing is permitted no sooner than 8 weeks postsurgery. The actual time is determined by careful monitoring of the radiographic status and consideration of the stability of the construct. One must be cognizant of the mechanism of bone graft physiology in that the replacement phenomena renders the graft soft even though this situation is radiographically inert. Therefore, caution and conservatism should prevail when weight bearing is considered. When weight bearing is initially permitted, it is best to use a removeable short leg walking cast for 2 weeks followed by unprotected weight bearing. Range of motion exercises are continued throughout.

If closed reduction techniques have been used, the same guidelines for mobilization and weight bearing are followed. However, one must realize that it is highly unlikely that rigid fixation would result, and only gentle range of motion should be done. Protruding pins should be left intact for a minimum of 6 weeks unless persistent drainage or marked loosening hastens their removal.

Closed Treatment

Closed treatment of intra-articular calcaneal fractures is a viable alternative to the surgical approach.[20,42–44] It is primarily indicated when the other methods would not likely yield a better result. Situations in which this might occur would be the elderly patient with a grossly comminuted fracture pattern. Here fixation would be difficult at best and the patient's presumably altered physiologic status would preclude an optimal surgical result.

Because the intra-articular calcaneal fracture has such high variability in its presentation, it is possible to confuse the average surgeon who might not deal with this injury more than a few times. Because of the complex arrangement of the facets and the difficult task of anatomic restoration, closed treatment is preferred when the surgeon has limited experience in these injuries.

The psychological profile of the patient is also important to assess when deciding on the type of treatment. Patients who are poorly motivated or would have difficulty following the postoperative regimen should be treated conservatively.

The proponents for closed treatment rightly contend that the calcaneus always heals owing to its abundant blood supply.[45] Therefore, immobilization of the bone is unnecessary to obtain union. The accumulation of edema and blood escapes into the soft tissues, which in turn evokes an inflammatory reaction about the tendons and joints. Immobilization in the face of this leads to clot organization, scar formation with acceptance of the malpositioned fragments, and resultant stiffness and pain. This same scar formation decreases lymphatic and venous return, predisposing to chronic swelling.

We believe that the best conservative approach is one that favors early mobilization.[3,37,45] When closed treatment is chosen, the involved extremity is gently compressed with an Ace bandage. Contrast baths are employed on the second or third postinjury day. Aggressive active and passive range of motion exercises are begun at the same time. Non-weight bearing is enforced for at least 8 to 10 weeks. The patient is instructed to perform the exercise–contrast bath sequence three or four times a day. Analgesic support is often necessary and should be encouraged. Nonsteroidal anti-inflammatory agents will also be of benefit in many patients. A posterior splint or sugar tong splint is optional. The theory behind this treatment regimen is that the motion would serve to mold the articular facets into smooth yet incongruous surfaces.[45] The post-traumatic fibrosis would also be minimized.

We have had satisfying results with this method. Many of the patients attain excellent range of motion with little post-traumatic arthrosis in the middle to long term. Radiographic findings usually correlate poorly with the patient's clinical response.

Cast immobilization has been advocated in some circles for the intra-articular calcaneal fracture. Weight bearing is seldom recommended. It is our opinion that cast immobilization should not be an option for the reasons outlined above. The usual result is a very stiff, often painful heel and subtalar joint with chronic edema. The patient is better off with no treatment rather than this regimen because there is little hope for the restoration of motion after fibrosis has ensued.

Immediate arthrodesis is also included in the literature as a primary form of therapy.[46–48] We mention this for the sake of completeness only. It should be abandoned as a treatment option. It is surprising that many of these patients never require arthrodesis regardless of the type of treatment. Often the subtalar joint is so stiff that late arthrodesis would not be expected to provide benefits other than pain relief. Many patients are able to accept varying degrees of discomfort rather than submit to an arthrodesing procedure. Therefore, immediate arthrodesis should never be done. It can always be done at a later date.

The advantages of closed treatment are that no hospitalization is required. The complications of surgery, including anesthetic and wound infections, are avoided. However, we do not mean to imply that this is universally the best form of treatment. Each and every calcaneal fracture must be assessed on the basis of the entire patient, the skills of the surgeon, and a realistic expectation of the outcome. No patient should be denied the opportunity for more aggressive treatment if the ultimate outcome can be predictably better.

COMPLICATIONS

Complications from intra-articular calcaneal fractures can be separated into those problems that arise from the fracture itself and those that arise from surgical treatment. Those that the nature of the fracture is responsible for include subtalar joint stiffness, pain, degenerative joint disease, peroneal tendonitis or impingement, and varus or valgus deformities. Those arising from surgical manipulation of the fracture include primarily wound problems and sural nerve damage. The obvious risks of surgery in general are not included in this discussion but should be considered.

Subtalar joint incongruity can be expected to lead to a variety of problems. Because of the lack of a congruous surface, loss of motion is to be expected. This can be accentuated by long-term immobilization or postsurgical scarring. Regardless of the total range of motion, the residual absolute motion through an incongruous joint will lead to loss of joint space, periarticular spurring, and degenerative arthritis. The resultant loss of motion can also be expected to add to the patient's discomfort (Fig. 24-22). Treatment of this entity consists of the usual and customary therapies for any degenerative joint, ranging from injections, orthoses, nonsteroidal anti-inflammatory medications, and physical therapy to selective arthrodesis.

Pain in the hindfoot region is a common sequela. It must be carefully evaluated because of the many different etiologic factors. Heel pad pain is not a direct consequence of the articular component of the fracture but is a frequent residuum of these fractures that result from a vertical fall. The presumed cause is disruption of the heel pad septae and crushing of the fat pad.[37,41,49,50] This problem is difficult to deal with. Cortisone injections, soft tissue supplements such as PPT or Spenco, and orthotics are indicated with varying levels of success.[4,41]

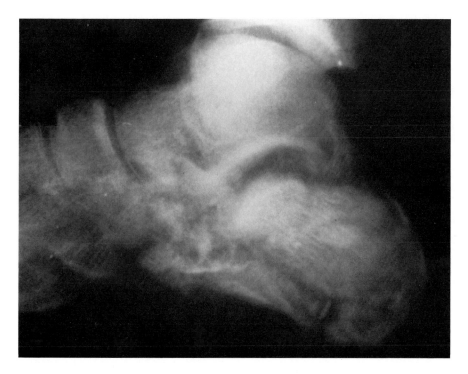

Fig. 24-22. Nineteen-month postoperative lateral view of malreduced calcaneal fracture. Note the incongruity of the subtalar joint and loss of height of the calcaneus.

Post-traumatic degenerative joint disease can be expected whenever the articular facets have not been accurately restored or the complex three-dimensional relationships between the facets have been altered. The mechanism of arthritic development is the same for any joint that has articular incongruity, but is probably accelerated in the case of calcaneal fractures because of the multifaceted subtalar joint. In fact, articular step-offs of 2 mm are probably more morbid than highly comminuted, grossly displaced fractures. This is probably due to the fact that fractures that result in loss of motion, presumably highly comminuted ones, produce less abrasive forces. On the other hand, those less displaced fractures are less likely to limit motion and cause more rapid joint space narrowing from repetitive grinding. Although the majority of the time the most significant changes are in the posterior facet, this is only due to the higher percentage of weight

borne by this facet. Certainly the incongruity can emanate from the middle or anterior facet in decreasing probability. The interdependence of the three facets predisposes any and all of the articulations when even one is disrupted. Treatment is along the same lines as for subtalar incongruity.

Peroneal tendonitis or constriction is usually a result of the widened lateral wall of the body of the calcaneus.[4,51] Because the tendon sheaths and their resultant course is fixed between the lateral malleolus and the lateral calcaneal wall, any narrowing or alteration of this space will interfere with normal tendon gliding. The peroneal tubercle can become damaged during the fracture, and subsequent hypertrophy or displacement serves to impinge in this area. This is a frequent location for peroneal dysfunction. Similarly when the foot is immobilized without periodic and aggressive mobilization of the tendons, then the resultant scar will further serve to tether the function. Symptoms of instability of the ankle or subtalar joint are possible when significant displacement of the tendons occurs.

Lateral decompression and peroneal retinaculoplasty are often necessary if conservative measures fail. Generous bony resection is required to reestablish the normal anatomic tunnel. Aggressive early range of motion exercises will optimize the surgical result.

Frontal plane deformities are uncommon following intra-articular calcaneal fractures. The natural valgus collapse of the calcaneus during the injury makes the likelihood of a varus deformity rare. Many of the valgus frontal plane deviations are a result of the loss of motion in the fixed valgus position. Frontal plane deviations are somewhat more likely following open reduction if there has been inaccurate restoration of the articular components. Varus angulations may be created by surgical manipulation.

REFERENCES

1. Rockwood CA, Jr, Green DP: Fractures in Adults. JB Lippincott, Philadelphia, 1984
2. Slatis PK, Kiviluoto O, Santavirta S: Fractures of the calcaneum. J Trauma 19:939, 1979
3. Lance EM, Carey EJ, Wade PA: Fractures of the os calcis. A follow-up study. J Trauma 4:15, 1964
4. Clisham MW, Berlin SJ: The diagnosis and conservative treatment of calcaneal fractures. A review. J Foot Surg 20:28, 1981
5. Spector EE: Fractures of the calcaneus. J Am Podiatry Assoc 65:789, 1975
6. Cave EF: Fracture of the os calcis. The problem in general. Clin Orthop 30:64, 1963
7. Essex-Lopresti P: The mechanism, reduction technique and results in fractures of the os calcis. Br J Surg 39:395, 1952
8. Wilson OW: Functional capacity following fractures of the os calcis. Can Med Assoc J 95:908, 1966
9. Matteri RE, Frymoyer JW: Fractures of the calcaneus in young children. J Bone Joint Surg 55A:1091, 1973
10. Schmidt T, Weiner DJ: Calcaneal fractures in children. Clin Orthop 171:150, 1982
11. Schuberth JM: Principles of fracture management in children. Clin Pod Surg 4:267, 1987
12. Wiley JJ, Pofitt A: Fractures of the os calcis in children. Clin Orthop 171:150, 1982
13. Manter JT: Movements of the subtalar and transverse tarsal joints. Anat Rec 80:397, 1941
14. Inman VT: Joints of the Ankle. Williams & Wilkins, Baltimore, 1976
15. Sarrafian SK: Anatomy of the Foot and Ankle. JB Lippincott, Philadelphia, 1983
16. Cavaliere RG: Ankle and rearfoot-calcaneal fractures. In McGlamry ED (ed): A Comprehensive Textbook of Foot Surgery. Williams & Wilkins, Baltimore, 1987
17. Hermann OJ: Conservative therapy for fracture of the os calcis. J Bone Joint Surg 19:709, 1937
18. Wong PCN: Vertebral column and os calcis fracture patterns in a confined community (Singapore). Acta Orthop Scand 37:357, 1966
19. Gaul J: Calcaneal fractures involving the subtalar joint. South Med J 59:605, 1966
20. Rowe CR, Sabellarides HR, Freeman PA: Fractures of the os calcis: a long term study of 146 patients. JAMA 184:98, 1963
21. Watson-Jones R: Fractures and Joint Injuries. 4th Ed. Churchhill Livngstone, Edinburgh, 1962
22. Bohler L: Diagnosis, pathology and treatment of fractures of the os calcis. J Bone Joint Surg 13:75, 1931
23. Broden B: Roentgen examination of the subtaloid joint in fractures of the calcaneus. Acta Radiol 31:85, 1949
24. McReynolds IS: The case for operative treatment of fractures of the os calcis. In Leach RE, Hoaglund FT, Riseborough EJ (ed): Controversies in Orthopedic Surgery. WB Saunders, Philadelphia, 1982
25. Carey EJ, Lance EM, Wade PA: Extra-articular fractures of the os calcis. J Trauma 5:362, 1965
26. Norfray JF, Rogers LF, Adams GP: Common calcaneal avulsion fracture. AJR 134:119, 1980
27. Degan TJ, Morrey BF, Braun DP: Surgical excision for anterior process fractures of the calcaneus. J Bone Joint Surg 64A:519, 1982
28. Gellman M: Fracture of the anterior process of the calcaneus. J Bone Joint Surg 33A:382, 1951
29. Piatt AD: Fracture of the promontory of the calcaneus. Radiology 67:386, 1956
30. Dachtler HW: Fractures of the anterior superior portion of the os calcis due to indirect violence. AJR 25:629, 1931
31. Bachman S, and Johnson SR: Torsion of the foot causing fracture of the anterior calcaneal process. Acta Chir Scand 105:460, 1953

32. Lowry M: Avulsion fractures of the calcaneus. J Bone Joint Surg 51B:494, 1969

33. Lungstadaas S: Treatment of avulsion fractures of the tuber calcanei. Acta Chir Scand 137:579, 1971

34. Palmer I: The mechanism and treatment of fractures of the calcaneus. J Bone Joint Surg 30A:2, 1948

35. Soeur R, Remy R: Fractures of the calcaneus with displacement of the thalamic portion. J Bone Joint Surg 57B:413, 1975

36. Burdeaux BD: Reduction of calcaneal fractures by the McReynolds medial approach technique and its experimental basis. Clin Orthop 177:87, 1983

37. O'Connell F, Mital MA, Rowe CR: Evaluation of modern management of fractures to the os calcis. Clin Orthop 83:214, 1972

38. Stephenson JR: Displaced fractures of the os calcis involving the subtalar joint: the key role of the superomedial fragment. Foot Ankle 4:91, 1983

39. Stephenson JR: Treatment of displaced intra-articular fractures of the calcaneus using medial and lateral approaches, internal fixation and early motion. J Bone Joint Surg 69A:115, 1987

40. Harding D, Waddell JP: Open reduction in depressed fractures of the os calcis. Clin Orthop 199:124, 1985

41. King RE: Axial pin fixation of fractures of the os calcis (method of Essex-Lopresti). Orthop Clin North Am 4:185, 1973

42. Lindsay WRN, Dewer FP: Fractures of the os calcis. Am J Surg 95:555, 1958

43. Omoto H, Kazuyuki S, Mototsugu S: A new method of manual reduction for intraarticular fractures of the calcaneus. Clin Orthop 177:104, 1983

44. Shannon FT, Murray AM: Os calcis fractures treated by non-weightbearing exercises. J R Col Surg Edinb 12:40, 1978

45. Parkes JC, II: The nonreductive treatment for fractures of the os calcis. Orthop Clin North Am 4:193, 1973

46. Harris R: Fractures of the os calcis. Treatment by early subtalar arthrodesis. Clin Orthop 30:100, 1963

47. Pennal GF, Yadav MP: Operative treatment of comminuted fractures of the os calcis. Orthop Clin North Am 4:197, 1973

48. Thompson KR: Treatment of comminuted fractures of the calcaneus by triple arthrodesis. Orthop Clin North Am 4:189, 1973

49. Miller WE: Pain and impairment considerations following treatment of disruptive os calcis fractures. Clin Orthop 177:82, 1983

50. Miller WE, Lichtblau PO: The smashed heel. South Med J 58:1229, 1965

51. Deyerle WM: Long term followup of fractures of the os calcis. Diagnostic peroneal synoviagram. Orthop Clin North Am 4:213, 1973

25

Foot and Ankle Fractures in Children

Steven DeValentine, D.P.M.

When dealing with fractures of the foot and ankle in adults, one tends to think in relatively static terms. When something is broken, the surgeon's primary objective is to restore that part as near as possible to its preinjury condition without much regard for future events. We must think in more dynamic terms when dealing with fractures of the foot and ankle in children. The management of a particular type of ankle fracture in a 5-year-old child may vary significantly from the management of that same fracture in a 12-year-old child. In choosing a specific treatment approach, one must consider the child's age, sex, fracture type, blood supply, the presence of angular or rotational deformity, and local and systemic factors that affect growth. A functional knowledge of anatomy and physiology of growing bone is essential to proper management of these injuries. Only long-term follow-up will determine whether the outcome is a success or failure.

The intent of this chapter is to provide a useful review of functional anatomy and physiology of growing bone as it relates to the management of foot and ankle fractures in children as well as provide practical methods of dealing with some specific fracture types. The Salter-Harris classification system is used because of its wide acceptance, ease of applicability, and prognostic value. I prefer the Dias-Tachdjian classification system for pediatric ankle fractures because it is based on the Lauge-Hansen mechanistic classification system, which is currently widely used in the management of adult ankle fractures.

FUNCTIONAL ANATOMY AND PHYSIOLOGY OF GROWING BONE

Limb Development and Bone Formation

The extremities of the human fetus are first identifiable as limb buds at about the fifth week of gestation. The central portion of the limb bud is composed of primitive undifferentiated mesenchymal cells that are able to differentiate into muscle, hyaline cartilage, and the cartilaginous precursor of bone. The central portion of what will become the long bone is the first cartilage to be converted to bone. This process is referred to as endochondral ossification. Ossification of this cartilaginous precursor of bone is stimulated by an increase in PaO_2 brought about by development and invasion of the nutrient artery. The axial and appendicular skeletal bones are formed through this process of endochondral ossification. In contrast, cranial and fascial bones are ossified directly from the primitive fibrous mesenchymal precursor without the intermediary formation of cartilage. This process of direct ossification is referred to as membranous bone formation. The terms endochondral ossification and

473

membranous bone formation refer only to primary bone development. Once primary bone formation has occurred, both endochondral ossification and membranous bone formation contribute to continuing bone growth. Long bones grow in length through endochondral ossification of physeal cartilage and in diameter through metaphyseal remodeling of this endochondral bone. The diaphyseal portion of long bones also grows in diameter by periosteal new bone formation. Periosteum forms bone through direct ossification of noncartilaginous fibrous tissue that is really a type of membranous bone formation. Primary membranous bones (i.e., cranial, fascial, clavicle) also exhibit some endochondral ossification characteristics at their periphery where cartilaginous growth plate areas undergo ossification. Endochondral ossification within the central portion of the long bone (diaphysis) produces the primary ossification center that is always present at birth. Endochondral ossification at the end of the long bone, which occurs in response to the invasion of the epiphyseal arteries, produces the secondary ossification center of the epiphysis. Secondary ossification centers of long bones may or may not be present at birth. The growth plate or physis is made up of various layers of cartilaginous cells within a matrix ground substance that undergo proliferation and gradual endochondral ossification with formation of new bone on the metaphyseal side of the physis.

The metaphysis of immature long bones is composed of a loosely woven spongiosa bone that has greater porosity, vascularity, and elasticity than mature bone. The metaphyseal spongiosa bone is gradually converted to a denser diaphyseal lamellar bone through endosteal remodeling. The lamellar cortex of immature diaphyseal bone is much less dense (greater porosity) and has a much greater elasticity than adult diaphyseal cortical bone. As bone matures it becomes denser (less porous) and harder. The comparative lack of cortical strength in growing bone is to some extent compensated by a much thicker and more biologically active periosteum. The periosteum is very firmly attached in the metaphyseal and epiphyseal region but is more easily separated from the diaphysis. Thus, when a fracture occurs, the periosteum is usually left intact. This helps decrease displacement and provides a soft tissue hinge that is very useful in achieving reduction. The greater osteogenic potential of immature periosteum is one factor that results in the much faster healing rate of pediatric fractures. The greater porosity and more abundant vascularity of pediatric bone are also significant factors in producing a more rapid healing response. In general, the younger the child, the more rapid the healing rate, with fractures in infants and young children healing in about one-half the time required for the some fracture in an adult.

Hyaline articular cartilage is thought to differentiate from the same cartilaginous precursor cells that form the physis and the epiphysis. Once formed, however, hyaline cartilage will not undergo ossification. This partially explains the failure of rotated or inverted osteochondral fracture fragments to become incorporated and ossified.

The small irregular cancellous bones that compose the greater and lesser tarsal area are also formed through endochondral ossification. A primary ossification center usually forms in the center of the bone as a result of nutrient artery invasion and increase in local PaO_2. The primary ossification centers of the calcaneus, talus, and cuboid are present at birth. The primary ossification center of the lateral cuneiform appears at about 1 year of age and those of the navicular and medial cuneiforms between 3 and 4 years of age. Gradual ossification of the tarsal bones' cartilaginous precursor occurs from centrally outward in a circumferential manner following the pre-existing cartilage template.

The small tubular metatarsals and phalanges develop in a manner similar to that of the long bones, with their primary ossification centers being present at birth. A physis is initially present at both ends of the metatarsals and phalanges but decreases in size at one end to form a small spherical portion of cartilage between the hyaline articular cartilage surface and the metaphysis (pseudoepiphysis). No secondary ossification center or ephiphysis forms at this end of the bone. A true secondary ossification center (epiphysis) does form at the other end of the bone but is usually not radiographically visible until about 3 years of age. The true physis that is the primary contributor of growth to the small tubular bones is found at the base of the phalanges and first metatarsal. The lesser metatarsal true physis is at its distal end. A metatarsal or phalanx may on occasion appear to have a physis and secondary ossification center at both ends. This is especially common in the first metatarsal. The distal spherical physis (pseudoepiphysis) is of secondary importance and does not contribute to longitudinal growth. Ossification of the growth plate occurs during adolescence when the metaphyseal vascular channels invade the physis. This results in bone union between the metaphysis and epiphysis and cessation of growth at skeletal maturity. The sequence of events that results in growth plate closure is an orderly and fairly predictable process, although the initiation of the process may vary from child to child. Radiographic measurement of a child's skeletal age may be compared with chronologic age to better predict the outcome of physeal injuries.

The Physis

The physis is composed of layers of cells embedded in a matrix of ground substance composed of collagen fibers in chondroitin sulfate (Fig. 25-1). Salter likened this substance to reinforcement rods in concrete.[1] The layer of chondrocyte cells nearest the epiphysis is embedded in an abundant amount of strong matrix and is referred to as the germinal (or resting) cell layer or zone. The next layer of cells is composed of columns of cells undergoing rapid mitosis and is referred to as the zone of proliferation. The third layer is composed of chondrocytes that hypertrophy to as much as five times their normal size. Because of the greater size and number of cells within the zone of hypertrophy, there is a corresponding decrease in the amount of cementing matrix substance. The hypertrophic cells gradually "disintegrate" to form a fourth layer of endochondral ossification where bone is laid down at the metaphyseal side of the plate. This disintegration of the hypertrophic cells results in an invasion of metaphyseal blood vessels that increases the local oxygen tension and promotes

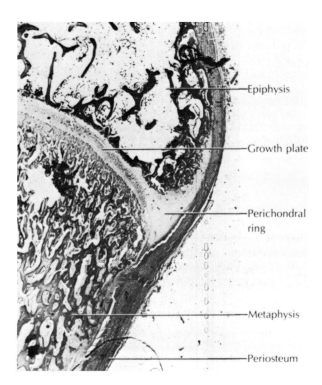

Fig. 25-1. The peripheral edge of a rodent long bone. (From Rockwood,[4] with permission.)

ossification of the matrix ground substance. The area between the zone of hypertrophying cells and the zone of ossifying cells is the weakest part of the physis because of the reduced concentration of cementing ground substance, and this is the area where cleavage is most likely to occur (Table 25-1). As long as the layers of proliferating and hypertrophying cells remain attached to the epiphysis with its epiphyseal blood supply undisturbed, there is no reason why growth disturbance should occur. The metaphyseal bone produced by endochondral ossification is spongiosa bone that gradually remodels to form the denser and stronger cortical bone of the diaphysis. The width of the metaphysis and physis of a long bone is approximately twice the diameter of the diaphysis. This greater cross-sectional area increases resistance to separation and helps compensate for the metaphysis' lesser ability to resist stresses compared with cortical bone. The spongiosa bone of the metaphysis also functions as a shock absorber. The ability of the physis to resist

Table 25-1.   Applied Histology of the Epiphyseal Plate

Epiphysis	Resting cells	Matrix abundant
↑	Proliferating cells	Plate strong
	Hypertrophying cells	Matrix scanty
		Plate weak
	Zone of provisional calcification	Matrix calcified
↓		Plate stronger
Metaphysis	Endochondral ossification	

separation is also increased by the mountainous convolutions and small interdigitating mamillary processes that increase its surface area and increase its resistance to shear stress.

The lateral portion of the plate forms a structure referred to as the perichondrial ring, which is contiguous with the epiphyseal cartilage and the metaphyseal periosteum (Fig. 25-1). The perichondrial ring adds lateral growth to the plate and increases its strength. Because the perichondrial ring area has a separate blood supply, it is possible to have injuries that will cause central but not peripheral growth arrest or vice versa.

Two anatomic types of epiphyses have been described. Pressure epiphyses are subject to the compressive forces of muscular contraction and weight bearing and are associated with the articular ends of long bones. The proximal and distal tibial epiphyses are typical pressure epiphyses. Traction epiphyses are nonarticular and are often referred to as apophyses. Traction epiphyses are usually subject to tensile forces from muscle attachments. The tibial tubercle, calcaneal apophysis, and styloid process of the fifth metatarsal are good examples of traction epiphyses. Injuries to traction epiphyses are fairly rare, but even when they occur, concern over anatomic alignment need not be as great since traction epiphyses do not contribute to overall long bone growth. Pressure epiphyses can be subdivided into intracapsular epiphyses such as the femoral head and extracapsular epiphyses such as the distal tibial, fibular, and metatarsal epiphyses.

There are three primary sources of blood supply to the ends of long bones (Fig. 25-2A). The nutrient artery is the major source of blood sup-ply to the diaphysis and the metaphyseal sinusoids that supply the metaphyseal side of the growth plate (zone of endochondral ossification). The epiphyseal vessels that enter through joint capsule supply the majority of the germinal and proliferative cell layers. In addition, periosteal and perichondrial vessels supply the peripheral portion of the growth plate. When separation of an extra-articular epiphysis occurs, both the epiphyseal and metaphyseal blood supplies are usually maintained. If the separation is between the hypertrophic and ossifying layer of cells, where the plate is structurally weakest (where separation occurs at least 50 percent of the time) and if the epiphyseal blood supply to the growing part of the physis remains intact, the likelihood for growth disturbance is extremely low.[1,2] The epiphyseal blood vessels of intra-articular epiphyses must enter through joint capsule on the metaphyseal side of the physis and then traverse over the surface of the plate to enter the epiphysis (Fig. 25-2B). When separation of intra-articular epiphyses occurs, epiphyseal vessels are very easily damaged. This explains the high incidence of avascular necrosis that occurs in intracapsular epiphyses, such as the capital femoral epiphysis. Fortunately, most epiphyses, including all in the foot and ankle, are of the extracapsular type.

A multitude of local and systemic factors may affect epiphyseal growth (Table 25-2). The most important of the systemic factors is probably genetic and the most important nongenetic factor is probably nutrition. Nutritional differences are probably greatly responsible for increases in height in the general population over the last

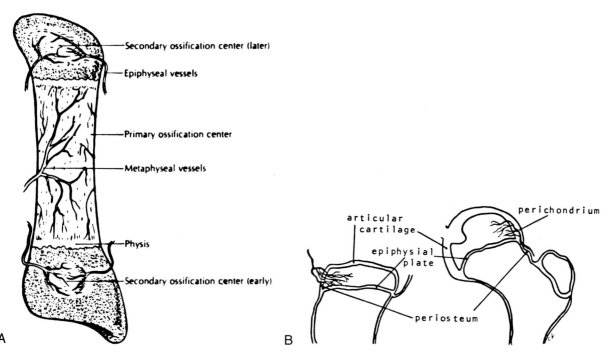

Fig. 25-2. **(A)** The primary sources of blood supply to the ends of long bones. (From Rockwood,[4] with permission.) **(B)** Two basic patterns of blood supply to the epiphysis. With disruption of the intracapsular epiphysis (femoral head), epiphyseal vessels are frequently sheared off, resulting in loss of vascular supply to the epiphysis and germinal cell layers, and causing avascular necrosis. (From Salter and Harris,[1] with permission.)

Table 25-2.   Factors Affecting Epiphyseal Growth

Factors	Effect on Growth
Systemic factors	
Genetic	↑ ↓
Nutrition	↑ ↓
Growth hormone (GH)	↑ GH → gigantism
	↓ GH → dwarfism
Thyroid hormone (TH)	↑ TH → ↑ rapidity
	↓ TH → cretinism
Androgens	↑ growth → eventual closure
Estrogens	↑ growth → early closure
Local factors	
Compression	slight ↑ → ↑ growth
	large ↑ → ↓ growth
Nearby fracture	↑ growth
Infection	↓
Injury	↓
Interference with circulation	↓

several centuries. The lower incidence of epiphyseal injuries in girls was formerly attributed to less physical activity, but the effect of estrogen may be a more important factor. Estrogen stimulates an increased rapidity of growth in girls during adolescence, but also results in early physeal closure, causing girls to be shorter than boys at maturity.

We know that a differential growth rate occurs among different epiphyses. It is unclear what systemic or local factors are responsible for the different rates of growth that occur in different epiphyses, but proximal epiphyses are usually responsible for a much greater percentage of extremity growth than are distal epiphyses. This becomes important in dealing with potential limb length discrepancies from epiphyseal injuries. Injuries about the ankle, for example, are of much less consequence in determining overall limb length than injuries about the knee joint. There also exists a potential for a differential growth rate within any individual epiphysis. A primary local factor affecting differential growth within any individual epiphysis is compression. A slight increase in compression stimulates physeal growth, whereas a larger increase in compression may retard physeal growth. Bright et al.[3] have pointed out that physiologic tibial and genu varum spontaneously correct as a result of differential physeal growth stimulated by slight increases in compression from angular deformity.[4] The child with tibial or genu varum in infancy responds to slightly increased compression of the medial epiphyses about the knee by increasing the growth rate of the medial physis compared with the lateral physis, resulting in reduction of the physiologic varus deformity. An understanding of this concept becomes extremely important in evaluating the ability of an individual epiphyseal injury to undergo spontaneous correction.

In general, spontaneous correction of angular deformities of less than 15 to 20 degrees will occur, with greater deformities correcting faster if adequate growth remains prior to skeletal maturity. In some cases, it may be more prudent to accept a slight deformity that will probably correct spontaneously rather than risk growth plate damage from too forcible manipulation. One should also be aware that rotational deformities will not spontaneously reduce and always require anatomic realignment.

BIOMECHANICAL PROPERTIES OF GROWING BONE

A great deal of valuable and interesting experimental work concerning mechanical properties of growing bone has been done. Most of this work has been done in animal models, and a comprehensive discussion is beyond the scope of this chapter. A basic knowledge of the biodynamics of bone and physeal function as well as failure is not only relevant but imperative for appropriate clinical management of pediatric skeletal injuries.

Mature (adult) bone is physiologically and mechanically in a relatively static state compared with immature (pediatric) bone. Immature bone is in a much more dynamic state of activity, which results in a much greater variability of fracture pattern. The variable nature of these injuries is determined by both extrinsic and intrinsic factors. Extrinsic factors such as magnitude, direction, and rate of application of force are important in determining the location and way in which bone or physis will fail. These extrinsic factors are constantly changing in children with growth and with increase in body weight and size and increasing physical activity with age. Intrinsic factors such as bone structure, density, elasticity, and energy-absorbing capacity are also important in determining bone's response to applied loads. Trabecular patterns are changing in accordance with Wolff's law much more rapidly in children in response to extrinsic forces. As a result, failure patterns will change in a corresponding manner. The trabecular or spongiosa bone of the epiphysis and metaphysis has a greater flexibility than mature spongiosa or cortical bone and thus acts as a very effective shock absorber in transmitting loads from articular surfaces to diaphyseal bone. Articular and physeal cartilage also provides a shock-absorbing function. Both diaphyseal and metaphyseal immature bone has a much greater elasticity than mature bone, which allows greater energy absorption capacity. This greater elasticity is probably a function of less density (greater porosity). Immature bone is not less ossified, just less in volume. As bone matures, density increases (porosity decreases) and bone becomes less elastic.

When external loads are applied to bone, the force concentrations are referred to as *stresses*. Stresses can be measured as force per unit area. Bone responds to stress by developing microscopic deformations in its physical structure. This response to stress (applied force) is defined as *strain*, which can be measured as stretch per unit of length. The strain produced by constant or repetitive low-grade stresses results in normal remodeling (reorientation of structure and trabecular patterns) in accordance with Wolff's law. When stress applied to bone increases beyond strain, microscopic deformations coalesce to become macroscopic fractures and bone fails.

Different types of stresses occur when loads are applied from different directions. Stresses that culminate in longitudinal strains of bone are referred to as compression or tension (elongation). Forces applied at oblique angles to bone result in shear stress, and rotational force causes torsional stress. Each type of stress tends to cause certain types of strain failure. Stresses that are applied to bone in other than longitudinal directions tend to produce *transverse* or *oblique* fractures through areas of bone with the least strain resistence; that is, metaphysis, physis, and epiphysis. These fracture patterns may vary significantly with the changing structure of these dynamic areas of pediatric bone. Torsional stresses result in *spiral fractures*, which usually involve the diaphysis of long bones (i.e., tibia, fibula) or occasionally short tubular bones (i.e., metatarsals, phalanges). *Compression* or *crush fractures* occur as a result of a direct compression stress and occur most commonly in the metaphyseal area. *Comminuted fractures* occur as a result of stresses applied in several directions. The younger the child, the less common is fracture comminution owing to the greater capability of immature porous bone to absorb energy.

Although the location and frequency of the preceeding types of fractures vary considerably more in children than in adults, the mechanism and the mode of failure are basically the same.

The strain response of immature bone to longitudinal compression force is much different from that of mature bone. When a longitudinal compression force is applied to the more elastic, tubular, naturally curved long bone of a child, a slight bending occurs. A compression strain occurs on the concave side and tensile strain occurs on the convex side. Below a certain stress point the bone responds by bending and then, when the stress is removed, returns to its prior shape. The greater elasticity of immature bone allows greater deformation than would be possible in mature bone. Beyond that stress point, immature bone may undergo a permanent bowing without returning to its prestress shape. This phenomenon is called *plastic deformation* and has been demonstrated in long bones of children. In the lower extremity, plastic deformation or bowing of the fibula is usually seen in combination with a tibial fracture and may make reduction of the tibial fracture difficult. With an increasing compression load, failure will occur on the tensile side of the bone causing a *greenstick fracture* (Fig. 25-3). A portion of the periosteum and cortex is left intact on the compression side of the bone and aids in reduction. Greenstick fractures are less common as children approach adolescence and bone density increases and elasticity decreases. Another type of fracture that occurs only in children primarily as a result of immature bone's ability to undergo plastic deformation is the *torus fracture*. This is a compression fracture of metaphyseal bone in which the thinner cortical metaphyseal bone of a child fails on the compression side first, leaving the tensile side intact. Torus fractures are by nature very stable but do require protection since one can assume that plastic deformation and probable microfracture have occurred even on the undisrupted tensile side of the metaphysis.

Physeal Biomechanics

Bright and co-workers describe the physis as a nonhomogeneous, anisotropic, viscoelastic substance.[3] This can be defined as a physical material that reacts differently to physical stresses along different axes and in which stress increases

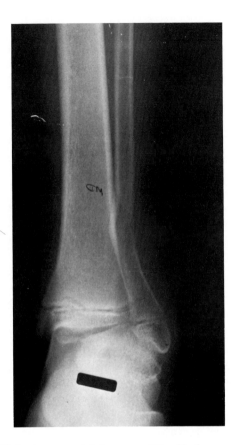

Fig. 25-3. A greenstick fracture of the fibula associated with a Salter-Harris type III medial malleolar pull-off fracture and lateral ankle dislocation in a pronation-external rotation injury in an adolescent.

relative to the rate of strain increase. The growth plate is subjected to a combination of compression, tension, and shear forces in most activities. (Those forces that increase shear stresses are more likely to cause disruption.) The likelihood of disruption is greatest with torsional loading and least with axial loading, with bending forces being intermediate.[3] Because of its viscoelastic nature, the physis is better able to withstand forces applied at a rapid rate than forces applied at a slower, continuous rate. In addition, the physis and underlying metaphyseal bone are thought to provide some shock absorption to sudden loading. All of these characteristics help to protect against physeal disruption with the usual sudden loading types of forces that occur in pediatric injuries.

The physis is the second most rigid musculoskeletal structure, with bone being the most rigid. Because of this, the physis is more likely to absorb force than surrounding soft tissue structures and physeal disruption normally occurs before soft tissue injury. Once the physis slips, the surrounding soft tissue structures (periosteum, joint capsule, ligaments, etc.) undergo loading. Most researchers believe that physeal disruption can occur without displacement. These injuries may be easily mistaken for sprain, and one should always maintain a high index of suspicion with injuries near epiphyses. Injuries that may cause ligament tears, tendon rupture, or joint dislocation in adults may produce physeal injuries in children. The only signs of physeal injury without disruption may be distinct local tenderness over the epiphysis or slight widening of the physis on radiographs compared with the normal side. Follow-up radiographs in 2 to 3 weeks should demonstrate evidence of bone healing if disruption has occurred.

Salter and others, on the basis of their experimental work, stated that classical physeal disruption always occurs between the hypertrophying layer and ossifying layer, leaving the germinal cell layer intact.[1] Bright et al. suggested, on the basis of their experimental work, that physeal fractures may take a circuitous course through other layers of the plate, including the germinal cell layer, as often as 50 percent of the time.[3] This points out that the possibility of growth disturbance should be considered with any physeal injury. It is particularly important to discuss this with parents even though the likelihood of growth disturbance may be very low.

INCIDENCE

The majority of injuries in children do not involve fractures. Hanlon and Estes found the incidence of fracture or dislocation in children seen at St. Luke's Hospital, Bethlehem, Pennsylvania, for injuries over a 3-month period to be about 15 percent.[5] They then analyzed 698 pediatric patients (birth to 18 years) with fractures seen over a 10-year period at the same institution. The upper extremity was affected in 65 percent and the lower extremity in 31 percent, with the remainder of fractures involving the trunk or skull. Approximately 80 percent of fractures involved the major long bones of the extremities and the clavicle. About 7 percent of fractures involved the small bones of the hand and about 6 percent involved the small bones of the foot. The highest incidence of fracture was found during adolescence, with fractures very rarely occurring before the age of 2 years. Athletic activities were the most common cause of injury.

Only about 15 to 20 percent (2 to 3 percent of all injuries) of pediatric fractures involved the physis. The distal physes of the extremities have the highest incidence of injury. In a review of 118 epiphyseal injuries, Rogers found that the distal tibial and fibular physes were injured in 25 percent of the patients.[6] Only the distal radius is more frequently injured. Peterson, in a retrospective review of 330 epiphyseal injuries over a 20-year period, found that boys were affected greater than two times more often than girls, with the peak incidence in girls being between years 8 and 13 and in boys between years 12 and 16.[7] (Fig. 25-4). The peak incidence of physeal inju-

ries during adolescence is probably due to a variety of factors. The growth plate becomes much thicker as the individual approaches skeletal maturity, and experimental studies have shown that thicker physes are much more susceptible to mechanical failure. As the child nears skeletal maturity, the perichondrium and periosteum become much thinner and provide less stability. In addition, the increased weight of the individual predisposes to mechanical failure.

The age of the child at the time of injury is an important factor in predicting the outcome. Fortunately, most epiphyseal injuries occur near skeletal maturity. Premature closure of the growth plate at this age, particularly of the distal extremity epiphyses, usually does not result in significant leg length discrepancy. However, the older child has less ability to correct angular deformity. Growth arrest in the younger child is a much more serious problem, but the prognosis for correction of angular deformity is usually much more favorable than in an adolescent. It is easy to see that one must carefully consider both the age of the patient and the type of deformity (angular versus growth arrest) to determine an appropriate course of treatment.

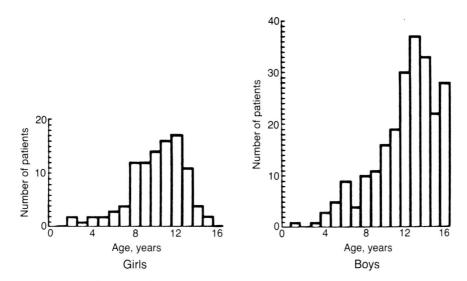

Fig. 25-4. Distribution of 330 epiphyseal injuries over a 20-year period reveals a peak incidence in girls between the ages of 8 and 13 years and in boys between the ages of 12 and 16 years. (From Peterson,[7] with permission.)

CLASSIFICATION OF PHYSEAL INJURIES

Categorization of physeal injuries is the first and most important step in the determination of an appropriate course of treatment. A classification system allows one to subdivide a general category of problems to identify individual variations and then, through adequate follow-up, to determine more individually appropriate types of treatment and prognoses. Classification systems for physeal injuries have been proposed by Poland,[8] Salter and Harris,[1] Aitken,[9] and Weber,[10] and Ogden.[11]

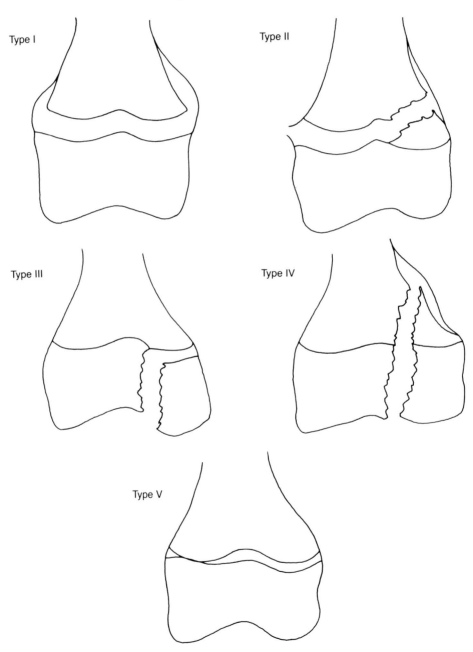

Fig. 25-5. Salter-Harris classification of epiphyseal injuries.

All of these classification systems are based on radiographic appearance and prognosis and are fairly similar. The classification system proposed by Salter and Harris is the most widely used in the United States and consists of five types (Fig. 25-5). Types I and II are extra-articular injuries and, in general, carry the best prognosis. A type I injury is a simple transverse slipping of the growth plate. It is most common in infancy or early childhood and may be associated with some pathologic diseases, such as rickets or scurvy. Type I injuries are also the most common injury of the distal fibular physis and may occur without displacement.

Type II injuries involve a metaphyseal fracture on the compression side of the injury; the radiographic appearance of the metaphyseal fragment may be referred to as the Thurston Holland sign. Type II injuries are the most common type of epiphyseal injury and are more common in older children (usually older than age 10). Both type I and II injuries usually have an intact periosteal hinge on the compression side of the injury that facilitates closed reduction and helps to prevent over reduction. Open reduction is usually unnecessary with type I and II injuries, and less than anatomic reduction may be acceptable in some situations. Since type I and II injuries involve primarily cartilaginous tissues, healing usually occurs in approximately one-half to two-thirds the time required for type III or IV injuries.

Type III physeal injuries are characterized by an intra-articular fracture as well as growth plate separation. In the foot and ankle, type III injuries most often involve the medial malleolus. Anatomic alignment is essential not only to avoid growth disturbance but also to restore joint surface congruity and prevent eventual joint arthroses. Type IV injuries involve a vertical fracture through the metaphysis, physis, and epiphysis and into the joint. These fractures are usually unstable and tend to migrate proximally, resulting in vertical displacement of the physis and articular surface. Vertical physeal displacement tends to promote fusion of the metaphysis on one side of the vertical fracture with the epiphysis on the other side of the fracture, which causes an angular deformity to develop. In contrast, transverse displacement (of the physis) alone may result in growth arrest but usually does not cause angular deformity. Anatomic alignment is essential to restore integrity of the growth plate as well as joint congruity. Type III and IV injuries usually require open reduction to restore anatomic alignment. Salter and Harris originally described a type V physeal fracture as compression of the growth plate without displacement. This is the least common type of traumatic physeal injury and may be impossible to diagnose at the time of injury. A more common cause of type V injury may be from compression of the epiphysis by the trailing edge of the metaphysis during other Salter-Harris type I through IV injuries or from overzealous closed reduction. Type V injuries may also have nontraumatic causes such as metaphyseal osteomyelitis or epiphyseal aseptic necrosis, both of which usually cause central growth arrest.

In 1969, Rang proposed a sixth type of growth plate injury that is often used along with the Salter-Harris classification system.[12] Rang's type VI injury is described as a bruising of the peripheral growth plate that usually occurs as a result of blunt trauma and may cause the development of a peripheral osseous bridge that would cause an angular deformity.

FRACTURES OF THE FOOT

Fractures of the small bones of the foot are much more common in adolescents than in younger children. Most fractures in younger children are the result of a direct injury such as dropping a heavy object on the foot. Injuries in older children tend to be indirect owing to athletic activities. A clear understanding of anatomic development of the pediatric foot is of paramount importance in evaluating injuries in younger children.

Primary ossification centers are present in the phalanges, metatarsals, cuboid, talus and calcaneus at birth (Fig. 25-6). The primary ossification centers of the navicular and cuneiforms are not radiographically visible until between 1 and 4 years of age. A secondary ossification center (epiphysis) develops at the proximal end of each phalanx and at the distal end of the lesser four

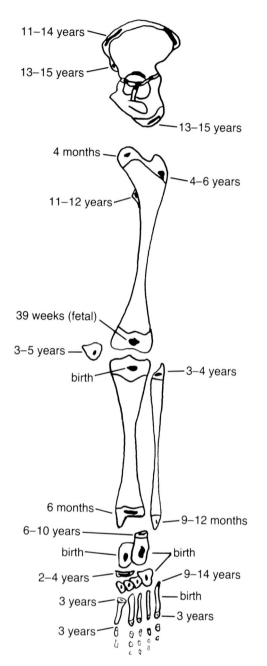

11–14 years

13–15 years

13–15 years

4 months

4–6 years

11–12 years

39 weeks (fetal)

3–5 years

birth

3–4 years

6 months

9–12 months

6–10 years

birth

birth

2–4 years

9–14 years

3 years

birth

3 years

3 years

Fig. 25-6. Age of radiographic appearance of secondary ossification centers of the major bones of the leg and foot. (Adapted from Ogden,[22] with permission.)

pseudoephysis that sometimes develops at the distal end of the first metatarsal for a fracture. Secondary ossification centers (epiphyses) also develop in other areas and can easily be mistaken for avulsion fractures if the clinician is not familiar with their location and the time when they first become radiographically apparent. The epiphysis at the base of the fifth metatarsal becomes evident between about 9 and 14 years of age. The calcaneal apophysis usually appears between age 6 and 10. A secondary ossification center may also form at the navicular tuberosity (os tibiale externum) or at the posterior aspect of the talus (os trigonium tarsi), first becoming radiographically visible between age 8 and 12. These may or may not fuse to their primary ossification centers (navicular and talus). Although avulsion, slipping, or fracture of any of these secondary centers can occur, careful clinical correlation is necessary to avoid over diagnosis of these injuries. When injuries to traction epiphyses (apophyses) of the foot occur, displacement is usually minimal and reduction is usually not necessary since these growth plates do not contribute to overall foot length. In the rare event of complete avulsion, reduction and pinning should be performed since these traction epiphyses are the site of tendon insertions (i.e., Achilles and peroneus brevis tendons).

Physeal injuries of the foot are far less likely to cause significant length disturbance or functional impairment than growth plate injuries of the leg. This is in part because the foot grows relatively slowly after the age of 5. Thus, the window period of susceptibility to significant growth disturbance is greatly reduced. Blais et al., in a review of 512 children, found that the average increase in foot length is only about 0.9 cm/year after the age of 5.[2] Completion of foot growth also occurs earlier than completion of leg growth. The average foot has achieved 96 percent of its total length in girls and 88 percent of its total length in boys by the age of 12. Of course, one should keep in mind that skeletal age can vary significantly in different individuals of the same chronologic age. When a significant discrepancy is suspected, one should obtain hand films to determine skeletal age. Physeal injuries of the foot are much less common than physeal ankle injuries and are

metatarsals by about 3 years of age. In contrast an epiphysis develops at the proximal end of the first meatarsal at about the same time. One should be careful not to mistake the spherical more likely to result from direct trauma. These injuries most commonly involve the distal metatarsal and proximal phalangeal epiphyses and are likely to be the result of direct trauma to the foot (i.e., dropping a heavy object on or stubbing the foot). Lawn mower, bicycle spoke, and motorcycle injuries are common causes of pedal epiphyseal fractures.[13,14] Open fractures are also common, and soft tissue damage may be extensive. When open fractures are present, one should adhere to standard principles in the management of open fractures[15] (see Chap. 3).

Digital Fractures

Most phalangeal fractures are nondisplaced and can be treated with immobilization for 3 to 6 weeks. Taping digital fractures together and use of a stiff-soled shoe for 3 weeks is usually adequate in adolescents, as it is in adults. I prefer a short leg walking cast for 3 weeks in younger children. A cast offers better protection, and cast stiffness is not a problem in children. Displaced fractures can almost always be reduced by closed techniques with distal traction (Fig. 25-7). If angulation is involved, a pencil can be placed at the web space level to be used as a fulcrum against the proximal fragment while distal traction and reversal of displacement is applied to the distal fragment. Reduction is followed by use of a short leg weight-bearing cast for 3 to 6 weeks. Percutaneus pinning with a small Kirschner wire is necessary only when the reduction is unstable.

Metatarsal Fractures

Isolated metatarsal fractures are rare in children and tend to be the result of direct injury. They may occur at any location. Indirect injuries are more likely to involve more than one metatarsal. The distal metatarsal necks are most frequently involved probably because the smaller cross-sectional area and location at the distal end of the "lever arm" makes this location weakest. The next most common location for fracture is the metatarsal bases. These fractures are usually multiple undisplaced fractures and result from a direct blow (Fig. 25-8).[16] Diaphyseal fractures are

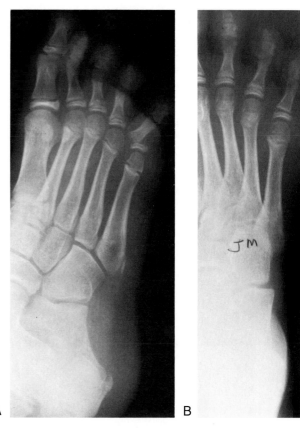

A   B

Fig. 25-7. (**A**) A displaced Salter-Harris type II fracture of the small toe in a 10-year-old girl sustained in a "stubbing" injury. (**B**) Closed reduction of the injury was performed with distal traction, using a pencil in the web space as a fulcrum under local digital block.

the least common, but when they occur are often displaced, unstable, and the result of more violent injuries.

Undisplaced metatarsal fractures, even if multiple, are very stable owing to thick periosteal and ligament attachments and can be treated with a short leg weight-bearing cast for 3 to 6 weeks, depending on the child's age. Displaced metatarsal neck fractures usually occur proximal to the physis, although Salter-Harris type II fractures involving the physis are common. One or two displaced fractures can usually be reduced by closed methods by application of distal traction to the involved digit(s) with reversal of displacement. Application of finger traps for 5 to 15 minutes may be helpful. Reduction can often be

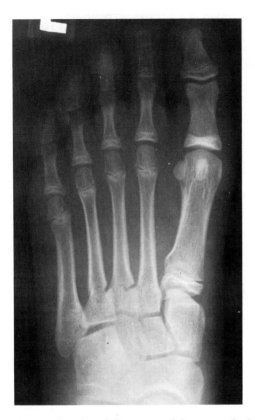

Fig. 25-8. Undisplaced fractures of the second, third, and fourth metatarsal bases in a 9-year-old girl that occurred as the result of dropping a heavy object on the midfoot.

performed in older children in an outpatient setting under local nerve block with sedation. Multiple displaced fractures are usually unstable and require reduction under general anesthesia (Fig. 25-9). Closed reduction can be attempted and, if possible, percutaneous pinning can be performed with the use of image intensification fluoroscopy. Frequently, however, these fractures require open reduction. If open reduction is necessary, one must be very careful to preserve capsular and periosteal soft tissue attachments to the metatarsal head to preserve epiphyseal and physeal blood supply. Smooth, small-caliber Kirschner wires placed from distal plantar through the metatarsal head or retrograde from the fracture site should be used for fixation. Reduction is followed by a short leg non-weight-

bearing cast for 3 to 6 weeks until the Kirschner wires are removed.

One should keep in mind, however, that spontaneous correction of angular deformity is much more likely to occur in children under the age of 10 than would be expected in an adult (Fig. 25-10). Anatomic alignment of nonarticular metatarsal fractures is usually not necessary in this age group. The most important consideration is to maintain anatomic alignment of the metatarsal heads, especially in the sagittal plane. Also, rotational deformity will not usually correct spontaneously.

Midfoot Fractures

Midfoot fractures in children are relatively uncommon. The navicular is probably the bone that is most often involved. Although delayed union or nonunion of tarsal (and carpal) navicular fractures is a significant potential problem in adults, it has not been identified as a problem in children. These fractures are usually caused by direct blunt trauma to the dorsum of the foot and are usually undisplaced. I was unable to find any reports of midfoot fractures in children in a recent review of the world literature. This attests to the rarity as well as the relative ease with which these fractures are usually handled. Immobilization in a short leg walking cast for 4 to 6 weeks is usually all that is necessary.

The only exception is the tarsometatarsal (Lisfranc's) fracture-dislocation. This can be caused by a direct injury to the dorsum of the foot (dropping a heavy object on the foot), but the most common cause is usually an indirect mechanism. The tarsometatarsal joints usually fail when an axial load is applied with the foot in the plantar-flexed position. The most common scenario is a child who is injured from a jump or fall from a height of several feet, landing with the foot in the tiptoe position. The injury has also been reported when an axial load is applied to the heel with the foot in the plantar-flexed position (dropping heavy objects on the back of the heel). Another indirect type of injury may occur when the forefoot is trapped (e.g., run over by an automobile tire) and the child falls backward.

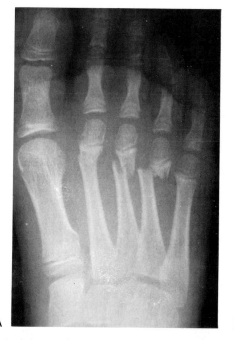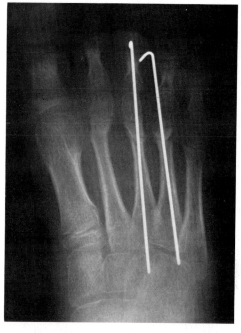

A   B

Fig. 25-9. **(A)** Displaced metatarsal neck fractures of the second, third, and fourth metatarsals in an 8-year-old girl. **(B)** Open reduction and pinning of the metatarsal neck fractures. The second metatarsal fracture is minimally displaced and stable, and adequate remodeling can be expected.

The injury is most common in adolescents. Wiley reported 18 cases in children under 17 years of age, collected over an 11-year period.[17] The average age at the time of injury was 12 years, ranging from 6 to 16 years of age. Eleven patients in Wiley's study had no significant displacement and were treated with a short leg walking cast. Seven patients underwent closed reduction, and four had percutaneous pinning. Fourteen of the 18 patients were asymptomatic at 3 to 8 months postinjury. Four patients had continuing pain at 1 year postinjury, and two of the four had radiographic evidence of incomplete reduction. These results emphasize the need for anatomic reduction when dislocation is present in this critical weight-bearing joint.

The types of fracture patterns that occur in children are similar to those that have been described for adult injuries. The dislocation may be convergent with all five metatarsals displaced dorsally and laterally, or divergent, with the first metatarsal displaced medially and the second through fifth metatarsals displaced dorsolaterally. In some cases, only the second through

fifth metatarsals may be displaced. Intra-articular fractures of the metatarsal cuneiform joints are common, and intra-articular fragments often prevent adequate reduction. In some cases spontaneous partial reduction may occur after injury, making identification difficult. Multiple oblique views at various angles are very helpful. Closed reduction under general anesthesia should be attempted for fresh injuries. However, tarsometatarsal fracture-dislocations are often unstable, and my preference is to use percutaneous pins medially and laterally even with closed reduction. If anatomic reduction cannot be achieved by closed methods, open reduction should be performed. I prefer two parallel linear incisions, one between the first and second metatarsals and a dorsolateral incision over the fourth metatarsal. I have successfully reduced missed fracture-dislocations as long as 3 to 4 weeks after injury. Following reduction, a non-weight-bearing cast should be applied for 4 to 6 weeks, followed by a weight-bearing cast for 3 to 4 weeks. Athletic activities should be avoided for 3 to 4 months.

Midfoot trauma very often involves severe

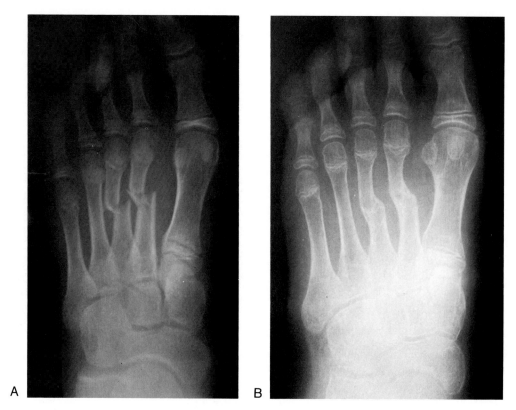

Fig. 25-10. **(A)** Displaced diaphyseal fractures of second and third metatarsals in a 9-year-old boy from a skateboard injury. Note that metatarsal head alignment is reasonably good. **(B)** Fractures 1 year later showing substantial remodeling and satisfactory metatarsophalangeal joint alignment. Further remodeling can be expected. Note that remodeling will not compensate for sagittal plane or rotational malalignment.

blunt trauma or contusion with massive soft tissue injury. The classic example is the child whose foot is run over by an automobile. The clinician should always be concerned about the development of a compartment syndrome. One or more of the classic signs of severe pain, pulselessness, paresthesia, and pallor may be present. A number of simple devices are available to check compartment pressure. Fasciotomy should be performed early if compartment syndrome is suspected.

Talar Fractures

Talar fractures in children are relatively rare compared with fractures in adults. Canale and Kelly, in a review of 71 talar neck fractures seen at the University of Tennessee over a 32-year period from 1942 to 1974, found only 12 cases involving patients under the age of 17.[18] Six of 12 patients were 15 or 16 years old at the time of injury. Only four patients were younger than 10 years old. Marti found only five talar fractures in children under the age of 17 over a 10-year period from 1961 to 1971.[10] A much greater proportion of the talus in children is composed of cartilage, which is very elastic, and pediatric spongiosa bone is capable of absorbing much greater force than adult spongiosa bone. When fractures do occur, they usually result from violent injuries such as falls from extreme heights or motor vehicle accidents that generate considerable force.

The talus is a very unique bone that resembles the femoral head in that three-fifths of its surface area is covered by articular cartilage and is devoid of periosteum. The remaining surface area provides attachment for ligaments and leaves few areas for nutrient artery entry. The talus has no muscular attachments. This renders the talus especially vulnerable to vascular embarrassment (as is the femoral head). The major blood supply to the talar body enters inferiorly through the arteries of the tarsal canal and sinus (branches of the posterior tibial and peroneal arteries). Some blood supply to the talar head and neck enters dorsally from branches of the dorsalis pedis artery. Undisplaced talar fractures rarely result in significant disruption of blood supply. The greater the degree of dislocation, the more likely is complete loss of circulation to the talar body. Thus, a progressively higher incidence of avascular necrosis occurs as one progresses from Hawkins type I to II and III injuries. The high incidence of avascular necrosis of the talus in adult fractures is well known and has been discussed thoroughly in Chapter 23. The incidence of avascular necrosis in children has not been adequately described in the literature, but is probably much lower. In the five juvenile talar fractures described by Marti, which included two type I, two margin fractures, and one type II, none developed avascular necrosis.[10] Some investigators have reported a higher than expected incidence of avascular necrosis in Hawkins type I undisplaced talar neck fractures in children.[18] The reason for this is not known, but the clinician should maintain a high index of suspicion even in these seemingly benign injuries. Younger children (under the age of 19) are much less likely to develop avascular necrosis, probably because the talus is primarily composed of cartilage with a relatively small proportion of ossified bone. Delayed development or permanent damage to the ossification center is more likely to occur than collapsing avascular necrosis. As a greater proportion of the talus becomes ossified, avascular necrosis becomes an increasing probability. All children with talar fractures should be observed closely for potential avascular necrosis. Serial radiographs must be compared for signs of increasing sclerosis, which indicates lack of normal bone resorption and remodeling secondary to interruption of blood supply. The development of a subchondral radiolucent line (Hawkin's sign) after adult talar fractures is considered evidence of a patent vascular supply. This presumably occurs because of disuse after injury. Although Hawkin's sign is useful in children, if present, its absence does not necessarily indicate avascular necrosis. Technetium 99 bone scanning may be useful in evaluating patients for potential avascular necrosis or in assessing progress in revascularization.

Medial, lateral, or posterior marginal fractures may occur. These are of minimal significance unless they are intra-articular. Fractures of the talar neck are the most common and are usually caused by forced dorsiflexion with impingement of the talar neck against the anterior tibia. They are described by Hawkin's classification as with adult fractures. Undisplaced fractures should be treated with a non-weight-bearing cast (usually long leg) for 4 to 6 weeks followed by a short leg walking cast for 3 to 4 weeks. Immobilization should be continued until radiographic evidence of fracture union is apparent. Hawkin's type II fractures should be treated with closed reduction by manipulating the foot into plantar flexion. If anatomic reduction cannot be achieved or if the fracture is unstable after closed reduction, percutaneous Kirschner wires can be inserted from anterior to posterior with the use of an image intensifier. Open reduction may be necessary, but it is best to minimize soft tissue dissection and avoid further potential vascular compromise.

Hawkin's type III fractures are extremely rare in children and would probably require open reduction and internal fixation with pins. Open reduction is best performed through a medial incision extending across the inferior aspect of the medial malleolus and forward along the talar neck just medial to the extensor hallucis longus tendon. Postoperative treatment of type II or III fractures would be similar to that of nondisplaced fractures with 4 to 6 weeks without weight bearing followed by 3 to 4 weeks of weight bearing. Some radiographic evidence of fracture healing should be present before weight bearing is allowed. If signs of avascular necrosis develop, the patient should theoretically not bear weight until radiographic or bone scanning evidence of revascularization occurs. This is extremely difficult with a child. A reasonable alternative might be a patellar tendon-bearing cast.

Transchondral Talar Fractures

The largest series of transchondral talar fractures was reported by Berndt and Harty in 1959.[19] Their report included 214 cases—24 cases of their own with the remainder gathered from a review of the literature.[19] Fifteen cases (7 percent) involved children less than 16 years old. The largest number of transchondral fractures in this review occurred between the ages of 20 and 30 (about 45 percent), with about 18 percent occurring between ages 10 and 20. Twelve of the 14 pediatric cases occurred between the ages of 11 and 15, the remaining 2 patients being 5 and 9 years old, respectively. The most common presentation is an adolescent with a history of a minor to moderate ankle sprain. In some cases no antecedent history of trauma may be present. Symptoms may range from minimal swelling with mild tenderness along the joint line to moderate swelling with diffuse pain. Lateral collateral ligament injury is frequently associated. Many patients do not seek medical attention at the time of initial injury. Chronic symptoms may include minimal recurrent swelling and diffuse aching and stiffness in the joint. The mechanism of injury is identical to that of adult transchondral fractures and probably involves inversion-dorsiflexion for anterolateral lesions and inversion-plantar flexion for posteromedial lesions.[19,20] The pathophysiology and classification of these injuries has been thoroughly described in Chapter 23. Prior to Berndt and Harty's report,[19] most transchondral fractures were treated nonoperatively. Pediatric fractures were thought to be especially amenable to nonoperative treatment since less mature cartilage was believed to have better healing potential. Generally recommended treatment had been a non-weight-bearing cast for up to 6 months. All 15 of Berndt and Harty's patients were treated nonoperatively.[19] Results were good in 3 patients, fair in 1 patient, and poor in 11 (73 percent) of the patients. Nine of the 11 patients eventually had surgery, yielding 8 good and 1 poor result.

The trend since Berndt and Harty's report has been toward earlier surgical treatment of transchondral fractures in both children and adults, although there is considerable disagreement among some investigators. Pediatric transchondral fractures should probably be managed by the same criteria as adult fractures. Stage I and II fractures should be treated with non-weight-bearing immobilization initially. I think it is reasonable to convert to a patellar tendon-bearing cast after 4 to 6 weeks. Healing may require several months. Stage II and III lesions have a high likelihood of not healing. This should be explained to parents, and excision of the fragment with drilling of the subchondral bone should be performed if resolution of symptoms does not occur within a few months. Stage IV lesions will not heal and require early surgical excision. One cannot determine the prognosis of transchondral fractures on the basis of classification alone. In a review of 31 transchondral fractures with an average follow-up of 11.2 years, Canale and Belding found degenerative joint arthrosis in 50 percent of patients.[20] Results were similar for patients who had surgery and those who did not (although these results were not compared by stage). Although all patients with symptoms had radiographic evidence of joint arthroses, many patients with radiographic degenerative changes did not have symptoms.[20] It is not unusual to see large stage I or II lesions in adolescents that don't heal but remain completely asymptomatic. It is doubtful that the long-term prognosis in these cases is affected by excision and drilling. These patients should be observed and treated only if symptomatic.

Surgical excision and drilling of lateral lesions can usually be performed through an anterolateral arthrotomy. Medial lesions are usually located more centrally or posteriorly along the talar dome (Fig. 25-11). Tomograms or a CT scan should be obtained to determine the exact location of the lesion. The traditional approach to the posteromedial lesion is through a transmalleolar osteotomy. This approach is reasonable in an adolescent approaching skeletal maturity.[21] If the physis is open, the medial malleolar fracture should be fixed with smooth parallel Kirschner wires. Motion should be started to stimulate fi-

Fig. 25-11. (**A**) Stage III medial transchondral fracture in a 13-year-old child as the result of an inversion "ankle sprain." (**B**) Lateral tomogram of fracture shows extent of defect and posteromedial location that would make anterior approach difficult. (**C**) Six months after excision of fragment and drilling of subchondral bone through a medial transmalleolar approach.

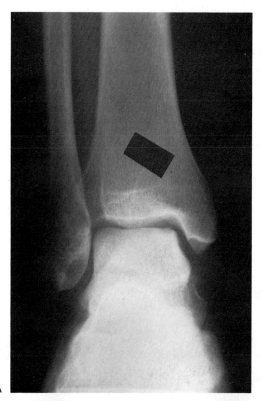

A

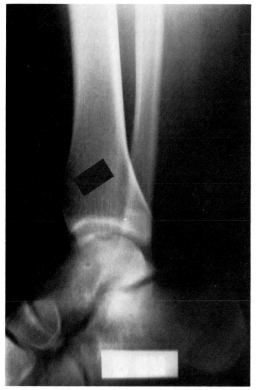

B

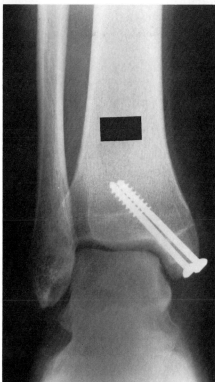

C

brocartilage remodeling as soon as the osteotomy shows evidence of healing. Once physeal closure has occurred, rigid lag screw fixation of the malleolus allows immediate early motion. An alternative approach would be arthroscopic excision of the fragment with curettage of bleeding subchondral bone. I have no experience with this procedure, but it could present a significant advantage in a child with an open physis with considerable remaining growth.

Calcaneal Fractures

Fractures of the calcaneus in children are probably even more unusual than talar fractures. They are extremely uncommon in children under the age of 10, with the vast majority occurring during adolescence when the foot is skeletally mature. Marti reported seeing only three calcaneal fractures in his large Amsterdam clinic over a 10-year period. All three children were between age 12 and 13 years and all injuries resulted from a fall from a height greater than 6.5 feet (2 m). All three fractures were of the intra-articular type. Only one intra-articular fracture in a child under the age of 10 has been seen in my clinic over a 4-year period. As with injuries to the talus in children, when calcaneal fractures occur they usually result from violent injuries. The most common mechanism by far is a fall from an extreme height. Spinal and other extremity fractures are frequently associated with calcaneal fractures. The more elastic nature and greater cartilaginous composition of the child's calcaneus together with less body weight makes fractures much less likely to occur than in adults. Displacement of calcaneal fractures is infrequent, probably because the force of injury is less and because the thicker periosteum in children helps prevent separation of fragments. Fracture patterns are similar to those in adult calcaneal fractures. Classification of calcaneal fractures has been thoroughly described in Chapter 24. Most classification systems divide fractures into extra-articular and intra-articular injuries. I prefer the Essex-Lopresti classification system for use in pediatric fractures. Extra-articular injuries include marginal fractures such as anterior process and beak fractures. One must be careful not to mistake the fragmented appearance of the calcaneal apophysis for fracture. The areas within the epiphysis that are frequently mistaken for fractures simply represent incomplete areas of epiphyseal ossification. Extra-articular fractures can almost always be treated nonsurgically. Marginal fractures that do not compromise the weight-bearing integrity of the calcaneus can usually be treated with immobilization in a short leg weight-bearing cast for 4 to 6 weeks depending on the child's age. Tuberosity fractures should be treated with a non-weight-bearing cast for 4 to 8 weeks depending on the child's age and evidence of radiographic healing. Displaced beak fractures resulting from Achilles tendon avulsion may require open reduction and should be treated with a long leg cast to neutralize the gastrocnemius-soleus muscle group.

Intra-articular calcaneal fractures in children occur by the same mechanism that occurs in adults. An axial loading force drives the posterior and lateral ridge of the talus into the calcaneus in a wedgelike manner. This causes a primary fracture line obliquely across the body of the calcaneus that may occur anterior to, through the middle of, or posterior to the posterior facet of the calcaneus. The primary fracture line tends to run obliquely from anterolateral to posteromedial and in some cases may run almost longitudinally. The primary fracture line frequently exits anterolaterally into the calcaneocuboid joint, and usually exits through the midportion of the medial wall. If the axial loading continues, a secondary fracture occurs. This may produce the tongue type of fracture described by Essex-Lopresti. With even greater force applied to the posterior facet, the facet is "driven" between the anteromedial and posterolateral fragments, forming a secondary fracture line that exits just posterior to the posterior facet. The posterior facet is depressed, "falling" anterior and inferior between the two main calcaneal fragments.

Most researchers have recommended nonoperative management of pediatric intra-articular calcaneal fractures.[4,22] Fractures with minimal or even moderate displacement in young children (under the age of 10) can be expected to undergo significant remodeling owing to the larger cartilaginous portion of the calcaneus that has not yet undergone ossification. These fractures would be treated with a non-weight-bearing cast for 4 to 6 weeks, until early radiographic evidence of fracture healing, followed by a short leg walking cast for 3 to 4 weeks. Displaced joint depression fractures in adolescents should be managed in the same manner that all other intra-articular fractures are treated. It is imperative to restore joint congruity to preserve function and prevent degenerative arthroses. Closed reduction is ineffective with these fractures. Open reduction requires considerable skill and operative experience with fractures. The operative approach is the same as with adult calcaneal fractures. A posterolateral incision is made inferior to the peroneal tendons. The tendons are freed from their sheath and retracted superiorly to expose the lateral wall of the calcaneus, subtalar joint, and sinus tarsi. The posterior facet is elevated and secured temporarily to the sustentaculum tali by one or two Kirschner wires. The primary fracture line is identified, irrigated, and cleared of depressed bone fragments. The tuberosity is then reduced with posterior and medial traction. In some cases, a medial incision may be necessary to expose the medial calcaneal wall fracture for adequate reduction. Fractures are secured with pins or pins and leg screws. Effort should be directed toward reducing all displaced fragments around the undisplaced sustentaculum fragment. Postreduction treatment consists of a non-weight-bearing cast for 6 weeks followed by a weight-bearing cast for 4 to 6 weeks.

Detailed radiographic examination is usually necessary to determine whether displacement is significant enough to warrant open reduction. Plain anteroposterior, lateral, and oblique radiographs of the foot may not be adequate. Axial views of the heel may show lateral displacement and help identify the medial wall fracture. Mortise views of the ankle often provide good visualization of the subtalar joint. CT provides the best visualization of the fracture and degree of displacement. CT scans are very useful in preoperative planning.

PHYSEAL INJURIES OF THE ANKLE

The Salter-Harris classification system provides information concerning the relative prognosis of various types of physeal injuries and is easy to apply on the basis of radiographic appearance. However, this classification system does not concern itself with the mechanism of injury or provide useful information that might aid in reduction or management of difficult fractures of the ankle. An understanding of the mechanism of injury has become an important standard in the management of ankle fractures in adults.[23] In 1950, Lauge-Hansen proposed a classification system that is now widely accepted as the standard in dealing with adult ankle fractures.[24] Although physeal fractures of the ankle can probably be adequately managed in most cases without the use of a Lauge-Hansen type of classification, a thorough understanding of the mechanism of injury not only aids in elucidating the most effective technique of closed reduction, but also provides a useful framework for a more physiologic approach to discussion and treatment of these injuries. In 1978, Dias and Tachdjian proposed a classification system for epiphyseal injuries of the ankle based on the Lauge-Hansen and Salter-Harris systems[25] (Fig. 25-12). They based their system on a review of 71 cases. Fifty-eight of the 71 cases (82 percent) could be classified using this system. Four major types of injuries are described in the Dias-Tachdjian classification that correspond to the Lauge-Hansen system: supination-adduction; supination-plantar flexion; supination-external rotation; and, pronation-external rotation. As in the Lauge-Hansen system, each type of fracture is described by two terms. The first describes the position of the foot at the time of the injury. The second term refers to the direction that the talus is driven by the injuring force. Thus, in a supination-external rotation injury, the foot remains supinated at the time of the injury while the foot is forcefully externally rotated. Since the foot is usually fixed to the supporting surface, this movement is equivalent to internal rotation of the leg. Individual stages of injury within each mechanism type are defined

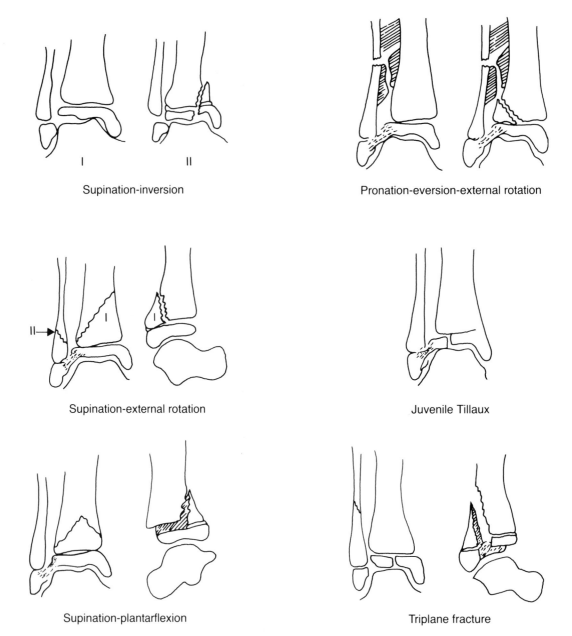

I   II

Supination-inversion

Pronation-eversion-external rotation

II→   I   I

Supination-external rotation

Juvenile Tillaux

Supination-plantarflexion

Triplane fracture

Fig. 25-12. Dias-Tachdjian adaptation of Lauge-Hansen classification for pediatric ankle fractures.

in terms of the Salter-Harris system. Thus, a stage I supination-adduction fracture is characterized by a Salter-Harris type I or II fracture of the distal fibula, whereas a stage II supination-adduction fracture is characterized by a Salter-Harris type III or IV fracture of the distal tibia. With the addition of the juvenile tillaux fracture and the tri-

plane fracture originally described by Marmor in 1970, a logical, complete, and useful classification system for epiphyseal ankle fractures is formed.[26,27] The vast majority of epiphyseal ankle injuries fit into one of these six categories (96 percent of the fractures in the Dias study[25] could be classified). The Dias-Tachdjian system provides a unified approach to the management of ankle injuries in children, using the same logical approach that is now applied to ankle injuries in adults. It provides a logical approach to closed reductions and appropriate immobilization as well as long-term prognosis and pitfalls.

The first step in classification is a careful radiographic analysis. Initial radiographs should include at least three views, including an anteroposterior, lateral, and mortise view with the leg in about 20 degrees of internal rotation. Inversion stress or internal or external rotation stress radiographs may be helpful in determining the type or extent of injury once plain films have been evaluated. Some fractures, for example, transitional fractures (juvenile tillaux and triplane), may be difficult to evaluate on plain films and may require tomograms or CT scans for further evaluation. Once the injury has been classified, a treatment plan can be developed. Many physeal ankle fractures are undisplaced and can be treated by immobilization alone. Closed reduction of displaced Salter-Harris type I and II fractures is almost always adequate even if slight displacement persists, and open reduction is rarely indicated. Closed reduction should be performed with the knee flexed 90 degrees while applying distal traction to the foot and first exaggerating and then reversing the mechanism of injury. A post-reduction radiograph should confirm an adequate reduction and should be repeated at 1-week intervals for 1 to 3 weeks to ensure maintenance of reduction. General anesthesia is usually preferred for maximum muscle relaxation to minimize the possibility of physeal damage from overly forcible manipulation.

After a retrospective review of 184 ankle fractures in children from 1970 to 1977, Spiegel et al. divided patients into two groups on the basis of the risk of developing complications of growth arrest, joint incongruity, or angular deformity.[28] The low-risk group, which consisted of 89 patients with type I or II fibular fractures, type I tibia fractures, and type III or IV tibia fractures with less than 2 mm of displacement, had a complication rate of 6.7 percent. The high-risk group, which consisted of 28 patients with type III or IV tibia fractures with greater than 2 mm of displacement, juvenile tillaux fractures, triplane fractures, and comminuted distal tibia fractures, had a complication rate of 32 percent. Spiegel and colleagues recommended open reduction of any type III or IV tibia fracture, juvenile tillaux fracture, or triplane fracture with greater than 2 mm of displacement.[28] They also identified a third group that consisted of 66 patients, all of whom had Salter-Harris type II distal tibia fractures. This group had a 16.7 percent complication rate, but individual complications occurred with equal frequency whether or not anatomic reduction was obtained. This points out a higher than expected complication rate for type II tibial injuries with the likelihood of complication being unpredictable in any individual case.

Some additional points worth remembering concerning management of these injuries include the following: (1) supination-adduction injuries usually result in medial or posteromedial dislocation of the foot, whereas supination-external rotation and pronation-external rotation injuries cause posterolateral foot dislocation, just as in adult ankle fractures; (2) a long leg cast is usually necessary for the initial 3 weeks following closed reduction of an external rotation injury to prevent rotation; (3) a non-weight-bearing short leg cast may be used for the initial 3 weeks following an open reduction with fixation.

Supination-Adduction Fractures

In Dias' study, 39 percent of the 71 juvenile ankle fractures were of the supination-adduction type.[25] This was the single most common type of injury. One would presume that the majority of these injuries were isolated distal fibular physeal fractures, although this was not mentioned in the study. Stage I of the supination-adduction injury consists of a Salter-Harris type I or II fracture of the distal fibular physis (Fig. 25-13). The corresponding injury in the adult would be either a lateral collateral ankle ligament rupture or a distal fibular pull-off fracture. Although a lateral ligament tear may occur in a child, a physeal injury is more likely. The younger child is much more likely to have a physeal injury, whereas ligament injuries become more common as the child approaches skeletal maturity. The type I injury of

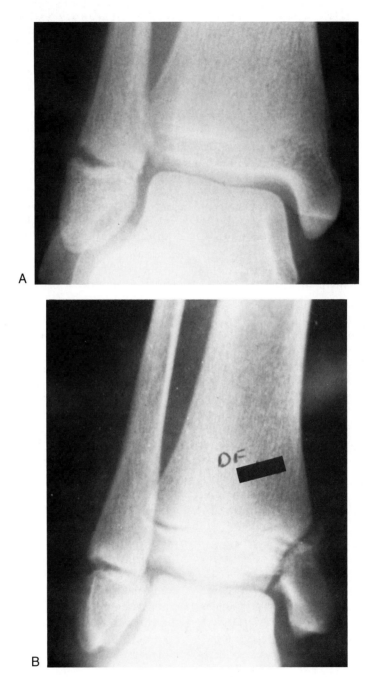

Fig. 25-13. **(A)** Stage I supination-adduction injury with Salter-Harris type I fracture of fibula. **(B)** Stage II supination-adduction injury with a Salter-Harris type I fracture of the fibula and a Salter-Harris type IV fracture of the medial tibia. (*Figure continues.*)

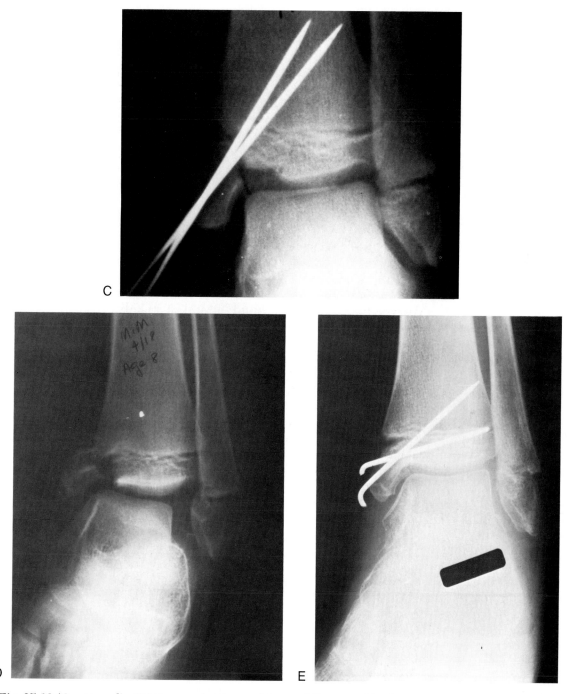

Fig. 25-13 (*Continued*). (**C**) Open reduction and internal fixation of the fracture shown in panel **B**. (**D**) Stage II supination-adduction injury with a Salter-Harris type I fracture of the fibula and a Salter-Harris type III fracture of the medial tibia. (**E**) Open reduction and internal fixation of the fracture in panel **D**.

the distal fibula is the most common pediatric physeal ankle injury, and one should be aware that it can occur without displacement and can easily be misdiagnosed as an ankle sprain. The only sign of this injury may be localized tenderness and swelling about the physis with or without slight separation or notching of the physis on radiographs. Comparison radiographs of the uninjured ankle may be helpful. Unlike an ankle sprain, minimal or no tenderness is usually present directly over the lateral ankle ligaments. A child presenting with this history and these physical findings should be treated with immobilization even if no displacement is observed on a radiograph. Open reduction of this type I or II fibular injury is virtually never necessary. Closed reduction can be performed by gentle eversion of the foot with counterpressure against the fibula. Immobilization with a short leg walking cast for 3 to 4 weeks is usually adequate.

As in the supination-adduction injury in the adult, a continuation of supination force results in a push-off fracture of the medial tibial malleolus of either the Salter-Harris III or IV type. The average age at the time of injury for Salter-Harris type III and IV injuries has varied with different studies. Kling found the average age for type III injuries to be between 8 and 10 years, whereas type IV injuries were more frequently seen between 10 and 13 years.[29] Some investigators have found the average age of patients with these injuries to be slightly older.[7,30,31] While the stage I fibular injury is fairly benign, the type III or IV tibial injury can have serious consequences. Closed reduction is performed as described above for stage I injuries but is less likely to result in anatomic reduction. Open reduction and internal fixation should be considered for displacement of Salter-Harris type III or IV tibial fractures with greater than 2 mm of displacement. Kling pointed out that those patients with displaced Salter-Harris type III and IV distal tibial fractures that received closed reduction, all of which were nonanatomic, had an 85 percent complication rate compared with those that received open reduction and internal fixation (all of which were anatomic after reduction), which had only a 5 percent complication rate.[29] Transmetaphyseal or epiphyseal Kirschner wires or screws

that do not cross the physis are preferable but smooth, small-caliber Kirschner wires crossing the physis at close to 90 degrees are acceptable. A short leg non-weight-bearing cast is used for 3 weeks, followed by a short leg walking cast for 3 weeks. A significant potential complication of the stage II supination-adduction injury is asymmetric fusion of the medial distal tibial growth plate, resulting in a progressive varus ankle joint deformity.

Supination-Plantar Flexion Fractures

The supination-plantar flexion injury described by Dias and Tachdjian results in a Salter-Harris type II fracture of the distal tibial physis with the metaphyseal fragment being posterior. The injury occurs as the result of a plantar flexion force exerted on a supinated foot. This usually results in a posterior displacement of the distal tibial epiphyseal fragment along with the foot. There is usually not an associated fibular fracture. Eight percent of juvenile ankle fractures in Dias' study were of the supination-plantar flexion type,[25] making this one of the least common mechanisms. As with most Salter-Harris type II fractures, closed reduction is usually adequate. Closed reduction should be performed by first applying distal and posterior traction with the foot in plantar flexion to disengage the metaphyseal fragment and then gently pulling the foot anterior with countertraction against the anterior tibia. Following closed reduction, a non-weight-bearing long leg cast is used for 3 weeks, followed by a weight-bearing cast for 3 weeks. Slight posterior displacement is acceptable, since displacement is in the plane of joint motion (which is easily compensated) and because transverse displacement of less than one-third of the metaphyseal cross sectional area has been shown to remodel well in the younger child.[1,3]

Supination-External Rotation Fractures

The supination-external rotation fracture pattern occurs primarily in the younger child (preadolescent). During adolescence, the differential strength characteristics of the metaphysis, physis, and epiphysis tend to alter the fracture pattern to produce transitional fractures, which will be described later. The incidence of supination-external rotation fractures is about 18 percent.[25] The supination-external rotation injury in children occurs by the same mechanism as in the adult injury. The main difference is that stage I in the child involves a tibial fracture instead of a fibular fracture as it does in the adult. The distinguishing feature of stage I is a Salter-Harris type II fracture with a large posterior metaphyseal fragment similar to that which occurs in the supination-plantar flexion injury. The characteristic

feature in the supination-external rotation stage I injury, according to Dias, is that the distal tibial metaphyseal fracture line on anteroposterior views runs from distal-lateral-inferior to proximal-medial-superior in an oblique fashion (Fig. 25-14).[25] The second stage of the supination-external rotation fracture involves a short oblique fibular fracture just above the distal fibular physis secondary to progression of the external rotation force of the talus within the ankle mortise. As in the adult, the foot is displaced posterolaterally. Closed reduction through reversal of the mechanism of injury is usually adequate if displacement is present. It is important to fully disengage the fibular fragment by accentuating the deform-

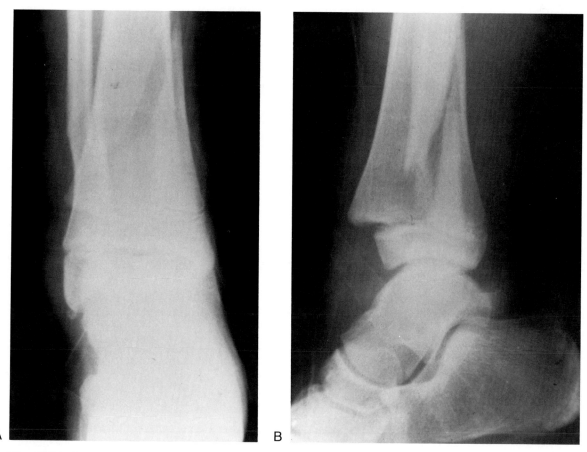

A   B

Fig. 25-14. Supination-external rotation Salter-Harris type II fracture of the distal tibial epiphysis. Note the long oblique tibial fracture from distal-lateral to proximal-medial on (**A**) the anteroposterior view and the typical long posterior metaphyseal spike with posterior displacement on (**B**) the lateral view. A long spiral fracture of the distal fibula that is characteristic of supination-external rotation injuries is also present.

ity along with distal traction before attempting reduction to obtain complete reduction of the rotational portion of the deformity. Slight valgus angulation secondary to fibular shortening is acceptable in the younger child (less than 10 years old), unlike in adult ankle fractures, because this angulation will reduce with growth. Because this is a rotationally induced injury, a long leg cast should be applied for 3 weeks initially to prevent rotation, followed by a short leg walking cast for another 3 weeks.

Pronation-External Rotation Fractures

Pronation-external rotation fractures accounted for approximately 15 percent of injuries in Dias' study.[25] Supination and supination-external rotation are far more common mechanisms than pronation, just as in adult ankle fractures. Pronation-external rotation injuries usually occur when the foot is "trapped" in the pronated position while the body falls to the contralateral side. This results in a relative external rotation movement of the talus with the foot fixed in the pronated position. Stage I is either a Salter-Harris type I or type II injury of the distal tibial physis. If a Salter-Harris type II injury occurs, the metaphyseal fragment is either lateral or posterolateral. Stage II of this injury is a fibular fracture above the level of the tibiotalar joint. This high fibular fracture is definitive of a pronation-external rotation injury, as in the adult pronation-external rotation ankle fracture (Fig. 25-15).

As with most Salter-Harris type I or II injuries, this fracture is usually amenable to closed reduction. After the deformity is increased slightly with distal traction, the foot should be internally rotated and inverted. One must attempt to restore fibular length, as with the adult pronation-external rotation injury; however, slight shortening and valgus angulation are acceptable in the younger child and should correct with growth. More than slight valgus angulation, especially in the older child with limited growth potential, deserves anatomic reduction by closed or open means to prevent a residual valgus ankle deformity. Any pronation-external rotation fracture re-

quiring closed reduction should be placed in a long leg cast for 3 weeks, followed by a short leg walking cast for 3 weeks.

Juvenile Tillaux Fractures

The so-called juvenile tillaux fracture was originally described by Sir Astley Cooper in 1822. Kleiger and Mankin redescribed this fracture in 1964 and referred to it as the juvenile tillaux fracture because of its similarity to the tillaux fracture in the adult (avulsion fracture of the distal lateral tibial tubercle by the anterior tibiofibular ligament as a result of an external rotation force).[26] The juvenile tillaux fracture appears radiographically on anteroposterior view as a Salter-Harris type III fracture of the lateral distal tibial epiphysis that usually involves from 20 to 50 percent of the width of the epiphysis[32] (Fig. 25-16).

The central or medial one-half of the distal tibial physis usually closes about 18 months earlier than the lateral one-half, the medial closure beginning at about age 12 to 14.[32,33] The juvenile tillaux fracture normally occurs only during this period, after closure of the medial tibial physis but before closure of the lateral physis. Numerous researchers believe that this fracture occurs as the result of an external rotation force that results in avulsion of the lateral epiphysis by the distal anterior tibiofibular ligament.[26,32–34] Dias studied nine patients with this fracture, all of whom were between the ages of 12 and 14, and found the anterior tibiofibular ligament to be intact in all four patients that had open reduction.[32] I have confirmed this in an additional four cases. Dias found that external rotation increased the displacement and internal rotation reduced the fracture in all cases.[32] The only physical sign of this injury may be localized tenderness and swelling over the anterolateral portion of the ankle. If the fracture is nondisplaced or minimally displaced, the only radiographic sign may be a vertical fracture line through the distal epiphysis on anteroposterior or oblique views. Multiple oblique views or tomography may be necessary to adequately demonstrate the degree of articular disruption or displacement (Fig. 25-17). If dis-

Fig. 25-15. (**A**) A stage II pronation-external rotation injury in a younger child with a Salter-Harris type I fracture of the distal tibial physis and the typical transverse fracture of the fibula characteristic of pronation injuries. (**B**) A pronation-external rotation injury in an adolescent (age 14) with a pattern that is more characteristic of an adult pronation-external rotation stage IV fracture pattern. Note the high transverse fibular fracture characteristic of pronation-external rotation injuries. Rupture of the tibiofibular syndesmosis is present from the joint level to the level of the fibula fracture. The distal fibular physis is open, but the distal tibial physis is almost closed. (**C**) Open reduction and internal fixation of injury in panel **B**.

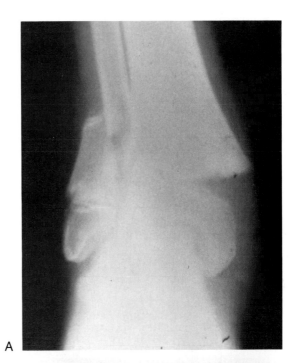

A

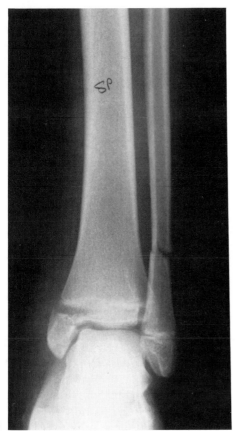

B

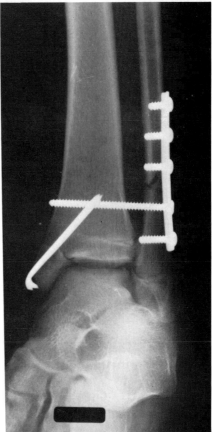

C

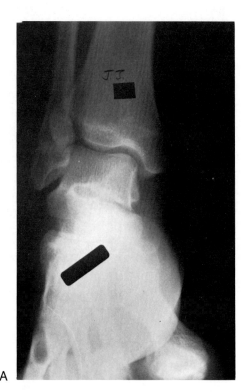

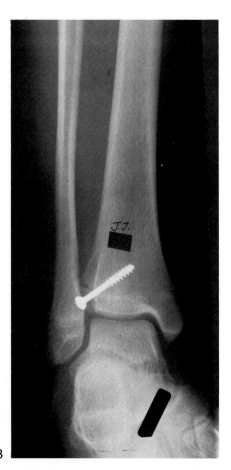

Fig. 25-16. (A) A juvenile tillaux fracture of the distal lateral tibial epiphysis. The fracture is always intra-articular and only occurs in adolescents near skeletal maturity. (B) Open reduction and internal fixation of fracture.

placement does occur, the fragment moves anterolaterally. This fracture never causes growth arrest or angular deformity since complete physeal closure must be imminent for this injury to occur, but significant long-term complications can occur owing to joint incongruity that can result in ankle joint arthritis. The adolescent tillaux fracture was included within the high-risk group in the study of Spiegel and colleagues, and anatomic reduction recommended.[28] Closed reduction can be attempted with distal traction followed by internal rotation of the foot but is usually not adequate. If closed reduction is performed, it should be followed by a long leg cast for 3 to 4 weeks and then a short leg walking cast for 3 to 4 weeks. One should be prepared to perform an open reduction if closed reduction proves inadequate. Displacement greater than 2 mm requires open reduction. The preferred method is with a lag screw from distal-lateral to proximal-medial. The screw can cross the physis since growth is already complete. Open reduction with rigid fixation should be followed by a non-weight-bearing short leg cast for 3 weeks, followed by a short leg walking cast for 3 weeks.

Triplane Fractures

Marmor first reported this injury in the English literature in 1970[27] as "an unusual fracture of the tibial epiphysis" but Lynn was the first to apply

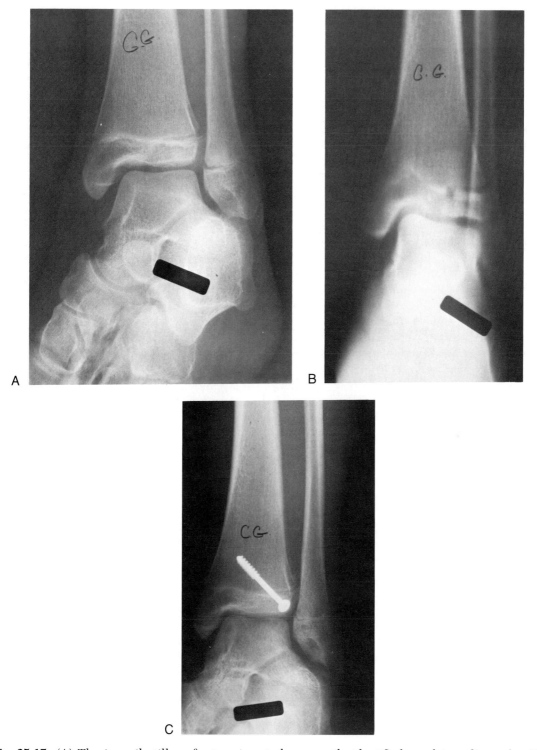

Fig. 25-17. (**A**) The juvenile tillaux fracture is not always easily identified on plain radiographs. (**B**) Frontal plane tomography of the patient demonstrates a displaced tillaux fracture. (**C**) Open reduction and internal fixation of fracture.

the descriptive term of triplane fracture in 1972.[35] The term transitional fracture is sometimes also used to refer to both juvenile tillaux and triplane fractures because these injuries only occur during the transitional period of adolescent and skeletal maturity.[36] The term triplane fracture is used because the fracture interface courses through all three body planes. Unlike typical fractures in more homogeneous areas of bone that tend to travel in a linear or spiral fashion, the triplane fracture assumes a circuitous course following the path of least resistance through the epiphysis, physis, and metaphysis (Fig. 25-18).

When the fracture is viewed in the anteroposterior direction, it starts as a vertical separation of the epiphysis and courses along the physis for a variable distance before exiting proximally and posteriorly through the distal tibial metaphysis. The point at which the physeal separation (transverse plane) stops and the metaphyseal (frontal plane) and epiphyseal (sagittal plane) fractures begin depends on the degree of closure or stability of the central, medial, and posterior part of the growth plate. The greater the skeletal maturity (and thus the greater the strength of the central, medial, and posterior growth plate), the more lateral the vertical (sagittal plane) epiphyseal fracture occurs.[37]

Most experimental and clinical evidence indicates that triplane fractures are the result of a supination-external rotation injury.[32,36,38] Supination-external rotation injuries in the adult produce a uniform fracture pattern and are responsible for 40 to 60 percent of all adult ankle fractures. Karrholm et al. in a retrospective review of 457 cases of ankle fractures in children found 39 percent to be supination-external rotation injuries, making supination-external rotation the most common mechanism in children also.[34] Thirty-one percent of fractures in Dias' study were of the external rotation type (supination-external rotation, 18 percent); juvenile tillaux, 4 percent; triplane, 9 percent.[32] Unlike in the adult, supination-external rotation fractures in children will produce drastically different types of fracture patterns on the basis of the degree of differential strength and maturity of various parts of the distal tibial physis. The spectrum of supination-external rotation injuries in order of as-cending age includes the supination-external rotation fracture pattern described by Dias,[32] the three- or four-fragment triplane fracture, the two-fragment triplane fracture, and the juvenile tillaux fracture. Dias' supination-external rotation injuries are most common in children under the age of 10. Van Laer in a review of 32 transitional fractures (which included juvenile tillaux and triplane fractures) found the average age at the time of injury to be 13.9 years, with a range of 11 to 16 years.[36] The average age for girls was 13.3 years and that for boys was 14.7 years, which would be expected because of the earlier physeal closure in girls (approximately 1 year).[36]

Two basic types of triplane fractures have been described. The three-fragment triplane fracture originally described by Marmor[27] occurs only before complete fusion of the medial tibial physis. The lateral epiphyseal fragment is very similar to the juvenile tillaux fracture. The second fragment consists of the medial and posterior epiphysis together with a posterolateral metaphyseal spike. The third fragment consists of the distal tibial metaphysis. The second type of triplane fracture, which was originally reported by Cooperman consists of only two fragments and only occurs after complete closure of the medial tibial physis[28] (Fig. 25-19). The distal fragment consists of the distal lateral portion of the epiphysis together with the posterior epiphysis and a posterior metaphyseal spike. The proximal fragment consists of the distal tibial metaphysis together with the medial portion of the distal tibial epiphysis. When the anteroposterior radiograph alone is viewed, the two-fragment triplane fracture, and sometimes even the three-fragment triplane fracture, cannot be distinguished from the juvenile tillaux fracture. The key to identification of the triplane fracture is the posterior metaphyseal spike seen on the lateral projection. Triplane fractures have the radiographic appearance of a Salter-Harris type III fracture on the anteroposterior view and a Salter-Harris type II fracture on the lateral view. For completeness, it should also be mentioned that a four-fragment triplane fracture was described by Karrholm et al. in 1981.[38] This fracture differed from the three-fragment fracture in that the distal medial epiphyseal fragment was separated from the posterior epiphysis

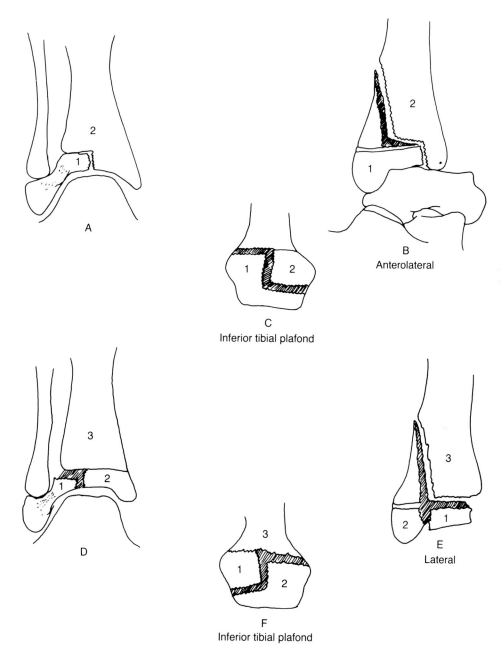

Fig. 25-18. (A–C) Typical two-fragment triplane fracture. The medial distal tibial physis is closed. Fragment 1 consists of the distal lateral tibial epiphysis, together with a posterior metaphyseal spike that remains attached to the distal fibula (cut away in diagram **B**). Fragment 2 consists of the medial distal tibial epiphysis together with the tibial shaft. (**D–F**) Typical three-fragment triplane fracture. The medial distal tibial epiphysis is open. Fragment 1 is the distal-lateral-anterior tibial epiphysis (tillaux fragment), which remains attached to the distal fibula by the anterior tibiofibular ligament. Fragment 2 consists of the distal medial tibial epiphysis, which remains attached to the posterior epiphysis and metaphysis. Fragment 3 is the tibial shaft. (Adapted from Tachdjian,[33] with permission.)

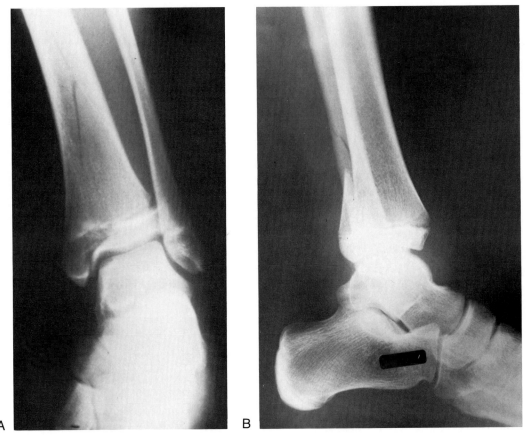

Fig. 25-19. **(A)** Two fragment triplane fracture with the vertical epiphyseal fracture line at the medial corner of the tibial plafond. **(B)** Lateral radiograph of fracture in panel **A.** Note the large posterior metaphyseal spike that may be mistaken for a Salter-Harris type II fracture.

to become the fourth fragment. As with other supination-external rotation injuries in the child, if the external rotation force continues after disruption of the tibial physis, a short oblique fibular fracture at the level of the syndesmosis will occur. This fibular fracture is similar to that which occurs in supination-external rotation injuries in the adult and is characteristic of an external rotation force. In adult supination-external rotation ankle fractures, the fibular fracture always occurs first, whereas in pediatric (epiphyseal) supination-external rotation ankle fractures, the fibular fracture occurs only after disruption of the distal tibial physis. The physis is biomechanically weaker than cortical bone and thus fails earlier.

Transitional fractures (juvenile tillaux and triplane) usually do not result in clinically significant growth arrest or angular deformity because the injuries only occur at an age when physeal closure is imminent.[36] However, any displacement of the articular surface of the tibial plafond will most likely result in joint arthrosis, leading to degenerative arthritis. In addition, widening of the ankle mortise is associated with significant long-term morbidity and must be reduced.[40] The degree of displacement of the articular surface may be difficult to assess on plain radiographs, and if reduction is borderline, a tomogram or CT scan should be obtained. In addition, it is almost impossible to distinguish between two- three-, and four-fragment triplane fractures on plain radiographs.

Many triplane fractures are undisplaced and can be treated with a long leg cast with the foot in internal rotation for 3 to 4 weeks, followed by a short leg walking cast for 3 to 4 weeks. Any displacement greater than 2 mm requires closed reduction under general anesthesia.[28,31,36] Closed reduction should be performed with the knee flexed 90 degrees, followed by internal rotation and supination of the heel with distal distraction. One should be prepared to perform open reduction if necessary. The three-fragment triplane fracture should be reduced by first fixing the tillaux fragment and then attempting closed reduction. If closed reduction is successful, the remainder of the fracture can be secured by anteroposterior pins or screws through the metaphysis. Open reduction of the two-fragment triplane fracture may require a medial approach. An associated fibular fracture may make reduction difficult because the distal fibular fragment, together with any attached distal tibial fragments, will be displaced posteriorly owing to the external rotation force. Disengagement of the fibular fragment and restoration of fibular length must be accomplished before tibial reduction can be achieved. Open reduction with fixation should be followed by a short leg non-weight-bearing cast for 3 to 4 weeks and then a short leg walking cast for 3 to 4 weeks.

COMPLICATIONS OF PHYSEAL INJURIES

Foot

Clinically significant complications from physeal injuries of the foot are relatively rare. This is probably due to a variety of factors, not the least of which is that foot growth does not contribute to overall lower extremity length. After the ages of 4 to 5, the foot grows at approximately one-half the rate of the distal tibia. Foot growth is generally complete by age 12 in girls and age 14 in boys, approximately 2 years earlier than completion of distal tibial growth. Because physeal foot injuries are most common in older children who have very limited remaining foot growth, growth cessation is rarely a problem. Most physeal foot injuries are also of the Salter-Harris type I or II vari-

ety, which are rarely associated with premature physeal plate closure. Occasionally, premature growth cessation of a single metatarsal may result in a transfer metatarsalgia and an overriding short toe. When this problem is not amenable to change of shoegear or accommodative support, the best treatment is lengthening of the short metatarsal after skeletal maturity. A plantar or dorsiflexion angular deformity of the metatarsal heads may also develop as a result of a partial physeal arrest or inadequate reduction. Minimal angular deformities of 15 degrees or less should correct spontaneously if adequate growth remains (at least 1 to 2 years). Anatomic reduction of metatarsal head deformity is critical in the older child with limited growth potential for spontaneous correction. Corrective proximal or distal metatarsal wedge osteotomy for residual angular deformity is rarely needed.

Ankle

Complications from physeal injuries of the ankle are usually of greater clinical significance and can be categorized as follows: angular deformities, rotational deformities, leg length discrepancy, degenerative arthritis of the ankle, and avascular necrosis of the distal tibial epiphysis.[11] Salter-Harris type I fractures rarely result in growth arrest. The high-risk group defined by Spiegel included juvenile tillaux, triplane, and Salter-Harris type III and IV tibia fractures with greater than 2 mm of displacement. Salter-Harris type II distal tibial fractures were unpredictable in terms of frequency of complications.

Angular deformities usually develop from a partial growth arrest of the distal tibial physis. The stage II supination-adduction injury is the most common cause of varus ankle joint deformity because of the vertical growth plate malalignment that frequently occurs with the Salter-Harris type IV fracture of the medial malleolus. Valgus ankle deformity caused by partial growth arrest is usually associated with pronation-external rotation injuries (Fig. 25-20). The best prevention of the residual varus or valgus ankle deformity is anatomic reduction at the time of injury. Some investigators have reported im-

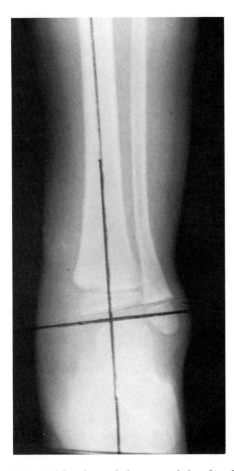

Fig. 25-20. Mild valgus deformity of the distal tibia and fibular in a 7-year-old child following a pronation-external rotation injury with a Salter-Harris type I fracture of the tibia and associated fibular fracture at age 5. The physis remains open, and spontaneous correction is expected.

provement of progressive angular deformities caused by partial physeal arrest after resection of the osseous bridge with interposition of an autogenous fat or a Silastic plug to prevent recurrent fusion of the growth plate.[3,33,41] Dias states that osseous bridge resection may be considered if the bridge involves less than 40 to 50 percent of the physis and at least 1 year of growth remains. If the osseous bridge involves greater than 40 to 50 percent of the growth plate, then epiphysiodesis should be performed. Angular ankle joint deformity may also require supramalleolar wedge

osteotomy. Opening wedges with bone graft are preferred to prevent shortening.

Rotational deformities result from external rotation injuries that are inadequately reduced. Unlike sagittal or frontal plane deformities, rotational deformities usually do not correct spontaneously. Clinically significant external rotation deformities have been specifically associated with triplane fractures. Derotational tibial osteotomy is the only effective treatment.

Limb length discrepancy may result from central or peripheral growth plate arrest and may not occur all at once. A gradual retardation of growth may be followed by a complete growth arrest. The younger child has greater potential for developing significant limb length discrepancy but also has greater growth potential for spontaneous correction of angular deformities. All children with growth plate injuries should be observed with serial radiographs every 6 to 12 months for at least 2 years postinjury and preferably to skeletal maturity. Potential limb length discrepancies of greater than 2 cm may require epiphysiodesis of the contralateral proximal tibial epiphysis at the appropriate age.

SUMMARY

A thorough knowledge of functional anatomy and physiology of growing bone is essential to proper management of pediatric foot and ankle fractures. The ability to classify foot and ankle fractures according to the Salter-Harris anatomic and radiographic classification provides useful prognostic information that may affect treatment. The Dias-Tachdjian mechanistic classification system for pediatric ankle fractures provides useful information about the extent of osseous and soft tissue injury and the best method of closed reduction and correlates well with the Lauge-Hansen system that is widely used for adult ankle fractures. Most epiphyseal foot fractures involve the metatarsals or phalanges and can usually be managed with closed reduction. Considerable spontaneous correction of deformity can be expected in the younger child (under the age of 10), but one should be aware that sagittal plane and rotational malalignment of the metatersal heads may cause significant problems. Fractures of the midfoot and rear foot are relatively rare in children and are usually the result of violent injuries. Somewhat less than anatomic alignment may be acceptable in very young children who have significant growth and remodeling potential. Midfoot and rear-foot fractures in adolescents should be treated the same as adult injuries. Anatomic restoration of articular surfaces is essential.

Salter-Harris type I and II fractures of the ankle can usually be managed with closed reduction. Salter-Harris type III and IV ankle fractures with greater than 2 mm of displacement require open reduction and internal fixation. One must also have a high index of suspicion for juvenile tillaux and triplane transitional fractures that may not be obvious on plain radiographs. Although these fractures usually do not produce significant limb length discrepancies, they are intra-articular fractures and ankle joint arthritis can result. Finally, younger children (under the age of 10) have a better prognosis for spontaneous correction of angular deformities not caused by growth arrest but a much poorer prognosis with growth arrest injuries than do older children, in whom growth arrest does not usually cause a significant problem. All children with growth plate injuries should be observed at regular intervals for at least 2 years or to skeletal maturity in the case of physeal disturbance. Treatment of epiphyseal fractures of the foot and ankle must be individualized but should always be based on a thorough knowledge of anatomy, bone growth physiology, classification, potential pitfalls, and prognosis.

REFERENCES

1. Salter RB, Harris MD: Injuries involving the epiphyseal plate. J Bone Joint Surg 45:587, 1963
2. Blais MM, Green WT, Anderson M: Lengths of the growing foot. J Bone Joint Surg 38A:998, 1956
3. Bright RW, Burstein AH, Elmore SM: Epiphyseal-plate cartilage. J Bone Joint Surg 56A:688, 1974
4. Rockwood C: Fractures in Children. JB Lippincott, Philadelphia, 1984
5. Hanlon CK, Estes WL, Jr: Fractures in childhood—a statistical analysis. Am J Surg 87:312, 1954
6. Rogers LF: The radiography of epiphyseal injuries. Radiology 96:289, 1970
7. Peterson C: Analysis of the incidence of injuries to the epiphyseal growth plate. J Trauma 12:275, 1972
8. Poland J: Traumatic Separation of the Epiphyses. Elder and Company, London, 1898
9. Aitken AP: Fractures of the epiphyses. Clin Orthop 41:19, 1965
10. Weber BC: Treatment of Fractures in Children and Adolescents. Springer-Verlag, New York, 1980
11. Ogden JA: Injury to the growth mechanisms of the immature skeleton. Skeletal Radiol 6:237, 1981
12. Rang M: The Growth Plate and Its Disorders. Williams & Wilkins, Baltimore, 1969
13. Letts RM, Mardirosian A: Lawnmower injuries in children. Can Med Assoc J 116:1151, 1977
14. Izant RJ, Rohmann BF, Frankel VH: Bicycle spoke injuries of the foot and ankle in children: an underestimated "minor" injury. J Pediatr Surg 4:654, 1969
15. Gustillo R: Management of Open Fractures. WB Saunders, Philadelphia, 1982
16. Figura MA: Metatarsal fractures. Clin Podiatry 2:247, 1985
17. Wiley JJ: Tarsometatarsal joint injuries in children. J Pediatr Orthop 1:255, 1981
18. Canale T, Kelly F: Fractures of the neck of the talus. J Bone Joint Surg 60A:143, 1978
19. Berndt A, Harty M: Transchondral fractures (osteochondritis dissecans) of the talus. J Bone Joint Surg 41A:988, 1959
20. Canale T, Belding R: Osteochondrial lesions of the talus. J Bone Joint Surg 62A:97, 1980
21. Alexander H, Lichtman D: Surgical treatment of transchondral talar-dome fractures (osteochondritis dissecans). J Bone Joint Surg 62A:646, 1980
22. Ogden, JA: Skeletal Injury in the Child. Lea & Febiger, Philadelphia, 1982
23. MacNealy GA, Rogers LF, Hernandez R et al: Injuries of the distal tibial epiphysis. AJR 138:683, 1982
24. Lauge-Hansen N: Fractures of the ankle: II: Combined experimental surgical and experimental roentgenologic investigations. Arch Surg 60:957, 1950
25. Dias LS: Physeal injuries of the ankle in children. Clin Orthop 136:230, 1978
26. Kleiger B, Mankin HJ: Fracture of the lateral portion of the distal tibial epiphysis. J Bone Joint Surg 46A:25, 1964

27. Marmor L: An unusual fracture of the tibial epiphysis. Clin Orthop 73:132, 1970

28. Spiegel PG, Cooperman DR, Laros GS: Epiphyseal fractures of the distal ends of the tibia and fibula. J Bone Joint Surg 60A:1046, 1978

29. Kling TF: Distal tibial physeal fractures in children that may require open reduction. J Bone Joint Surg 66A:647, 1984

30. Salter RB: Injuries of the ankle in children. Orthop Clin North Am 5:147, 1974

31. Cooperman DR, Spiegel PG, Laros GS: Tibial fractures involving the ankle in children. J Bone Joint Surg 60A:1040, 1978

32. Dias LS: Fractures of the distal tibial epiphysis in adolescence. J Bone Joint Surg 65A:438, 1983

33. Tachdjian M: The Child's Foot. WB Saunders, Philadelphia, 1985

34. Karrholm J, Hansson LI, Laurin S: Supination-eversion injuries of the ankle in children: a retrospective study of radiographic classification and treatment. J Pediatr Orthop 2:147, 1982

35. Lynn MD: The triplane distal tibial epiphyseal fracture. Clin Orthop 86:187, 1972

36. Van Laer L: Classification, diagnosis and treatment of transitional fractures of the distal part of the tibia. J Bone Joint Surg 67A:687, 1985

37. Peiro A, Avacil J, Martus F et al: Triplane distal tibial epiphyseal fractures. Clin Orthop 160:196, 1981

38. Karrholm J, Hansson LI, Laurin S: Computed tomography of intra-articular supination-eversion fractures of the ankle in adolescents. J Pediatr Orthop 1:181, 1981

39. DeValentine SJ: Evaluation and treatment of ankle fractures. Clin Podiatry 2:325, 1985

40. Ramsey PL, Hamilton W: Changes in tibiotalar area of contact caused by lateral talar shift. J Bone Joint Surg 58A:356, 1976

41. Bright RW: Operative correction of partial epiphyseal plate closure by osseous bridge resection and silicone rubber implant. J Bone Joint Surg 56A:655, 1974

26

The Acute Ankle: Differential Diagnosis

Gerard V. Yu, D.P.M.
Jeffrey S. Boberg, D.P.M.

Raymond Cavaliere, D.P.M.
Kieran T. Mahan, D.P.M.

DIAGNOSIS OF INVERSION INJURIES

Inversion injuries to the ankle and foot are a highly common presentation in both the emergency room and the practitioner's office. Because of the frequency of this presentation, it has been historically underdiagnosed and undertreated. Most commonly, the individual presents with a swollen, tender, and occasionally ecchymotic ankle after having twisted the ankle in an inversion direction. The most common injury that occurs because of this inversion mechanism is damage to the lateral ankle ligaments. However, there are a variety of other injuries that can occur with this mechanism. Unless the practitioner carefully examines for other types of injuries, the proper diagnosis may be missed (Table 26-1).

All too often these injuries are initially only given a cursory evaluation and treated symptomatically. Frequently, these patients return 2 to 3 months later when they still have significant pain and disability in the ankle joint. The purpose of this chapter is to identify the types of injuries that can be sustained other than lateral ligamentous injuries as a result of the inversion mechanism.

In the evaluation of patients with an inversion injury, the presenting history may give vital clues as to the type of injury. First, it is important to take into account the elapsed time between the time of injury and the time of presentation. An ankle may not appear grossly swollen and may, therefore, look like an insignificant injury. However, if the elapsed time between injury and presentation has been small, and if the patient has already treated the ankle with ice, the visible edema and ecchymosis may be minimal. On the other hand, a grossly swollen and ecchymotic ankle may appear far worse than the true extent of damage if the patient has treated the ankle with heat and if there has been a significant time delay between injury and presentation. In addition, during the history, the patient may recall the exact type of mechanism that resulted in the injury. Information such as whether or not the foot was fixed with the ankle then turning over or whether the patient experienced an audible snapping sensation may help determine areas of injury. The amount of pain that the patient experiences at the time of injury is variable and may not necessarily correlate with the extent of injury. An initial neuropraxia may cause the area to be temporarily anesthetic.

The most important technique for evaluating other areas of the ankle–foot complex is inspection and palpation. This should be done in a sys-

TABLE 26-1. Differential Diagnosis of Inversion Injuries

Ankle fractures
Anterior calcaneal beak fractures
Ligamentous ankle disruptions
Extensor digitorum brevis avulsion
Cuboid fractures (traction and crush)
Fifth metatarsal fractures (tuberosity and base)
Osteochondral fractures of the ankle
Peroneal subluxation
Lateral talar process fractures
Sinus tarsi syndrome
Entrapment neuropathies and neuritis

tematic and clockwise fashion, beginning with the anteroinferior talofibular ligament. Next the anterior talofibular ligament is inspected and palpated. In sequence, the dorsal calcaneocuboid area, fifth metatarsal base and tuberosity, and inferior calcaneocuboid area are palpated. Next the inferior fibular area is palpated including the fibula itself as well as the insertion of the calcaneofibular ligament on the calcaneus. Last, the entire fibula is palpated including the course of the peroneal tendons.

With the history of an inversion injury, initial ankle radiographs are obtained, with additional foot radiographs as needed, based on the initial inspection and palpation. A variety of additional techniques can be utilized. These are most commonly utilized in the patient who presents with a chronically painful foot and ankle some months following an ankle injury. These techniques may include arthroscopy, technetium scans, tomograms, computed tomography (CT) scans, and various arthrographic techniques (Table 26-2).

TABLE 26-2. Approach to the Acute Ankle

History
Inspection
Palpation
Ankle radiographs
Foot radiographs
Stress views, arthrography
Other imaging techniques

Just as important as the initial diagnosis is follow-up examination of patients with inversion ankle injuries. It is possible to miss one type of injury, particularly when it may be overshadowed by a larger initial injury. Periodic follow-up of these patients is critical to ensure a return to full function.

The inversion injury of the foot and ankle is most commonly labeled "ankle sprain." Our purpose here is to identify the variety of different conditions that can occur under the same presentation. Competent evaluation of the foot and ankle inversion injury requires a thorough knowledge of foot and ankle anatomy and mechanics, as well as experience in treating traumatic conditions of the foot and ankle. Success in the management of these conditions requires a thorough initial evaluation as well as consistent follow-up examinations and treatment.

OSTEOCARTILAGINOUS LESIONS OF THE TALAR DOME

Osteocartilaginous lesions of the talar trochlear surface are known to occur following inversion ankle injuries, yet frequently go undiagnosed. The incidence of osteochondral fractures is about 0.9 percent of all fractures and approximately 0.1 percent of all talar fractures.[1]

The first loose body removed from the ankle was reported by Munro in 1856.[2] Since then, a great diversity of terms have been used to describe this lesion. This confusion in labeling has been primarily due to controversy in etiology. Konig, in 1888,[3] observed loose bodies in the knee joint and referred to them as corpora mobile. He theorized, without evidence, that they were a result of spontaneous necrosis of bone. Hence, the term *osteochondritis dissecans* was introduced into the literature. In 1922, Kappis introduced this same descriptive term to lesions of the ankle joint.[4] Other terms used to describe this talar dome lesion include intra-articular fragmentary fracture of the talus,[5] flake fracture, chip fracture, joint mice, loose bodies, and osteocartilaginous body. Berndt and Harty, in 1959, have been credited for correctly describing this lesion from both an etiologic and anatomic standpoint.[6] Through fresh cadaveric studies, they were able to reproduce these lesions traumatically and then describe the lesion as a transchondral fracture. By definition, this term describes a fracture through the articular cartilage of the talus to the subchondral trabeculae of the underlying cancellous bone.

Other proposed etiologic factors have been presented that include embolic phenomena, accessory ossicle formation, and endocrine disorders.[7] A hereditary factor has been favored by many, including Wagoner and Cohn,[8] Gardiner,[9] Pick,[10] and Hanley et al.[11]

Most authorities agree that trauma is the apparent cause of these injuries.[1,12] Besides the work of Berndt and Harty,[6] Roden et al. in 1953 reported a traumatic etiology in 54 out of 55 osteochondritis-dissecans-like lesions.[13] Others, including Naumetz and Schweigel,[14] Davidson et al.,[15] and O'Donoghue,[16] have further substantiated the traumatic etiology of these lesions. Recently, Canale and Belding reported on 29 patients with 31 ankle lesions. Of these lesions, 25 had traumatic origins; however, the remaining 6 lesions presented without any history of trauma.[17] This occasional finding, a transchondral talar fracture unassociated with a specific episode of trauma, has also been supported by Naumetz and Schweigel[14] and Flick and Gould.[12]

Mechanism of Injury and Classification

In 1959, Berndt and Harty classified the lesion of osteochondritis dissecans or transchondral fractures into four different stages (Fig. 26-1): stage I, a small area of compression of subchondral bone; stage II, a partially detached osteochondral fragment; stage III, a completely detached osteochondral fracture fragment remaining in the defect; and stage IV, a displaced osteochondral fragment.[6] They found approximately 44 percent of these lesions anterior and lateral and 56 percent posterior and medial on the talar trochlear surface (Fig. 26-2).

Using refrigerated and fresh lower extremity specimens, Berndt and Harty classically repro-

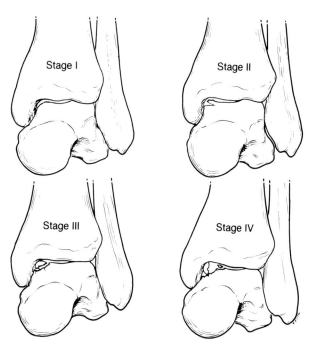

Fig. 26-1. The four stages of talar osteochondral fracture according to the classification of Berndt and Harty. (From Cavaliere,[19] with permission.)

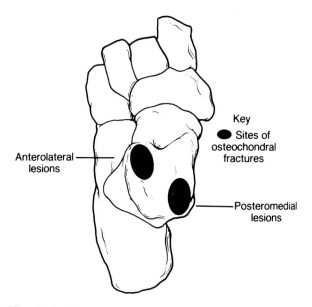

Fig. 26-2. Diagrammatic representation of usual sites of talar injury according to Berndt and Harty. (From Cavaliere,[19] with permission.)

duced both medial and lateral talar lesions.[6] The medial lesions were produced in the posterior third of the talus and resulted after an inversion-plantar flexion ankle injury in association with lateral rotation of the tibia on the talus (Fig. 26-3). Lateral lesions, occurring centrally, were reproduced after an inversion injury to a dorsiflexed ankle (Fig. 26-4). Berndt and Harty thought that the principal force causing both types of lesions was torsional impaction. In the medial talar dome lesion, with plantar flexion of an inverted foot and with lateral rotation of the tibia on the talus, the posteromedial edge of the talar dome is forcibly compressed against the inferior lip of the tibia (stage I). As these forces continue to drive the talus into the tibia, the compressed and impacted posteromedial talar margin may progress through its stages (stages II through IV). This progression can occur only after rupture of the posterior fibers of the deltoid ligament or anterior fibers of the lateral collateral ligament. In the lateral talar dome lesions, as the foot is strongly dorsiflexed and inverted, the lateral superior talar process is compressed and impacted against the medial articular portion of the fibula (stage I). As the force continues, the shearing force may be great enough to cause distortion and displacement of the talar lesion (stages II through IV). This progression can only occur after rupture of the lateral collateral ligaments.

Diagnosis

There are no pathognomonic signs or symptoms of transchondral talar dome fracture.[6] In fact, the injury is often elusive and misdiagnosed; and because of this, its incidence highly under-reported.[18,19] In a retrospective review of patients with osteochondral lesions by Thompson and Loomer, only 3 of 11 were initially properly diagnosed.[20] Flick and Gould reported on a group of patients, 43 percent of whom were erroneously labeled as having a "sprained ankle."[12]

The index of suspicion should be high on the part of the examining physician when assessing anyone who has sustained an ankle injury, especially when inversion has been a major component.[15] Stage I injuries are often misdiagnosed owing to lack of radiographic evidence of injury and to intact collateral ankle ligaments. Ankle range of motion is usually full and unrestricted, and the lesions are painless because of the absence of sensory fibers in articular cartilage. These injuries are usually labeled ankle sprains. Viability of the cartilaginous injury is excellent, and a confirmed radiographic diagnosis should be sought in anyone with a history of previous inversion-plantar flexion injury who continues to complain of exercise-related ankle pain, sensations of clicking or catching, or persistent swelling (Fig. 26-5). Repeat radiographic examinations

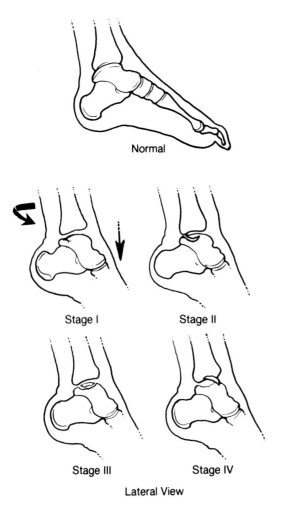

Normal

Stage I   **Stage II**

Stage III   **Stage IV**

Lateral View

Fig. 26-3. Mechanism of medial transchondral talar dome lesions according to Berndt and Harty. (From Cavaliere,[19] with permission.)

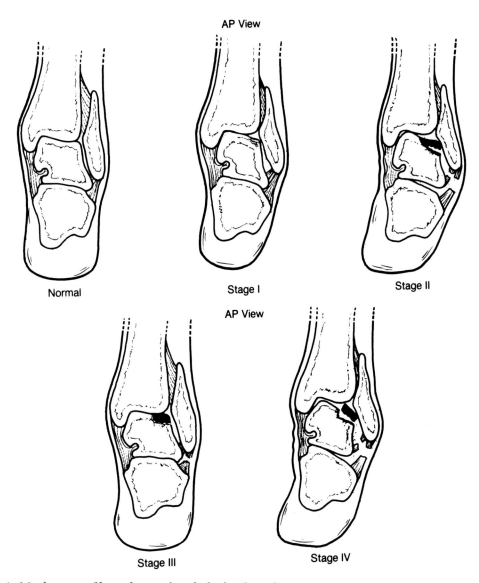

AP View

Normal   Stage I   Stage II

AP View

Stage III   Stage IV

Fig. 26-4. Mechanism of lateral transchondral talar dome lesions according to Berndt and Harty. (From Cavaliere,[19] with permission.)

should occur in approximately 2 weeks when clinical suspicion is high[19]; however, confirmation of the lesion may occur as late as 5 months after initial injury. Flick and Gould hypothesized that transformation of stage I (or any other stage lesion) to a more severe lesion may occur. This progression is believed to be due to post-traumatic resorption and avascular necrosis of the fracture fragment, combined with repeated and mild ankle inversion stresses.[12]

Stage II and greater lesions are painful secondary to associated ligamentous damage and subchondral injury. The symptoms of osteochondral lesions are classically either acute or chronic. Acute phase symptoms include ankle swelling, ecchymosis, and limited active and passive ankle motion due to synovitis. These symptoms usually predominate for approximately 3 to 6 weeks[18] but may not dissipate for several months, being dependent on the severity of the initial ankle

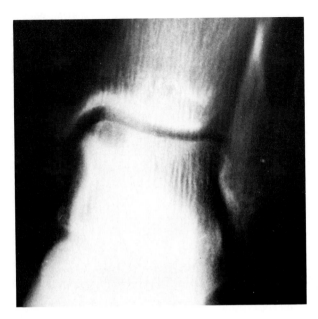

Fig. 26-5. Medial circular lucency of the talar dome with a surrounding sclerotic border identified with tomography in this 32-year-old woman with continued complaints of ankle pain and swelling. Patient is 10 months post ankle injury.

derness in the intrasyndesmotic space between the talus and tibiofibular syndesmosis.

Radiographic study of the ankle joint should include a minimum of three views: anteroposterior, mortise or medial oblique, and lateral. Although the anteroposterior ankle view shows the medial talar dome clearly, the lateral dome is obscured by the lateral malleolus. In the medial oblique or mortise ankle view, with the ankle internally rotated 10 to 15 degrees, the medial and lateral malleoli are parallel, and the talofibular space is visible. The lateral talar dome is therefore more visible. The lateral ankle view allows for clear observation of the relative anteroposterior position of the lesion; however, superimposition of the malleoli at times will obscure the view. Owing to these difficulties encountered radiographically, additional internal oblique ankle views are recommended with the ankle in plantar flexion, neutral flexion, and dorsiflexion to examine the talar trochlear surface in different planes. In this way, both anterior and posterior medial and lateral lesions are identified. This procedure may also be employed with the lateral films, should the need arise.

If these radiographs fail to identify a suspected lesion, then the clinician should order tomograms.[22–24] These should be performed in sagittal and frontal planes in 5-mm sections. Should the lesion appear chronic, then bone scanning may provide more information. Other tests that could yield additional information include arthrography, CT scans, and even nuclear magnetic resonance imaging (Fig. 26-6A–C). Arthroscopy can play a role in the diagnosis and perhaps treatment of many anterolateral talar dome lesions.

Treatment

According to Berndt and Harty, the pathologic events in osteochondral fractures begin with trauma, leading to fracture, followed by disruption of blood supply to the avulsed or compressed fragment.[6] The cartilaginous portion remains viable because of low metabolic demand and synovial nutrition of the chondrocytes. The osseous portion of the fragment becomes avascular and undergoes aseptic necrosis. The fracture

sprain. The chronic phase begins as the acute phase ends and is dependent on the initial treatment of the injury and the extent of trauma. Symptoms will now include those of osteoarthritis with pain and swelling aggravated with activity and relieved with rest: stiffness, deep aching sensations, crepitations, limitation of motion, and possible feelings of ankle instability. This chronic phase may last indefinitely and, in fact, may progress to more advanced lesions should surgical treatment be postponed. Interestingly, a delay in treatment for several months to a year has not been shown to affect adversely the surgical results.[6,12,21] Other clinical findings may include joint locking and documented instability of the collateral ankle ligaments. Obviously, in the acute phase, the magnitude of the signs and symptoms is relative to the degree of fracture and ligamentous disruption. Chronic phase symptoms would be more corroborated with the degree of ankle joint degeneration and the fracture fragment size. Finally, in anterolateral lesions, patients may have demonstrable localized ten-

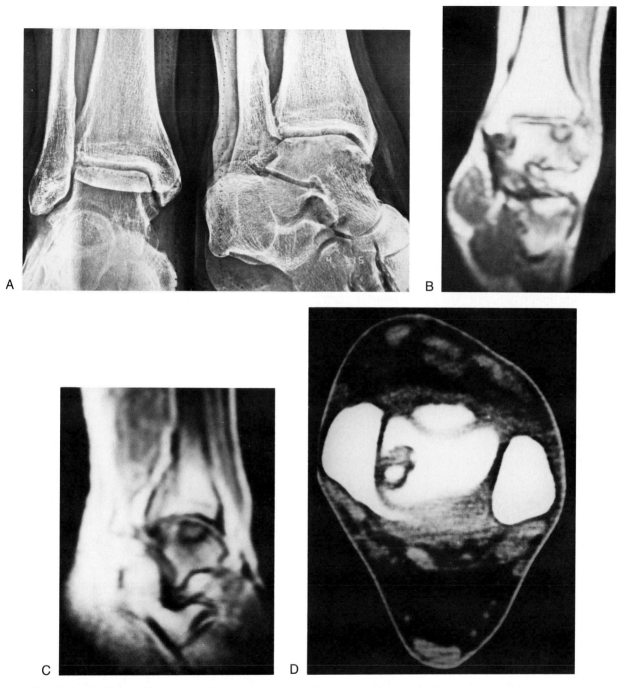

Fig. 26-6. (**A**) Xeroradiographs of a suspected osteochondral ankle injury. This imaging technique was chosen because of its superior cortical bone enhancement; however, no fracture could be delineated with certainty. (**B & C**) Coronal and sagittal magnetic resonance images of the same ankle that clearly demonstrate size and extent of this central and medial osteochondral fracture. (**D**) Further documentation of this injury was possible as seen on this transverse section by CT.

literally becomes a "dead prisoner in a sterile cell."[6] The subsequent healing process requires absolute immobilization to allow capillary ingrowth across the fracture line from the body of the talus. This process, known as creeping substitution, is possible with stage I, II, and III lesions. Should motion shear off this capillary ingrowth, then sequestration or nonunion of the fracture fragment results. Stage IV lesions, being totally separated from their nutrient bed and possibly rotated 180 degrees within their bed, do not have this potential to heal as described.

Important radiographic and morphologic differences between the medial and lateral talar dome lesions have been reported by Canale and Belding.[17] This morphologic variation explains why lateral lesions are often more advanced and symptomatic than the medial ones and why they may further progress in lesion stage or severity with improper treatment. They found that the lateral lesions were more shallow and wafer-shaped, therefore having a greater width than depth. This factor is responsible for a greater degree of displacement found with lateral lesions. Medial lesions were described as being morphologically deep and cup-shaped, therefore having

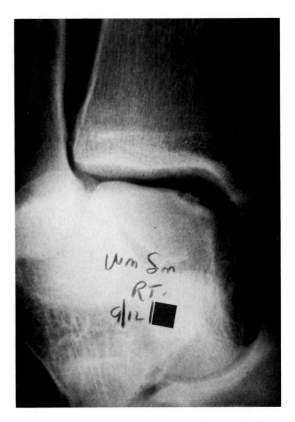

Fig. 26-8. Medial oblique ankle radiograph demonstrating a posteromedial stage II osteochondral fracture. Stability and repair of this injury would best be achieved through extended non-weight-bearing casting.

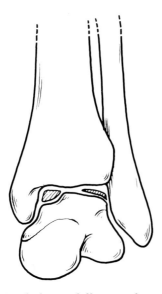

Fig. 26-7. Morphologic difference between medial and lateral transchondral fracture fragments according to Canale and Belding. (From Cavaliere,[19] with permission.)

a greater depth than width. This shape undoubtedly is responsible for less frequent medial fragment displacement (Fig. 26-7).

Treatment of these lesions is generally conservative or surgical and depends on the stage, size, and location of the lesion. In general, stage I and stage II lesions should be treated conservatively regardless of location. This is also true for medial stage III lesions (Fig. 26-8). Lateral stage III lesions, as well as all stage IV lesions, should be treated by early operative repair.[17] Furthermore, surgical intervention is recommended for symptomatic patients who have undergone adequate conservative care of their initial lesions, regardless of their stage (Fig. 26-9).

Conservative treatment regimens have been described and range from rest, physical therapy,

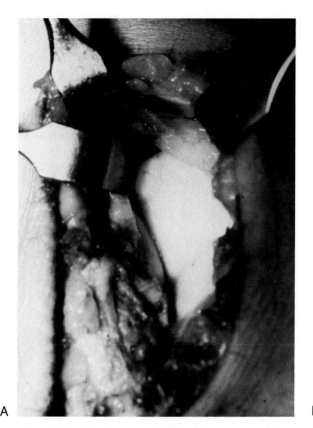
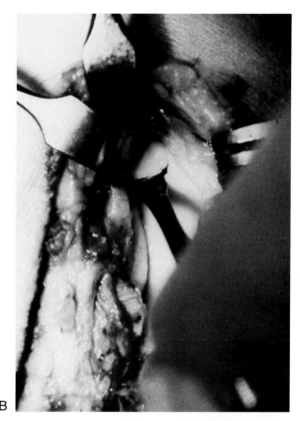

A   B

Fig. 26-9. (A) Chronically painful anterolateral stage II lesion seen here intraoperatively. (B) Surgical extirpation of the partially attached osteochondral fracture fragment is performed in an effort to control pain and limit lesion progression and ankle deterioration.

supportive dressings, and support stockings to patellar weight-bearing braces, arch supports, and cast immobilization, all for various periods of time. There has been no stated optimal length of time for casting, although there is some evidence that short periods of immobilization are associated with poor results. In a short review of casting times correlated with good results by Flick and Gould,[12] they found that longer periods of casting gave better results. It is therefore prudent to advocate casting of the short leg type for 2 to 4 months for optimal results. The goal of cast immobilization should be relief of symptoms and not radiographic healing, since this rarely occurs with conservative treatment.[17] Cameron reported a period of 7.5 months prior to radiographic evidence of healing and stated that immobilization was the only effective means to achieve union prior to the onset of a nonunion.[25]

There is sufficient evidence supporting the contention that operative lesions do better with early operation than with conservative care. Berndt and Harty reported superior results with operative therapy in adults and children versus those treated conservatively.[6] These results supporting early operative treatment are also advocated by Davidson and associates,[15] Alexander and Lichtman,[21] O'Farrell and Costello,[18] and Blom and Strijk.[22]

Operative approaches for anterolateral talar lesions are usually conducted through an anterolateral incision over the ankle joint with a corresponding anterolateral ankle arthrotomy. Owing to the usual position of the lateral fracture fragment, the anterolateral to posteromedial obliquity of the talus in the transverse plane, the posterior position of the fibula, and the large surface area of the anterior talar trochlear surface, the

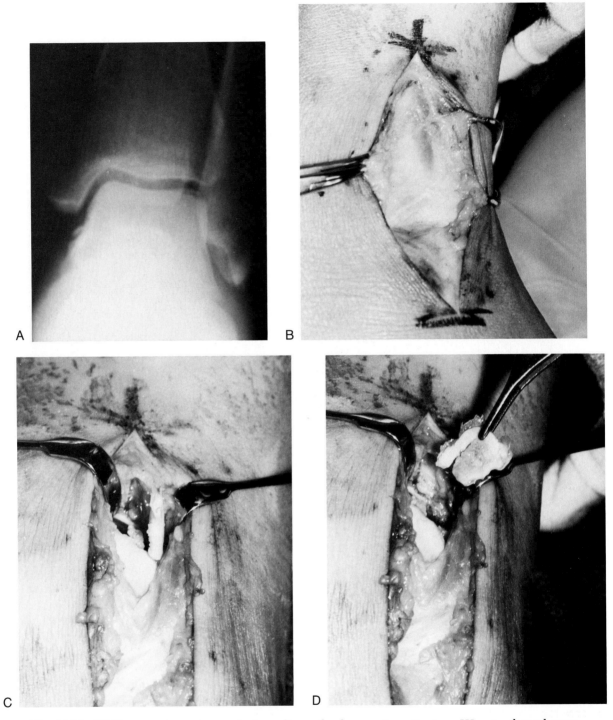

Fig. 26-10. (**A**) Preoperative anteroposterior radiograph of a symptomatic stage III anterolateral osteochondral fracture. Note the mild superimposition of the lateral malleolus. (**B**) The deep fascia is seen, and the arthrotomy will be made just medial to the talofibular syndesmosis. All encountered lateral tarsal and lateral malleolar arteries and veins are identified, clamped, cut, and ligated. (**C**) After arthrotomy into the tibiotalar joint is complete, the foot is plantar flexed and the osteochondral fracture is easily seen. (**D**) The underside of the fracture fragment is seen as it is removed from the talar dome. The surrounding cartilaginous surfaces are then sharply debrided. (*Figure continues.*)

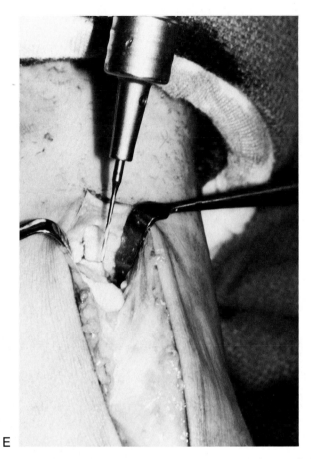

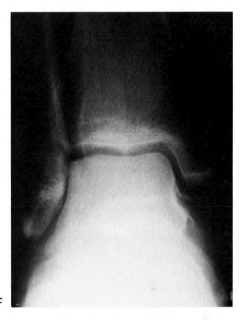

E   F

Fig. 26-10 (*Continued*). (**E**) The remaining defect is drilled repeatedly with a fine drill or Kirschner wire to stimulate fibrocartilaginous ingrowth. (**F**) Immediate postoperative radiograph demonstrating complete removal of the lesion.

lateral trochlear surface is easily accessible. Lateral transchondral fracture fragments are therefore easily exposed and treated; however, occasionally one may need to divide the anterior talofibular ligament and forcibly invert the ankle joint to gain access to more central lesions. The lateral collateral ligament is then primarily repaired. Rarely is there a need for a lateral malleolar osteotomy or syndesmotomy (Fig. 26-10).

Medial transchondral dome lesions present a more difficult surgical approach because of their more posterior location. One surgical approach involves the creation of a medial malleolar osteotomy. Prior to the creation of such an osteotomy, the medial talotibial articulation should be iden-

tified through an anteromedial arthrotomy to avoid inadvertent osteotomy into the talus. Prior to creation of the osteotomy, it is recommended that drill holes or, in fact, final screw fixation be accomplished with two 4.0-mm cancellous compression screws or one 6.5-mm and one 4.0-mm cancellous screw. The fixation can then simply be retracted enough to allow osteotomy and reflection of the malleolus. Exposure and treatment of the transchondral lesion is then accomplished, and rigid anatomic internal compressive fixation of the malleolus is achieved (Fig. 26-11). This technique allows excellent exposure as well as excellent postoperative rigidity without worry of rotational instability of the malleolus. Early and

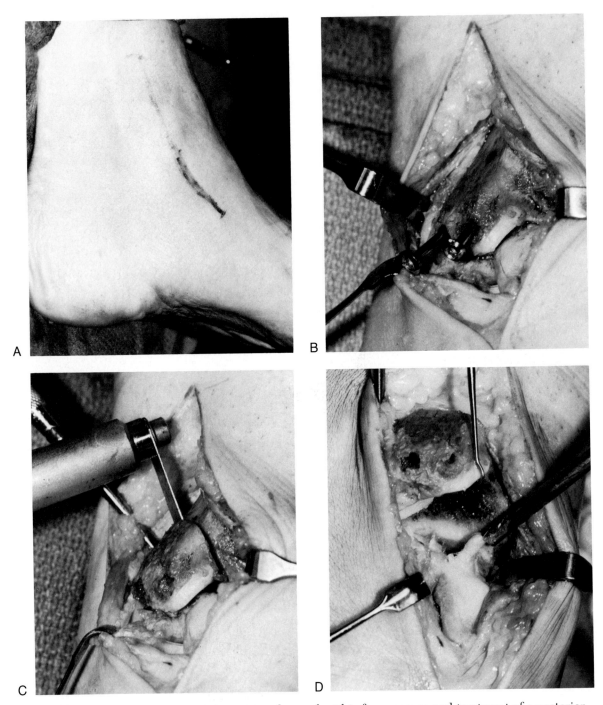

Fig. 26-11. (A) Preoperative incision centered over the tibia for exposure and treatment of a posterior and medial transchondral talar fracture. **(B)** An anteromedial arthrotomy is made and subcapsular and subperiosteal dissection completed about the medial tibiotalar articulation. The deep posterior fibers of the deltoid ligament are left intact as they insert into the medial malleolus. The tibiotalar articulation is identified and protected medially while cancellous compression screws are placed across the proposed medial malleolar osteotomy, prior to its execution. The screws are subsequently distracted. **(C)** The osteotomy is completed. **(D)** The medial malleolus is retracted superiorly and the foot is maximally plantar flexed at the ankle, allowing subsequent full visualization of the posterior and medial osteochondral fracture. (*Figure continues.*)

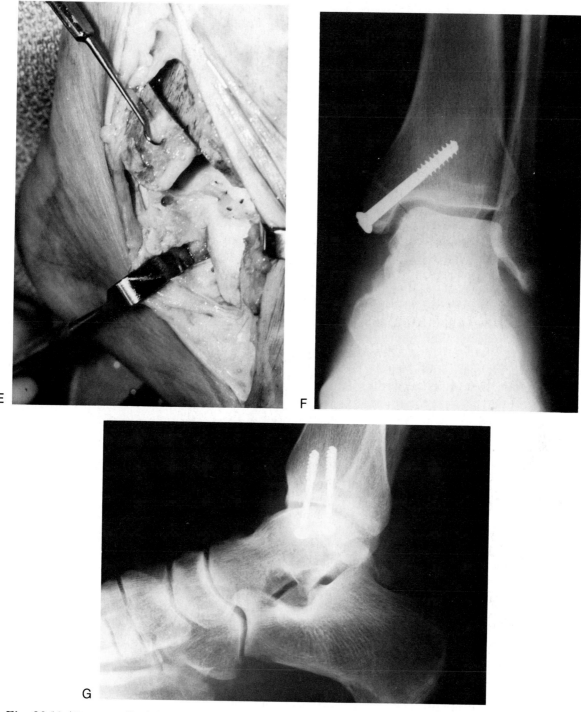

Fig. 26-11 (*Continued*). (**E**) The fragment is removed, and the base of the lesion is sharpened and drilled with a small smooth Kirschner wire. (**F**) The medial malleolus is then anatomically and rigidly fixated. Intraoperative radiographs confirm proper alignment with resolution of the lesion. (**G**) Postoperative lateral radiograph demonstrating proper alignment and fixation in both planes.

aggressive range of motion exercises and physical therapy should be properly executed for optimal results.

Thompson and Loomer described an excellent surgical approach which allows for inspection of the entire medial trochlear surface of the talus without the need for a transmalleolar osteotomy.[20] They described a 10-cm incision curved convex posteriorly, posterior to the medial malleolus, exposing the medial capsule. A 2-cm longitudinal anteromedial ankle arthrotomy is performed, and with maximal plantar flexion of the foot, the anterior one-half to two-thirds of the superior rim of the talus is inspected. If proper exposure is not attained, then an incision is placed over the tibialis posterior tendon sheath posteriorly and the tendon is retracted anteriorly, and the remainder of the tarsal tunnel is gently retracted posteriorly. An incision is then placed in the deep surface of the flexor retinaculum, effecting a posteromedial arthrotomy, and with maximal ankle dorsiflexion, the posterior one-half of the talus is exposed, examined, and treated. The postoperative regimen would again consist of early range of motion, weight bearing, and return to function as tolerated.

Occasionally, an anteromedial ankle arthrotomy may be sufficient to reach medial lesions that are not too posterior. The surgical approach involves a curvilinear incision placed lateral to the tibialis anterior tendon that is deepened to the level of the deep fascia. The tibialis anterior tendon sheath is then incised laterally and the tendon is retracted medially. Care should be taken to identify, clamp, and tie off encountered branches of the medial malleolar and medial tarsal arteries and veins. The arthrotomy is then performed deep to the tibialis anterior tendon sheath, exposing the medial anterior talar dome lesions. Should plantar flexion of the ankle not allow adequate exposure of the lesion, then the anteromedial articular surface of the tibia overlying the talar lesion is grooved with a narrow gouge as described by Gould[26] and later by Flick and Gould.[12] The area of the distal tibial articular surface removed is approximately 4 to 5 mm wide anteriorly by 6 to 8 mm deep. It is not replaced, and active, early range of motion ankle exercise is instituted. Flick and Gould report no increased

radiographic evidence of ankle arthrosis at 24 months in six of eight patients requiring this approach.[12]

The actual surgical procedure or procedures involved after exposure of the fracture fragment usually entail excision of the fragment with curettage of its articular borders and drilling of the defect with small Kirschner wires. These maneuvers encourage bleeding into the defect with subsequent fibrocartilaginous metaplasia and filling of the defect. Cartilaginous remodeling should be done with a sharp curette or surgical blade and at 90 degrees to the crater defect to minimize the defect size. Should the transchondral fracture fragment be large (greater than 2 cm), then replacement of the fragment with minifragment screw fixation should be attempted. In all surgical cases, early and active postoperative ankle range of motion exercises will further encourage the degree and quality of fibrocartilaginous repair. Filling of the defect by fibrous tissues occurs over months and years and has been noted to take as long as 7 years.[27] Therefore, one should look for resolution of symptoms versus radiologic cure in postoperative patients, as well as in those treated conservatively.

Summary

Transchondral fractures of the talus are often elusive injuries with no pathognomonic signs or symptoms. They are usually associated with trauma; however, they may be found on routine radiographic examination in asymptomatic patients without any history of a traumatic episode.[12] Their presence must therefore be sought by a suspicious examiner, especially following any ankle injury with which an inversion component is described. In this way, acute lesions can be treated either conservatively or surgically immediately according to the protocols presented. Early, appropriate surgical treatment, as well as adequate early conservative care, has been documented to yield good results. Should initial conservative care fail, then operative treatment should follow prior to the development of posttraumatic arthrosis.[15] Alexander and Lichtman[21] and Flick and Gould[12] state that a delay in several months will not adversely affect the surgical result. O'Farrell and Costello concluded that early surgery gives the best results, with 12 months being the critical delay time.[18]

Prior to surgery and again intraoperatively, the surgeon should assess the integrity of the lateral collateral ligaments. Should they be unstable, a delayed primary repair or lateral ankle stabilization should be performed.[15] As stated earlier, there is some evidence to acknowledge the fact that stage I through III symptomatic osteochondral lesions may progress to a more aggressive lesion should inadequate or suboptimal treatment be rendered. The end of this progress would result in a stage IV transchondral lesion that could predictably lead to degenerative arthrosis should surgical treatment be delayed further. The association of subchondral cysts adjacent to the osteochondritis dissecans lesion has also been observed (Fig. 26-5).

In addition to misdiagnosis and delay in treatment, the physician should also be aware of concomitant injury including lateral ligamentous disruption, associated fracture, and peroneal dislocation. Prognosis concerning these injuries should improve and is dependent on initial accurate diagnosis combined with early, adequate treatment.

ANTERIOR PROCESS FRACTURES OF THE CALCANEUS

The orthopedic literature dealing with the subject of fractures of the calcaneus is quite extensive, and the mere suggestion of the words "calcaneal fracture" immediately impart images of severe and extensive disruption of the architectural configuration, alterations of the articular relationships, and gross disturbance or loss of normal function. The largest of the bones in the foot, the calcaneus is fractured more often than any other tarsal bone and thus has received widespread recognition and study. The results have been an impressively detailed orderliness to several classifications for calcaneal fractures; however, most have placed little emphasis on the potential disability of fractures to the superior distal

portion of the calcaneus.[28–32] Textbooks of anatomy have failed to give a specific name to this anatomic portion of the calcaneus.[33–35] This dorsal or superior distal protuberance has arbitrarily been referred to as the anterior process or superior beak most commonly[36–44] and the calcaneal promontory[45] or anterior lip[46] less often.

The true incidence of fractures of this portion of the calcaneus has been difficult to determine, although some reports indicate that it may be one of the most common types of calcaneal fractures but is frequently overlooked.[39,42,47] Several reports have indicated that the injury represents from 3 to 23 percent of all calcaneal fractures.[30,40,48] Although Dachtler is credited with the first major article drawing attention to this fracture in 1920 with a review of 20 cases,[36] the fracture was briefly described in the Scandinavian literature prior to that.[49] During the 1950s, several investigators provided additional detailed descriptions of the fracture and their experience with various treatment modalities.[38,41–43,45,46]

Classification

Rowe et al. classified the fracture as type Ic, along with fractures of the tuberosity (type Ia) and fractures of the sustentaculum tali (type Ib).[40] Based on a review of 154 fractures, the overall incidence was determined to be 21 percent. Only central depression fractures with various degrees of comminution and other fractures involving the subtalar joint accounted for a higher incidence.[40] The Watson-Jones classification designates this fracture as a type 4 injury.[28,29,32] Essex-LoPresti referred to this injury as a "parrot nose" type fracture with an overall incidence of about 5 percent and identified the failure of Bohler to include this injury in his original classification of calcaneal fractures.[31] We believe, as do other researchers, that fractures of the anterior process of the calcaneus are the most common of the extra-articular fractures of the calcaneus, extra-articular being defined as fractures not involving the subtalar joint proper.[39,47]

In 1982, Degan et al. reported on a classification of this particular fracture based on the size and location of the fracture line.[39] Type I is an undisplaced fracture involving only the tip of the process itself. Type II is a displaced fracture that does not involve the articular surface, and type III is a large displaced fragment involving the calcaneocuboid joint itself.

Anatomically, the dorsal distal portion of the calcaneus is continuous with the distal articular saddle-shaped surface that articulates with the cuboid. A portion of it may also articulate with the navicular. The architectural configuration of this structure varies considerably in its development; it may be broad and blunt or beak-shaped and prolonged.[42,44] It is well developed between the age of 7 and 10 years. A detailed anatomic description of this process was recently published by Jahss and Kay,[44] and the reader is referred to this reference for greater detail. When well developed, it may possess a medial cartilaginous articular surface that articulates with a corresponding portion of the talus. We suggest that perhaps an enlarged anterior process of the calcaneus is related to the formation of calcaneonavicular coalitions, although this has not been previously reported. The bifurcate ligament is a strong ligament with a narrow origin from the lateral aspect of the anterior calcaneal process. It goes forth to attach medially to the navicular as the calcaneonavicular ligament and laterally to the cuboid as the calcaneocuboid ligament. The calcaneocuboid portion of the bifurcate ligament is wider; it appears weaker and tears more readily than the calcaneonavicular portion, based on anatomic studies.[44]

Mechanisms of Injury

Fractures of the anterior process of the calcaneus have been associated with industrial accidents,[36] motor vehicle accidents,[37,39] and misadventures while climbing or descending stairs.[42,44] Although they may occur in any age group, there appears to be greater frequency of injury in individuals between the ages of 30 and 60 years.[38,41,47] The fracture not infrequently occurs in sedentary individuals, especially housewives and wearers of high-heeled shoes, which, it is believed, predispose the wearer for twisting injuries.[38,45] The fracture may occur as a result of a direct or indirect blow to the area.[36,42] In other cases, twisting is reported by patients, although they are usually uncertain of the precise direction.[38]

Investigators generally agree that fractures of the anterior process of the calcaneus occur by one of two different mechanisms. Most fractures are believed to represent an avulsion fracture and occur as a result of a severe twisting or sprain injury in which the foot is suddenly placed in a position of plantar flexion and inversion. This results in a sudden increase in tension on the bifurcate ligament with an avulsion fracture of the calcaneus.[30,37,39,41,42,44–47] Rarely does this fracture fragment originate from the navicular bone. Because the mechanism of injury so closely resembles the mechanism responsible for rupture of the anterior talofibular ligament of the ankle joint, it is often referred to as a sprain fracture (Fig. 26-12).

A second, less common mechanism is a shearing or impaction fracture that occurs as a result of a sudden dorsiflexion and eversion force against the forefoot, resulting in a compression fracture of the anterior process of the calcaneus by the cuboid bone.[39,41,45,46] Misadventures while climbing stairs, falls from a height, and stepping into unsuspected holes may result in this type of fracture (Fig. 26-13).

As one might suspect, fractures of the remaining bones of the foot and ankle could also occur as a result of the same mechanisms of injury described above. Associated soft tissue structures might also be injured.

Diagnosis

The clinical characteristics of this injury closely mimic those of the typical ankle sprain; however, there are several specific findings that readily distinguish it from an injury to the lateral collateral ligaments of the ankle joint (Fig. 26-14). Like ankle fractures, a cracking sensation may be reported by the patient and result in a severe limp or hop. Immediate pain develops and persists for several days. The focal point of maximum tenderness is identified 2 to 3 cm ante-

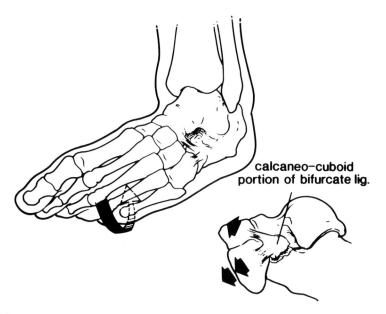

calcaneo-cuboid
portion of bifurcate lig.

Fig. 26-12. Diagrammatic representation of the avulsion fracture mechanism of injury.

rior and 1 to 2 cm inferior to the lateral malleolus. This is a striking feature, both visually and upon digital palpation of both areas. A hematoma may form. Ecchymosis is usually present in the area, both on the dorsum and, less often, on the plantar

aspect of the foot. Pain is significantly increased by simultaneous plantar flexion and adduction-inversion of the forefoot or simultaneous dorsi-flexion and abduction-eversion of the forefoot when the subtalar joint and ankle joint are immo-

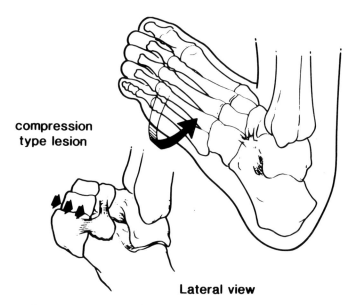

compression
type lesion

Lateral view

Fig. 26-13. Diagrammatic representation of the less common mechanism of sheering or impaction, resulting in a compression fracture.

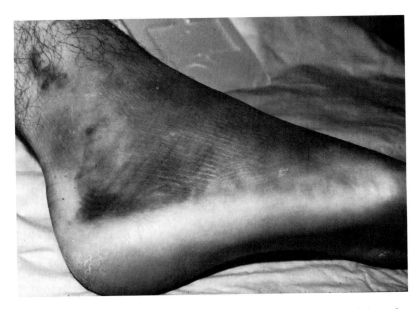

Fig. 26-14. Typical clinical presentation following anterior process fractures of the calcaneus. Note the clinical similarity in presentation to that of a typical ankle sprain injury or other injury discussed in this chapter. Ecchymosis and edema cover the entire lateral aspect of the foot and ankle; however, clinical examination and radiographic findings all substantiate and confirm the specific diagnosis.

bilized. Pronatory and supinatory movements of the subtalar joint and active dorsiflexion or plantar flexion of the ankle joint are comparably much less uncomfortable. This is another striking feature that differentiates this injury from the typical ankle sprain. Manipulation of the midtarsal joint and forefoot may also result in muscle spasm. The development of a peroneal spastic flatfoot has been reported as a result of this injury.[38,39] Walking or weight bearing is not infrequently virtually impossible for patients with fractures of the anterior process of the calcaneus. The patient is usually unable to stand on the affected limb without contralateral limb support.

Associated injuries of the same extremity include fractures of the remaining tarsal bones in the ankle itself and have received attention in the medical literature.[39,42,50] Fractures of the calcaneus and ankle may occur if sufficient supinatory or rotatory forces are present and have been confirmed by experimental studies.[42] Fractures of the navicular, cuboid, and fifth metatarsal, as well as dislocations of the talonavicular joint and talocalcaneal joint, have also been reported.[30,47,50] Because of the potential and possibility of simul-

taneous injury, the clinical examination must include a comprehensive and detailed scrutiny of both the osseous and soft tissue structures of the ankle joint and rearfoot complex (Fig. 26-15).

The diagnosis of fracture of the anterior process of the calcaneus requires multiple foot radiographs. Because of the possibility of other fractures, a series of ankle radiographs should be obtained. The medial oblique radiograph (standard oblique) is most useful for visualization of this fracture (Fig. 26-16). We are in agreement with several investigators who suggest obtaining the medial oblique radiograph at several different angles of projection to allow for variation in the size and shape of the anterior process of the calcaneus.[38,42] The fracture line runs obliquely across a variable portion of the distal superior portion of the calcaneus at its articulation with the cuboid. At times, the fracture may present itself as only a faint linear shadow or lucency. The fragment itself may be displaced or nondisplaced (Fig. 26-17).

Lateral views may also be helpful, but overlap of the talus with the anterior process of the calcaneus frequently obscures clear visualization of

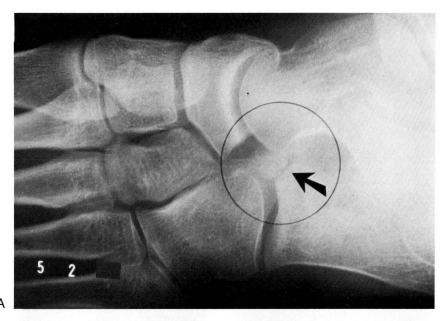

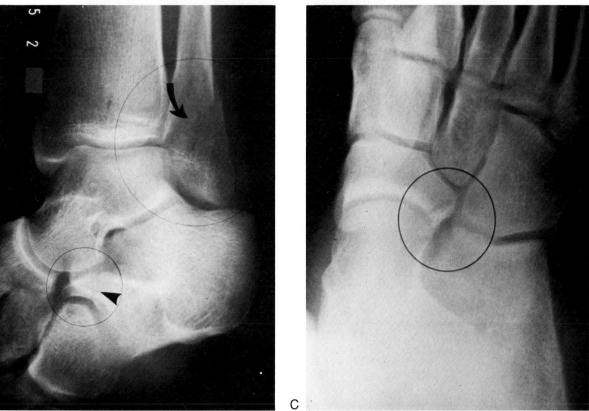

Fig. 26-15. **(A)** A medial oblique and **(B)** mortise view of the left ankle in a patient who suffered a severe ankle sprain injury. Note concomitant fractures of the anterior beak of the calcaneus as well as a spiral oblique fracture of the fibula occurring in the same individual with one mechanism of injury. **(C)** Medial oblique radiograph demonstrating an unusual avulsion fracture of the lateral aspect of the navicular body. This fracture represents an avulsion fracture of the bifurcate ligament at its attachment to the navicular bone. This fracture is rarely seen but is believed to occur by the avulsion fracture mechanism previously discussed.

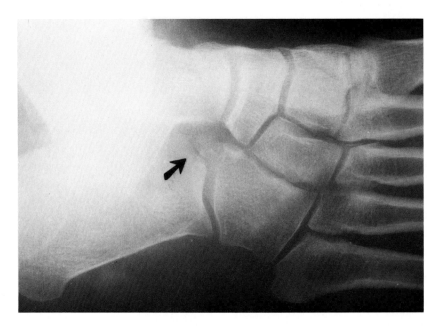

Fig. 26-16. Standard medial oblique radiograph demonstrating minimally displaced anterior beak fracture of the calcaneus.

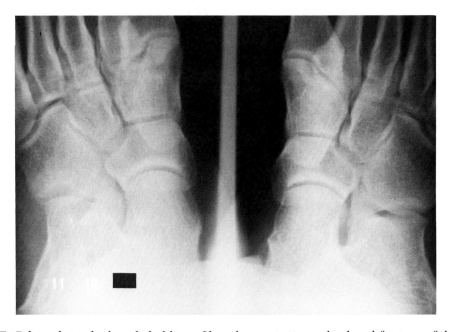

Fig. 26-17. Bilateral standard medial oblique films demonstrating a displaced fracture of the anterior beak of the calcaneus of the left foot. Note the significant change in contour to the midtarsal joint and in particular the calcaneocuboid joint of the left foot in comparison with the right foot.

the fracture lines, especially if no significant displacement is present (Fig. 26-18). A non-weight-bearing lateral or an oblique lateral radiograph may be helpful in visualizing the full extent of the fracture line (Fig. 26-19).[46] The use of a magnifying glass has been reportedly helpful in evaluating radiographs of this fracture.[38] Post-traumatic amorphous calcifications may also occur.

On rare occasions, we have found it helpful to use specialized radiographic techniques to identify and confirm this fracture. These may include lateral tomography (Fig. 26-20), CT, or magnetic resonance imaging. When prolonged disability is present and strong suspicion for osseous pathology cannot be confirmed on standard radiographs, a conventional bone scan may prove helpful in confirming or excluding such a diagnosis (Fig. 26-21). Because of their prohibitive cost, such studies should not be ordered indiscriminately or injudiciously.

It is important to distinguish this fracture from the supernumerary bone, os calcaneus secundarius, which generally has smooth edges, a rounded appearance, and a thin cortical sheath.[39,45,46,50,51] The configuration of the os calcaneus secundarius, however, may be variable.[34,52] The suggestion of an un-united epiphysis has also been reported.[45]

Treatment

Appropriate treatment will vary depending on the size and degree of comminution of the fracture fragment, as well as the amount of displacement. Recommended treatments have ranged from adhesive strappings and elastic bandages[42] to short leg casting[38–40,45–47] to surgical intervention.[39,40,43,46,52] The initial treatment consists of rest, ice, compression, and elevation. We routinely use a Jones compression bandage as the initial treatment to minimize and resolve edema. If the fracture is incomplete, a compression bandage for 4 to 6 weeks may be adequate with partial weight bearing as tolerated (Fig. 26-22). This may be followed by a course of aggressive physical therapy for range of motion, ultrasound, or phonophoresis and cross-fiber massage to decrease fibrosis and improve mobility. Complete undisplaced fractures should be casted for 5 to 8

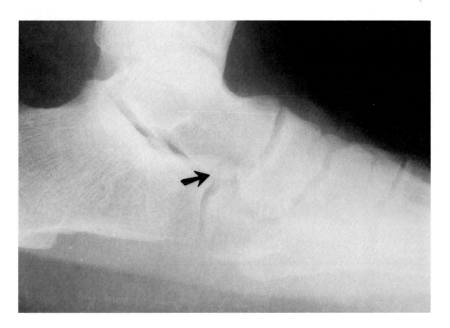

Fig. 26-18. Lateral radiographic view demonstrating fracture of the anterior process of the calcaneus. Unless this injury is strongly suspected, it is easily overlooked on a lateral film. Medial oblique radiographs confirm the diagnosis.

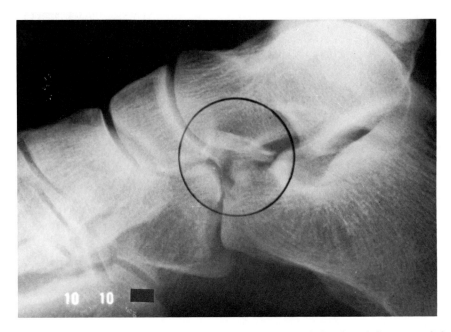

Fig. 26-19. Lateral radiograph demonstrating a large comminuted displaced fracture of the interior process of the calcaneus. This fracture subsequently was surgically excised but owing to other concomitant injury of the calcaneocuboid joint developed severe tarsal arthritis. Note compaction fracture of the cuboid in the middle and inferior aspects of the joint.

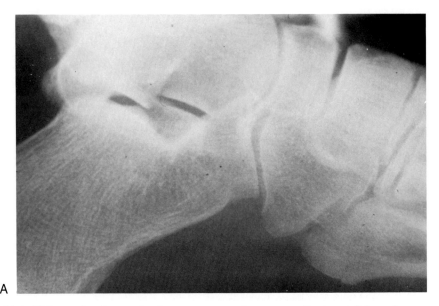

A

Fig. 26-20. **(A & B)** Lateral radiograph of a suspect anterior process fracture of the calcaneus confirmed by lateral tomography. Note the clear delineation of the fracture fragment in the lateral tomogram. This detail is difficult to appreciate in standard lateral radiographs. (*Figure continues.*)

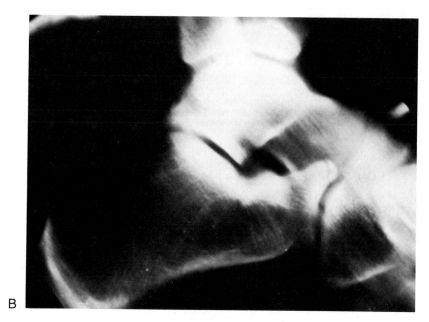

B

Fig. 26-20 (*Continued*).

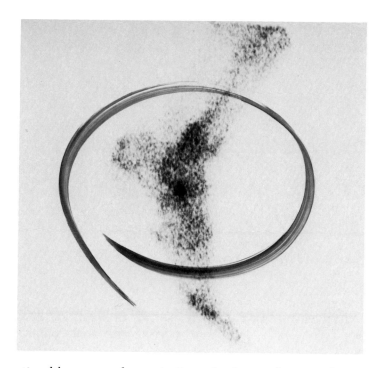

Fig. 26-21. Conventional bone scan demonstrating a focal area of increased uptake in the midtarsal region. Surgical exploration subsequently confirmed an old small fracture of the interior process of the calcaneus.

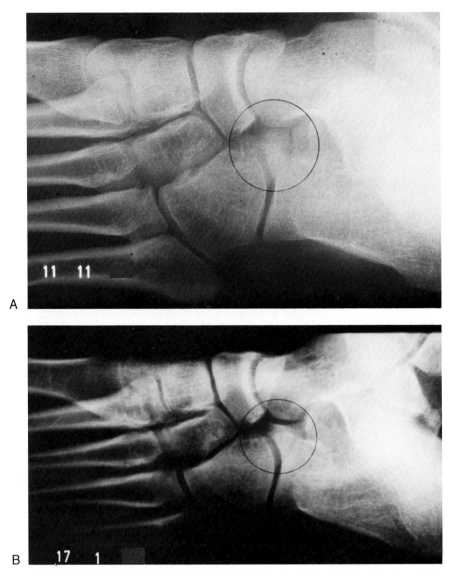

Fig. 26-22. (A & B) Standard medial oblique radiographs demonstrating a nondisplaced fracture of the anterior process of the calcaneus treated by cast immobilization for 6 weeks. Follow-up radiographs show complete osseous union without evidence of degenerative arthritis in the calcaneocuboid joint or the articulation between the calcaneus and navicular.

weeks until radiographic consolidation is seen. We recommend an initial nonweight-bearing period of 4 weeks, followed by weight bearing for the balance of the time of cast immobilization. Simple displaced fractures deserve an attempted manipulation and closed reduction under fluoroscopic control. When the fracture fragments fail to unite and prolonged disability occurs, surgical excision is highly recommended. If a displaced fracture fragment cannot be reduced anatomically by closed manipulation, open reduction with internal fixation employing compression screws is indicated.[53] If anatomic reduction with appropriate internal fixation cannot be attained,

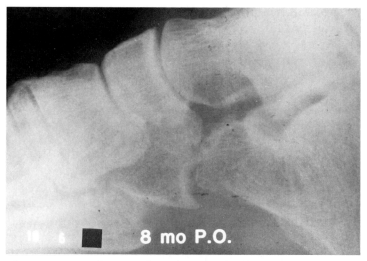

8 mo P.O.

Fig. 26-23. Severe degenerative arthritis in the calcaneocuboid joint 8 months following surgical excision of the comminuted displaced fracture fragment shown in Figure 26-19. This patient subsequently required a triple arthrodesis with excellent resolution of symptomatology.

consideration should be given to primary excision. Delayed surgical excision is more likely to result in a poor clinical result and prolonged disability (Fig. 26-23).[39] When severe degenerative changes develop, isolated arthrodesis of the calcaneocuboid joint, or more commonly triple arthrodesis, will be necessary. In our experience, triple arthrodesis has proved more successful than isolated midtarsal joint fusions.

Unless the correct diagnosis is established and early, appropriate treatment is rendered, prolonged disability is likely. Disability periods ranging from 3 weeks to 60 months have been reported,[36,38,39,42,45,46] and it is not uncommon for total disability to persist for periods of 6 months or longer with residual discomfort and swelling present to various degrees.[36,39,42,45] It is our belief that this injury, although now recognized and diagnosed more commonly than in the past, continues to be misdiagnosed or even undiagnosed in a great number of cases. It is a definite clinical entity deserving of recognition and close scrutiny whenever a significant traumatic injury of the foot or ankle is sustained. A high index of suspicion is paramount for successful diagnosis and treatment.

OS TRIGONUM

Trauma to the posterior lateral process of the talus is known alternatively as fractured os trigonum or Shepherd's fracture. Rosenmuller[54] was first credited with describing the os trigonum (named for its characteristic triangular appearance) in 1804. It is one of 38 different accessory bones of the foot.[55] Shepherd,[56] following postmortem examination of three specimens, thought that this was not an accessory bone, but an avulsion fracture from the foot being twisted in some manner, though he has never able to reproduce the fracture with cadaveric specimens. He believed there was only one center of ossification to the talus, dismissing the idea this could be an ununited apophysis. That same year, in the same journal, Shepherd's theory was refuted. Referencing both Gruber (1864) and Stieda (1869), Professor Turner stated that the origin of the ossicle was due to the presence of a secondary epiphysis that failed to unite with the body of the talus, not from injury.[57] Considerable debate still exists among clinicians and anatomists as to whether the accessory ossicle is independently formed or an un-united fracture of the posterior lateral process. Clinical and histologic findings of surgically excised fragments have not been able to differentiate between the two.[58–60] It would seem, then, appropriate to use the term os trigonum syndrome for all symptomatology, be it from fracture or developmental anomaly.

In early childhood the posterior border of the talus is rounded. By age 8 to 11, a secondary center of ossification appears posteriorly and rapidly unites with the main body of the talus. As the size, time of appearance, and union are so variable they may be overlooked. McDougall found evidence of secondary ossification centers in 29 of 35 unselected radiographs of young children. Occasionally, an additional ossification center was noted, corresponding with the posteromedial tubercle.[61]

The posterolateral process of the adult talus is quite variable in size. When it is enlarged or elongated, some have considered this a fused os trigonum. The percentage of feet with a separate os trigonum ranges from 3 to 15 percent, with 7 percent being the accepted average.[62–66] The ossicle may be attached to the talus by fibrous, fibrocartilaginous, or cartilaginous tissue.[34]

The posterolateral process forms the lateral wall of the groove on the posterior talus for the flexor hallucis longus tendon. The inferior surface articulates with the posterior facet of the calcaneus, while the dorsal surface is nonarticular. The posterolateral process also serves as attachment for the posterior talofibular ligament.

That separate ossicles are found in some adult ankles is an established fact. McDougall proposed several theories to explain their presence.[61] The first is detachment by repeated minor trauma. With the ankle in extreme plantar flexion, the posterior talar process directly impinges on the posterior tibial plafond. Case reports involving soccer players and ballet dancers[67] support this mechanism. Moeller theorized that excessive subtalar joint pronation presents the opportunity for mechanical microtrauma.[60] During subtalar joint pronation, the talus advances anteriorly, directing the posterolateral tubercle against the posterosuperior articular facet of the calcaneus, creating either compressive or shearing forces. A second method is detachment by

sudden violence. Most commonly this results from extreme plantar flexion injuries as previously described. Excessive dorsiflexion may also cause avulsion the posterior process by fibers of the post-talofibular ligament.[68] The third theory is persistence of a second center of ossification.

Presenting signs and symptoms vary with the mechanism of injury. Acutely injured ankles are quite painful and swollen. Patients ambulate with a discernible limp or remain non-weight bearing on the injured side. An enlarged area of ecchymosis is usually present anterior to the Achilles tendon. The entire posterior ankle is tender to palpation, making it difficult to pinpoint the exact site of injury. Pain may be reproduced in the posterior ankle by passive dorsiflexion of the hallux with the foot held perpendicular to the leg or by applying resistance as the patient actively plantar flexes the hallux. However, this test is difficult to interpret and diagnostically inaccurate in the acutely traumatized ankle. Included in the differential diagnosis are transchondral talar dome fractures, lateral talar process fractures, calcaneal or fibular fracture, ruptured lateral collateral ankle ligaments, subluxed peroneal tendons, and partial or complete rupture of the Achilles tendon.

The typical patient with os trigonum syndrome, however, presents with chronic pain in the posterior ankle and heel. The initial symptoms are insidious and progressive.

A history of trauma is usually absent, but occasionally these symptoms result as late sequelae of inversion ankle sprains. Visual examination of the ankle fails to reveal any edema or ecchymosis. Pain can be elicited by palpation deep within the posterolateral ankle. Pain upon active or passive motion of the hallux, as previously described, is more specific for the chronic than the acute injury, although it is not usually present. Ankle range of motion is usually restricted, with reproduction of pain upon passive plantar flexion of the foot.

Although the os trigonum is usually found unilaterally[65,66] lateral radiographs should be taken of both ankles. If a fused os trigonum is present on the contralateral ankle identical in shape, size, and position to the symptomatic side, one might conclude that a fracture is present.

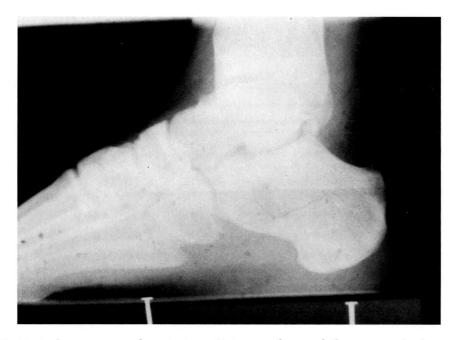

Fig. 26-24. Typical appearance of os trigonum. Note smooth, rounded contour and sclerotic margins.

The free os trigonum is usually round and smooth, whereas a fractured fused os trigonum appears serrated, especially in the acute injury (Fig. 26-24). Eventually the roughened edges become smooth and sclerotic as a nonunion forms. Occasionally no fracture or a questionable fracture is seen, despite strong clinical evidence to the contrary. This may be due to obliquity of the fracture line or from the fibula obscuring the fracture line. If repeat lateral radiographs taken at slightly differing angles are unsatisfactory, tomograms or CT scans should be employed (Fig. 26-25). A Tc 99m bone scan should be ordered in all suspected cases. Its effectiveness in pinpointing the os trigonum as the cause of pain has been documented.[69] However, a negative scan should not rule out the os trigonum from the differential diagnosis. A disruption of the fibrous or fibrocartilaginous bar that attaches the os trigonum to the talus will produce symptoms, yet yield a cold scan for lack of osseous involvement.

Other diagnoses to consider in chronically painful ankles include stenosing tenosynovitis of the flexor hallucis longus, Achilles tendinitis, Achilles and calcaneal bursitis, tarsal tunnel

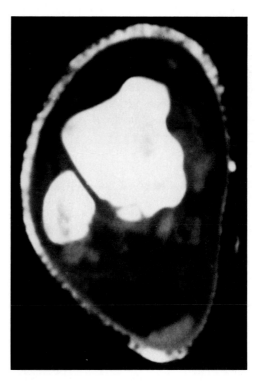

Fig. 26-25. The os trigonum can be clearly visualized with CT scanning.

syndrome,[70] talofibular arthritis, and calcaneal apophysitis.

Conservative care should be offered initially. Acute fractures should be treated with an non-weight-bearing cast for 6 weeks. Although union of the fracture is uncommon, an asymptomatic nonunion is not. Those patients with chronic symptoms may respond to one or more injections of local anesthetic and steroid into the painful area, or immobilization in a cast. In persistently painful os trigonum syndrome, surgical excision is the treatment of choice. The procedure offers uniformly excellent results with minimal morbidity.[60,71-73]

FRACTURES OF THE LATERAL PROCESS OF THE TALUS

Acute or persistent pain about the lateral aspect of the ankle and foot may be due to an overt fracture of the lateral process of the talus. This fracture injury, which may occur as an isolated entity or in combination with other soft tissue or osseous injury of the foot or ankle, is more common than previously thought. It has received increased attention in more recent years.[53,74-76] Most of the English literature emphasizes the need for greater recognition of this fracture as a potentially disabling entity if undiagnosed, ignored, or mistreated.

Fractures of the talus themselves are rare and estimated to comprise only about 1 percent of all fractures.[77] Fractures of the lateral process itself are much more common than considered and have been estimated to represent 24 percent of all fractures of the body of the talus. In 1965, Hawkins reported on 50 consecutive fractures of the talus and on 13 cases of lateral process fractures.[76] These fractures were the second most common fractures seen in the talus. In the same year, Mukherjee and associates independently reported on 13 cases seen over a period of 13 months from approximately 1,500 cases of ankle sprains and fractures, an incidence of 0.86 percent. Prior to these two major publications, we are able to document only 24 other cases of this injury based on an extensive review of the litera-ture.[73,74,77-82] Marottoli is credited with the first reported cases (10 total) in 1942.[78]

Anatomy

Anatomically, the lateral surface of the talus is triangular in outline and forms an apex on its inferior aspect referred to as the lateral process of the talus (Fig. 26-26). It extends from the lower margin of the articular surface of the talar dome to the posteroinferior surface of the talus. It has both articular and nonarticular surfaces. Both the lateral and inferior surfaces of this portion of the talus are coated with hyaline cartilage, and these form components of both the ankle joint and the subtalar joint (Fig. 26-27). Specifically, the lateral surface articulates with the medial or inner surface of the fibula, while the inferior surface articulates with the superior surface of the calcaneal posterior facet, the major component of the subtalar joint complex. Fractures of the lateral process of the talus are thus intra-articular fractures in nature, and patients are subject to the disabling afflictions of such fractures. Although no ligamentous structure is attached directly to the apex of the process itself, a number of ligaments surround this process, including the lateral collateral ligaments of the ankle (anterior talofibular ligament, posterior talofibular ligament, and calcaneofibular ligament) and the lateral ligaments of the subtalar joint. In anatomic studies performed to define the lateral process of the talus, Hawkins found that the latter talocalcaneal ligament lies deep to, parallel with, and slightly anterior to the calcaneofibular ligament.[76] This is a fairly small band of tissue that restricts separation of the adjacent surfaces of the talocalcaneal joint. The calcaneofibular ligament, by its anatomic position and orientation to the subtalar joint, also assists in this restraining action.

Hawkins also studied the trabeculation pattern of the lateral process of the talus.[76] Although there is little trabeculation seen at the apex of the process itself, it is clear that there is adequate provision made for the transmission of forces between the superolateral and inferolateral surface near the root of the process. The opposing surfaces of the posterior subtalar joint are normally

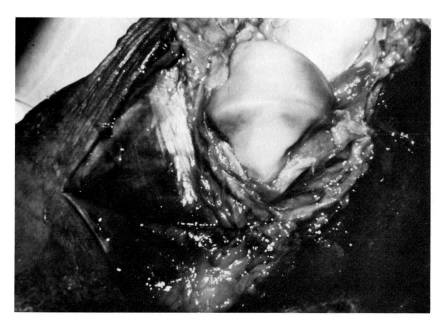

Fig. 26-26. Cadaveric specimen demonstrating the lateral process of the talus. Notice the triangular outline of the lateral surface with a well-defined apex inferiorly. The dome of the talus is also shown.

in close apposition to each other. In inversion, the lateral part of the posterior talar facet migrates superiorly on the posterior calcaneal facet, causing separation as well as an increase in compression force transmission on the lateral process itself.

Mechanisms of Injury

Several mechanisms of injury have been postulated. The most popular theory is based on anatomic cadaveric research that suggests that the fracture occurs with a fall from a height with the

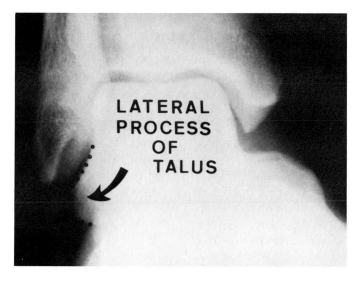

Fig. 26-27. Anteroposterior view of the ankle demonstrating the lateral process of the talus (arrow). This surface articulates with both the fibula laterally and the posterior subtalar joint inferiorly.

ankle in a dorsiflexed position and the foot supinated or inverted in the rear-foot complex.[74] Fjeldborg referred to this as a "supination-dorsal flexion fracture," in which the incongruence of the talocalcaneal joint resulted in fracture of the lateral process because of its weakness.[74] The incongruity results in compression or shearing of the lateral process by the underlying calcaneus. The lateral portion of the talus is thus wedged between the calcaneus and tibia primarily, with the fibula playing a secondary or passive role. Hawkins[76] and Mukherjee et al.,[75] in attempting to correlate their 13 cases each, agreed with the theory proposed by Fjeldborg. They were able to establish that their patients suffered an "inversion injury" and in many instances had dorsiflexion of the foot at the time of injury. A fall from a height or unexpected stepping into a hole, frequently reported by patients, is consistent with the proposed mechanism.

Fjeldborg describes the three stages to this injury: fissure (stage I), fracture with displacement of the lateral process of the talus (stage II), and finally, fracture with displacement of the fragment and subtalar joint dislocation (stage III).[74] He presented three cases as clinical evidence to support his staging and proposed mechanism of "supination-dorsal flexion fracture."

Cummino has suggested that such fractures represent an avulsion fracture of the tip of the lateral process produced by pull of the lateral talocalcaneal ligament or a direct compression or direct blow to the process itself.[77] This has not been confirmed clinically to any significant degree and therefore, although possible, these are not commonly accepted mechanisms.

Diagnosis

The physical findings are frequently unremarkable and often indistinguishable from those of a severe ankle sprain. The immediate disability, pain and swelling just anterior and inferior to the lateral malleolus, is typical. Pain on direct palpation of the fibular malleolus itself is not remarkable, while direct palpation just inferior and anterior to the malleolus may be excruciating, especially in the acute injury period. Ecchymosis and edema may be seen and will generally develop sometime later if not within the first few hours. Pain upon active or passive range of motion of both the ankle and subtalar joint may be severe and help distinguish this injury from others described in this chapter. Crepitus of one or both joints is not infrequently present, especially if the injury is undiagnosed or mistreated. Chronic, unexplained, and persistent pain on motion are clues to the diagnosis of this fracture. Post-traumatic arthritis results when the condition persists for years without appropriate treatment.

An accurate diagnosis requires radiographic evaluation and should include anteroposterior, lateral, and mortise views of the ankle. Placement of the foot in slight plantar flexion may prove helpful in improving visualization of the fracture. Three types of distinct fracture patterns have been described.[76] The first is a simple fracture of the lateral process of the talus that extends from the talofibular articular joint surfaces inferiorly to the posterior talocalcaneal articular surfaces of the subtalar joint (Fig. 26-28). This type of fracture is easily recognized on the previously mentioned radiographs. The second type is the comminuted fracture that involves both the fibula and the posterior calcaneal articular surface with the articular surface of the talus and the entire lateral process (Fig. 26-29). The third type is a chip fracture of the anterior and inferior portion of the posterior articular process of the talus. This fracture is best seen on the lateral radiograph in close proximity to the sinus tarsi and does not involve the talofibular articulation itself, as do types I and II.

Adequate visualization of this anatomic area is usually accomplished with the standard radiographic views discussed above. In a limited number of cases, tomograms, or preferably CT scans or magnetic resonance imaging will be helpful in further delineating the extent of injury and status of the ankle joint or subtalar joint complex.

Treatment

There is general agreement that early treatment is likely to produce the best results and may

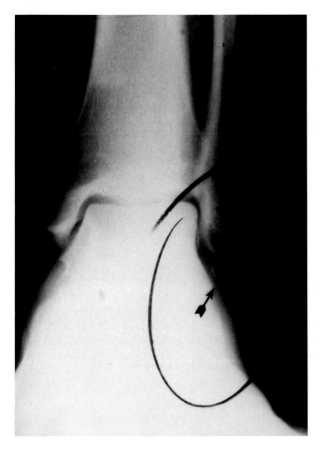

Fig. 26-28. Anteroposterior view of the left ankle demonstrating a simple fracture (arrow) of the lateral process of the talus.

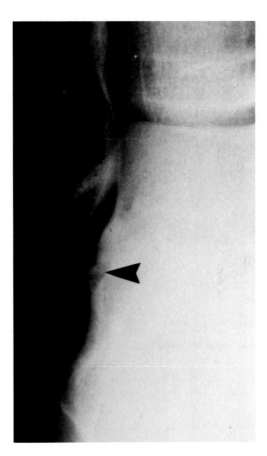

Fig. 26-29. Anteroposterior view of the right ankle demonstrating a comminuted fracture (arrow) of the lateral process of the talus. Notice the irregular contour to the lateral process with evidence of comminuted bone fragments between the fibula and talus as well as at the inferior aspect of the lateral process.

be either conservative or surgical, depending on the nature and type of fracture. Displaced fractures must be reduced by either closed or open reduction techniques. Closed reduction should be confirmed radiographically. If successful, the extremity is immobilized in a non-weight-bearing cast for 4 to 6 weeks, followed by a weight-bearing cast for an additional 2 to 3 weeks. The foot should be placed in a neutral position in the sagittal plane with slight eversion of the subtalar joint. Fractures that remain displaced should be considered for open reduction and internal fixation.[74–76] The use of two small Kirschner wires has been shown to be effective in maintaining

alignment and position of the fracture fragments.[75] Whenever possible, however, small compression screws are preferred over Kirschner wires and have been shown to be extremely effective.[53,83] The commonly used screws are the 2.0- or 2.7-mm cortical screws; small fractures may be fixated with a 1.5-mm cortical screw, and larger fractures involving a substantial portion of the lateral process of the talus are fixated with one or more cortical or one or more 4.0-mm cancellous screws. A small metallic washer is occasionally employed. Primary surgical excision should be a strong consideration whenever comminuted fractures are present. The results of

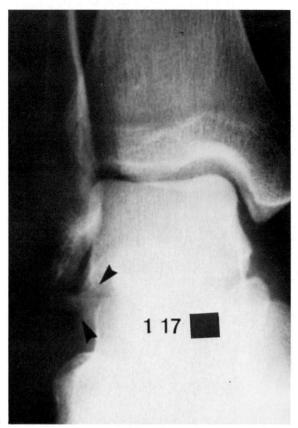

A

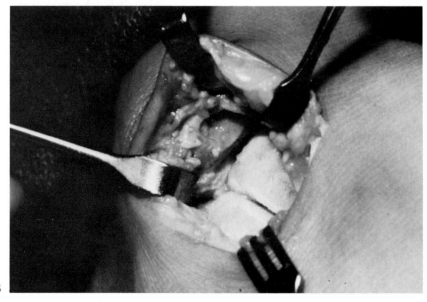

B

Fig. 26-30. (A) Preoperative anteroposterior view of the right ankle of a patient who sustained a fracture of the lateral process of the talus (arrow). Owing to significant disability, surgical exploration was performed consisting of a cheilectomy and arthroplasty of the lateral aspect of the ankle joint and the posterior facet of the subtalar joint. (B) Intraoperative picture demonstrating the fibula articulation with the lateral aspect of the talus and the posterior facet of the subtalar joint following arthroplasty and cheilectomy. (*Figure continues.*)

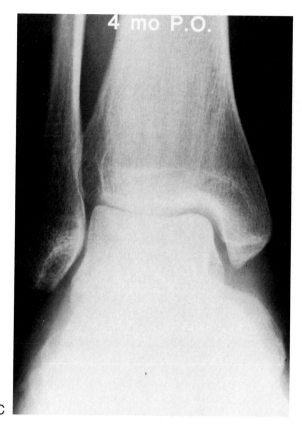

C

Fig. 26-30 (*Continued*). (**C**) Anteroposterior radiograph of the right ankle 4 months following surgical exploration with cheilectomy and arthroplasty.

early excision have been far superior to nonoperative treatment and treatment by later excision for these fractures.[75,76,82,83]

Persistent disability and chronic pain are frequently seen due to malunion, nonunion, or posttraumatic degenerative changes involving the talofibular component of the ankle joint or posterior facet of the talocalcaneal joint. These will usually require surgical intervention, which may consist of excision of loose fragments or cheilectomy or arthroplasty procedures. The surgical approach consists of a lateral incision inferior to the tip of the lateral malleolus and lying within the natural skin lines. Not only does this approach provide excellent exposure to the lateral aspect of the ankle joint and posterior facet of the subtalar joint, it also results in a very cosmetically acceptable and barely perceptible postsurgical scar. The surgical technique requires

meticulous dissection and preservation of the ligamentous structures and joint capsule. Failure to preserve these structures may result in chronic ankle instability. Detailed attention to identification of the sural nerve posteriorly and the intermediate dorsal cutaneous nerve anteriorly is important to avoiding postsurgical entrapment neuropathies. A small surgical drain system should be used whenever less than ideal hemostasis has been achieved. The extremity is placed in a Jones compression dressing for 3 to 5 days; then the surgical site is redressed and examined and then immobilized for 4 to 6 weeks in a short leg non-weight-bearing cast) (Figs. 26-30 and 26-31).

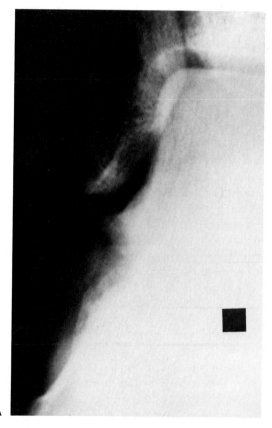

A

Fig. 26-31. (**A**) Preoperative radiograph demonstrating a comminuted fracture with secondary degenerative changes of the lateral process of the talus. This patient sustained a severe inversion sprain injury 9 months prior to surgical exploration, with remodeling and excision of the fracture fragment. (*Figure continues.*)

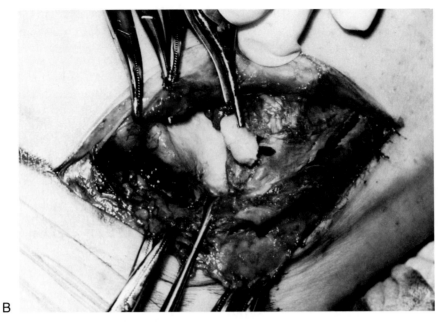

B

Fig. 26-31 *(Continued)*. **(B)** Intraoperative picture showing the large fracture fragment that was excised. The lateral process of the talus was remodeled. The patient had an excellent recovery without the need for surgical fusion.

In a small number of patients, severe degenerative arthritis of the subtalar joint, and to a lesser degree the ankle joint, may develop. These may not be amenable to the surgical approaches outlined above. Not infrequently, a subtalar joint arthrodesis is necessary to resolve the patient's complaints of pain and loss of normal function. When fusion is necessary, subtalar joint arthrodesis is accomplished with a single 6.5-mm cancellous bone screw. Resection of the articular surface of the posterior facet is performed through a lateral incisional approach, and a compression screw is inserted through a medial incision just anterior to the medial malleolus. It is not necessary to resect the middle and anterior facets of the subtalar joint in such cases. If severe valgus of the subtalar joint is present, an appropriately fashioned allogenic cortical cancellous bone graft is inserted within the posterior facet prior to insertion and tightening of the cancellous screw. Rigid internal compression fixation is readily achieved and permits an accelerated postoperative care program, precluding the necessity of cast immobilization, although the patient is still maintained in a non-weight-bearing status for 8 to 12 weeks. If severe degenerative arthritis involving the ankle joint or the midtarsal joints of the foot develops, an ankle, triple, or pantalar arthrodesis may be necessary. In severe cases requiring major arthrodesis of one or more tarsal joints, the clinical and radiographic results have been extremely gratifying to both the patient and surgeon.

SUBLUXING PERONEAL TENDONS

A thorough examination of the ankle following injury should always include the peroneal tendons. Anterior subluxation of the peroneal tendons from the retromalleolar groove, or peroneal subluxation, occurs approximately once in every 200 ski injuries. Other recent reports show subluxation of peroneal tendons to occur in activities as diverse as dancing, running, basketball, cycling, and diving and from a direct blow.[84–86]

The peroneal tendons arise in the lateral compartment of the leg and pass behind the fibular malleolus in a common synovial sheath, with the longus slightly lateral and posterior to the brevis tendon. At this level the tendons are in effect contained within a fibro-osseous tunnel (Fig. 26-32). The anterior wall is formed by the lateral malleolus, and the medial border is formed by the posterior talofibular and calcaneofibular ligaments. The posterior wall is formed from elements of the calcaneofibular ligament and peroneal retinaculum. The superior peroneal retinaculum, a thickening of the deep fascia extending from the lateral malleolus to the calcaneus, forms the lateral wall.

The anatomy and function of the peroneal groove is controversial. Edwards' dissection of 170 fibulae found 82 percent to have a definite sulcus, 11 percent to be flat, and 7 percent to be

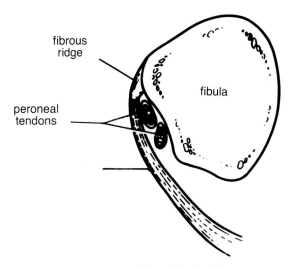

Fig. 26-33. Cross section of distal fibula showing peroneal tendons in their groove, secured by the superior peroneal retinaculum.

convex.[87] The average width of the sulcus was 6 mm, with a depth of 3 mm. In 70 percent of the specimens, a cartilaginous ridge augmented the lateral edge of the groove. The absence or shallowness of the groove is thought to be a major predisposing factor to injury. Muralt demonstrated that if the superior peroneal retinaculum was severed, no dislocation would be possible unless there was a special configuration to the distal fibula.[88]

However, Edwards believed that "even when augmented by cartilage, it is not of sufficient properties to retain the tendons in the groove."[87] This theory is supported by Ekert and colleagues' recent anatomic dissection of 25 amputated limbs.[89] They found the posterior fibular surface to be flat, and when a shallow groove was present, its depth was so "variable," that a "usual" could not be described. More recently, CT has been reported useful in evaluating the peroneal groove.[90]

One consistent finding reported by Eckert et al. was a ridge of fibrocartilaginous tissue along the lateral lip of the groove, loosely connected with the underlying periosteum (Fig. 26-33).[88] The superior peroneal retinaculum does not have any strong connection to the ridge, but blends

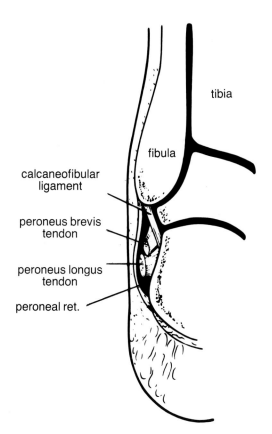

Fig. 26-32. Demonstration of fibro-osseous tunnel through which the peroneal tendons pass.

with the periosteum on the lateral aspect of the fibula. Peroneal subluxation has been classically attributed to a tear of the retinaculum, allowing anterior subluxation of the peroneal tendons. However, in Eckert and co-workers' report of 73 cases, rupture of the retinaculum was rare. Instead, the retinaculum is stripped from the periosteum overlying the lateral malleolus and occasionally avulses a thin cortical shell. Surgical findings revealed three patterns of injury (Fig. 26-34):

Grade I—the retinaculum and periosteum were separated from the fibrocartilaginous lip (51 percent).

Grade II—the fibrous lip was elevated along with the retinaculum (33 percent).

Grade III—a thin fragment of bone along with the fibrous lip was elevated (16 percent).

Other anatomic features of lesser importance that may predispose a patient to peroneal dislocation include congenital absence of the retinaculum, post-traumatic laxity of the retinaculum,[91] and laxity that may develop in calcaneovalgus foot types.[92,93]

Mechanisms of Injury

Although Alm and associates cite two cases of tendon dislocation following a direct blow,[85] all other cases involve some type of indirect trauma to the ankle. The precipitating event appears to be a rapid dorsiflexion of the ankle followed by a sudden, massive reflexive contraction of the peroneals and other ankle plantar flexors. In fact, Achilles tendon ruptures have occurred concomitantly.[91] Subtalar joint position is generally everted, giving the peroneals a greater mechanical advantage. Conversely, Stover and Bryan[91] propose that as the feet invert, the calcaneofibular ligament tenses, thus diminishing the size of the tunnel and forcing the tendons against the retinaculum.

Diagnosis

The acute injury is easily misdiagnosed as a sprained ankle. Edema and ecchymosis make the correct diagnosis difficult unless the examiner is

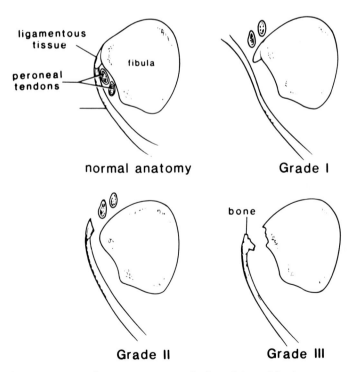

Fig. 26-34. Three patterns of injuries commonly found in subluxing peroneal tendons.

aware of certain key signs and symptoms. A snap is often heard during the fall followed by moderate to severe pain. Edema will often be localized posterior and superior to the lateral malleolus. The tendons are often dislocated at the initial examination. If not visualized, they are readily palpable. Passive ankle plantar flexion will cause the tendons to reduce, while active contraction of the peroneals will result in spontaneous dislocation. Patients with chronic dislocation will complain of a popping or snapping and a feeling of uneasiness or giving way of the ankle. On examination, however, no instability of the ankle or subtalar joint is evident. Subluxation of the tendons can be recreated by repetitive active ankle dorsiflexion, then plantar flexion (Fig. 26-35). An alternative method is to have the patient flex the knee while externally rotating the foot. Many times the dislocation yields an audible click. Crepitus can often be palpated along the tendon's course, especially as it passes over the lateral malleolus. Examination of the contralateral ankle is important to rule out congenital laxity of the peroneal retinaculum.

Radiographs will typically demonstrate an increase in soft tissue volume and density over the lateral malleolus. A fracture lying parallel to the lateral malleolus is pathognomonic for peroneal subluxation.[94] This correlates with a grade III injury. It is best seen on internal oblique or mortise views. Reported incidences range from 10 to 50 percent.[85,91,94-96]

Treatment

Several investigators recommend treating all acute cases conservatively.[89,91,96-98] Stover and Byran[91] found excellent results if a non-weight-bearing cast was applied for 6 weeks. Strapping, weight-bearing casts, heel lifts, crescent pads behind the malleolus, or other forms of conservative therapy demonstrate less than 60 percent success rate.[97]

Owing to ease of repair, predictability of results, and low morbidity, most authorities now recommend surgical repair in all acute and chronic cases.[84,85,96,99]

A multitude of surgical procedures have been devised, reflecting not only the ingenuity of many surgeons but the various philosophies regarding the importance of the peroneal groove and retinaculum.

All reparative procedures can be divided into three categories: (1) direct retinaculum repair[84-86,89]; (2) creation of a new retinaculum[96,100-102]; (3) groove deepening.[100,101]

Direct repair involves opening the peroneal sheath, roughening the malleolus, and direct fasciodesis by suture. Beck reattached the retinacu-

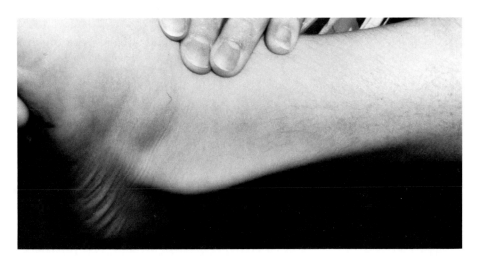

Fig. 26-35. Resistance is applied as the foot is actively everted against that resistance, causing the peroneal tendons to sublux.

lum using an Arbeitgemeinshaft für Osteosynthesisfragen (AO) cancellous screw with a washer.[86] When direct repair is properly performed, no cast is necessary, a clear improvement over other methods.

The classic procedure to recreate a new retinaculum was described by Jones.[92] A slip of the Achilles tendon is freed, leaving the calcaneal insertion intact. The tendon is routed through a drill hole in the fibula from posterior to anterior and then sutured back onto itself, surrounding the peroneal tendons. A non-weight-bearing short leg cast is applied for 4 to 6 weeks.

In cases associated with chronic lateral ankle instability, a new retinaculum may be created by the tendon graft used to recreate the calcaneofibular ligament. Such a procedure is described by Garevitz,[103] who performs a split peroneus brevis stabilization procedure. When the new ligament is passed from the fibula to the calcaneus, it is passed over the peroneal tendons rather than beneath them.

A groove-deepening procedure was originally described by Kelly (Fig. 26-36).[101] A veneerlike graft is cut from the inferior lateral half of the fibular malleolus. The graft is rotated obliquely posterior and fixated with two screws.

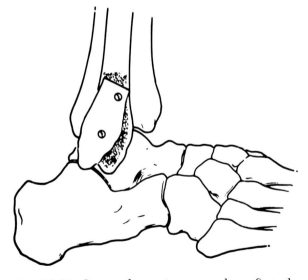

Fig. 26-36. Groove-deepening procedure first described by Kelly.

EXTENSOR DIGITORUM BREVIS AVULSION FRACTURES

An avulsion fracture of the superolateral aspect of the calcaneus at the site of origin of the muscle extensor digitorum brevis has been seen by us in the emergency room setting on several occasions following what is described as a typical ankle sprain injury. An exhaustive review of the medical literature, however, reveals only two articles to date dealing with this specific entity.[51,106] Kohler made reference to this injury and demonstrated such a fracture.[51] Norfray and associates discussed the details of the injury in a publication in 1980 and estimated the frequency of this injury following ankle sprains to be 10 percent, based on a review of 100 consecutive ankle injuries seen during one winter period in a hospital emergency room.[106]

The extensor digitorum brevis muscle is a thin muscle originating on the dorsum of the foot, from the dorsal or superior aspect of the calcaneus, the interosseous talocalcaneal ligament, and a portion of the stem of the inferior extensor retinaculum. The origin of the muscle is just proximal and slightly lateral to one of the attachments of the bifurcate ligament. It attaches to the calcaneus at the lateral expanded edge of the tarsal canal. Thus, the origin of this muscle lies in close proximity to a number of soft tissue structures that support the intertarsal joints of the rear foot and major extrinsic tendons to the foot. The muscle divides distally into four distinct bellies that insert into the hallux and second, third, and fourth toes. There is no attachment to the fifth toe. The muscle serves as an extensor during foot function.

Mechanism of Injury

Norfray and associates have suggested that during forced inversion of the foot, as can occur during the common ankle sprain, the extensor digitorum brevis is rapidly stretched beyond its physiologic limits, resulting in a tear of the muscle at its origin, along with an avulsion fracture of the calcaneus.[106] We suggest that this may also occur with sudden relfex contracture of the muscle, along with other extrinsic musculature, in an attempt to halt aggressive inversion or supination movement of the foot and ankle in an acute ankle sprain injury. This injury most probably involves significant strain across the midfoot region and, in particular, the midtarsal and subtalar joints in the direction of the supination. This would be consistent with the injuries reported by Norfray and associates that involved slipping on ice, falling over snow-covered obstacles, falling off a porch, or twisting the foot and ankle on stairs.

Diagnosis

Physical examination reveals an acutely swollen foot and ankle at the lateral aspect just anterior and inferior to the lateral malleolus and adjacent to the sinus tarsi. A finding is that of a well-demarcated hematoma directly over the substance of the muscle itself (Fig. 26-37). This can be easily confirmed by direct observation and comparison with the contralateral extremity. The area of hematoma is the site of both maximum tenderness and swelling, which is not infrequently well demarcated from the surrounding tissues. The lateral collateral ligaments of the ankle and the fibula itself are surprisingly nontender to direct palpation. Active contracture of the muscle to even mild to moderate amounts of resistance is extremely painful. In some cases, we have found the patient unable to voluntarily contract the muscle because of severe pain. Surprisingly, to both the patient and treating physician, passive inversion of the subtalar joint and dorsiflexion or plantar flexion of the ankle joint produced much less pain and discomfort than anticipated. Clinical differentiation of this injury and fractures of the anterior beak or promontory of the calcaneus may be difficult. Midtarsal joint and motion and weight bearing of the affected extremity cause increased symptomatology in the latter injury.

With the passing of several days, one may observe the appearance of ecchymosis extending distally into the hallux and lesser toes along the course of the individual muscle bellies, making the diagnosis easier (Fig. 26-38). Multiple radiographic views are usually necessary to confirm the clinical suspicion of an avulsion fracture caused by this muscle.

The avulsion fracture caused by this muscle can usually be readily identified on a series of

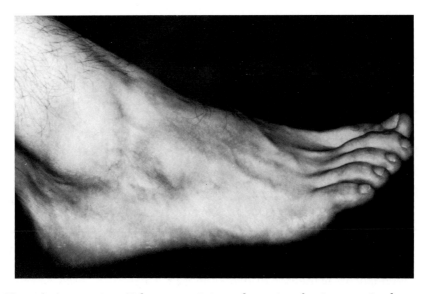

Fig. 26-37. Clinical presentation 48 hours postinjury of a patient having sustained an extensor digitorum brevis avulsion fracture. Note the well-demarcated hematoma and ecchymosis surrounding the extensor digitorum brevis muscle belly.

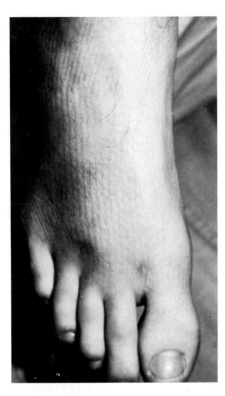

Fig. 26-38. Five days postinjury. Management with a Jones compression cast. Ecchymosis has proceeded along the course of the individualized tendons of the extensor digitorum brevis to the level of the digits.

foot and ankle radiographs. This avulsion fracture has a characteristic location on the dorsoplantar radiograph of the foot and anteroposterior radiograph of the ankle. Additional coned-down views may better delineate the small cortical fragments. Norfray and associates demonstrated the precise anatomic location of the extensor digitorum brevis muscle on a nonpreserved lower extremity amputation specimen by isolating its origin, covering it with a radiopaque substance, and visualizing the substance on a dorsoplantar view of the foot and anteroposterior view of the ankle.[106]

The anteroposterior view of the ankle usually demonstrates the fracture as a small cortical, somewhat linear, fragment well inferior to both the fibular malleolus and the lateral process of the talus (Fig. 26-39). Its distance from the tip of the fibular malleolus and presentation of a nor-

mal architecture of the fibula discourages the diagnosis of an avulsion fracture of the lateral collateral ligaments. The standard dorsoplantar view of the foot also demonstrates the fracture fragment along the lateral margins of the calcaneocuboid joint (Fig. 26-40). The larger the hematoma, the more easily visualized the fracture fragment owing to displacement of the avulsed cortical bone laterally away from the calcaneus. The hematoma itself will manifest as a well-demarcated increase in soft tissue volume and density inferior to and distal to the fibular malleolus (Fig. 26-41). We have found that a lateral oblique view of the foot (reverse oblique) may, on occasion, prove helpful in visualizing the avulsed cortical piece of bone displaced into the soft tissue structures (Fig. 26-42).

Other views of the ankle or foot are generally not beneficial in the diagnosis of this injury. Stress films and in-ankle arthrography, although useful in the diagnosis of ligamentous injuries of the sprained ankle, are not directly helpful in this injury, as this muscle is not related in an anatomic sense to the ankle joint proper. While specialized radiographic techniques such as CT, magnetic resonance imaging, and conventional bone scans may be helpful, their prohibitive costs preclude recommending their use on a routine basis.

The avulsion fracture may be confused with the accessory bones, secondary cuboid, secondary os calcis, and os peroneum; however, their contour and shape and ready visualization on multiple radiographic views helps distinguish these entities. An avulsion fracture of the calcaneofibular ligament, although presenting similarly on the anteroposterior view of the ankle, is not seen on the dorsoplantar view of the foot. The "nutcracker" fracture of the cuboid identified by the lateral, dorsoplantar, and medial oblique views of the foot has been well reported and will not be discussed here.[107]

Treatment

Treatment of the acute injury is generally conservative and consists of rest, ice, compression bandaging, and elevation. We frequently use a

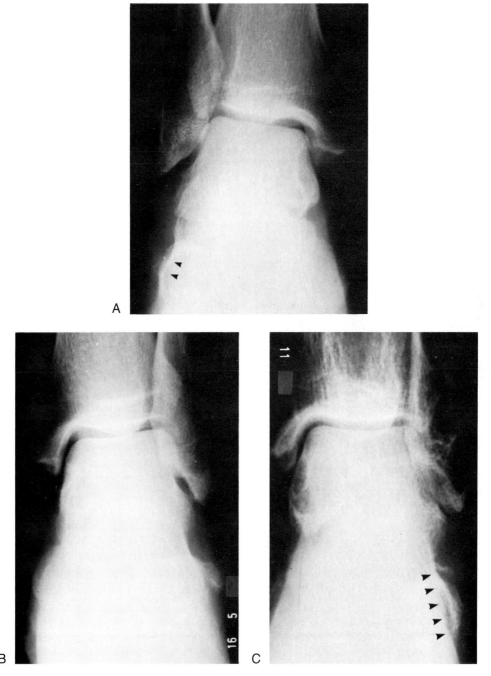

Fig. 26-39. (A) Anteroposterior view of the ankle showing a small avulsion of the extensor digitorum brevis (arrow) following an acute ankle sprain injury. Clinically, the ankle was unremarkable on physical examination. There was exquisite tenderness and an inability to actively contract the extensor digitorum brevis muscle. (B) Anteroposterior radiograph of an ankle showing a long-term follow-up of an individual who previously sustained an avulsion fracture of the extensor digitorum brevis. Notice the protuberance of bone that is now healed to the calcaneus. This fragment of bone caused irritation along the cutaneous nerves of the foot and subsequently required a surgical excision with remodeling of the calcaneocuboid joint. (C) Anteroposterior view of a left ankle demonstrating chronic changes about the ankle mortise as well as an old extensor digitorum brevis avulsion fracture injury (arrow). Most of the primary fragment has healed to the calcaneus. Note some small exostoses at the superior aspect of the avulsion fracture.

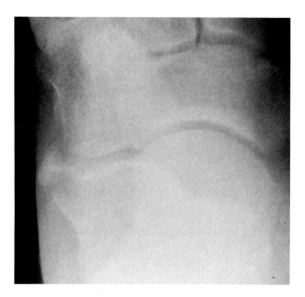

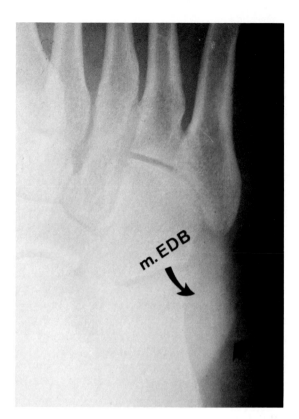

Fig. 26-40. Dorsoplantar view of the left foot demonstrating an extensive avulsion fracture of the extensor digitorum brevis with multiple smaller fragments. Clinically, the foot was exclusively tender to palpation and demonstrated ecchymosis in the area of the extensor digitorum brevis.

Fig. 26-41. Medial oblique radiograph of right foot demonstrating a large hematoma in conjunction with an injury to the extensor digitorum brevis muscle belly (arrow). Note the well-delineated margins of the hematoma.

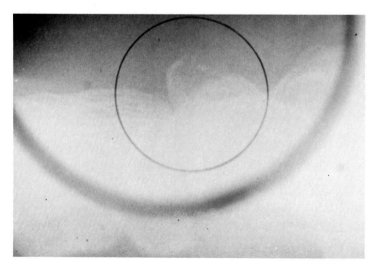

Fig. 26-42. Lateral oblique view of the right foot under magnification demonstrating a large avulsion fracture of the extensor digitorum brevis along with several smaller fracture fragments.

modified Jones compression dressing to control the edema and simultaneously immobilize the extremity for the first 24 to 72 hours. Evacuation of the hematoma to relieve pressure and local infiltration of a steroid, enzyme, and local anesthetic may prove helpful in controlling symptoms and disseminating the hematoma. Primary surgical repair of the torn origin with excision of the fracture fragment or fragments is rarely necessary. The limitation of weight bearing will be determined by the severity of the injury, the degree of symptomatology, and other concomitant injuries to the foot or ankle. In select cases, a short leg weight-bearing or non-weight-bearing cast may be required for 3 to 4 weeks. Within 5 weeks, most patients are able to return to near full activity with conventional shoegear. Follow-up radiographs not infrequently demonstrate resorption of the thin fracture fragments. Various physical therapy modalities, especially ultrasound, may prove helpful in the later stages to resolve symptoms. If pain persists, simple excision of the fracture fragments may be required at a later date. In such cases, one can expect to find significant atrophy and degenerative changes of the muscle itself during surgical exploration (Figs. 26-43 and 26-44). If left for a long time, the displaced fracture fragments may interfere with the movement of the tarsal joints and contribute to the formation of degenerative arthritis. In such cases, single or multiple joint arthrodesis may be required.

FIFTH METATARSAL BASE FRACTURES

Fractures involving the proximal aspect of the fifth metatarsal bone are quite common. They can be separated into two distinct fracture patterns: (1) a fracture of the tuberosity, and (2) a fracture of the proximal metatarsal shaft at the metaphyseal-diaphyseal interface. This latter group is known as the Jones fracture.

The mechanism of injury, choice of therapy, and prognosis depend on the accurate classification of these fractures. Although the direction of forces directed against the fifth metatarsal will vary, both the tuberosity fracture and the Jones fracture may result from inversion ankle injuries.

The base of the fifth metatarsal is projected laterally and posteriorly as the styloid process of tuberosity. The tendon of the peroneus brevis inserts here and expands to four times its diameter along the dorsolateral aspect of the base. Several other musculotendinous structures attach to the base. The flexor digiti minimi arises on the plantar surface and inserts into the fifth toe. The abductor digiti quinti arises from the plantar lateral tubercle of the calcaneus passing underneath the base, to which it is usually attached, and proceeds distally into the fifth toe. The tendon of the peroneus tertius inserts on the dorsolateral aspect of the metatarsal, just distal to the tuberosity, and is considerably less sturdy than that of the brevis. Dameon noted that only the peroneus brevis appeared strong enough to avulse a bone fragment (Fig. 26-45).[108]

The fifth metatarsal base is well secured to the adjacent cuboid and fourth metatarsal by both dorsal and plantar interosseous ligaments, making dislocation rare. This stability must be appreciated to understand the mechanisms of injury to the fifth metatarsal base and shaft.

There are several anatomic peculiarities associated with the base of the fifth metatarsal, the presence of which may be mistaken for a fracture. An anomalous epiphyseal plate located between the base and shaft has been noted,[108,109] but its incidence has never been recorded. More commonly, a secondary center of ossification, or apophysis, may be present. It has been reported as being seen in 22 percent of 164 feet[108] and in 26 percent of 1,000 foot radiographs.[66] The apophysis is most commonly visible between the ages of 9 and 16 years. The time of appearance to the time of ossification is usually under 2 years. It has not been reported as being present in children under the age of 8 years.[66,109]

The apophysis appears as a thin waferlike bone whose margins are sometimes scalloped, lying parallel or slightly oblique at the plantar lateral aspect of the styloid process (Fig. 26-46). It is often best visualized on a medial oblique foot radiograph. Pain and inflammation associated with the development of the apophysis was first described by Iselin.[66]

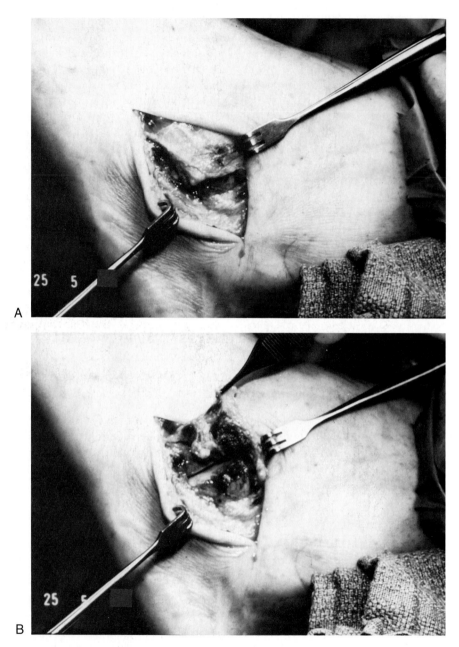

Fig. 26-43. **(A)** Surgical approach to exploration of the calcaneocuboid joint for persistent pain follow-ing an inversion sprain injury. Notice the atrophy present in the extensor digitorum brevis muscle belly, which has been incised in a reverse L fashion. **(B)** Dissection of the atrial thick extensor digitorum brevis muscle belly demonstrates several small cortical fragments of bone that failed to heal to the underlying calcaneus. Note the early degenerative arthritis present in the calcaneocuboid joint. This injury was caused by a sudden inversion ankle sprain injury.

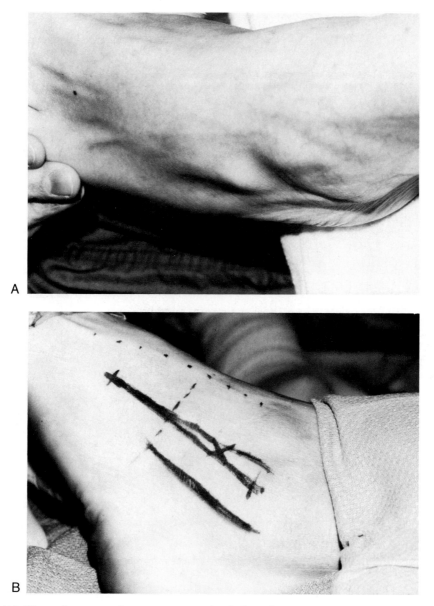

Fig. 26-44. **(A)** Clinical picture demonstrating a healed avulsion fracture of the extensor digitorum brevis of the lateral aspect of the left foot. This protuberance of bone was irritating the sural nerve and intermediate dorsal cutaneous nerve causing dysesthesias and paresthesias to the lesser digits. **(B)** Surgical incision planning for exploration of the area and remodeling of a malunion of a prior extensor digitorum brevis avulsion fracture. The inferior line represents the course of the sural nerve. The most superior line indicates the pathway of the intermediate medial dorsal cutaneous nerve. The longest line indicates the surgical incision with the X indicating the area of the sinus tarsi. (*Figure continues.*)

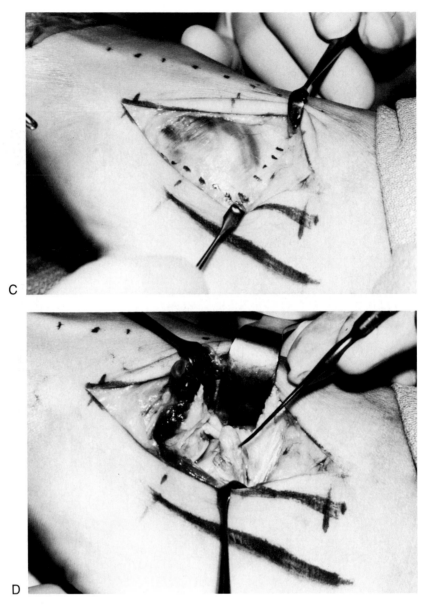

Fig. 26-44 (*Continued*). (**C**) Following incision and subcutaneous dissection, the deep fascia is preserved. Note the deep fascia preservation over the extensor digitorum brevis muscle belly. The extensor digitorum brevis muscle belly was then incised in a reverse **L** fashion and dissected superiorly and distally to expose the underlying malunited avulsion fracture. (**D**) Following reflection of the overlying extensor digitorum brevis muscle belly, a large malunited avulsion fracture was identified originating from the area of origin for this intrinsic muscle. Deep to this malunited fracture is the bifurcate ligament spanning the calcaneocuboid and calcaneonavicular joint complexes. Note preservation of the ligament structures of the sinus tarsi just proximal to the malunited fracture fragment. Significant degenerative arthritis of the calcaneocuboid joint was not evident. (*Figure continues.*)

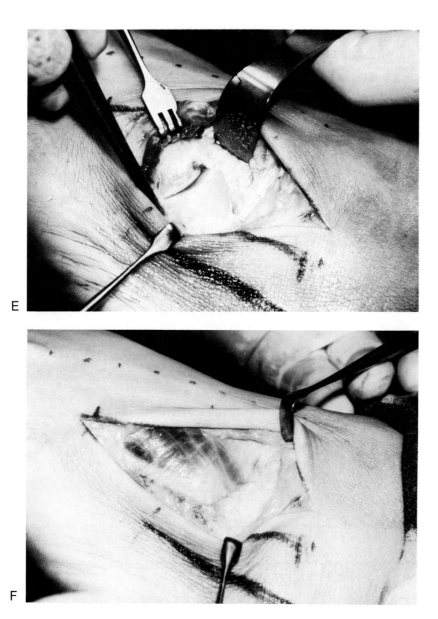

Fig. 26-44 (*Continued*). (**E**) Presentation of the joint complex following resection of the malunited fracture fragment and remodeling of the dorsal superior aspect of the calcaneus. The extensor digitorum brevis muscle belly was then replaced and sutured, and subcutaneous tissue and skin was closed in an anatomic manner. (**F**) Presentation following replacement of the extensor digitorum brevis muscle belly, which has been sutured along the original incisions. Note careful preservation of the overlying deep fascia at all times to minimize hematoma and postoperative swelling.

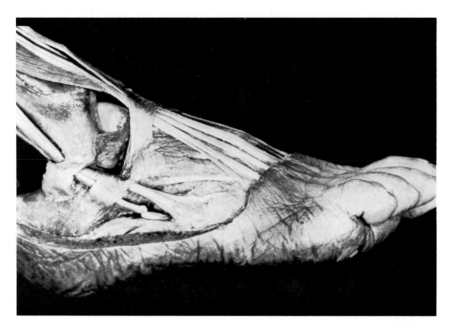

Fig. 26-45. Cadaveric dissection demonstrating the significant attachment of peroneus brevis to the fifth metatarsal.

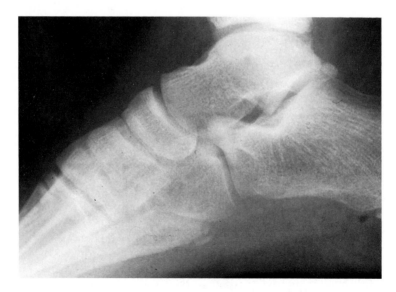

Fig. 26-46. Fifth metatarsal apophysis or os vesalianum pedis. Note the thin waferlike bone paralleling the metatarsal shaft.

Two accessory bones may be mistaken as fracture fragments, the os peroneum and os vesalianum pedis. The os peroneum is seen in approximately 15 percent of all adult feet.[66] It is a true sesamoid bone lying within the peroneus longus tendon, at the lateralmost aspect of the peroneal groove of the cuboid. The ossicle, usually smooth and round, may be bipartite. Careful examination of foot radiographs should easily exclude this sesamoid bone as a fractured base of the metatarsal (Fig. 26-47).

The os vesalianum pedis was first described in 1555 by Vesalius. Vesalius' initial description of the bone was contradictory, and since then the controversy has continued. Holland quotes Vesalius as saying "A small bone, opposite the outer side of the joint, and placed proximally to the little toe, and probably articulating with the cuboid."[110] A reproduction of the tracing from Vesalius demonstrates an apparent os peroneum on one view and a different ossicle on another view. For the os vesalianum pedis to be a true accessory bone three postulates must be met—that it is followed in the animal series, that it is present in the fetus, and that it is connected by hyaline cartilage with its supporting bone.[66] Based on this and the absence of the os vesalianum pedis in radiographs of adult feet, most believe that this bone does not exist but has been misidentified as a secondary epiphysis.[65,66,110]

The apophysis or os vesalianum pedis can be differentiated from a fracture fairly readily. The apophysis lies parallel to the styloid process, whereas a fracture is perpendicular to the metatarsal and usually involves the articulation with the cuboid or fourth metatarsal. Additionally, the apophysis is always plantar lateral, never near the cuboid or fourth metatarsal.

True fractures of the tuberosity are the result of either direct or indirect trauma. The most commonly described mechanism of injury is an indirect avulsion fracture by the peroneus brevis. While the individual is falling with the feet held in plantar flexion and inversion, the peroneals reflexively contract and avulse a portion of the tuberosity (Fig. 26-48). Occasionally the tuberosity may fracture by a direct blow, usually during a fall. The tuberosity, which can be quite large, is held so firmly in place that it lacks the ability to absorb shock and will break. This fracture pattern usually involves comminution. Although it is difficult to separate the exact mechanism by a patient's history, an avulsion fracture will produce only one fracture line, whereas direct injury may produce multiple fracture lines.

Displacement of the fracture fragment is rare owing to the strong ligamentous attachments, making open reduction unnecessary. In a review of 100 tuberosity fractures by Dameon, all but 1 healed, that becoming an asymptomatic nonun-

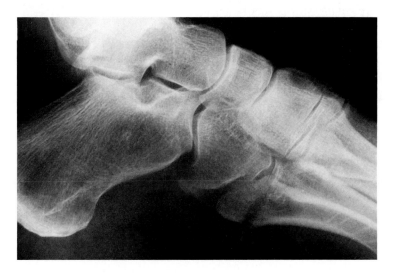

Fig. 26-47. The os peroneum can be seen clearly as a separate ossicle beneath the cuboid.

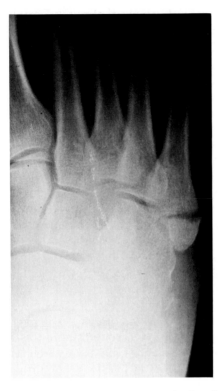

Fig. 26-48. Classic avulsion fracture. The break is perpendicular to the long axis of the metatarsal and proximal to the metaphyseal-diaphyseal juncture.

form of strenuous activity. Approximately 73 percent of all reported cases are the result of an acute injury. The remaining cases apparently arose as the result of a stress fracture (Fig. 26-49).[112,114,115]

Initial treatment by casting, strapping, or other forms of bandaging with partial weight bearing generally yield poor results, and when union does occur, refracture is likely. In 1984, Torg[113] and later Lehman et al.[117] developed a standardized classification system upon which treatment should be based. Type I fractures are acute with no previous history of pain and minimal cortical hypertrophy. These patients should all be treated with a short leg non-weight-bearing cast. Type II fractures include previous symptoms, a fracture line involving both cortices with periosteal bone elevation, and a widening of the fracture line with evidence of intramedullary sclerosis. This fracture may eventually heal if treated conserva-

ion.[108] Initial therapy with an elastic bandage or short leg cast produced the same results. All patients were clinically healed in 3 weeks and radiographically healed by 2 months. Dameon concluded that only symptomatic care was necessary. Anderson concurs, utilizing some form of immobilization with weight bearing.[111] Symptomatic nonunions are rarely if ever found with tuberosity fractures, no matter what the treatment rendered.

The Jones fracture occurs in the proximal diaphyseal region of the fifth metatarsal bone, approximately 1.5 cm distal to the flare at the base or 3 cm distal to the tuberosity. Previously reported cases have shown this to be a troublesome injury.[108,112–115] It differs from other metatarsal fractures in that it is slow to heal, predisposed to reinjury, and often leads to prolonged periods of disability. The typical patient is a young athletic male who injured his foot while engaged in some

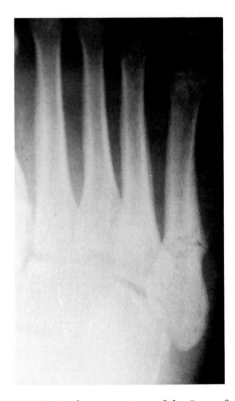

Fig. 26-49. Typical presentation of the Jones fracture. Note distal location and evidence of pre-existing stress fracture.

tively, but an active athlete would benefit most from surgical correction. Type III fractures were characterized by repeated trauma and symptoms, a wide fracture line, no periosteal bone, and complete obliteration of the medullary canal by sclerotic bone. Treatment is operative with curettage of the medullary canal and corticocancellous bone grafting.

Kavanaugh and colleagues extensively studied the mechanism of injury.[114] All patients were asked to detail specifically the position of their ankle and foot at the time of injury. Eleven of their patients underwent high-speed cinematography and force plate analysis, in which they mimicked the foot position at the time of injury. In not one case was inversion the mechanism of injury. The apparent inability of the foot to invert concentrates the vertical and mediolateral force over the fifth metatarsal base, resulting in fracture.

However, that mechanism of injury is diametrically opposed to the writings of Jones.[118] He believed that the history of injury was "sufficiently constant" to diagnose the injury. It is "caused by body pressure on an inverted foot while the heel is raised." He reported five cases, all involving inversion ankle trauma. These findings were recently confirmed by a retrospective review by Seitz of 53 patients with Jones fracture.[109] Thirty-nine patients clearly described an inversion injury, and 10 of 21 patients reviewed by Zelko related an inversion injury.[112] None of the patients observed by Seitz were athletic, and the average age was 35 years. No patient had prior symptoms, and all injuries were described as acute. Of the 36 patients who were observed, all were treated by casting with soft compressive dressings with weight bearing to tolerance. All patients healed without operative intervention. Average clinical healing time was 9.8 weeks, with only two people developing a delayed union.

These findings clearly separate proximal fractures of the fifth metatarsal into two categories. In the first category are those fractures occurring in a young athletic individual, showing evidence of stress fracture or of having prodromal symptoms. These patients are slow to heal and often require operative intervention. The second category includes those fractures that result from inversion ankle trauma and respond uniformly well to conservative care, a true Jones fracture.

ACKNOWLEDGMENTS

A special acknowledgment and expression of appreciation is extended to Pauli Jaffe, medical photographer of Meridia Huron Hospital, Cleveland, Ohio, for her generous efforts, expertise, and assistance with the medical photographs used in this chapter.

Special appreciation is also extended to Liz Amerson for her numerous hours in transcribing and editing this chapter.

REFERENCES

1. Lindholm TS, Osterman E: Osteochondritis dissecans of elbow, ankle, and hip: a comparison survey. Clin Orthop 148:245, 1980
2. Phemister DB: The cause and changes in loose bodies arising from the articular surface of the joint. J Bone Joint Surg 6:278, 1924
3. Konig F: Über Freie Korper in den Gelenken. Dtsch Z Chir 27:90, 1888
4. Kappis M: Weitere Beitrage zur Traumatisch-Mechanischen Entstehung der "Spontanen" Knorpelablosungen (Sogennante Osteochondritis Dissecans). Dtsch Z Chir 171:13, 1922
5. Rendu A: Fracture intra-articulaire parcellaire de la poulie astraglienne. Lyon Med 150:220, 1932
6. Berndt A, Harty M: Transchondral fractures (osteochondritis dissecans) of the talus. J Bone Joint Surg 41A:988, 1959
7. Arcomano JP, Kamhi E, Karas S, Moriarty VJ: Transchondral fracture and osteochondritis dissecans of the talus. NY State J Med 78:2183, 1978
8. Wagoner G, Cohn BNE: Osteochondritis dissecans. A resume of the theories of etiology and the consideration of heredity as an etiologic factor. Arch Surg 23:1, 1931
9. Gardiner TB: Osteochondritis dissecans in three members of one family. J Bone Joint Surg 37B:142, 1955
10. Pick MP: Familial osteochondritis dissecans. J Bone Joint Surg 37B:142, 1955

11. Hanley WB, McKusick VA, Barranco FT: Osteo-chondritis dissecans with associated malformation in two brothers. J Bone Joint Surg 49A:925, 1967

12. Flick AB, Gould N: Osteochondritis dissecans of the talus (transchondral fractures of the talus): a review of the literature and new surgical approach for medial dome lesions. Foot Ankle 5:165, 1985

13. Roden S, Tillegard P, Unander-Scharin L: Osteo-chondritis dissecans and similar lesions of the talus. Acta Orthop Scand 23:51, 1953

14. Naumetz VA, Schweigel JF: Osteocartilaginous lesions of the talar dome. J Trauma 20:924, 1980

15. Davidson AM, Steele HD, MacKenzie DA, Penny JA: A review of 21 cases of transchondral fracture of the talus. J Trauma 7:378, 1967

16. O'Donoghue DM: Chondral and osteochondral fractures. J Trauma 6:469, 1966

17. Canale T, Belding R: Osteochondral lesion of the talus. J Bone Joint Surg 62A:97, 1980

18. O'Farrell TA, Costello BG: Osteochondritis dissecans of the talus. J Bone Joint Surg 64B:494, 1982

19. Cavaliere RG: Talar fractures. p. 904. In McGlamry ED (ed): Comprehensive Textbook of Foot Surgery. Vol. 2. Williams & Wilkins, Baltimore, 1987

20. Thompson PJ, Loomer RL: Osteochondral lesions of the talus in a sports medicine clinic. A new radiographic technique and surgical approach. Am J Sports Med 12:460, 1984

21. Alexander A, Lichtman DM: Surgical treatment of transchondral talar dome fractures (osteochondritis dissecans). Long term followup. J Bone Joint Surg 62A:646, 1980

22. Blom JM, Strijk SP: Lesions of the trochlea tali. Osteochondral fractures and osteochondritis dissecans of the trochlear tali. Radiol Clin (Basel) 44:387, 1975

23. Newberg AH: Osteochondral fractures of the dome of the talus. Br J Radiol 52:105, 1979

24. Yvars MF: Osteochondral fractures of the dome of the talus. Clin Orthop 114:185, 1976

25. Cameron BM: Osteochondritis dissecans of the ankle joint. A report of a case simulating a fracture of the talus. J Bone Joint Surg 38A:857, 1956

26. Gould N: Technique tips. Foot Ankle 3:184, 1982

27. Burr RC: Osteochondritis dissecans. Can Med Assoc J 41:232, 1939

28. Kovesti JM, Jr: Management of fractures of the os calcis: a literature search. J Am Osteopath Assoc 75:94, 1975

29. Gage JR, Premer R: Os calcis fractures and analysis of 37. Minn Med 64:169, 1971

30. Jaekle RF, Clark AG: Fractures of the os calcis. Surg Gynecol Obstet 663, 1937

31. Essex-LoPresti P: The mechanism, reduction, technique, and result in fractures of the os calcis. Br J Surg 39:395, 1952

32. Wilson JN (ed): Watson-Jones Fractures and Joint Injuries. Vol. 2. 6th Ed. p. 1156. Churchill Livingstone, New York, 1982

33. McMinn RMH, Hutchings RT, Logan BM: A Color Atlas of Foot and Ankle Anatomy. Appleton-Century-Crofts, East Norwalk, CT, 1982

34. Sarrafian SK: Anatomy of the Feet and Ankle: Descriptive, Tomographic, Functional. JB Lippincott, Philadelphia, 1983

35. Grant JC: Grant's Altas of Anatomy. 6th Ed. Williams & Wilkins, Baltimore, 1972

36. Dachtler HW: Fractures of the anterior superior portion of the os calcis due to indirect violence. AJR 25:629, 1931

37. Christopher F: Fractures of the anterior process of the calcaneus. J Bone Joint Surg 13:877, 1931

38. Gellman M: Fractures of the anterior process of the calcaneus. J Bone Joint Surg 33A:382, 1951

39. Degan TJ, Morrey DF, Braun DP: Surgical excision of anterior process fractures of the calcaneus. J Bone Joint Surg 64A:519, 1982

40. Rowe CR, Sakellarides HT, Freeman PA, Sorbic C: Fractures of the os calcis—a long term follow-up study of 146 patients. JAMA 184:98, 1963

41. Green W: Fractures of the anterior superior beak of the os calcis. NY State J Med 56:3515, 1956

42. Backman F, Johnson SR: Torsion of the foot causing fracture of the anterior calcaneal process. Acta Chir Scand 105:460, 1953

43. Levine J, Kenin A, Spinner M: Nonunion of a fracture of the anterior superior process of the calcaneus. J Bone Joint Surg 41A:178, 1959

44. Jahss MH, Kay DS: An anatomic study of the anterior superior process of the os calcis and its clinical application. Foot Ankle 3:268, 1983

45. Piatt AD: Fracture of the promontory of the calcaneus. Radiology 67:386, 1956

46. Bradford CH, Larsen I: Sprain-fractures of the anterior lip of the os calcis. N Engl J Med 244:970, 1951

47. Carey EJ, Lance EM, Wade PA: Extra-articular fractures of the os calcis: a follow-up study. J Trauma 5:362, 1965

48. Rosendahl-Jensen S: Fractura calcanei: prognosis of an insurance material. Acta Chir Scand 112:69, 1956

49. Ahlberg A: Studien uber 111 Nacuntersuchte Falle von Calcaneusfrakturen. TR Elander, Goteborg, Jordborg, 1940

50. Hunt D: Compression fracture of the anterior articular surface of the calcaneus. J Bone Joint Surg 52A:1637, 1970

51. Kohler A, Zimmer EA: Borderlands of the Normal and Early Pathologic in Skeletal Roentgenology. 3rd Ed. Grune & Stratton, Orlando, FL, 1968

52. Giannestras MJ, Sammarco GJ: Fractures and dislocations in the foot. p. 1400. In Rockwood CA, Jr., Green DP (ed): Fractures. JB Lippincott, Philadelphia, 1975

53. Heim U, Pfeiffer KM: Small Fragment Set Manual. 2nd Ed. Springer-Verlag, New York, 1982

54. Rosenmuller JC: quoted in Holland CT = On Rarer ossifications seen during x-ray examinations. J Anat 55:235, 1921

55. O'Rahilly R: A survey of carpal and tarsal anomalies. J Bone Joint Surg 35A:626, 1953

56. Shepherd RJ: A hitherto undescribed fracture of the astragalus. J Anat Physiol 17:79, 1882

57. Turner W: A secondary astragalus in the human foot. J Anat Physiol 17:82, 1882

58. Ihle C, Cochren R: Fracture of the fused os trigonum. Am J Sports Med 10:47, 1982

59. Lapidus P: A note on the fracture of os trigonum. Report of a case. Ball Hosp Joint Dis 33:150, 1972

60. Moeller F: The os trigonum syndrome. J Am Podiatry Assoc 10:491, 1973

61. McDougall A: The os trigonum. J Bone Joint Surg 37B:257, 1955

62. Galinski A, Crovo, Ditmais J, Jr: Os trigonum as a cause of tarsal coalition. J Am Podiatry Assoc 69:191, 1979

63. Keith A: In Moullin C: Br Med J 1:16, 1901

64. Shands A: The accessory bones of the foot: an X-ray study of the feet of 1,054 patients. South Med Surg 93:326, 1931

65. Geist E: Supernumerary bones of the feet—a roentgen study of the feet of 100 normal individuals. Am J Orthop Surg 12:403, 1914

66. Burman M, Lapidus P: The functional disturbances caused by the inconstant bones and sesamoids of the feet. Arch Surg 22:936, 1931

67. Hamilton W: Stenosing tenosynovitis of the flexor hallucis longus tendon and posterior impingement upon the os trigonum in ballet dancers. Foot Ankle 3:74, 1982

68. Parkes James, II: Injuries of the hindfeet. Clin Orthop 122:28, 1977

69. Johnson R, Collier B, Carreara G: The os trigonum syndrome. Use of bone scan in the diagnosis. J Trauma 24:761, 1984

70. Havens R, Kaloogian H, Thul J, Hoffman S: A correlation between os trigonum syndrome and tarsel tunnel syndrome. J Am Podiatr Med Assoc 76:450, 1986

71. Ecker M, Rilter M: The symptomatic os trigonum. JAMA 201:204, 1967

72. Pennal G: Fractures of the talus. Clin Orthop 30:53, 1963

73. Sneppen O, Christensen S, Kragsoe O, Lorentzen J: Fractures of the body of the talus. Acta Orthop Scand 48:317, 1977

74. Fjeldborg O: Fracture of the lateral process of the talus. Acta Orthop Scand 39:407, 1968

75. Mukherjee SK, Pringle RM, Baxter AD: Fracture of the lateral process of the talus—a report of 13 cases. J Bone Joint Surg 56B:263, 1974

76. Hawkins LG: Fracture of the lateral process of the talus—a report of 13 cases. J Bone Joint Surg 47A:1170, 1965

77. Cummino CV: Fracture of the lateral process of the talus. AJR 90:1277, 1963

78. Marottoli OR: Sobre laf fracturas de la aposfisis externa del astragalo. Anal Chir 8:58, 1942. (Cited in current literature, J Bone Joint Surg 25:225, 1943.)

79. Klieger B: Fractures of the talus. J Bone Joint Surg 30A:735, 1948

80. Bonin JG: Injuries to the Ankle. Grune & Stratton, Orlando, FL, 1950

81. Milch H, Milch RA: Fracture Surgery. Paul B. Hoeber, New York, 1959

82. Dimon JH: Isolated fractures of the posterior facet of the talus. J Bone Joint Surg 43A:275, 1961

83. McGlamry ED (ed): Comprehensive Textbook of Foot Surgery. Vol. 2. Williams & Wilkins, Baltimore, 1987

84. Earle AS, Meritz JR: Dislocation of the peroneal tendons of the ankle. Northwest Med 71:108, 1972

85. Alm A, Lamke LO, Liljechohl SO: Surgical treatment of dislocation of the peroneal tendons. Injury 7:14, 1975

86. Beck E: Operative treatment of recurrent dislocation of the peroneal tendons. Arch Orthop Trauma Surg 98:247, 1980

87. Edwards ME: The relations of the peroneal tendons to the fibula, calcaneus and cuboid. Am J Anat 42:213, 1981

88. Muralt V (cited in Arch Orthop Trauma Surg 98:247, 1980)

89. Eckert WR, Lakes M, Davis EA: Acute rupture of

the peroneal retinaculum. J Bone Joint Surg 58A:670, 1976

90. Szczukowski M, St Pierre RK, Fleming LL, Somogyi J: Computerized tomography in the evaluation of peroneal tendon dislocation. Am J Sports Med 11:444, 1983

91. Stover CN, Bryan DR: Traumatic dislocation of the peroneal tendons. Am J Surg 103:180, 1962

92. Jones E: Operative treatment of chronic dislocation of the peroneal tendons. J Bone Joint Surg 14:574, 1932

93. Miller JW: Dislocation of peroneal tendons—a new operative procedure. Am J Orthop 9:136, 1967

94. Church CC: Radiographic diagnosis of acute peroneal tendon dislocation. AJR 129:1065, 1977

95. Murr S: Dislocation of the peroneal tendons with marginal fracture of the lateral malleolus. J Bone Joint Surg 43B:563, 1961

96. Watson-Jones R: Fractures and Joint Injuries. 5th Ed. Vol. 2. p. 1140. Churchill Livingstone Edinburgh, 1976

97. McLennan JG: Treatment of acute and chronic luxations of the peroneal tendons. Am J Sports Med 8:432, 1980

98. Sarmineto A, Wolf M: Subluxation of peroneal tendons. J Bone Joint Surg 57A:115, 1975

99. Escalas F, Figueras JM, Merino JA: Dislocation of the peroneal tendons. J Bone Joint Surg 62A:451, 1980

100. Zoellner G, Clancy W: Recurrent dislocation of the peroneal tendons. J Bone Joint Surg 61A:292, 1979

101. Kelly RE: An operation for the chronic dislocation of the peroneal tendons. Br J Surg 7:502, 1920

102. Thompson FR (cited in J Bone Joint Surg 61A:292, 1979)

103. Gurevitz SL: Surgical correction of subluxing peroneal tendons with a case report. J Am Podiatr Med Assoc 69:357, 1979

104. Hanson R: Operative treatment of a case of laxatio-habitualis tendon peroneal bilaterally. Acta Orthop Scand 1:1937

105. Anderson LD: Campbell's Orthopedics. Vol. 2. CV Mosby, St. Louis, 1971

106. Norfray JF, Rogers LF, Adama GP et al: Common calcaneal avulsion fracture. AJR 134:119, 1980

107. Hermel MB, Cohen G: The nutcracker fracture of the cuboid by indirect violence. Radiology 60:850, 1953

108. Dameon TB: Fractures and anatomical variations of the proximal portion of the fifth metatarsal. J Bone Joint Surg 57A:788, 1975

109. Seitz WH, Jr: The Jones' fracture in the non-athlete. Foot Ankle 6:97, 1985

110. Holland CT: On rarer ossifications seen during X-ray examination. J Anat 55:235, 1921

111. Anderson LD: Injuries of the forefoot. Clin Orthop 122:18, 1977

112. Zelko RR, Torg JS, Rachan A: Proximal diaphyseal fractures of the fifth metatarsal—treatment of the fractures and their complications in athletes. Am J Sports Med 7:95, 1979

113. Torg JS, Balduini FC, Zelko RR et al: Fractures of the base of the fifth metatarsal distal to the tuberosity. J Bone Joint Surg 66A:209, 1984

114. Kavanaugh JH, Brower TD, Mann RV: The Jones fracture revisited. J Bone Joint Surg 60A:776, 1978

115. Delee JC, Evans JP, Julian J: Stress fracture of the fifth metatarsal. Am J Sports Med 11:349, 1983

116. Arangio GA: Proximal diaphyseal fractures of the fifth metatarsal (Jones fracture)—two cases treated by cross-pinning with review of 106 cases. Foot Ankle 3:293, 1983

117. Lehman RC, Torg JS, Pavlov H, Delee JC: Fractures of the base of the fifth metatarsal distal to the tuberosity, a review. Foot Ankle 7:245, 1987

118. Jones R: Fracture of the base of the fifth metatarsal bone by indirect violence. Am Surg 35:697, 1902

SUGGESTED READINGS

Clisham MW, Berlin SJ: The diagnosis and conservative treatment of the calcaneal fractures: a review. J Foot Surg 20:28, 1981

Jahss MH (ed): Disorders of the Foot. Vol. 2. WB Saunders, Philadelphia, 1982

Kalish SR: The conservative and surgical treatment of calcaneal fractures. J Am Podiatry Assoc 65:912, 1975

Mann RA (ed): Surgery of the Foot. 5th Ed. CV Mosby, St. Louis, 1986

McGlamry ED (ed): Comprehensive Textbook of Foot Surgery. Vol. 2. Williams & Wilkins, Baltimore, 1987

Parkes JC: Injuries of the hindfoot. Clin Orthop 122:28, 1977

Perlman M et al: Inversion lateral ankle trauma: differential diagnosis, review of the literature, and prospective study. J Foot Surg 26:102, 1987

Rynn M, Fazekas EA, Hecker RL: Osteochondral lesions of the talus. J Foot Surg 22:155, 1983

Spatt JF, Frank NG, Fox IM: Transchondral fractures of the dome of the talus. J Foot Surg 25:68, 1986

Trepal MJ, Cangiano SA, Anarella JJ: Transchondral fractures of the talar dome. J Foot Surg 25:369, 1986

Wells D, Oloff-Solomon: Radiographic evaluation of transchondral dome fractures of the talus. J Foot Surg 26:186, 1987

Wisotsky L: Compression fracture of the anterior articular surface of the calcaneus associated with avulsion fracture of the tuberosity of the navicular. Arch Podiatr Med Foot Surg 4:3, 1977

Wu K: Surgery of the Foot. Lea & Febiger, Philadelphia, 1986

27

Acute Soft Tissue Trauma of the Ankle

Joshua Gerbert, D.P.M.
Albert Burns, D.P.M.

This chapter describes the evaluation, diagnosis, and management of acute soft tissue injuries of the ankle. Deltoid ligament ruptures and lateral collateral ligament distortions or ruptures are described. The focus is primarily on a practical clinical approach to these problems and methods that we have found to provide satisfactory results during the past 10 years at the California College of Podiatric Medicine. The pertinent anatomic structures and literature reviewed are presented within each specific injury section.

DELTOID LIGAMENT RUPTURES

Anatomy

The deltoid or medial collateral ligament is a large, broad, and strong structure that has superficial and deep layers.[1-3] The deltoid originates from the medial malleolus, which ends structurally in two colliculi, one anterior and one posterior, which are divided by an intercollicular groove.[1,2] The superficial layer of the deltoid originates from the anterior colliculus and is divided into three separate ligaments (Fig. 27-1). The three superficial bands blend into one broad structure, and all three originate from the anterior colliculus. The naviculotibial ligament in-

serts into the navicular and the spring ligament; the calcaneotibial ligament inserts into the medial surface of the sustentaculum tali; and the superficial talotibial ligament inserts into the medial tubercle of the posterior process of the talus. The calcaneotibial ligament is the strongest band, and its fanlike shape gave the deltoid its name.

The deep layer of the deltoid ligament consists of two bands that originate from the posterior colliculus and intercollicular groove (Fig. 27-2). The two bands are the deep anterior talotibial ligament, which inserts into the medial surface of the neck of the talus, and the deep posterior talotibial ligament, which inserts into the medial tubercle of the posterior process of the talus.[1]

Mechanism of Injury, Signs, and Symptoms

Injury to the deltoid ligament is rarely solitary and is usually accompanied by other ligament injuries or fractures.[2-4] The most common associated injuries are fractures of the fibula and ruptures of the tibiofibular ligaments. The force applied to the foot to cause this injury is an external rotation or an abductory, everting, or pronatory force.[2,4,5] The deltoid may be found ruptured, therefore, in a supination-external

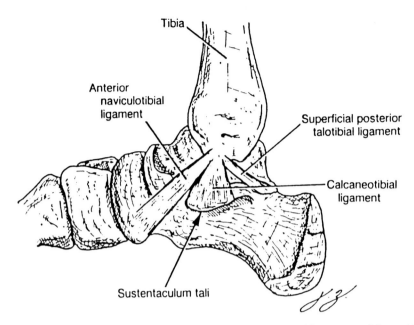

Fig. 27-1. Superficial parts of the medial collateral ligament or deltoid ligament of the ankle joint. Note the anterior naviculotibial ligament, the calcaneotibial ligament, and the (superficial) posterior talotibial ligament. (From Draves,[1] with permission.)

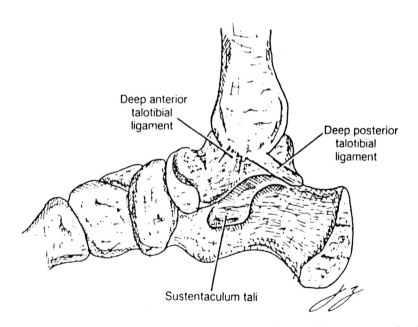

Fig. 27-2. Arthology of the deep parts of the deltoid ligament of the ankle joint. Note the deep anterior talotibial ligament and the deep posterior talotibial ligament. The deep posterior talotibial ligament is the major part of the medial collateral ligament that attaches to the intercollicular groove and the posterior colliculus of the medial malleolus. (From Draves,[1] with permission.)

rotation, pronation-external rotation, or pronation-abduction injury of the ankle.[4] For an isolated rupture of the deltoid ligament to occur, an initial pronation or abduction of the foot would have to occur.

Rupture of the deltoid will cause pain and swelling on the medial and anterior aspects of the ankle.[2-4] Tenderness will be present on palpation of the ligament, and a palpable defect may pinpoint which ligaments are involved.[6]

A rupture of the deltoid ligament is usually associated with other injuries. Because of this, the usual presentation is that of a completely edematous and ecchymotic ankle that is being splinted by surrounding musculature. Any injured ankle should, therefore, be evaluated for possible rupture of the deltoid ligament.

Diagnosis

With any ankle injury, scout radiographs should be obtained to rule out possible fractures. These would include anteroposterior, lateral, and mortise views of the ankle, taken weight bearing if possible. In children in whom you anticipate open epiphyses, the scout films should be taken bilateral to allow for comparison. In pronation injuries one should also take a high fibula view. In evaluating these scout radiographs not only does one look for fractures but also for increased joint space or clear space between the medial aspect of the talar body and the lateral or internal surface of the medial malleolus. In the mortise view one can best evaluate the clear space[2,3,5,6] as shown in Figure 27-3.

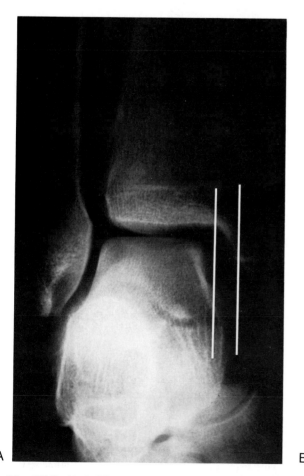 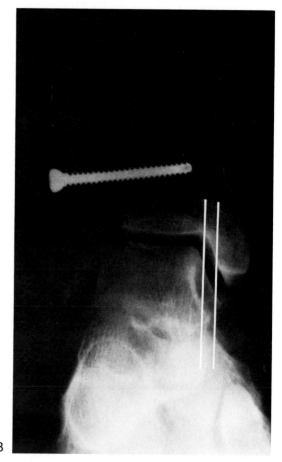

A   B

Fig. 27-3. (A & B) In a mortise view of the ankle, the distance between the medial malleolus and the talus is measured. Displacement of 3 mm or more demonstrates a tear of the deltoid ligament, and a clear space of 1 cm or more indicates a complete rupture of the deltoid ligament.

Close in 1956 demonstrated that unless the deltoid ligament was ruptured, lateral displacement of the talus in relation to the tibia would not excess 2 mm, even if all the tibiofibular ligaments were ruptured.[7] A clear space of 1 cm or greater is diagnostic of a complete rupture of the deltoid ligament. There have been attempts to correlate the millimeters of clear space with specific tears of the ligaments of the deltoid; however, the only consistent finding is that displacement or a clear space of 3 mm or more indicates a tear of part of the deltoid ligament.

For more accurate assessment of the integrity of the deltoid ligament one can perform an eversion stress maneuver provided that there were no fractures present.[3,4,6] As with stress films taken for inversion injuries, the ankle needs to be anesthetized. The stress film can either be performed manually as described for the inversion stress maneuver or by using the Telos apparatus. This test must be performed bilaterally in order to compare the talar tilt between the injured and the uninjured ankle. Due to the rarity of this isolated injury, there are no specific millimeters of talar tilt, as there are for the inversion stress maneuver, to indicate a rupture. However, it has been our experience that between the clinical signs and symptoms and the comparison stress views a diagnosis of deltoid rupture can easily be made as seen in Figure 27-4.

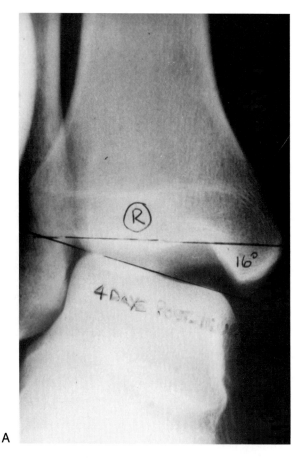
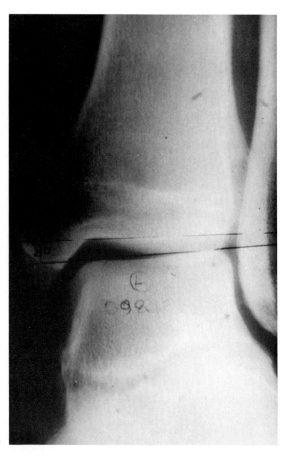

A   B

Fig. 27-4. (A & B) Eversion stress radiographs of suspected deltoid ligament rupture are taken bilaterally, and the angulation between the tibial plafond and talar dome is compared. This is done when routine radiographs are equivocal for the injury. These eversion stress radiographs show a marked difference on the injured right ankle and give a definitive diagnosis.

Treatment

Traditional treatment of the ruptured deltoid ligament has consisted of closed reduction and external casting.[3,5] Experience has shown that meticulous replacement of the deltoid ligament does not appear to be essential, and in most instances involving fibular fractures, the ruptured deltoid did not need to be repaired if the lateral side was anatomically and rigidly fixed.[3,5] Surgical repair of the deltoid ligament is clearly indicated if closed reduction does not replace the talus to its proper position. This could occur if the deltoid rolled up or inverted or if the posterior tibial tendon became trapped.[4] If there are concomitant fractures, the casting regimen would be dictated by the requirements of the specific fracture (see Chap. 28). After successful closed reduction or operative repair of the ruptured deltoid ligament, the patient is placed in a non-weight-bearing below-the-knee cast for 3 to 6 weeks. This is followed by a weight-bearing below-the-knee cast for another 3 to 6 weeks. The total casting regimen should range from 6 to 12 weeks, depending on the individual extent of injury, disruption, or fracture. This is followed by extensive rehabilitation with ankle range of motion and muscle-strengthening exercises.

LATERAL COLLATERAL LIGAMENT DISTORTION OR RUPTURE

Anatomy

The lateral collateral ligaments are composed of three small distinct ligaments that do not reinforce each other, as do the medial ankle ligaments. The anterior talofibular ligament is triangular or fan-shaped, intracapsular, and, among the three ligaments, considered to be the primary stabilizer of the ankle.[8] The calcaneofibular ligament is rather narrow and cordlike, lying outside the capsule, just beneath the peroneal tendon sheath. The third ligament that forms the lateral collateral arrangement and the rarest to be injured is the posterior talofibular ligament. This is thicker and stronger than the other two ligaments and is intracapsular.[1,9]

Mechanism of Injury, Signs, and Symptoms

The most common mechanism of injury is inversion and plantar flexion of the foot relative to the ankle, which will distort or rupture the anterior talofibular ligament. If the inversion portion if severe enough, the calcaneofibular ligament may also be damaged. Rarely, with only a true inversion maneuver, the calcaneofibular ligament may be singularly distorted or ruptured. Depending on the severity of the forces producing the injury, the time span since injury, and the initial self-treatment, one may encounter a variety of signs and symptoms. Usually the pain and the inability to place weight on the injured ankle will cause the patient to seek medical care. It has been our experience that the extent of edema or ecchymosis does not serve as a good indicator of the extent of ligamentous damage.

Diagnosis

After a careful history of the injury is obtained and a clinical examination of the foot and lower leg is performed, standard radiographs should be taken (see Chap. 26) to rule out osseous damage. When performing the clinical examination, one should begin palpation away from the most likely ligamentous injury and gradually work toward it. Palpation should begin with the head and neck of the fibula and progress distally. One must not forget to palpate the anterior aspect of the ankle joint for possible diastasis and the medial aspect for possible deltoid ligament or medial malleolar damage. Palpation of the foot should include the metatarsals, the anterosuperior process of the calcaneus, and the posterolateral tubercle of the talus, all of which can be fractured with an inversion ankle injury.

Once any osseous damage has been eliminated, the physician has an obligation in most cases to continue the evaluation to determine whether the lateral ligaments are intact. In patients who have a history of chronic lateral ankle instability or who live a very sedentary lifestyle, owing to age or medical condition, the need for additional evaluation may not be necessary.

If the evaluation is to continue, we recommend that stress views of the ankle be obtained as the next step in the diagnostic process. This would consist of an inversion stress test and a push-pull stress test, which must be performed bilaterally. The injured ankle must be adequately anesthetized prior to performing these maneuvers to prevent the peroneal tendons from going into spasm during the procedure, thereby invalidating the stress tests. A common peroneal nerve block and local ankle infiltration at the site of maximum tenderness generally offers appropriate anesthesia.

The use of Telos equipment for taking stress views has permitted better quality control, more reliable data on a reproducible basis, and greatly reduced radiation exposure to the examiner (Fig. 27-5).[10] One can also easily perform the necessary stress maneuvers manually; however, proper protective shielding must be worn by the examiner. When performing the inversion stress test manually, it is important to grasp the heel and invert the foot to maximize the force at the ankle. A standard anteroposterior ankle radiograph is taken and the degree of talar tilt is determined as shown in Fig. 27-6. A 5 to 6 degree difference between the injured and uninjured ankle generally signifies ligamentous rupture. In our experience, the extact degree of talar tilt is not a true indication of which ligament is ruptured.

The push-pull stress test (Fig. 27-7) or the anterior drawer sign specifically evaluates the integrity of the anterior talofibular ligament. The evaluation of this test is demonstrated in Fig. 27-8.

In the following situations, one cannot use stress tests to evaluate the integrity of the ligaments: genetic ligamentous laxity; history of chronic ankle instability of the uninjured ankle; inability to achieve adequate anesthesia of the injured ankle; and inability to properly maneuver the uninjured ankle for a valid stress test. In

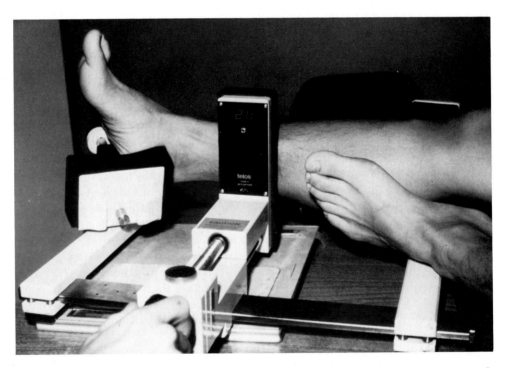

Fig. 27-5. The Telos apparatus as used to perform the inversion stress test. It is necessary to place the pad that holds the heel in such a way that it internally rotates the leg. There is a stationary pad positioned laterally on the upper leg, and the pressure pad is positioned just above the medial malleolus. Pressure is applied to 20 units, and this forcibly inverts the foot.

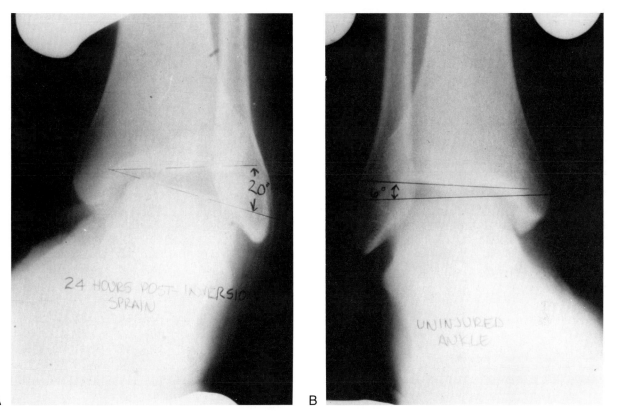

Fig. 27-6. Comparison of (**A**) injured and (**B**) uninjured ankles subjected to stress. A difference of greater than 5 degrees between ankles is definitive for a tear of the lateral collateral ligaments.

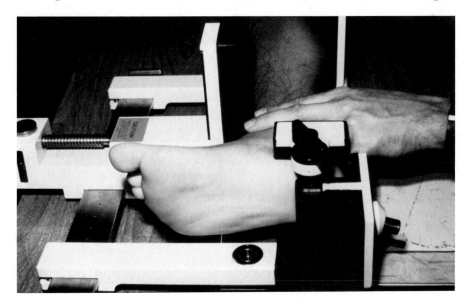

Fig. 27-7. Push-pull stress test as demonstrated on Telos equipment. The leg is placed with the lateral side down on the apparatus, so that the heel is secured in the pad and the stationary pad is posterior to the upper leg. The pressure pad is placed anteriorly just above the level of the ankle joint and advanced to a pressure of 20 units.

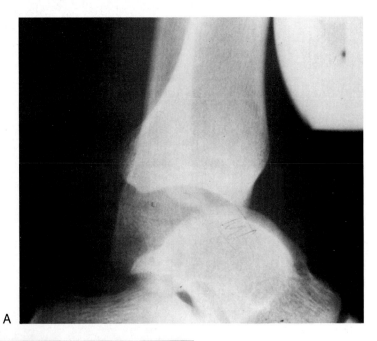

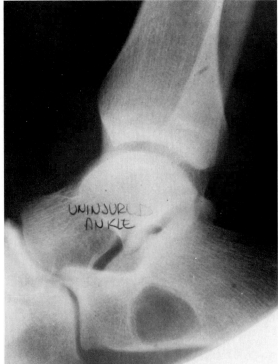

Fig. 27-8. Comparison between the (**A**) injured and (**B**) uninjured ankles that were stressed for anterior displacement. This specifically evaluates the integrity of the anterior talofibular ligament, and if it is intact there should be no displacement of the talus anteriorly out of the ankle mortise. This is a subjective evaluation based simply on whether there is displacement.

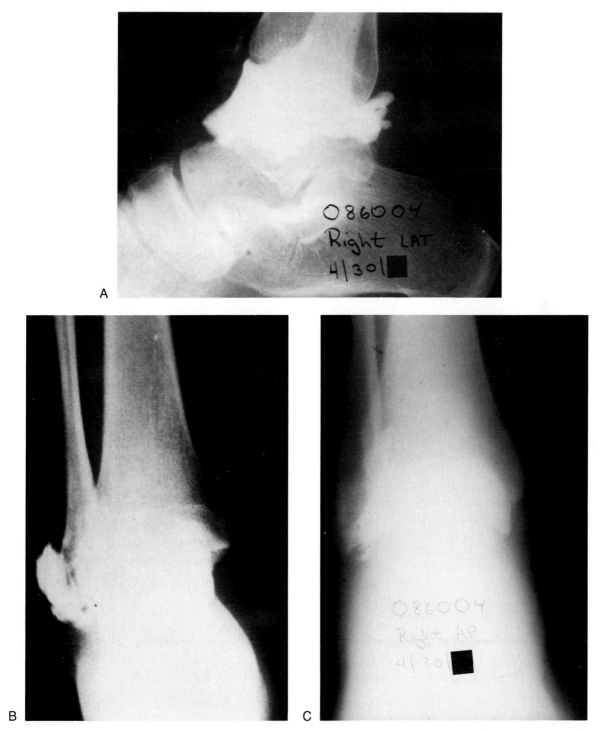

Fig. 27-9. Arthrography of the ankle. **(A)** Dye within the normal confines of the ankle joint, showing a stretched anterior capsule and pouching of the posterior capsule because the foot is plantar flexed. **(B)** Dye shown escaping to the lateral side of the lateral malleolus, which is definitive for a tear of the lateral collateral ligaments. For the anatomic variant in which the peroneal tendon sheath is connected with the ankle joint, dye would appear behind the lateral malleolus, not lateral to it. **(C)** Dye shown passing superiorly through the syndesmosis of the ankle, which is definitive for a diastasis.

these rare circumstances, arthrography of the ankle would be the next diagnostic test. In our experience, the main indication for ankle joint arthrography in a soft tissue ankle injury is to evaluate for a possible ankle diastasis.[11]

In performing ankle joint arthrography to evaluate the collateral ligaments, one must consider the following. (1) The patient must have no allergy to iodine. (2) The injection should be administered at the anteromedial aspect of the ankle. This will prevent any confusion in interpreting the radiograph if dye was injected into the soft tissue during administration. (3) The test must be performed within the first 5 to 7 days following the injury. This is necessary because the synovial tissue of the capsule heals very rapidly and could prevent any dye from leaking out even though there was a tear in the capsule and the ligament had been ruptured. (4) Dye that is found within the normal anatomic confines of adjacent tendon sheaths and not within the surrounding soft tissue should be considered a normal anatomic variant (Fig. 27-9).[12,13]

Peroneal tenography is also a diagnostic technique advocated by some for specifically evaluating the integrity of the calcaneofibular ligament. However in using this technique, one must remember that for some patients there is a normal connection between the peroneal tendon sheath and the ankle joint capsule. Therefore, if the dye injected into the peroneal sheath is seen in the ankle joint but there is no dye seen in the soft tissue surrounding the ankle, one should interpret this as a negative test. We normally utilize this test when evaluating the peroneal tendon sheath for a possible stenosis or distortion of the tendon itself.[14,15]

In the future the use of MRI without any invasive technique may provide more definitive information on the integrity of the ligaments.

Treatment

Treatment for a patient who has sustained a lateral collateral ligament distortion (sprain) or a true rupture depends on several factors. We manage this acute problem in one of the following ways.

Symptomatic Therapy

Symptomatic therapy treats the immediate signs and symptoms, supports the patient, and mobilizes the ankle joint as quickly as possible. The therapy includes elastic compression of the ankle, ice compresses, analgesics, weight bearing to tolerance, and physical therapy as needed. Full activity is permitted as soon as local signs and symptoms subside. We utilize this form of therapy in the following situations.

1. Patients with negative stress radiographs or negative ankle arthrogram.
2. Patients with a history of chronic ankle instability who will be evaluated at a later date for a possible stabilization procedure.
3. Patients with a significant medical history that contraindicates more definitive treatment.
4. Geriatric patients who lead a sedentary lifestyle or in whom prolonged disability would be detrimental.
5. Patients who present for treatment 3 or more weeks following the traumatic episode.

These patients should be forewarned that the treatment is aimed only at relieving the signs and symptoms and that the ankle will still be prone to some instability if, in fact, a ligament was ruptured.

Definitive Therapy

In reviewing the literature, one finds many articles proposing either primary operative repair or plaster-type immobilization for patients with ruptured collateral ligaments. Ruth in 1961 found 90 percent success using surgical treatment versus 66 percent following immobilization.[16] Freeman in 1965 found only 25 percent success following surgery versus 53 percent success postimmobilization.[17] Brostrom in 1966 found 91 percent success following surgery versus 79 percent success after immobilization.[18] Staples in 1972 found 88 percent success following surgery versus 58 percent following plaster casting.[19] Chirls in 1973 treated 200 patients with plaster immobilization and had an 88 percent success rate.[20] Hansen in 1979 treated 144 patients with plaster casting and found a 70 percent success rate.[21] Niedermann in 1981 treated 102 patients surgically with an 80 percent success rate and

107 patients by casting with a 76 percent success rate.[22] Evans in 1984 treated 50 patients with surgical repair and 50 patients with cast immobilization and found that after a 2-year follow-up, instability occurred three times more often in the operative patient.[23] In our on-going study, we are finding no significant difference between primary repair and immobilization. Therefore, knowing that a surgical repair carries the risk of potential anesthetic complications, difficulties in wound healing, and infection, we elect to utilize immobilization therapy as our definitive therapy of choice in the majority of cases.

Immobilization Treatment

Initially, the patient's ankle is immobilized in a compression-type bandage to eliminate the edema. Then, within approximately 48 hours following the injury, a below-the-knee weight-bearing cast is applied. This can be in the form of a traditional plaster cast or, with a compliant patient, a removable synthetic cast. The length of casting varies from 3 to 6 weeks. With the compliant patient, the cast can be removed at 3 weeks followed by the use of an inflatable cast-type splint for an additional 3 weeks. For those patients who are very active, we utilize the inflatable cast-type splint for at least 6 to 9 weeks following the removal of the original cast-type immobilization. If stress radiographs were used to diagnose the rupture, then they should be repeated 3 to 6 months postinjury to determine the effectiveness of the treatment. Physical therapy modalities are used as needed to assist the patient in regaining full use of the ankle joint.

Surgical Treatment

The patients we select for surgery are young and very athletic and in need of complete ankle stability. Initially, the patient's ankle is immobilized in a compression-type bandage to reduce the edema. This has in some cases required hospitalization to maintain the optimum skin conditions for an operative procedure. Normally surgery will occur 2 to 3 days following the traumatic episode. However, we have on several occasions performed the procedure 6 to 12 months after the trauma and obtained good results. This is called delayed primary repair and may create another category for operative repair. For those patients who seek medical care 3 or more weeks after the injury and in whom one can demonstrate a ligamentous rupture with stress radiographs, this may offer an alternative therapy.

The torn ligaments and capsule are repaired with 2-0 nonabsorbable suture, and the ankle is then wrapped in compression bandages. Postoperative management is the same as described for the immobilization technique. In a delayed primary repair, the capsule has healed but appears loose. A section is removed in the area of the anterior talofibular ligament, and even if the ligament cannot be identified, the area is closed with 2-0 nonabsorbable suture. This tightens the area and enables scarring and contraction to provide the necessary stability. Once again, management is that described for the immobilization technique.

REFERENCES

1. Draves DJ: Anatomy of the Lower Extremity. Williams & Wilkins, Baltimore, 1986
2. Pankovich AM, Shivaram MS: Anatomical basis of variability in injuries of the medial malleolus and the deltoid ligament. Acta Orthop Scand 50:225, 1979
3. Staples OS: Injuries to the medial ligaments of the ankle. J Bone Joint Surg 42A:1287, 1960
4. Staples OS: Ligamentous injuries of the ankle joint. Clin Orthop 42:21, 1965
5. Souza LJ, Gustilo RB, Meyer TJ: Results of operative treatment of displaced external rotation-abduction fractures of the ankle. J Bone Joint Surg 67A:1066, 1985
6. Cox JS: Surgical and nonsurgical treatment of acute ankle sprains. Clin Orthop 198:118, 1985
7. Close JR: Some applications of the functional anatomy of the ankle joint. J Bone Joint Surg 38A:761, 1956
8. Johnson EE, Marklof KL: Contribution of the anterior talofibular ligament to ankle laxity. J Bone Joint Surg 65A:81, 1983
9. Sarrafian SK: Anatomy of the Foot and Ankle. JB Lippincott, Philadelphia, 1983
10. Christensen J, Dockery G, Schuberth J: Evalua-

tion of ankle ligamentous insufficiency using the Telos ankle stress apparatus. J Am Podiatr Med Assoc 76:527, 1986

11. Gordon R: Arthrography of the ankle joint. J Bone Joint Surg 52:1623, 1970

12. Brostrom L: Sprained ankles. II: Arthrographic diagnosis of recent ligament ruptures. Acta Surg Scand 129:485, 1965

13. Fulp M: Arthrography of the ankle. J Am Podiatry Assoc 63:502, 1973

14. Evans G, Frenyo S: The stress tenogram in the diagnosis of ruptures of the lateral ligament of the ankle. J Bone Joint Surg 61B:347, 1979

15. Teng M, Destouet J, Gilula L et al: Ankle tenography: a key to unexplained symptomatology. Part I: Normal tenographic anatomy. Radiology 151:574, 1984

16. Ruth CJ: The surgical treatment of injuries of the fibular collateral ligaments of the ankle. J Bone Joint Surg 43A:229, 1961

17. Freeman MAR: Treatment of ruptures of the lateral ligament of the ankle. J Bone Joint Surg 47B:661, 1965

18. Brostrom L: Sprained ankles. V: treatment and prognosis in recent ligament ruptures. Acta Chir Scand 132:537, 1966

19. Staples OS: Result study of ruptures of lateral ligaments of the ankle. Clin Orthop 85:50, 1972

20. Chirls M: Inversion injuries of the ankle. J Med Soc NJ 70:751, 1973

21. Hansen H, Damholt V, Termansen NB: Clinical and social status following injury to the lateral ligaments of the ankle. Acta Orthop Scand 50:699, 1979

22. Niedermann B et al: Rupture of the lateral ligaments of the ankle: operation or plaster cast? Acta Orthop Scand 52:579, 1981

23. Evans GA, Hardcastle P, Frenyo AD: Acute rupture of the lateral ligament of the ankle. J Bone Joint Surg 66B:209, 1984

28

Ankle Fractures*

George Gumann, D.P.M.

Ankle fractures have been described by numerous articles detailing their classification and treatment. There has been a gradual shift from conservative to the more aggressive operative treatment of these fractures. However, the treatment of ankle fractures still elicits enlightened debate.

ANATOMY

The ankle joint is a mortise in which the talus is constrained by the fibula laterally and the tibia both superiorly and medially. This configuration has also been referred to as the malleolar fork.[1] The distal aspect of the tibia flares and is quadrilateral in cross section, terminating in an articular surface. This articular surface faces not only inferiorly but also anteriorly about 15 to 20 degrees. This region of the tibia is known as the plafond. The anterior aspect of the plafond is wider than the posterior aspect. The posterolateral prominence is the posterior malleolus, also known as the third malleolus[2] or Volkmann's process.[3] The posterior aspect of the distal tibia is located more inferiorly than the anterior aspect. The anterolateral portion of the tibia extends more laterally than the posterolateral portion and is known as the tubercle of Tillaux-Chaput. Between the tubercle of Tillaux-Chaput and the posterior malleolus on the lateral aspect of the tibia is the fibular notch or fibular incisura. This is for the distal articulation between the tibia and the fibula, which is also referred to as the syndesmosis. There is actually an articular facet on the inferior aspect of the fibular notch. Medially, the tibia extends distally as the medial malleolus. The medial malleolus is divided into the anterior and posterior colliculi. They are divided on the lateral surface by the intercollicular groove. This lateral surface also contains a cartilaginous facet for articulating with the medial aspect of the talus. The anterior colliculus extends more distally. The posterior tibial tendon courses in a groove along the posterior aspect of the posterior colliculus.[1,4]

The distal fibula becomes triangular in cross section and is known as the lateral malleolus. There is a triangular facet that has its apex inferiorly, located on the medial surface, which articulates with the lateral surface of the talus. Posterior to this facet is the fibular fossa. The lateral malleolus extends about 1 cm lower than the medial malleolus and is located more posteriorly.

The talar body is wedge shaped, being wider anteriorly than posteriorly. It is also wedge shaped in the frontal plane, being wider inferiorly. The talus is covered over 60 percent of its surface with hyaline cartilage. There are no muscular attachments. The dorsal articular surface of the talus is concave in the frontal plane and convex in the sagittal plane. It is known as the dome of the talus and has a central sagittal groove that corresponds to a ridge on the inferior tibial pla-

---

* The opinions and assertions of the author are not to be construed as reflecting official U.S. Army/Army Medical Department policy.

fond. There is a comma-shaped facet on the superior aspect of the medial surface that articulates with the medial malleolar facet. The entire lateral surface is an articular facet that is triangular, with its apex directed inferiorly, which articulates with the lateral malleolus.

The ankle joint is invested with a complex arrangement of ligaments. The lateral collateral ligaments are composed of the anterior talofibular, calcaneofibular, and posterior talofibular ligaments. The anterior talofibular ligament is flat, intracapsular, and about 1 cm wide. This ligament is attached to the anterior aspect of the lateral malleolus and extends inferiorly, anteriorly, and medially to attach to the anterolateral edge of the talar body. It is relaxed in dorsiflexion and taut in plantar flexion. It prevents mainly anterior displacement of the talus out of the mortise as well as some slight degree of talar tilt. The calcaneofibular ligament is a cordlike structure extending from the inferior pole of the lateral malleolus and attaching to the lateral aspect of the calcaneus. It is directed inferiorly, medially, and posteriorly from the lateral malleolus. It controls the frontal plane movement of both the ankle and subtalar joints. The calcaneofibular ligament mainly prevents talar tilt in the ankle mortise. It is taut in dorsiflexion and relaxed in plantar flexion, thereby being reciprocal to the anterior talofibular ligament. It is extracapsular and deep to the peroneal tendons. The posterior talofibular ligament courses from the fossa on the lateral malleolus in a medial and posterior direction to attach to the posterolateral aspect of the talar body.[1] The anterior talofibular and calcaneofibular ligaments are the most commonly injured ligaments in ankle sprains. The fibular collateral ligaments are not commonly injured in ankle fractures.

The deltoid ligament is clinically divided into superficial and deep portions. The superficial deltoid ligament is attached to the anterior colliculus and is composed of the naviculotibial, calcaneotibial, and superficial talotibial ligaments. The deep deltoid ligament is more important. It is attached to the posterior colliculus and intercollicular groove, extending laterally to attach to the medial surface of the talus. It is composed of the deep anterior talotibial and deep posterior talotibial ligaments.[4]

However, the most important ligaments stabilizing the ankle joint are the syndesmotic ligaments composed of the anterior inferior tibiofibular (anterior syndesmosis), interosseous, and posterior tibiofibular (posterior syndesmosis) ligaments. The anterior syndesmosis is attached to the tubercle of Tillaux-Chaput and extends inferiorly, laterally, and posteriorly to attach to the anterior aspect of the fibula. It is about 2 cm wide and is the most commonly ruptured ligament in ankle fractures. The interosseous ligament attaches the distal fibula to the distal tibia and is posterior to the midpoint of the fibula. This ligament is highly variable, and as it extends superiorly, it becomes the interosseous membrane.[5] The posterior syndesmosis extends from the posterior malleolus laterally to attach to the fibula. Some consider the inferior portion of this ligament to be the inferior transverse tibio-fibular ligament.[1]

Which structures therefore, are most important for ankle stability? Yablon et al. demonstrated on fresh cadaveric specimens that the lateral malleolus was the key in maintaining ankle stability.[6,7] When only the deltoid ligament was severed, no ankle instability ensued, either valgus tilt or rotational. The medial malleolus was osteotomized at the level of the plafond and only 10 degrees of rotational instability was noted, but no talar tilt. Isolated division of the fibular collateral ligaments revealed 10 degrees of varus talar tilt and 30 degrees of rotational instability. Finally, osteotomy of the fibula below the level of the anterior syndesmosis produced the greatest amount of instability. There were 20 degrees of varus talar tilt and 40 degrees of external rotational instability.

However, the work of Yablon and colleagues has recently been somewhat contradicted by Harper.[8] In fresh cadaveric specimens, he found that valgus tilt of the talus could occur if both the superficial and deep deltoid ligaments were transected. Yet no valgus tilt occurred if one of the ligaments remained intact. But he did confirm Yablon's conclusion that the lateral malleolus was the primary restraint to lateral talar displacement. If the lateral malleolus was removed, the talus could subluxate laterally 3 mm even in the presence of an intact deltoid ligament. The deep deltoid ligament was confirmed as the secondary restraint against lateral talar displacement.

The anterior syndesmosis, of all the syndesmotic ligaments, is best positioned to resist external rotation. In cadaver experiments with an isolated transection of the anterior syndesmosis, the anterior tibiofibular distance was increased by 4 to 10 mm with external rotation of the foot.[9] This reflects an anterior diastasis and also may cause a slight increase in the space between the talus and medial malleolus. Yablon et al. noted that with an oblique fibular osteotomy accompanied by division of the anterior syndesmosis, they could produce valgus tilt of the talus on external rotation of the foot.[7]

The ankle joint has been considered a hinge-type joint, but this is an oversimplification. The ankle is externally rotated 15 to 20 degrees from the axis of the knee. Two axes of rotation have been described by Barnett and Napier.[10] One axis is for dorsiflexion and one is for plantar flexion. Also, the talus has a larger radius of curvature on the lateral dome that produces movement more like a cone than a cylinder. Consequently, with dorsiflexion there is external rotation and posterior gliding of the talus, whereas plantar flexion produces inversion and anterior gliding. Also, the ankle works in combination with the subtalar and midtarsal joints. However, for clinical expediency, the ankle is considered to dorsiflex and plantar flex around a single axis oriented along the inferior poles of the malleoli. Normal dorsiflexion is considered from 10 to 20 degrees, while plantar flexion is from 30 to 50 degrees. Also, as the talus dorsiflexes, the ankle mortise can widen up to 1.5 mm to accommodate the wider anterior aspect of the talus. During this motion, the fibula externally rotates and may slide proximally. Consequently, the malleoli are in firm contact with the talus throughout the ankle range of motion.[11]

CLASSIFICATION

Historically, Hippocrates discussed ankle fractures in about 300 BC. However, it was Sir Percivall Pott, in the 18th century, who really attempted to describe some of the pathologic findings.[12] He observed a fracture of the fibula slightly above the ankle joint with rupture of the deltoid ligament and lateral subluxation of the talus caused by abduction. It has been stated that this fracture actually does not occur, as Pott believed that the distal syndesmotic ligaments remained intact. This is interesting because his name has been commonly applied to the bimalleolar fracture. The first person to attempt to delineate ankle fracture mechanisms was Dupuytren.[13] He developed a classification system based on cadaveric experiments that recognized the forces of adduction and abduction. His name has also been attached to the fracture described by Pott, especially by the French. He has also been linked to a fracture involving a diastasis. Ashley Cooper, in 1822, described many different fracture configurations.[14] It was Earle who described posterior malleolar fractures in 1823.[15] In 1840, Maisonneuve proposed that external rotation was an additional force producing ankle fractures.[16] He indicated that this force produced an oblique fracture of the fibula and that differences occurred depending on the involvement of the syndesmosis. His name has been classically applied to the fracture of the proximal fibula with diastasis between the distal tibia and fibula. In 1872, Tillaux described fractures of the anterolateral margin of the tibia implicating the anterior syndesmotic ligament.[17] Then, in 1875, Wagstaffe described two cases of vertical fracture of the anterior fibula.[18] A similar experience was noted in 1886 when LeFort reported three cases of isolated fracture of the anterior portion of the lateral malleolus.[1] Although von Volkmann also described fractures of the anterolateral aspect of the tibia in 1875,[3] his name has been attached to posterior malleolar fractures. Ashhurst and Bromer, in 1922, published a classic study on the classification of ankle fractures by mechanism of injury.[19] They divided the fractures into categories of adduction, abduction, external rotation, and compression. Each category of fracture was further subdivided into degrees of injury. Ashhurst and Bromer were the first to use anatomic, surgical, and radiographic studies to postulate their classification scheme, but they emphasized the bony components while ignoring the concomitant ligamentous injuries.[19] In 1932, Hendersen used the term trimalleolar fracture, but this fracture was actually reported by Cotton in 1915.[15] He described an injury with both malleoli fractured along with the posterior margin of the tibia and posterior dislocation of the talus. The name Cotton has been attached to the trimalleolar fracture. In 1947, Bosworth reported on an irreducible fracture-dislocation of the ankle.[1] The lateral malleolus was fractured and the proximal fibular fragment was entrapped behind the tibia. During the 1950s, Lauge-Hansen published a series of articles also describing mechanisms of injury.[20-22] In 1972, Weber proposed a classification[23] that was modified from that proposed by Danis and which is accepted by the Association for the Study of Problems of Internal Fixation (AO/ASIF) group.

Ankle fractures have also been classified by their anatomic location, disregarding their mechanism of injury. This was popularized by Quénu, who divided the fractures into unimalleolar and bimalleolar with trimalleolar being added later.[15] This was an easy way to describe the radiographic findings but again emphasized the osseous component over the ligamentous structures. Also, the ability to compare these fractures is difficult since a unimalleolar fracture involving the tibia is quite different from a unimalleolar fracture of the fibula.

Presently, there are two commonly accepted classification schemes for fractured ankles, the Lauge-Hansen and Danis-Weber (AO) classifications. The Lauge-Hansen classification (Table 28-1 and Fig. 28-1) was derived experimentally but has been confirmed both radiographically and surgically.[20-22] It consists of two words and represents five general patterns of injury. The first word is either supination or pronation, referring to the position of the foot at the time of the injury. The second part refers to the direction the talus moves in the ankle mortise—adduction, abduction, or eversion (external rotation). The fracture pattern is based on the configuration and location of the fibular fracture. These mechanisms of injury are then subdivided into sequential stages representing the specific structures damaged and the order of damage. Thus, if a stage IV injury is present, then stages I to III must also have occurred. Lauge-Hansen recognizes both the ligamentous as well as the osseous structures injured, and 95 to 98 percent of all ankle fractures can be classified. Lauge-Hansen favored closed

Table 28-1. Lauge-Hansen Classification

Supination-adduction
 Stage I: transverse fracture of the fibula at or below the ankle joint or rupture of the fibular collateral ligaments.
 Stage II: superiorly oriented fracture of the medial malleolus.

Supination-eversion (external rotation)
 Stage I: rupture of the anterior inferior tibiofibular ligament or bony avulsion off the tibia or fibula.
 Stage II: spiral fracture of the fibula at the level of the syndesmosis.
 Stage III: rupture of the posterior inferior tibiofibular ligament or fracture of the posterior malleolus.
 Stage IV: rupture of the deltoid ligament or fracture of the medial malleolus.

Pronation-abduction
 Stage I: rupture of the deltoid ligament or fracture of the medial malleolus.
 Stage II: rupture of the anterior and posterior inferior tibiofibular ligaments or their bony avulsion.
 Stage III: oblique fracture of the fibula at the level of the syndesmosis.

Pronation-eversion (external rotation)
 Stage I: rupture of the deltoid ligament or fracture of the medial malleolus.
 Stage II: rupture of the anterior inferior tibiofibular ligament or its bony avulsion with rupture of the interosseous ligament-membrane.
 Stage III: spiral fracture of the fibula above the level of the syndesmosis.
 Stage IV: rupture of the posterior inferior tibiofibular ligament or fracture of the posterior malleolus.

Pronation-dorsiflexion
 Stage I: fracture of the medial malleolus.
 Stage II: fracture of the anterior lip of the tibia.
 Stage III: fracture of the supramalleolar aspect of the fibula.
 Stage IV: a relatively transverse fracture of the posterior aspect of the tibia.

reduction of ankle fractures and believed that if the mechanism of injury could be established, then the reduction could be accomplished by reversing the original injury mechanism. Two problems with the Lauge-Hansen classification are its complexity and the somewhat confusing terminology.

The Danis-Weber (AO) classification is far simpler (Fig. 28-2).[23] It is divided into three types depending on the level of the fibular fracture in

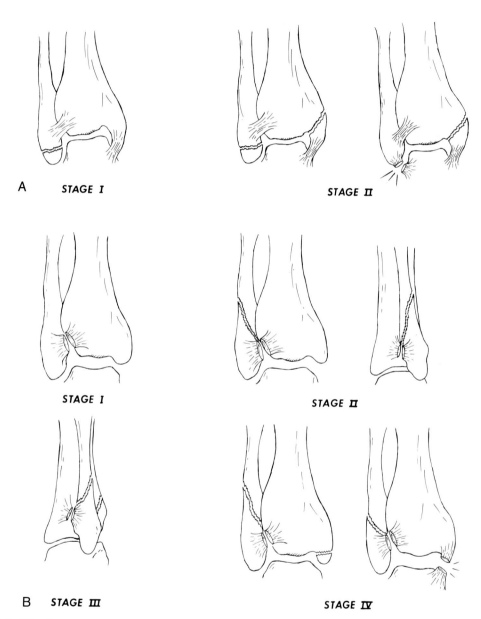

Fig. 28-1. The Lague-Hansen classification. (**A**) Supination-adduction. (**B**) Supination-external rotation. (*Figure continues.*)

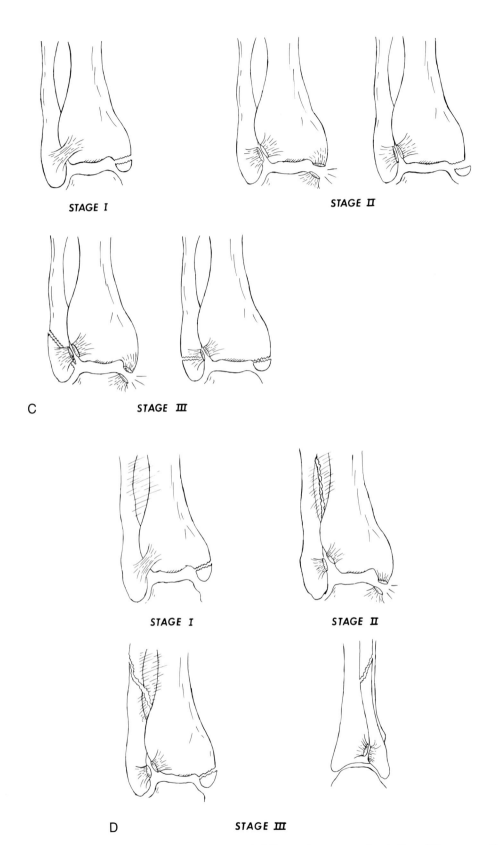

STAGE I

STAGE II

C   STAGE III

STAGE I

STAGE II

D   STAGE III

Fig. 28-1 (*Continued*). (**C**) Pronation-abduction. (**D**) Pronation-external rotation. (*Figure continues.*)

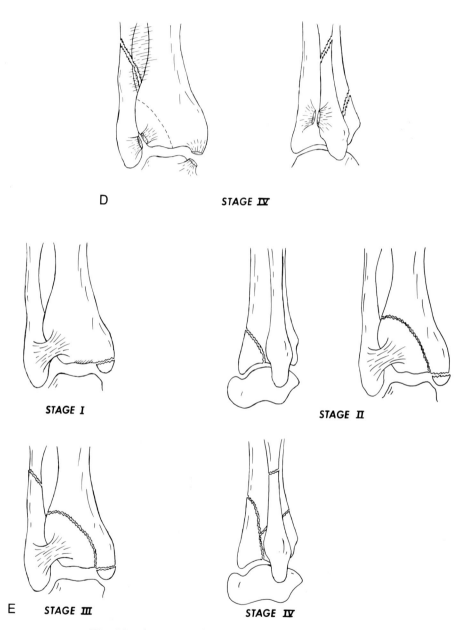

D   STAGE **IV**

STAGE *I*

STAGE *II*

E   STAGE *III*   STAGE *IV*

Fig. 28-1 (*Continued*). (**E**) Pronation-dorsiflexion.

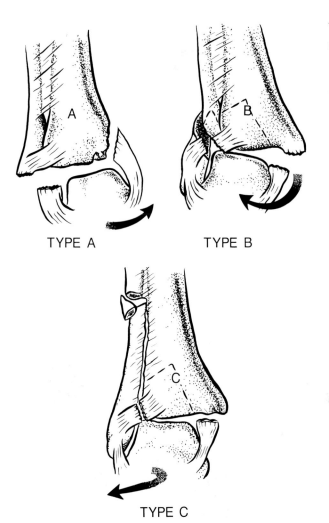

TYPE A   TYPE B

TYPE C

Fig. 28-2. (A–C) The Danis-Weber (AO) classification. (Redrawn from Mueller et al.,[57] with permission.)

relationship to the distal syndesmosis. It also takes into account both ligamentous and osseous injuries. However, it does not explain the mechanism of injury as well as the Lauge-Hansen classification. Consequently, for this article, the Lauge-Hansen classification is presented first and in the greatest detail, with later comparison with the Danis-Weber classification.

Supination-Adduction Fractures

Supination-adduction fractures occur from an inversion force applied to the foot and ankle.

With the foot supinated, the fibular collateral ligaments are taut and the injury starts on the lateral side. There are two stages to this type of fracture. Stage I classically presents as a transverse fracture of the fibula, usually at or below the level of the joint (Figure 28-3), or as an injury to the fibular collateral ligaments. With a transverse fibular fracture, the syndesmotic ligaments are usually not involved because the fracture usually is below the level of the joint. However, if the fracture occurs at the level of the tibial plafond, then both the anterior and posterior syndesmotic ligaments may be ruptured. In this case, there would be no instability of the syndesmosis because the interosseous ligament remains intact. If an isolated fibular collateral ligament injury occurs, this is a sprained ankle, not a fracture, and it is treated according to the degree of stability. If the talus continues to invert in the ankle mortise, it im-

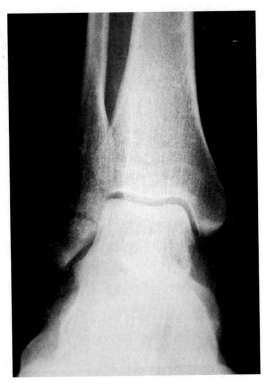

Fig. 28-3. Supination-adduction stage I injury with a nondisplaced transverse fracture of the fibula below the ankle joint as seen on an anteroposterior radiograph.

pacts against the medial malleolus and results in a push-off fracture. This produces a stage II injury, which is seen radiographically as a superiorly oriented fracture of the medial malleolus (Fig. 28-4). It may even be completely vertical. If no fibular fracture is seen on the radiograph in a stage II injury, it can be inferred that some damage to the fibular collateral ligaments has occurred.

Yde studied 488 ankle fractures over 8 years, and the incidence of supination-adduction fractures was 20.1 percent.[24] Of this number, 80.6 percent were stage I, with 70.5 percent of the transverse fractures being below the level of the ankle joint. Gudas reports a study of 803 ankle fractures at St. Gallen, Switzerland, that revealed an incidence of 10 percent supination-adduction fractures, of which 64 percent were stage II.[15] A variation in the supination-adduction fractures

was observed by Ashhurst and Bromer[19] as well as by Magnussen.[25] They noted occasional medial malleolar fractures that were transverse. Hamilton reports that this is explained by having two varieties of supination-adduction injury.[1] The most common is the classic adduction injury, which produces a superiorly oriented medial malleolar fracture, whereas a rare adduction injury occurs with rotatory talar subluxation, producing either a transverse medial malleolar fracture or a ruptured deltoid ligament.

The stage I transverse fracture of the fibula is many times nondisplaced. Consequently, it can be treated in a weight-bearing short leg cast for 6 weeks. Although it is usually stable, radiographs must be obtained for 2 to 3 weeks on a weekly basis to check the fracture position. If it is displaced, an attempt at closed reduction can be made by applying a valgus force after first in-

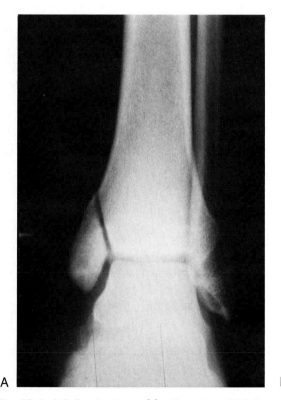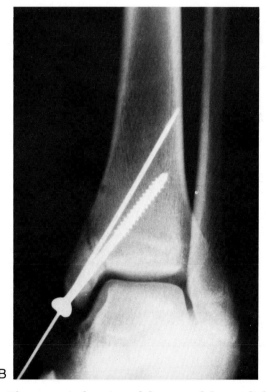

Fig. 28-4. (A) Supination-adduction stage II injury with a superiorly oriented fracture of the medial malleolus demonstrated on an anteroposterior radiograph. If there is no evidence of a fibular fracture, the presence of fibular collateral ligament damage is indicated. (B) Mortise view of surgical reduction with fixation by a 4.5 mm malleolar screw and Kirschner wire.

creasing the deformity in the adduction direction followed by the application of a short leg cast. If an anatomic reduction is accomplished, then the treatment can be the same as above. If it is not satisfactorily reduced, operative fixation can be accomplished by a tension-band wire if the lateral malleolar fragment is small. If the fragment is large (at the level of the plafond), a one-third tubular plate can be used as an alternative form of fixation. The plate will provide only neutralization, while the tension-band wire will create interfragmental compression. The fibular fracture is more likely to be displaced in a stage II injury.

If the medial malleolar fracture is nondisplaced (with or without a nondisplaced fibular fracture) in a stage II injury, it is treated in a long leg cast with the knee flexed from 45 to 90 degrees to prevent weight bearing. This is because the more vertical the fracture, the less the buttressing effect of the tibial plafond and the greater the likelihood of proximal migration of the fracture fragment with weight bearing. This fracture is kept non-weight bearing for the initial 5 to 6 weeks, at which time the cast is converted to a walking short leg cast for the final 2 to 3 weeks. Radiographs are obtained for the first 3 to 4 weeks on a weekly basis to check for loss of fracture position.

If the medial malleolar fracture is displaced, it is fixated with two 4.0-mm cancellous screws (4.5-mm malleolar or 6.5-mm cancellous screws can also be used). It may be necessary to use a washer with the screw to prevent the screw head from penetrating the thin cortex on the medial aspect of the distal tibia. Orientation of the screws perpendicular to the fracture prevents proximal migration of the fractured medial malleolus while the screws are tightened (Fig. 28-5). The more superiorly oriented the fracture, the more transverse the placement of the screws until a vertical fracture is reached so that the screws are perpendicular to the long axis of the tibia. In this type of fracture, the use of a tension-band wire also tends to cause proximal migration of the fracture fragment. If a fibular fracture is present in a stage II injury in which the medial malleolus is fixated, the fibula is fixated as described above whether it is displaced or not (Fig. 28-5). If the

radiographs demonstrate an isolated displaced stage II medial malleolar fracture without evidence of fibular fracture that is to undergo open reduction with internal fixation, the stability of the fibular collateral ligaments must be assessed. After the patient is anesthetized, stress testing can be performed clinically and confirmed, if necessary by stress radiography. Also, the stability of the fibular collateral ligaments can be confirmed under direct visualization through the anteromedial incision used to expose the medial malleolus. Although the fibular collateral ligaments should be ruptured in this case, it is interesting to note that many times they are not. If there is an indication of rupture, the ligaments are explored and primarily repaired.

Supination-Eversion (External Rotation) Fractures

One of the confusing aspects of the Lauge-Hansen classification is the word *eversion*, which is used to describe external rotation. Since the foot is supinated at the time of the injury and usually on the ground, it is really internal rotation of the leg that produces a relative external rotation of the talus out of the ankle joint. Again, since the foot is supinated, the injury pattern starts laterally and is divided into four stages. Stage I is usually a rupture of the anterior syndesmosis. It can also occur as a bony avulsion off the anterior lateral aspect of the tibia (tubercle of Tillaux-Chaput) or off the anterior aspect of the lateral malleolus (Wagstaffe lesion). Stage II produces the hallmark of this injury pattern, which is the spiral fracture of the fibula at the level of the syndesmosis. This fracture starts at or slightly below the ankle joint and extends in a spiral manner in a superior posterior direction. Stage III is a rupture of the posterior syndesmosis or a fracture of the posterior malleolus. Stage IV is a medial injury involving either a ruptured deltoid ligament or a fractured medial malleolus.

The supination-external rotation fractures are the most common ankle fractures encountered. In reported series, they compose from 40 to 75 percent.[1] Yde, in his study of 488 ankle fractures, encountered this type of fracture pattern in 57.4

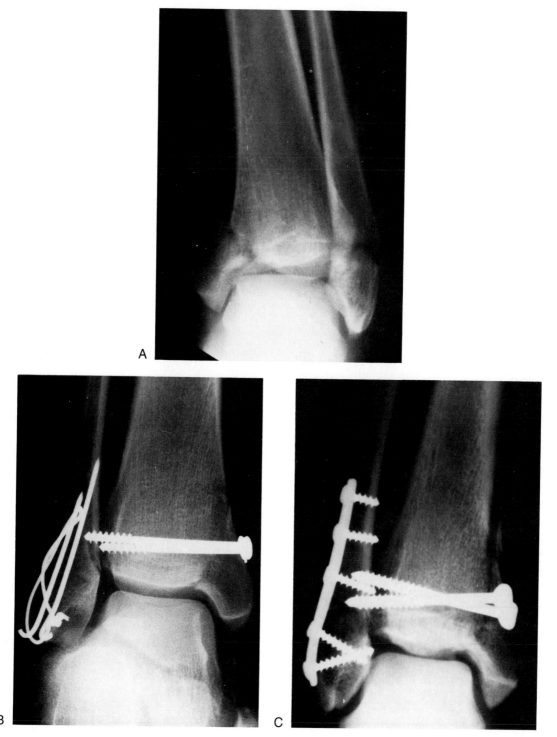

Fig. 28-5. (**A**) Anteroposterior view of a supination-adduction stage II injury demonstrating both a transverse fracture of the fibula and a vertical fracture of the medial malleolus. (**B**) Stage II injury in which the fibula is fixated with a tension-band wire and the medial malleolus is fixated with two 4.0-mm cancellous screws. (**C**) Stage II injury in which the fibula is fixated with a one-third tubular plate and the medial malleolus is fixated with two 4.5-mm malleolar screws.

percent.[24] The St. Gallen study of 803 fractures reported an incidence of 54.9 percent.[15] Lauge-Hansen reported an incidence of 71 percent in 228 fractures.[20–22]

An isolated stage I injury is somewhat rare. Hamilton reports an overall incidence of 5 percent in supination-external rotation fractures.[1] In the surgical exploration of 405 supination-external rotation fractures, Cedell reported that stage I occurred in 96 percent of cases, with midsubstance tear of the anterior syndesmosis accounting for 65 percent of the injuries.[26,27] He also indicated that the Wagstaffe lesion occurred more often than avulsion of the anterolateral tibia. An isolated anterior syndesmosis rupture is treated conservatively, but a large displaced bony avulsion may require open reduction with internal fixation.

The stage II spiral fibular fracture is the most common ankle fracture according to Lauge-Hansen (Fig. 28-6).[20–22] Yde[24] and Cedell[26,27] believe that they compose 50 to 60 percent of all supination-external rotation fractures and 30 percent of all ankle fractures. Yet Hamilton states that they represent only 34 percent of supination-external rotation fractures.[1] The stage II fracture is also probably the most controversial in regards to treatment. If it is nondisplaced, the treatment consists of a weight-bearing short leg cast for 7 to 8 weeks, with radiographs obtained weekly for the first 3 weeks to check for loss of position. A displaced stage II fracture can produce a difference in treatment depending on the preference of the attending physician. This fracture has been treated to a large extent by just cast immobilization with good long-term results.[28] Kristensen and Hansen reported on 94 conservatively treated cases of stage II fractures over 16 to 25 years that caused minimal complaints and whose late results compare equally well with Cedell's surgical treatment.[29] Other investigators advocate open reduction with internal fixation for any displacement.[23,30] I always attempt to improve the position of a displaced stage II fracture by using a modified Charnley mold and a two-stage long leg cast. It has been noted that the distal fibular fragment is usually externally rotated and shortened.[6] To correct this deformity, the closed manipulation is performed by first externally ro-

tating the foot to increase the deformity, followed by inversion and internal rotation of the foot. A short leg cast is applied. Then a three point mold is used with one hand over the lateral malleolus and the other over the medial aspect of the distal tibial metaphysis above the medial malleolus. A third hand is placed by the cast technician over the proximal fibula. This is the principle of ligamentotaxis in which an attempt is made to manipulate the distal fibular fragment through the fibular collateral ligaments and direct pressure. The short leg cast is then converted to a long leg cast with the knee flexed 15 to 20 degrees and the leg internally rotated. This attempt at closed reduction may not be successful because the distal fibular fragment becomes impinged on the proximal fragment. Postreduction radiographs are obtained to ascertain the position of the fracture. If the reduction is deemed satisfactory, the patient is held in this cast (non-weight bearing) for 3 weeks with radiographs obtained weekly. At 3 weeks, the fracture is sticky and the cast is changed to a weight-bearing long leg cast with the foot in a neutral position for the next 3 weeks. The cast is converted to a short leg cast for the final 2 weeks. At 8 weeks the cast is removed and the fracture is radiographed for signs of union. If healing, the patient starts weight bearing to tolerance in an elastic anklet and undergoes physical therapy. An alternative course of treatment is early weight bearing after the initial reduction on the theory that the stability of the reduction should be tested. If it displaces, this will be detected on the weekly radiographic examination. The fracture can then be either remanipulated or more likely have an open reduction with internal fixation.

What constitutes a satisfactory reduction? A satisfactory reduction is less than 1 mm of lateral displacement with no shortening. If greater than 1 mm of displacement or shortening is present, then consideration is given to open reduction with internal fixation if the patient is a surgical candidate and desires surgery. A greater discussion of reduction criteria is found in the section on treatment options. At surgery, the spiral fracture of the fibula is anatomically reduced and fixated with one or more cortical lag screws (either 3.5 or 2.7 mm) depending on the length of the

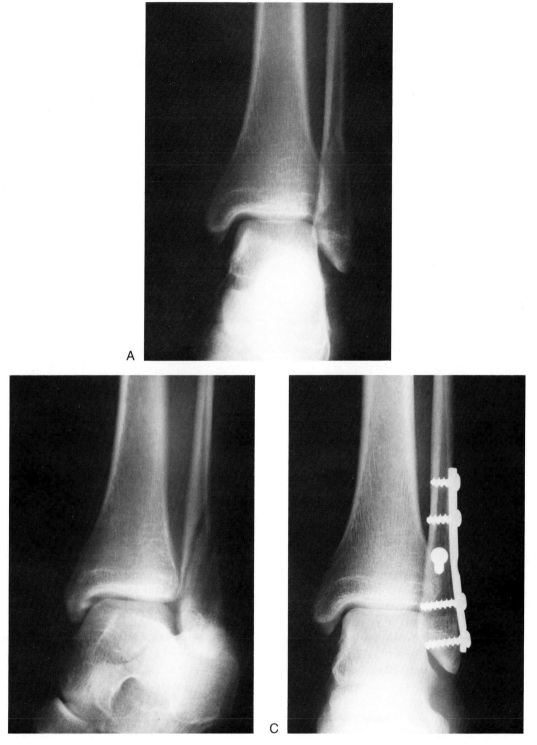

Fig. 28-6. (A) Anteroposterior and (B) oblique, views of a supination-external rotation stage II injury demonstrating a spiral fibular fracture at the level of the syndesmosis. (C) Anteroposterior view of open reduction and internal fixation. A 3.5-mm cortical lag screw has been employed for interfragmental compression and a one-third tubular plate has been applied for neutralization. The anterior syndesmosis was primarily repaired.

fracture. A 4.0-mm cancellous screw can also be utilized as a lag screw in this region. The lag screws are placed from anterior to posterior and used to produce interfragmental compression, which is one of the cardinal principles of the AO/ASIF group. A one-third tubular plate is applied for neutralization to the lateral aspect of the fibula (Fig. 28-6). In elderly patients with osteoporosis, one may encounter difficulty in obtaining screw purchase in the lateral malleolus. In this case, it may be necessary to apply the plate along the posterior surface of the fibula in an anti-glide position. It thus may be possible to obtain a lag screw across the fracture by placing it through the plate going from posterior to anterior and angled superiorly. The holes in the lower end of the plate corresponding to the lateral malleolus may not even have to be used. If the fibular fracture is a long spiral, it can be fixated with multiple lag screws alone. The anterior syndesmosis, which is usually ruptured in its midsubstance, is repaired primarily with sutures. Sometimes drill holes are necessary if the ligament will not hold the suture or if the ligament has been avulsed directly off the bone. If the anterior syndesmosis is intact but there has been a bony avulsion off the tibia or fibula, it is fixated with a lag screw. If the avulsed piece of bone is small, it may need to be fixated with a Kirschner-wire instead of a screw. Although Lauge-Hansen believed that tibial avulsion is most common, my experience is similar to Cedell's[26,27] that midsubstance rupture is the most common means of failure for the anterior syndesmosis. Weber[23] has indicated that the anterior syndesmosis is ruptured in 50 percent of cases, but my experience indicates a much higher percentage. Occasionally, the spiral fracture will begin below the ankle joint and there will be no anterior syndesmotic disruption or bony avulsion. In other words, stage I was bypassed. This has been described as the mixed oblique fracture of Destot and occurs with an incidence of 2 to 4 percent.[1] If the patient is not a surgical candidate or refuses surgery, then the best attempt at a closed reduction is made and a greater amount of displacement is accepted.

It is unusual for the supination-external rotation injury to stop at stage III. This end-stage fracture was present in 4 percent of cases in Yde's study.[24] It usually proceeds to stage IV, producing medial injury that significantly reduces the stability of the ankle. However, Hamilton states that it represents 23 percent of supination-external rotation fractures.[1] The posterior malleolus is fixated only if it represents 25 to 30 percent of the tibial articular surface. In Yde's series, only 14 percent of posterior malleolus fractures in supination-external rotation injuries were greater than 25 percent of the surface and required fixation.[24] The fixation of the posterior malleolus is detailed in another section.

A stage IV fracture configuration usually requires open reduction with internal fixation. This is because of the difficulty in obtaining an anatomic reduction by closed means, especially with a medial malleolar fracture, and the increased degree of instability preventing the maintenance of the reduction. At surgery, if there is a medial malleolar fracture, both sides of the ankle are opened to evaluate the fractures. The fibula is fixated as described above and takes priority. Then the medial malleolus is fixated with two 4.0-mm cancellous screws if possible (Fig. 28-7). Two other techniques for fixation include using one cancellous screw and one Kirschner-wire or a tension-band wire. The tension-band wire is reserved for a small fragment, a comminuted fracture, osteoporotic bone, or if the screws fail to obtain good purchase. When the deltoid ligament is ruptured, it is not necessarily repaired (Fig. 28-8). The medial side is opened and the deltoid ligament primarily repaired only if it is trapped in the joint space preventing reduction, an osteochondral fragment is in the medial joint space, or there has been a dislocation of the ankle. Experience has shown that many fracture-dislocations produce osteochondral damage on the medial talar dome that may not be apparent radiographically. If the deltoid ligament is to be explored, the medial side is opened first, followed by the lateral side. After the medial joint space is explored, sutures are preplaced in the deltoid ligament but left untied. This prevents the deltoid ligament from slipping back into the joint space and facilitates primary repair later. After the fibula is reduced and fixated along with stabilization of the syndesmosis, then the deltoid liga-

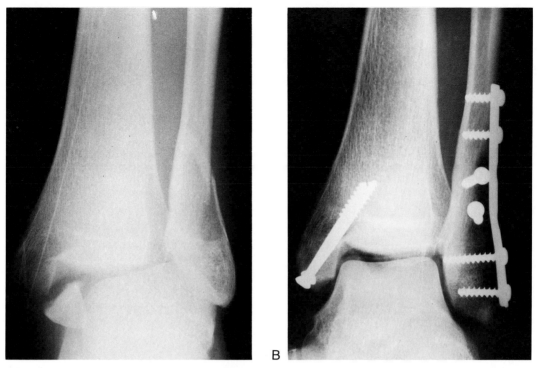

Fig. 28-7. (A) Anteroposterior view of a supination-external rotation stage IV fracture-subluxation demonstrating a spiral fracture of the fibula at the syndesmosis, a small posterior malleolus fracture, and a transverse fracture of the medial malleolus. (B) Mortise view of open reduction with internal fixation with the fibula fixated with lag screws and a neutralization plate, while the medial malleolus is fixated with two 4.0-mm cancellous screws. The anterior syndesmosis was primarily repaired.

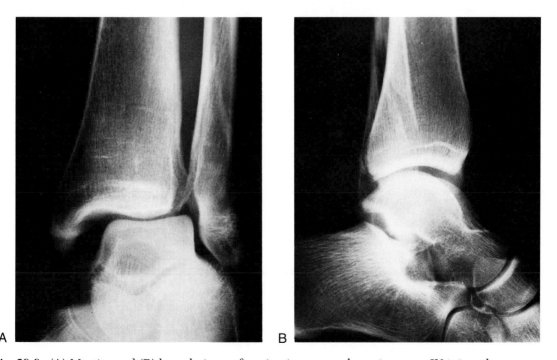

Fig. 28-8. (A) Mortise and (B) lateral views of supination-external rotation stage IV injury demonstrating a spiral fracture of the fibula and lateral talar subluxation indicating rupture of the deltoid ligament. (*Figures continues.*)

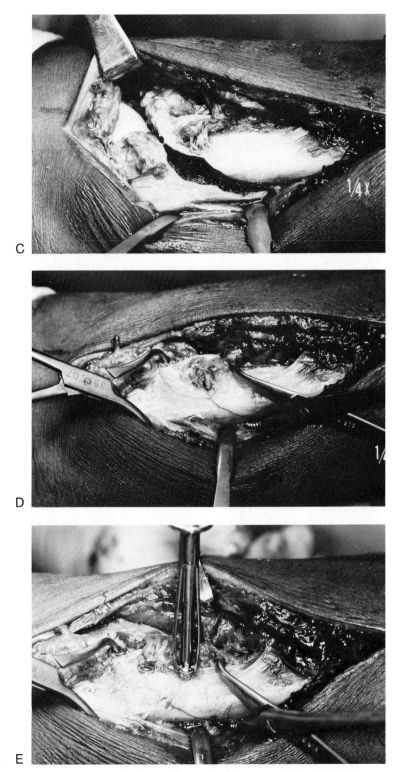

Fig. 28-8 (*Continued*). (**C**) Spiral fracture of the fibula is seen with midsubstance rupture of the anterior syndesmosis. No articular damage is noted on the talus. (**D**) Fracture is anatomically reduced and held with bone reduction clamps. (**E**) Two 3.5-mm cortical screws are employed for interfragmental compression utilizing AO lag technique. (*Figure continues.*)

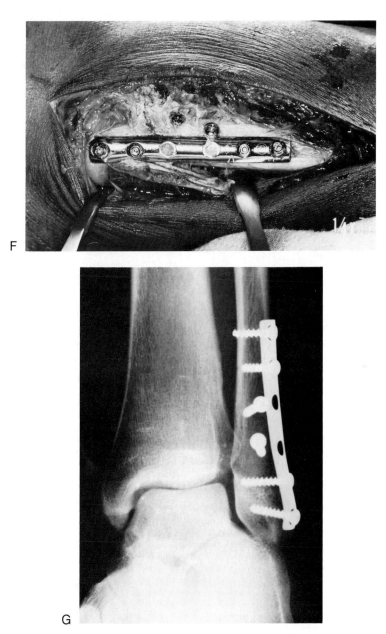

Fig. 28-8 (*Continued*). (**F**) Rigid internal fixation complete with cortical lag screws and neutralization plate. The anterior syndesmosis is primarily repaired. (**G**) Mortise view of open reduction with internal fixation in which the deltoid ligament was not primarily repaired.

ment is primarily repaired. The deltoid ligament is not repaired if the ankle is only subluxated and reduction of the fibula reduces the talus anatomically in the mortise. Yablon et al. have demonstrated that a ruptured deltoid ligament produces no instability in the presence of an anatomically reduced and fixated fibula with a stable syndesmosis.[6] This view is further supported by Denham,[31] Mast and Teipner,[32] and Baird and Jackson.[33] Usually with a stage IV injury, there is either a fractured medial malleolus or a ruptured deltoid ligament as individual lesions. However, on occasion, it is possible to have a combined injury in which only the anterior colliculus is fractured and there is also rupture of the deep deltoid ligament.[4] Last, the anterior syndesmosis is addressed and repaired as indicated previously. With supination-external rotation stage III or IV fractures, there is supposed to be no true diastasis. The fibular fracture at the level of the syndesmosis may rupture both the anterior and posterior syndesmosis but spares the interosseous ligament. Consequently, the distal tibiofibular relationship is not disturbed and a transyndesmotic screw is not indicated. Rarely, one may encounter a patient who has also ruptured the interosseous ligament or does not have one, which produces total syndesmotic instability. The stability of the syndesmosis is always tested after repair to check for this rare variation which would require transyndesmotic fixation.[5]

Pronation-Abduction Fractures

The fracture mechanism causing pronation-abduction fractures occurs in the frontal plane without a rotational component and has three stages. Since the foot is pronated, causing the medial structures to be taut, the injury starts medially. Stage I involves either a fracture of the medial malleolus or a rupture of the deltoid ligament (Fig. 28-9). In clinical practice, an isolated complete rupture of the deltoid ligament may not occur if Yablon's explanation is correct. As the talus is forced laterally, it pushes against the fibula, rupturing the anterior and posterior syndesmosis simultaneously (stage II). A bony avulsion of either ligament is also possible but less common. It is also occasionally possible to simultaneously rupture all three syndesmotic ligaments. Stage III produces an oblique or transverse fracture of the fibula, usually at the level of the syndesmosis (Fig. 28-10). The oblique fracture is much more common and is the hallmark of this mechanism. The fracture proceeds from the medial aspect of the fibula to the lateral aspect in a superior direction. There is no indication of a spiral configuration. On the lateral radiograph, the fibular fracture may appear almost transverse or as if coming to a point. Although this fracture usually occurs at the syndesmosis, it sometimes occurs above it, which produces a greater ligamentous instability as all three syndesmotic ligaments may be ruptured. It is reported that pronation-abduction fractures represent less than 5 percent of all ankle fractures.[20] Yde's incidence was 1.96 percent,[24] and Lauge-Hansen found 11 fractures in 228 cases.[20-22] Hamilton states that depending on the series, this mechanism accounts for 5 to 20 percent of all fractures.[1]

An isolated fracture of the medial malleolus in a stage I injury is treated in a walking short leg cast for 7 to 8 weeks if nondisplaced. Closed reduction of a displaced medial malleolus fracture is difficult. It may be attempted by everting the foot first, followed by inverting and pushing up on the inferior aspect of the fractured fragment. If displaced and surgically approached, the fracture is fixated as previously described (Fig. 28-9). The stage II pronation-abduction injury is unusual and, if all three syndesmotic ligaments are ruptured, can result in a diastasis. This mechanism of injury can produce a subluxation of the ankle without fracture. The resulting instability of the syndesmosis can be difficult to control in a cast and may require a transyndesmotic screw.

The fibular fracture in stage III, while usually oblique, can occasionally be transverse. It is treated in a long leg cast if nondisplaced and the ankle mortise is anatomic. The cast is applied with the foot inverted and adducted. The extremity is kept non-weight bearing because of associated medial injury, which promotes instability. The same protocol is followed as outlined above for supination-external rotation fractures. If the fracture is displaced, an attempted closed reduction is performed by first increasing the valgus

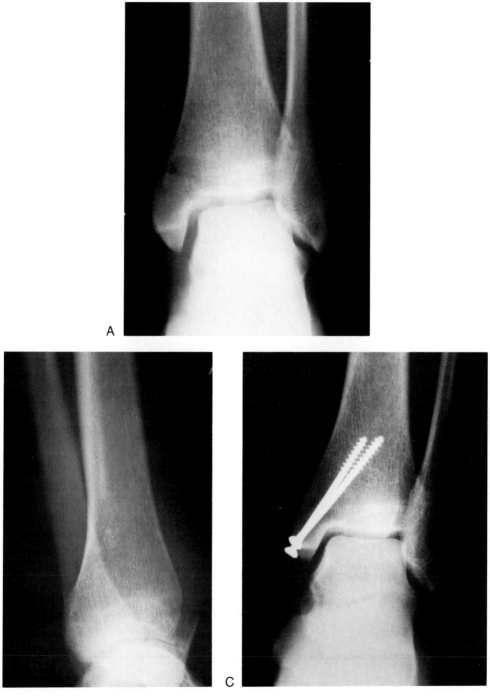

Fig. 28-9. (**A**) Anteroposterior and (**B**) lateral views of a pronation stage I injury. This could be either a pronation-abduction or a pronation-external rotation fracture but has not progressed far enough to declare itself. (**C**) Anteroposterior view of open reduction with internal fixation utilizing two 4.0-mm cancellous screws.

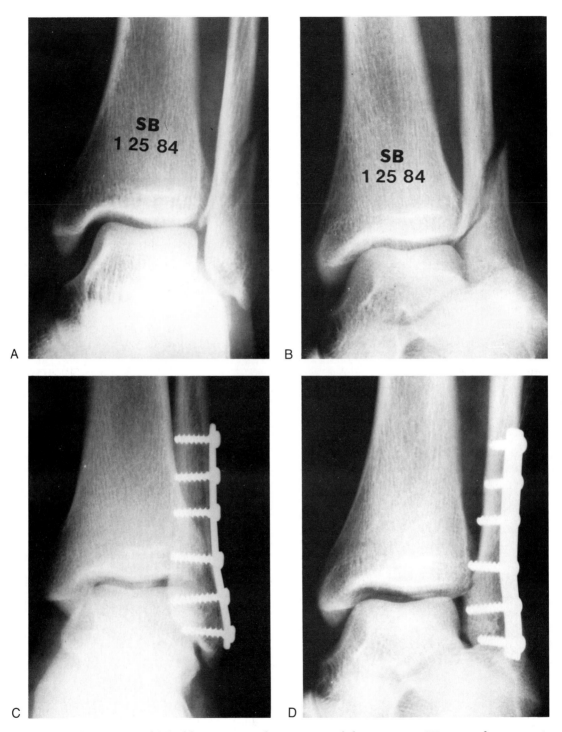

Fig. 28-10. (**A**) Mortise and (**B**) oblique views of a pronation-abduction stage III injury demonstrating an oblique fracture of the fibula with lateral talar subluxation. There is no evidence of a spiral configuration. (**C**) Anteroposterior and (**D**) mortise views of open reduction with internal fixation with cortical lag screws employed through a one-third tubular plate which is in an anti-glide and neutralization position.

deformity and then inverting and adducting the foot with no internal rotation, using a modified Charnley mold with a two-stage long leg cast. However, it is difficult to obtain an anatomic reduction by closed means, and the fracture pattern is unstable.

Stage III fractures usually require open reduction with internal fixation. The oblique configuration of the fibular fracture makes it difficult to use a lag screw from anterior to posterior or in the opposite direction. Instead, a one-third tubular plate is applied to the lateral aspect of the fibula for neutralization and a 3.5-mm cortical lag screw is incorporated through the plate to provide interfragmental compression (Fig. 28-10). The plate, by being on the lateral aspect of the fibula, is also in an anti-glide position for this particular fracture complex. The anterior syndesmosis is primarily repaired or treated as described previously for bony avulsions. Usually a transyndesmotic screw is not required to stabilize the syndesmosis because the level of the fracture at the syndesmosis spares the interosseous ligament. As in the supination-external rotation fractures, there is no true diastasis. However, if the fibular fracture is located above the syndesmosis, then a transyndesmotic screw should be used if indicated, since all the syndesmotic ligaments may be ruptured, producing a diastasis. The specific use of a transyndesmotic screw is described in the next section. With a stage III injury, an associated medial malleolar fracture or ruptured deltoid ligament is treated as described previously.

Pronation-Eversion (External Rotation) Fractures

As with pronation-abduction fractures, the pronation-eversion mechanism of injury starts medially and proceeds in a lateral direction but with an external rotation component. This injury mechanism has four stages. If the foot is fixated on the ground, the external rotation is actually produced by internal rotation of the leg, just like supination-external rotation fractures. Stage I is the same as for the pronation-abduction injuries, producing a fractured medial malleolus or a ruptured deltoid ligament. It is not possible to dis-

tinguish between these two mechanisms because the injury has not proceeded far enough to declare itself. Stage II is the rupture of the anterior syndesmosis and interosseous ligament-membrane. Again, there can be bony avulsion off either the tibia or fibula instead of ligamentous disruption. Although the stage II injury involves slightly different ligaments in the pronation-abduction and the pronation-external rotation injuries, it is difficult to distinguish between them clinically. Stage III is a spiral fracture of the fibula above the level of the syndesmosis which is the hallmark of this mechanism. This fracture is classically described as occurring 5 to 7 cm above the syndesmosis, but can occur anywhere from just above the syndesmosis proximally up to the fibular neck, as described by Maisonneuve[16,34] (Fig. 28-11). Stage IV is a rupture of the posterior

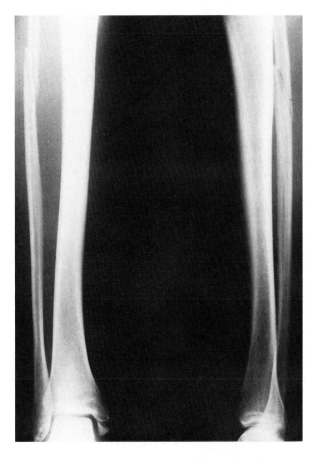

Fig. 28-11. Anteroposterior and lateral radiographs demonstrating a Maisonneuve fracture.

syndesmosis or fracture of the posterior malleolus (Fig. 28-12). Hamilton reported that pronation-external rotation fractures composed 7 to 19 percent of all ankle fractures.[1]

In an interesting study, Pankovich indicated that fibular fractures above the syndesmosis could have three mechanisms: (1) supination-external rotation, (2) pronation-abduction, and (3) pronation-external rotation.[35] The difference is the configuration of the fibular fracture. He stated that a supination-external rotation mechanism produces a short spiral fracture going from the anterior fibular cortex in a posterosuperior direction. The pronation-external rotation mechanism produces a short oblique fracture going from the anterior cortex of the fibula in a posteroinferior direction. Finally, as indicated previously, a pronation-abduction mechanism can produce a transverse or an oblique fracture above the syndesmosis. Hamilton also states that he has seen supination-external rotation fractures above the syndesmosis without medial injury.[1] Although this is academically interesting, it does not alter the closed reduction technique or the operative approach for the two external rotation injuries. I still treat all spiral fibular fractures above the syndesmosis as pronation-external rotation fractures. Another interesting fact is that Yde believes that the fibular fracture is stage IV of the pronation-external rotation mechanism while the posterior syndesmosis rupture/posterior malleolus fracture is stage III.[24]

It is uncommon to see this fracture configuration nondisplaced. It represents the maximum ligamentous instability in ankle fractures as there may be a true diastasis. It has been demonstrated that this fracture pattern can be easy to reduce but that reduction is difficult to maintain. Closed reduction is performed by first increasing the deformity with external rotation and pronation, then inverting and internally rotating the foot while the short leg cast is applied. A three-point Charnley mold is applied as described previously. The short leg cast is then converted to a long leg cast with the knee flexed 15 to 20 degrees and the leg internally rotated. The same course is followed after casting as described for supination-external rotation fractures.

However, it is more likely that pronation-external rotation fractures will be displaced and require open reduction with internal fixation. If the fracture is located in the lower half of the fibula, it is fixated as described previously with a combination of cortical lag screws and a one-third tubular plate for neutralization (Fig. 28-12). The medial malleolus or deltoid ligament injury is treated as previously described. The anterior syndesmosis is repaired, and the posterior malleolus is fixated if it approaches 25 to 30 percent of the articular surface.

The difference encountered with pronation-external rotation fractures is the amount of syndesmotic instability. After fixation of the fibula and repair of the anterior syndesmosis, the stability of the syndesmosis is checked by the hook test and by externally rotating the foot. In the hook test, a bone hook is used to grasp the fibula and pull it laterally while observing for opening of the syndesmosis. If the syndesmosis is unstable, a transyndesmotic screw is utilized. A stage III injury with an intact posterior syndesmosis will usually be stable after fixation of the fibula and repair of the anterior syndesmosis. However, a stage IV injury usually requires a transyndesmotic screw if there is a rupture of the posterior syndesmosis. If a large posterior malleolus fracture is present and fixated, then a transyndesmotic screw may not be necessary. If the posterior malleolus fracture is small, the broad attachment of the posterior syndesmosis may still be intact and stabilize the posterior aspect of the syndesmosis negating the need for a transyndesmotic screw. The transyndesmotic screw is utilized as a positional screw, so a cortical screw is utilized and tapped its full length to prevent compression. A cancellous screw or an overdrill lag technique with a cortical screw is not to be used. This is to prevent overtightening of the mortise, which could limit dorsiflexion, damage the articular facet on the lateral aspect of the tibia, or promote synostosis. Also, if a lag screw is utilized and it begins to back out, the reduction of the syndesmosis may be lost. The transyndesmotic screw is ideally placed 2 to 3 cm above the syndesmosis and should be oriented from posterolateral to anteromedial. It should be perpendicular to the long axis of the tibia and fibula. The foot should be in a neutral position or slightly dorsiflexed while

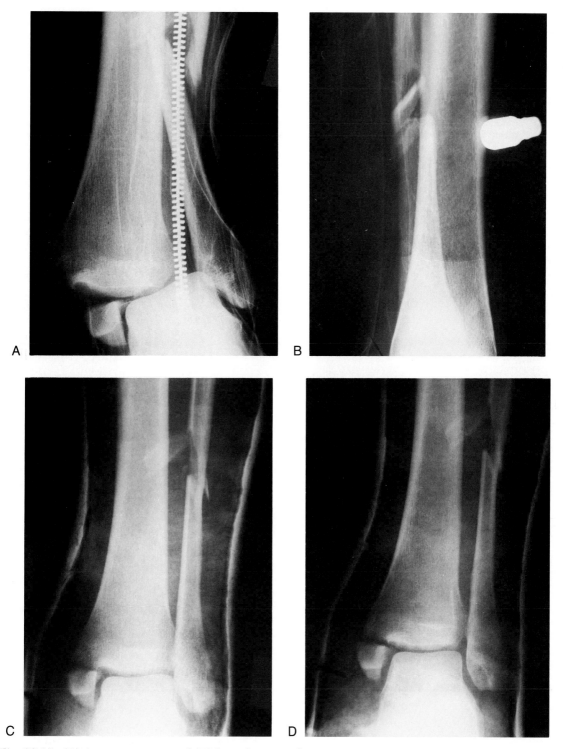

Fig. 28-12. **(A)** Anteroposterior and **(B)** lateral views of a pronation-external rotation stage IV fracture-dislocation demonstrating a comminuted fracture of the fibula above the syndesmosis, a diastasis, and a transverse fracture of the medial malleolus. **(C)** Anteroposterior, **(D)** mortise. (*Figure continues.*)

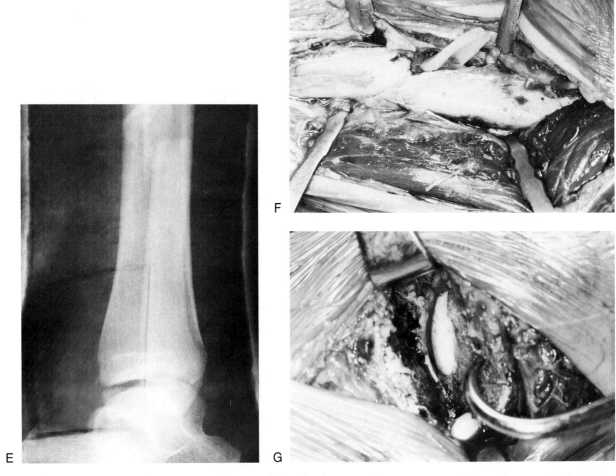

Fig. 28-12 (*Continued*). (**E**) Lateral views of closed reduction. The surgery was delayed because of skin complications. (**F**) Comminuted fibular fracture is visualized. (**G**) The medial malleolus is distracted inferiorly to reveal excoriations on the medial talar dome. (*Figure continues.*)

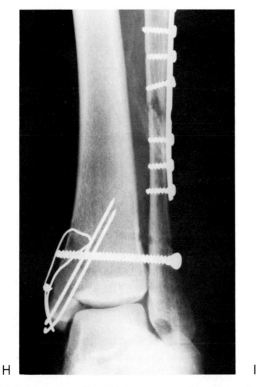
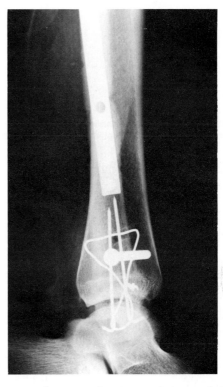

H   I

Fig. 28-12 (*Continued*). (**H**) Mortise and (**I**) lateral views of open reduction with internal fixation showing the fibula fixated in the usual manner while the medial malleolus has been fixated with a tension-band wire. A transyndesmotic screw has been employed to stabilize the distal tibia and fibula. A cancellous bone graft was harvested from the distal medial tibia and placed in the defect in the fibula.

the screw is being placed to prevent limitation of dorsiflexion. The transyndesmotic screw can be employed through a plate, below a plate, or as the only means of fibular fixation depending on the fracture configuration.

Fractures of the upper half of the fibula are reduced indirectly (Fig. 28-13). An incision is made about the anterolateral aspect of the ankle, and the distal fibular fragment is grasped with a bone reduction forceps with points. It is pulled to length and derotated. Provisional stabilization is obtained with a Kirschner-wire placed above the ankle joint, and radiographs are taken to confirm the reduction. If the reduction is anatomic, a transyndesmotic screw is placed and the Kirschner-wire is removed. A second set of radiographs are taken to confirm the reduction. I prefer to use a 4.5 mm cortical screw that engages four cortices (through both cortices in the fibula and tibia).

This prevents proximal migration of the fibula. Another technique is to use two 4.5-mm cortical screws and engage only three cortices (two in the fibula and the lateral cortex of the tibia). If the transyndesmotic screw is used through a plate, it needs to engage only three cortices as the plate will prevent proximal migration of the fibular fracture. One can use either 3.5- or 4.5-mm cortical screws. Willenegger, instead of screws, uses two Kirschner wires driven obliquely upward through the fibula into the tibia.[30] There is debate on which fixation technique is best, but the only absolutely wrong choice is to fixate a Maisonneuve fracture with a single cortical screw engaging only three cortices.

The posterior malleolus is reduced and fixated only if it represents 25 to 30 percent of the tibial articular surface as seen on the lateral radiograph (Fig. 28-14). Isolated fractures of the posterior

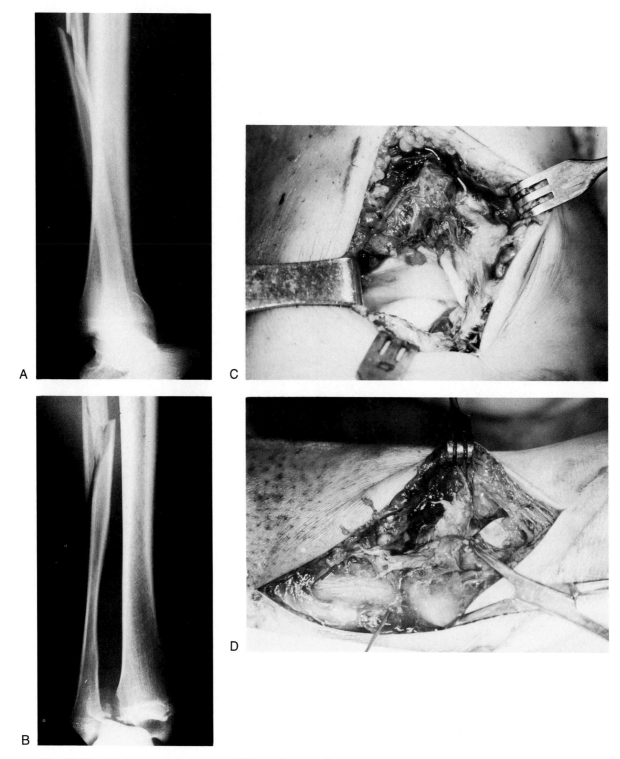

Fig. 28-13. (A) Anteroposterior and (B) lateral views demonstrating a comminuted high fibular fracture and a dislocation of the talus. There is a fracture of the posterior malleolus. (C) Rupture of both the superficial and deep portions of the deltoid ligament with lateral displacement of the talus. (D) The fibula is reduced indirectly with the aid of a towel clip and provisionally stabilized with a Kirschner wire followed by radiographs. (*Figure continues.*)

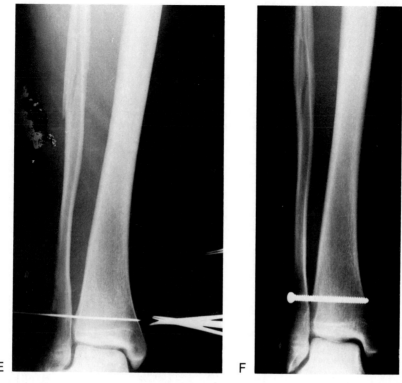

E   F

Fig. 28-13 (*Continued*). (**E**) Mortise view of reduction. (**F**) Mortise view of the final reduction and fixation.

malleolus do occur. At Fort Benning, this fracture is more common because of parachute training, in which soldiers land with their feet plantar flexed and have an axial loading force. The talus is pushed posteriorly and superiorly, fracturing the posterior malleolus. If the fracture is less than 25 percent of the tibial articular surface, treatment is a walking short leg cast for 4 to 6 weeks, even if the fracture is displaced. Displacement is usually minimal and in a superior direction. If the fracture is large and nondisplaced, treatment is a non-weight-bearing short leg cast with close radiographic follow-up. If large and displaced, the fracture is approached from a posteromedial incision behind the medial malleolus and reduced under direct visualization. The difficulty in this reduction is that the cortical margins are used for the reduction landmarks as the articular surface cannot be seen. Any comminution present makes the reduction difficult to evaluate. It is fixated with lag screws from anterior to pos-

terior through small anterior incisions. Either cortical or cancellous screws can be used. When placed from anterior to posterior, 3.5-mm cortical lag screws are preferred. This is because it is sometimes difficult to tell if the threads of a cancellous screw have completely crossed the fracture site. If the fracture extends along the entire posterior aspect of the tibia to include the medial malleolus, it is fixated through the posteromedial incision with 4.0-mm cancellous screws placed from posterior to anterior. If the reduction is not certain, it can be provisionally stabilized with Kirschner wires and radiographed prior to screw fixation. An alternative approach is from posterolateral behind the fibula, but this approach is difficult and offers no advantage.

More commonly, the posterior malleolus is part of a fracture complex (usually trimalleolar). In this case, the fibula is reduced and fixated first. This helps to reduce the posterior malleolus through the intact posterior syndesmosis. This

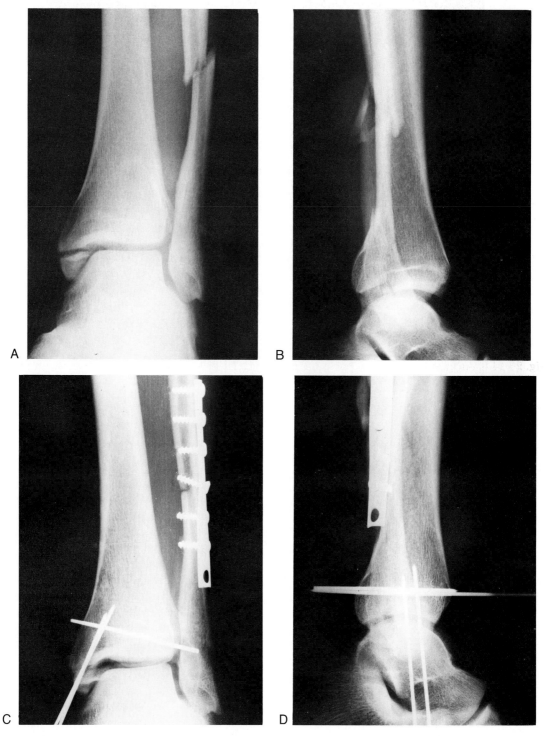

Fig. 28-14. (**A**) Mortise and (**B**) lateral views of a pronation-external rotation stage IV injury in which the posterior malleolus is large enough to require fixation. (**C**) Mortise and (**D**) lateral views of the initial reduction with the fibula reduced and fixated. The posterior malleolus and medial malleolus are reduced and provisionally stabilized. (*Figure continues.*)

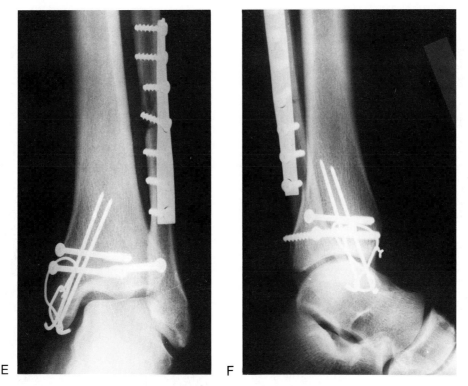

Fig. 28-14 (*Continued*). (**E**) Anteroposterior and (**F**) lateral views of the final reduction and fixation.

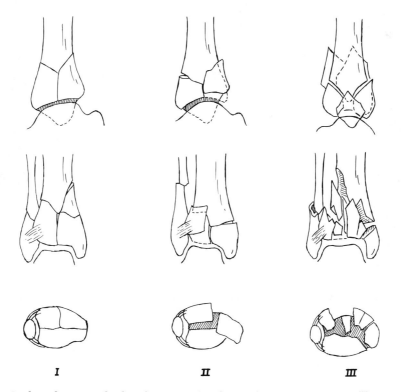

Fig. 28-15. AO classification of pilon fractures. (Redrawn from Mueller et al.,[57] with permission.)

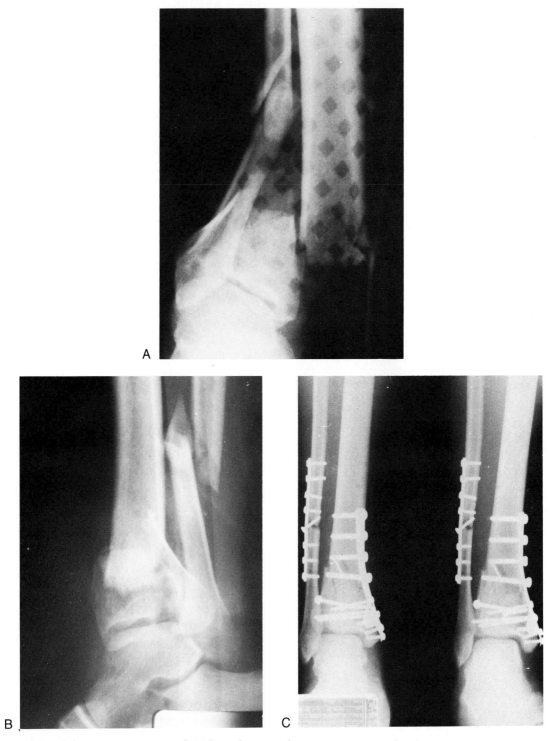

Fig. 28-16. **(A)** Anteroposterior and **(B)** lateral views of an open type III pilon fracture. **(C)** Anteroposterior and mortise views of open reduction with internal fixation.

reduction may not be anatomic, and any additional manipulation is done through the posteromedial incision. If a fractured medial malleolus is present, it can be distracted inferiorly, allowing direct visualization of the tibial articular surface for reduction of the posterior malleolus. The posterior malleolus may be provisionally stabilized with a Kirschner wire, and radiographs are obtained to confirm the reduction. If the reduction is anatomic, it can be fixated from anterior to posterior with a cortical lag screw, using the Kirschner wire as a guide. The Kirschner wire can be removed or left in place. If the fibular fracture is at the level of the syndesmosis, it is helpful to fixate the fibula initially with just a lag screw as a plate may obscure the posterior malleolus reduction on the lateral radiograph. After the position is confirmed, then the plate can be applied to the fibula and the medial injury addressed. A second set of radiographs are taken to assess the final reduction and fixation.

Pronation-Dorsiflexion Fractures

Pronation-dorsiflexion fractures are caused by high-velocity injuries and are the result of axial compression. Lauge-Hansen described four stages.[20–22] Stage I is a fracture of the medial malleolus. Stage II is a fracture of the anterior lip of the tibia. Stage III is a fracture of the supramalleolar part of the fibula. Stage IV is a fracture of the posterior tibia. In reality, this classification is not helpful. These injuries have been described as pilon fractures by the AO/ASIF group. This denotes a comminuted, intra-articular fracture of the distal tibia and fibula caused by the impaction of the talus. There are three types (Fig. 28-15). Type I is an intra-articular fracture of the distal tibia without significant articular incongruity. Type II is an intra-articular fracture of the distal tibia with significant articular incongruity. Type III is an intra-articular fracture of the distal tibia with displacement of the weight-bearing cancellous segments of the metaphysis (Fig. 28-16). These injuries are extremely complex and require great skill in their treatment. Treatment options include closed reduction and cast therapy, calcaneal pin traction, limited open reduc-

tion with internal fixation with or without the use of an external fixator, and open reduction with internal fixation. If open reduction with internal fixation is undertaken, the steps are as follows: (1) reconstruction of the fibula; (2) reconstruction of the distal tibial articular surface, using the talus as a template with provisional Kirschner-wire fixation; (3) cancellous bone graft; and (4) application of a buttress plate to the medial aspect of the tibia to prevent late varus deformity. Postoperatively, weight bearing must be delayed for 3 months to allow fracture consolidation.

DANIS-WEBER (AO) CLASSIFICATION

The Danis-Weber (AO) classification is divided into type A, type B, and type C, depending on the level of the fibular fracture (see Fig. 28-2). Type A is the fracture of the fibula below the level of the syndesmosis. It is usually transverse, and no instability of the syndesmosis occurrs. It may be associated with a superiorly oriented fracture of the medial malleolus. Type A represents the supination-adduction fracture pattern. Type B is the fracture of the fibula at the level of the syndesmosis. It may be spiral or oblique and indicates partial instability of the syndesmosis. It may be associated with a ruptured deltoid ligament or a fractured medial malleolus. Type B represents the supination-external rotation and most of the pronation-abduction fractures. Type C is the fracture of the fibula above the level of the syndesmosis. It always is associated with medial injury and has complete instability of the syndesmosis. It represents the Lauge-Hansen pronation-external rotation fractures.

EVALUATION OF THE TRAUMATIZED PATIENT

The usual course for a traumatized patient is to report to the nearest hospital emergency room. If the patient is brought by ambulance, the patient is usually evaluated at the injury site by an emergency medical technician and fractures are splinted. Injuries that occur at Fort Benning are usually initially evaluated by a medic, and patients are transported to our hospital by ground ambulance or helicopter. The patient is evaluated by the emergency room physician upon arrival at the hospital. If stable, the patient is sent for the appropriate radiographs. It is only after the emergency room physician reviews the radiographs that specialty consultation is called for. Since the majority of our patients have ankle fractures as their only injury, this is when we first see the patient. If the patient is polytraumatized, the emergency room physician may call for multiple specialty consults after the initial evaluation and while attempting to stabilize the patient to prevent shock. Life-threatening injuries to the head, chest, and abdomen must be evaluated and treated first. This is most commonly done by a general or trauma surgeon, who is the admitting physician. If there are multiple long bone fractures or fracture-dislocations, an orthopedic surgeon may be responsible for the overall care of the patient. Radiographs and other diagnostic tests, such as an abdominal tap, are performed in the emergency room while the patient is stabilized with fluids and packed blood cells. In consultation, the priority of the injuries must be established and a treatment plan formulated. Second priority goes to limb-threatening injuries and open fractures. Orthopedically, there is greater emphasis today on immediately fixating all major fractures as this may be the best shape the patient will be in for some time. Immediate fixation will allow mobilization of the patient, which will help prevent complications such as adult respiratory distress syndrome. Also, with open fractures or large skin defects, wound care can be made easier. Consequently, a thorough knowledge of the team approach to patient care is critical.

If the patient has an isolated ankle fracture, the extremity is usually splinted, iced, and elevated in the emergency room prior to evaluation. A thorough history is taken but rarely gives much useful information. The most common cause of ankle fractures at our institution is parachute training, followed by motor vehicle accidents, sports, and falls. The patient usually cannot remember the exact mechanism of injury, but some indication can be obtained of the level of violence. A complete physical examination is performed from head to toe to rule out potential life-threatening or other occult injuries. With this accomplished, the injured ankle is evaluated after the splint is removed. First, look for gross deformity, which indicates fracture-dislocation. It is rare to dislocate the ankle without fracture. Since most fractures are caused by external rotation, the foot is usually externally rotated with dislocations, sometimes up to 90 degrees. Also, inspection will reveal whether the fracture is closed or open. Considering how superficial the malleoli are, it is amazing that the percentage of open fracture is not higher. The Mayo Clinic reports an incidence of 4 percent.[1] The St. Gallen study showed open fractures in 25 of 803 ankle fractures for an incidence of 3.11 percent.[15] Next, the neurovascular status distal to the injury is evaluated. A fracture-dislocation has the potential for neurovascular embarrassment, and open fractures can transect a neurovascular element. Then, a very careful examination is performed, palpating from the knee to the toes to discover any concomitant injury. Palpation of the proximal fibula helps to rule out a Maisonneuve fracture. If there is an open fracture, a sterile dressing is applied and the patient is prepared for surgery. Patients with obvious open fractures may go straight from the emergency room to surgery, where the actual evaluation is performed in a sterile environment. In a closed fracture, careful palpation is made of the malleoli and ligaments. Attempted range of motion of the ankle is usually limited by pain and muscular splinting. Stress testing of the ankle, if indicated, is not performed until the radiographs are examined. Only after a thorough evaluation of the patient are the radiographs reviewed. If there is a question about a possible fracture on the radiograph, the patient can be evaluated again in regard to bony tenderness. It is important to correlate physical findings with the radiographs. An example would be a radiograph with a spiral fracture of the fibula at the level of the syndesmosis without obvious subluxation of the talus, perhaps indicating a supination-external rotation stage II fracture. However, clinical examination reveals deltoid ligament tenderness, indicating that the injury is really a stage IV fracture, which is more serious and unstable. This situation could be confirmed by stress external rotation testing.

Radiographic evaluation of any fracture requires a minimum of three views. The standard ankle views are the anteroposterior, mortise, and lateral. The anteroposterior view allows excellent study of the medial and lateral malleoli. It allows an assessment of the medial clear space between the medial malleolus and talus as well as the superior joint space between the tibia and the talar dome. These two joint spaces should be equidistant. The distance between the medial malleolus and the talus should not exceed 3 to 4 mm. If it does, there is disruption of the deltoid ligament with lateral talar subluxation.[1] The distal tibia and fibula in this view overlap, obscuring the lateral clear space between the lateral malleolus and the talus as well as the syndesmosis. A large posterior malleolus fracture may be visualized along the tibial metaphysis. Dislocations and subluxations are usually obvious. Osteochondral fractures within the joint space should also be looked for.

The mortise view is a specialized oblique view with the ankle internally rotated about 15 to 20 degrees. However, this is not a hard and fast rule. One should attempt to internally rotate the leg until the malleoli are parallel to the x-ray cassette. Once again, one sees the medial and lateral malleolar contour well. In this projection, all three joint spaces can be evaluated. Also, the syndesmosis can be analyzed for diastasis or bony avulsion. At times, this view may give the best indication of lateral talar subluxation. Dislocations are usually obvious. Again, look for a posterior malleolus fracture or osteochondral fractures within the joint. Additional oblique views, either internally or externally rotated, can be made to better visualize specific areas of the ankle. Specifically, the external oblique view (externally rotated 45 to 55 degrees) can be used to look for fractures of the anterior or posterior tibial lip and syndesmosis. The lateral view usually allows the best view of the fibular fracture configuration, especially if it is spiral. Also, a butterfly fragment may be visualized that is usually seen in pronation-external rotation fractures. This is the best view to visualize fractures of the anterior and posterior tibial lip. It will demonstrate anterior or posterior subluxation-dislocation of the talus. Although the fibula and tibia are superimposed, a medial malleolar fracture may be seen.

Radiographs of the leg, both anteroposterior and lateral views, may be obtained to rule out proximal fibular fractures. If there is a fractured medial malleolus or lateral talar subluxation on ankle films without a fibular fracture, a Maisonneuve fracture must be ruled out. Besides a Maisonneuve fracture, there can be a subluxation-dislocation of the fibular head or plastic deformation of the fibula. Radiographs of the foot are taken if indicated, requiring the dorsoplantar, oblique, and lateral views. An unusual fracture pattern may require the use of tomograms or a CT scan to help clarify the fracture pattern.

Stress radiographs can be useful in ankle fractures. They can be performed with supination-adduction fractures to test the fibular collateral ligaments. I find this unnecessary as their integrity can be detected clinically after the patient is anesthetized and confirmed intraoperatively as previously described. Another possible use of stress radiographs is to distinguish between a stage II and stage IV supination-external rotation fracture. Here one is attempting to detect a deltoid ligament rupture by observing lateral talar subluxation, which is indicated by an increased medial clear space on external rotation stress testing as described by Kleiger.[36] The integrity of the deltoid ligament and syndesmosis can be tested in a similar fashion for pronation injuries. In pronation injuries, if a fibular fracture is present, there should be little question that a deltoid ligament rupture has taken place if the radiographs show no medial malleolar fracture. Therefore, one should not need stress radiographs in this case. However, in stage II of both pronation injury mechanisms, it is possible to have a completely ligamentous injury that can produce subluxation (Fig. 28-17). If the pronation-abduction stage II injury has ruptured all three syndesmotic ligaments, lateral subluxation of the talus would be present on both stress abduction and stress external rotation testing. In pronation-external rotation stage II injuries, stress abduction will produce no talar subluxation, while stress external rotation will. This is because both the ante-

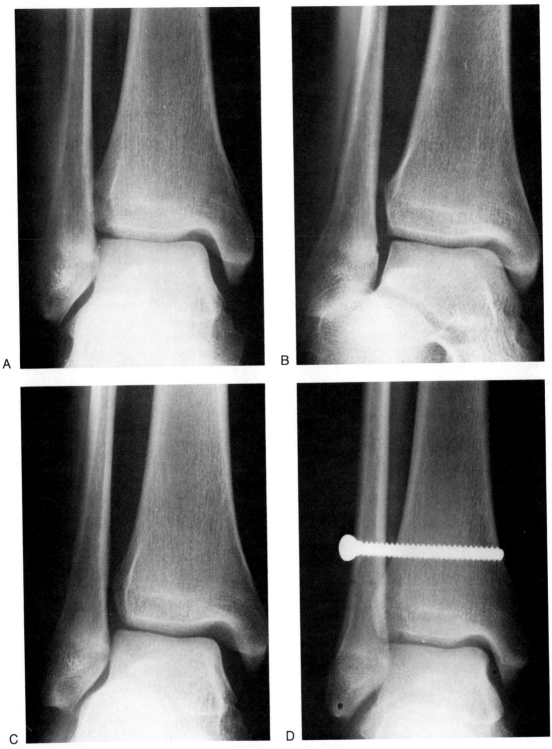

Fig. 28-17. (**A**) Anteroposterior and (**B**) mortise views of ankle injury with no apparent fracture from a parachute jump. On the mortise view there appears to be an increased distance between the distal tibia and fibula. (**C**) Stress external rotation view demonstrating lateral talar subluxation and diastasis. (**D**) Open reduction and internal fixation with transyndesmotic screw.

rior syndesmosis and the interosseous ligament are ruptured while the posterior syndesmosis remains intact. The problem is that a pronation-abduction stage II injury in which only the anterior and posterior syndesmoses are ruptured may produce the same findings because it has been demonstrated that a transected anterior syndesmosis can allow 1 to 2 mm of lateral talar displacement on external rotation even with an intact deltoid ligament.[7]

CLOSED REDUCTION

The best time to reduce a fractured ankle is as soon as possible after the injury. However, sometimes there is severe edema that precludes a reduction attempt until several days later. In this case, the ankle is placed in a modified compressive dressing (cast padding and elastic bandages) and an AO splint or short leg cast. The patient remains at bed rest with the extremity iced and well elevated. When the edema decreases, a closed reduction is attempted. The exception is a fracture-dislocation, which requires immediate reduction to prevent neurovascular embarrassment. Sedation is important for closed manipulation and can be administered either intramuscularly or intravenously. For intravenous sedation, 10 mg of diazepam followed by 100 mg of meperidine is routinely given. Both can cause respiratory depression and arrest, so care must be exercised. If sedation is given intramuscularly, 100 mg of meperidine is used. Other investigators have indicated the necessity of general anesthesia to accomplish an acceptable reduction.[1,7] If a fracture-dislocation is present, it is reduced by having the patient lie supine on the stretcher with the injured extremity over the edge flexed 90 degrees at the knee. Countertraction is applied by an assistant slowly pulling up on the thigh. The foot is manipulated by increasing the deformity followed by the application of longitudinal traction until the talus is pulled below the tibial plafond. At this point the foot is reduced in a direction opposite the injury mechanism. Since external rotation is the main injury mechanism, the foot is inverted and internally rotated. The

short leg cast is applied as described previously with a modified Charnley mold. The reduction maneuvers have been previously explained. The major principle of closed reduction is to reverse the original mechanism of injury. Consequently, a working knowledge of the Lauge-Hansen classification is indispensible.

If one decides to treat a fracture conservatively, it is imperative that radiographs be obtained weekly until there is no longer the danger of loss of reduction. If the fracture is unstable, an initial period of non-weight bearing is used. Cast treatment requires meticulous application of plaster and close follow-up. Multiple cast changes may be necessary as the edema subsides. The cast is also changed to position the foot in a neutral position at about 3 weeks if an exaggerated reduction position was initially necessary. A knowledge of cast therapy is important because not all patients are surgical candidates, even if they have a fracture that usually requires operative intervention. The patient's general medical condition or local skin conditions may preclude surgery. The goal of closed reduction is still to obtain as close to an anatomic reduction as possible (Fig. 28-18).

There is no universal agreement of what constitutes an acceptable reduction. Yablon et al. published their criteria for an acceptable closed reduction (Table 28-2).[7] This is in agreement with several other researchers. Joy et al. published an article on the evaluation of ankle fracture reduction and gave their radiographic assessment (Table 28-3).[37] Additionally, they indicated that a vertical line drawn down the center of the tibia should pass through the center of the talus on both the anteroposterior and mortise views. If it does not, then some shift, either medial or lateral, must be present in the talus. On the lateral view, a line drawn down the center of the tibia should pass through the most superior part of the talar dome. If it does not, the talus is either anteriorly or posteriorly displaced. They also indicated that a good reduction should have 0.5 mm or less of talar tilt. Denham has indicated that if the joint spaces are measured, they should differ by less than 2 mm.[31] Hamilton believes that the medial joint space is normally 3 to 4 mm and that anything greater than 4 mm indicates

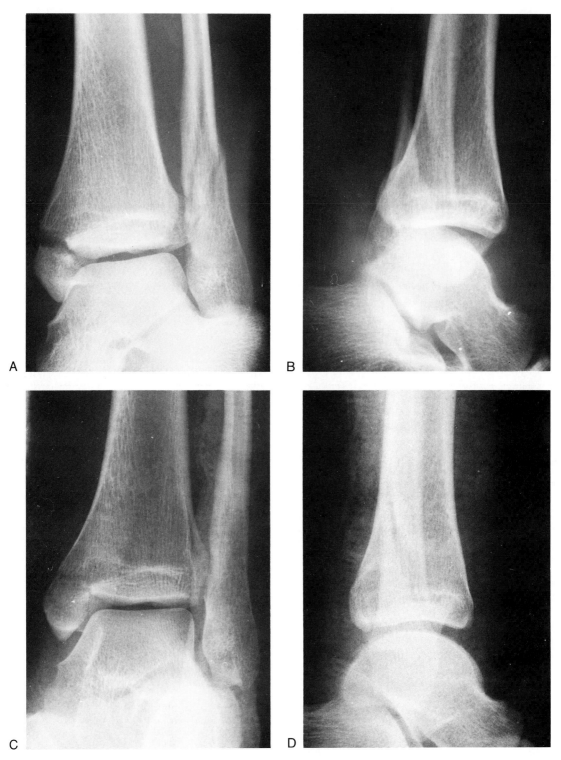

Fig. 28-18. (**A**) Mortise and (**B**) lateral views of a supination-external rotation stage IV fracture. (**C**) Mortise and (**D**) lateral views of closed reduction.

Table 28-2.   Closed Reduction Criteria

	Good	Fair	Poor
Lateral malleolus	Up to 1 mm of displacement in any direction Mortise widening ≤0.5 mm and talar tilt ≤0.5 mm	2–5 mm of displacement in any direction Mortise widening ≤2 mm and talar tilt ≤1.0 mm	>5 mm of displacement in any direction Mortise widening >2 mm and talar tilt >1.0 mm
Medial malleolus (at or above plafond)	≤2 of displacement in any direction Mortise widening ≤0.5 mm and talar tilt ≤0.5 mm	2–5 mm of displacement Mortise widening ≤2 mm and talar tilt ≤1.0 mm	Angulation rotation and displacement >5 mm Mortise widening >2 mm and talar tilt >1.0 mm
Medial malleolus (distal to plafond)	<2 mm of displacement laterally May be up to 5 mm of displacement in any other direction	≥2 mm of displacement laterally ≥5 mm of displacement in other direction	
Posterior malleolus	Posterior malleolus fracture ≤25% Proximal displacement <2 mm Mortise widening ≤0.5 mm and talar tilt ≤0.5 mm	Posterior malleolus fracture ≤25% Proximal displacement 2–5 mm Mortise widening ≤2 mm and talar tilt ≤1.0 mm	Posterior malleolus fracture >25% Proximal displacement >5 mm Mortise widening >2 mm and talar tilt >1.0 mm
Talus	Talar displacement ≤0.5 mm in any direction Talar tilt ≤0.5 mm	Talar displacement ≤2 mm Talar tilt ≤1.0 mm	Talar displacement >2 mm Talar tilt >1.0 mm

Table 28-3.   Criteria for Acceptable Closed Reduction

Score		Reduction Result
Good	Medial malleolus	Normal up to 2 mm of anterior, posterior, or distal displacement, if fracture is less than 3 mm distal to the plafond. Up to 5 mm of anterior, posterior, or distal displacement, if fracture is more than 3 mm distal to the plafond.
	Lateral malleolus	Up to 2 mm of displacement in any direction.
	Posterior malleolus	Not more than 2 mm in any direction.
	Talus	0.5 mm or less of talar tilt with other displacement of the talus less than 0.5 mm.
Fair	Medial malleolus	Anterior, posterior, or distal displacement of 2–5 mm if fracture is less than 3 mm distal to the plafond.
	Lateral malleolus	Displacement of 2–5 mm with medial, lateral, anterior, or posterior shift of the talus up to 1 mm.
	Other	Minimum or questionable joint damage noted on the radiograph or at surgery.
Poor		Any value worse than above. Any lateral tilt or shift of the medial malleolar fragment. Any definite axial rotation of the medial malleolar fragment. Severe joint damage. Any shift of the talus of more than 1 mm as measured by the weight-bearing line or medial clear space. Any tilt of the talus greater than 0.5 mm.

lateral subluxation of the talus and deltoid ligament rupture.[1] The tibia should overlap the fibula at the syndesmosis by 10 mm on the anteroposterior view. If it does not, then a diastasis exists. Lauge-Hansen has shown the inaccuracies of this measurement because it depends on the amount of rotation of the leg and the variability of the shape of the distal tibia.[1] I agree with this point and believe that a diastasis is best diagnosed by having an exact mortise view comparing both ankles and correlating it with the Lauge-Hansen classification. Because the talus will follow the fibula through the intact fibular collateral ligaments, an associated increase in the medial clear space should occur with diastasis. Ramsey and Hamilton have demonstrated that 1 mm of lateral talar displacement in the mortise reduces the contact area of the ankle joint 42 percent.[38] Reide et al. demonstrated experimentally that 2 mm of lateral displacement of the fibula can result in a 1 to 2 mm of lateral talar subluxation along with 1 to 2 degrees of talar external rotation, decreasing the contact between the tibia and talus by 51 percent.[39] Sarkisian and Cody measured the talocural angle, which is the intersection of a line drawn along the tibial articular surface and a line drawn between the tips of the malleoli.[40] They found that a variation of 2 degrees when compared with the uninjured ankle indicated significant displacement of the fibula in length or rotation and resulted in a greater rate of arthrosis. From the above discussion, it is easy to understand the importance of restoring both the correct length and rotation to the fibula.

TREATMENT CONSIDERATIONS

Deciding how to treat a specific fracture encompasses many factors. The fracture pattern, general health of the patient, local skin conditions, needs of the patient, and the capabilities of the surgeon are just some of these factors. The end results of treatment with either closed or open treatment have basically related to the adequacy of reduction.[41] Malka and Tillard found that open reduction gave an anatomic reduction in 80 to 85 percent of fractures, while closed treatment produced only 56 percent anatomic reductions.[42] They also reported that pronation-external rotation injuries gave the worst results regardless of treatment. Klossner observed 167 patients treated with closed reduction and had 65 percent good results.[43] Kristensen reported on 70 patients, with 64 percent good results obtained with cast treatment.[44] Cretskaja reported 60 percent good results with open reduction of 88 fractures.[15] Willenegger obtained 81 percent good results with operative treatment using rigid internal fixation.[30,45] Cedell[26,27] compared his results of 100 supination-external rotation fractures with those of Magnussen,[25] who used closed reduction techniques in 209 patients. Cedell had an arthrosis rate of 23 percent, and Magnussen had a rate of 49.8 percent. Bauer et al. have reported that ankle fractures are becoming more common and that there is a trend toward the more severe injuries.[46,47] This is especially marked in the supination-external rotation fractures, with stage IV increasing mainly in elderly women. Pronation injuries have shown only a slight increase. They found that 30 percent of patients had residual symptoms of discomfort more than 5 years after injury. Klossner reported a 27 percent rate of discomfort,[43] while Magnussen reported 33 percent.[25] In the fractures that Klossner treated with surgery, his rate was 28 percent,[43] while Cedell reported 27 percent.[26] Bauer et al. also showed that better anatomic results were obtained with operative reduction.[47,48] The operatively treated group had a more rapid decrease in edema and regained motion more rapidly. However, at an average of 7 years, traumatic arthritis was comparable between the treatment alternatives for similar type B fractures.

OPERATIVE TREATMENT

If surgical intervention is elected, then anything less than an anatomic reduction must be considered a failure. The principles of the AO/ASIF group are (1) atraumatic soft tissue technique, (2) anatomic reduction, (3) rigid internal fixation, and (4) early mobilization of the extremity. Additionally, surgery allows the evaluation of articular surfaces and the removal of osteochondral fractures. Operative treatment prevents loss of reduction, the necessity of remanipulation, and the need to immobilize the foot in an unphysiologic position and decreases the time of immobilization.[49] The goal of rigid internal fixation is to produce primary bone union, that is, bony union without the presence of callus. This is accomplished by using lag screws to obtain interfragmental compression, which prevents microscopic motion at the fracture site. At times, the lag screws need to be protected by one-third tubular plates for neutralization. The tension-band wire also creates interfragmental compression. Consequently, a thorough knowledge of AO technique is mandatory to obtain the above-stated principles.

The patient is given prophylactic antibiotics intravenously prior to surgery. A cephalosporin is utilized unless the patient has a documented allergy to penicillin, in which case vancomycin may be substituted. The antibiotics are continued for 24 hours postoperatively. The extremity is prepared and draped in the usual sterile manner. A rolled sheet is placed under the ipsilateral hip to internally rotate the leg and to facilitate access to the fibula. A pneumatic tourniquet is used for hemostasis and is applied at the midthigh level.

The fractures are approached through incisions illustrated in Figure 28-19. The anterolateral incision is used for exposure of the fibula and the anterior syndesmosis and for observing the lateral joint space. The posterolateral incision is used if the one-third tubular plate is to be applied to the posterior aspect of the fibula. The anteromedial hockey stick-shaped incision is used routinely to expose the medial malleolus, deltoid ligament, or medial aspect of the joint space. The posteromedial incision is used for large posterior malleolar fractures as well as fractures off the posterior aspect of the medial malleolus. The fractures are reduced anatomically and rigidly fixated as previously described. It is important that the internal fixation is adapted to the individual fracture pattern. The appropriate ligaments are primarily repaired. Intraoperative radiographs are always obtained to assess the quality of the reduction and to confirm the position of the internal fixation. This can be performed with a standard x-ray machine or an image intensifier. The image intensifier is faster but does not give good detail for finding osteochondral fractures or alignment of comminuted cortical margins. A suction drain is placed in the incision prior to closure. The tourniquet is not released until after the wound is closed and a dressing has been ap-

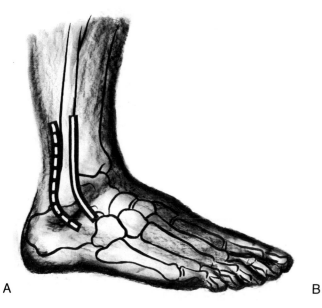

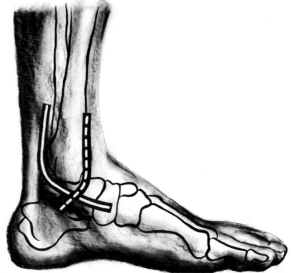

A   B

Fig. 28-19. **(A & B)** Surgical approaches to ankle fractures.

plied. If the tourniquet has been inflated for 2 hours, it is released and hemostasis is accomplished prior to closure. At the termination of surgery the patient is placed in an AO splint. However, if cartilaginous damage has occurred, the patient may be placed on a continuous passive motion machine. The suction drain is usually removed in 24 to 48 hours. The dressing is changed at 48 to 72 hours, and the patient begins active and passive range of motion exercises under physical therapy control. The goal is to regain motion that is equal to that of the uninjured ankle. At 7 days the sutures are removed and the incisions are reinforced with adhesive strips. The patient is subsequently placed in a weight-bearing short leg cast for approximately 4 to 5 weeks. If a transyndesmotic screw was used, then the short leg cast is non-weight bearing. An alternative is a splint or fracture brace, but the patient must not bear weight. This will allow the patient to remove the splint and perform range of motion exercises. There is a difference of opinion as to whether the patient should be kept non-weight bearing, but I prefer weight bearing whenever possible. Usually, primary bone union has occurred by 6 weeks, which will allow the patient to start unprotected weight bearing with the support of an elastic bandage. Physical therapy is instituted again. If a transyndesmotic screw was used, it is removed at 6 to 8 weeks under local anesthesia in a minor surgery room. When a transyndesmotic screw was used to fixate a Maisonneuve fracture, it is removed at 8 weeks.

OPEN ANKLE FRACTURES

Considering the subcutaneous position of the malleoli, it is surprising that the percentage of open ankle fractures is not higher. Obviously, open fractures increase the seriousness of any fracture with the risk of infection. This may lead to nonunion or to an infected nonunion. Also, the treatment of open fractures evokes great debate, especially regarding the placement of internal fixation.[1,50–53]

I utilize the classification of Gustilo and Anderson,[52] which is based on the length of the wound and the degree of associated soft tissue trauma. Type I is an open fracture with a wound of less than 1 cm. Type II is an open fracture with a wound greater than 1 cm without extensive soft tissue damage. Type III is an open fracture with extensive soft tissue damage, extensive skin flaps or skin loss, extensive contamination, bony comminution, and neurovascular injury. Obviously, the greater the severity of the wound, the higher the risk of infection. Gustilo and Anderson reported infection rates of 1 percent for type I injuries, 7 percent for type II injuries, and 44 percent for type III injuries.[52]

All open fractures are surgical emergencies and require debridement as soon as possible. After a thorough history and physical examination, the patient is transported to the operating room. The dressing is removed and cultures are obtained. After cultures are taken, therapeutic antibiotics are begun intravenously. The choice for type I and II injuries is a cephalosporin. If a type III fracture is present, the cephalosporin is supplemented with an aminoglycoside to provide gram-negative coverage. There is a difference of opinion as to the length of antibiotic coverage. I give antibiotics for 48 to 72 hours. The antibiotics and surgical debridement are best accomplished in the 6 to 8-hour "golden period," while the wound is contaminated but not infected. The debridement is the most important factor in the treatment of open fractures. Debridement is an art, with conservation of skin and bone but aggressive excision of dead adipose tissue and muscle. Part of the debridement process is copious irrigation with up to 5 to 10 liters of fluid.

The most controversial aspect in the treatment of open fractures is the implantation of metallic fixation devices.[1,51,54] Presently, type I and II open fractures are internally fixated at the initial debridement. In some type III open fractures, internal fixation may be used on a delayed basis at times. Franklin et al. have advocated a protocol that all ankle fractures should be internally fixated at the initial debridement regardless of type.[54] The greatest challenge is a type III open fracture of the ankle in which rigid internal fixation is not possible. In this case, an external fixator, stabilization with Kirschner wires, or a Steinmann pin driven through the calcaneus and talus into the tibia are alternatives. Elective incisions made at the time of the debridement are closed, but the area where the bone penetrated the skin is left open. Some type II and all type III open fractures have a second debridement in 48 hours. Additional debridements are performed as required. If the fracture was not internally fixated initially, delayed fixation is performed in 5 to 7 days at the time of the delayed primary closure. If a delayed closure cannot be performed, then a split-thickness skin graft is applied when the recipient site is ready. As stated above, the antibiotics are discontinued in 48 to 72 hours. If the wound then becomes infected, new cultures are taken and a new course of antibiotics is initiated along with incision and drainage. Antibiotic coverage is instituted on any return to the operating room. As with closed fractures, range of motion exercises are begun as soon as feasible after the operation.

COMPLICATIONS

The major complication of closed reduction and cast therapy is the failure to obtain an anatomic reduction. However, if an acceptable position is obtained, a second complication is loss of reduction. Consequently, close radiographic follow-up is mandatory. If loss of reduction occurs, the fracture can be remanipulated or surgically reduced and fixated. If the foot is held for a long period of time in an extreme position to maintain the reduction, it may be difficult to regain full motion. Cast treatment has been implicated with fracture disease (soft tissue atrophy, edema, osteoporosis, and restricted motion).

Another possible complication of closed treatment, at least initially, is compartment syndrome. This is an uncommon occurrence with ankle fractures, but it does happen. A compartment syndrome is an increase in the pressure within a closed osteofascial compartment. It can occur because of the external compression of the cast or an increase in the intracompartmental pressure of the leg. Since the first 3 days postinjury is the period of maximum edema, this is the time for close observation. Signs of a compartment syn-

drome are (1) pain out of proportion to the injury; (2) sensory changes, first subjective then objective; (3) muscular weakness; and (4) pain on passive motion of the digits. Pulses and capillary refill are poor indicators as they are usually normal in a compartment syndrome. The individual compartments that are involved will be tender and tense. What, therefore, makes this entity so difficult to diagnose? The fracture itself causes pain, and patients vary greatly in their ability to handle this pain. Sensory changes can occur from the edema alone or from direct contusion to a nerve at the time of injury. Patients may have muscular weakness and difficulty moving their toes because the tendons are gliding over fractured malleoli. The same rationale applies for pain elicited on passive movement of the toes. Another problem in diagnosis is that a compartment syndrome is slowly progressive. Thus, one must have a high index of suspicion and closely monitor patients at risk. The most common compartment syndrome is that of the anterior tibial compartment. The second most common in the leg is the deep posterior tibial compartment. However, any leg compartment can be involved.

The first goal of treatment is to recognize the syndrome. Initially, the cast should be monovalved or bivalved, including cutting the cast padding. The extremity is placed level in the bed since elevation decreases the arterial pressure. Sometimes, this is enough to prevent the compartment syndrome. One problem is that a precarious reduction may be lost when the cast is cut. If the compartment syndrome progresses, then decompression by fasciotomy is mandatory. If the diagnosis cannot be made from clinical presentation, then the intracompartmental pressure may be checked. Normally, the intracompartmental pressure is from 0 to 4 mmHg. Fasciotomy should be performed if the pressure is in the 30 to 40 mmHg range. The fasciotomy must be performed within 4 to 12 hours, or permanent neuromuscular damage will occur. I prefer a two-incision approach, with one incision anterolateral and the other posteromedial. All four compartments of the leg are released regardless of involvement. Others have advocated a one-incision parafibular approach. Fasciotomy, if in time, will resolve the compartment syndrome but presents new problems. It can convert a closed fracture to one that is open, and skin closure is difficult. Skin closure can be accomplished by delayed primary closure, progressive closure with adhesive strips, or split-thickness skin graft.

Closed treatment can result in nonunions, particularly of the medial malleolus (Fig. 28-20). This will occur in 4 to 18 percent of cases and is usually the result of periosteum becoming entrapped within the fracture site[1,41,55] If the nonunion is asymptomatic, no treatment is necessary. If symptomatic and small, the fragment can be excised. If the nonunion is large and symptomatic, a cortical window is cut across the nonunion site. The site is curetted, cancellous bone is brought down from the distal tibial metaphysis, and the cortical window is either slid down across the nonunion or it is rotated 180 degrees. Finally, the medial malleolus is internally fixated with either 4.0-mm cancellous screws or a tension-band wire. It may be difficult to obtain an anatomic reduction if the nonunion is displaced. Nonunion of the fibula is extremely rare and would be treated in a similar manner with fixation appropriate for the nonunion configuration, and a cancellous bone graft without a cortical component.

Nonunions have been divided into two types, hypertrophic and atrophic. The hypertrophic type is vascular with evidence of osteogenic activity and only requires stability to heal. The atrophic type is avascular with no evidence of healing and requires not only stability but also a bone graft to heal. The medial malleolar nonunion represents an atrophic type, but it is difficult to say this about the lateral malleolus as this is such an uncommon problem.

Besides nonunion, malunion of ankle fractures is another complication that can occur. Although it is more commonly associated with the closed treatment of fractures, it can also occur with surgery. A malunion will change the joint mechanics, resulting in traumatic arthritis. Malunion can occur to any of the malleoli, and attempting to correct the position is difficult. Any incongruity of the ankle joint is of great concern, including even small amounts of fibular rotation or shortening. One specific type of malunion that has received some attention recently is the sprung mortise as described by Weber.[56] This is the malunion of the fibula with an associated lateral talar subluxation (Fig. 28-21). The shortened and rotated malalignment prevents the fibula from sitting in the syndesmosis properly, producing lateral talar subluxation as the talus follows the fibula. Weber[56] recommended fibular osteotomy to correct this problem. A transverse fibular osteotomy is performed through the malunion. A dynamic compression plate is applied to the fibula along with an articulated tension device. This device can distract or compress the osteotomy. The distal fibular fragment is distracted to achieve length. It is also internally rotated to fit into the syndesmosis. A bone graft from the distal tibia is placed into the osteotomy site, and the articulated tension device is now used to compress the osteotomy. The plate is then rigidly secured to the fibula. This procedure has been recommended when there is no evidence of arthritic changes.

Complications of operative treatment are many. The inability to obtain an anatomic reduction or rigid internal fixation are just two. Of the two, lack of an anatomic reduction predisposes to traumatic arthritis along with all the inherent risks of an operation. This is the worst of all possible circumstances. There are several reasons why this could occur. Highly comminuted fractures may defy reduction because of loss of bony landmarks. The only way to handle this situation is to provisionally stabilize the fragments with Kirschner wires and take radiographs to confirm the position prior to final fixation. An anatomic reduction may be prevented by the entrapment of soft tissue or osteochondral fractures within the joint space. This is especially true of the deltoid ligament, which can become entrapped in the medial joint space, preventing repositioning of the talus even though the fibula is anatomically reduced. An anatomic reduction of the ankle is usually not possible if the medial malleolus is fixated but the fibula is not (Fig. 28-21). Fixation of only the medial malleolus was, at one time, traditional orthopedic teaching. Last, the talus can subluxate if a transyndesmotic screw is not used when indicated or it is used inappropriately. The inability to obtain rigid internal fixation can occur in comminuted fractures, when bony loss is present, and in elderly patients with

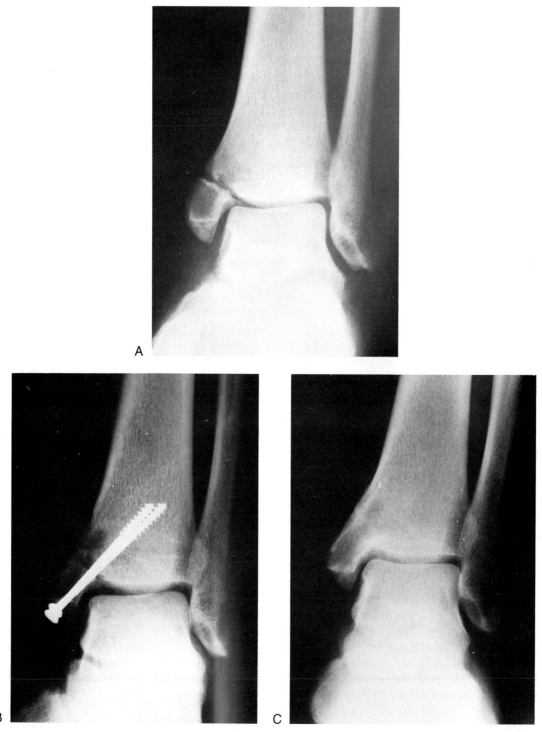

Fig. 28-20. (**A**) Mortise view of nonunion of the medial malleolus. (**B**) Surgical repair with curettage of nonunion site and tibial bone graft through a cortical window that was rotated 180 degrees followed by screw fixation. (**C**) Approximately 2 years postoperation with screws removed and nonunion healed.

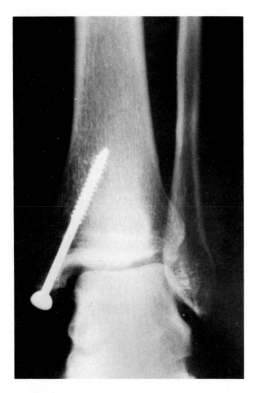

Fig. 28-21. Anteroposterior view of ankle fracture surgically repaired at another institution. The medial malleolus was fixated with a 4.5-mm malleolar screw, but the fibula was not fixated. Note the malunion of the fibula with residual talar subluxation producing a sprung mortise. This problem will require a fibular osteotomy.

severe osteoporosis. In these circumstances, a fractured medial malleolus might require the use of a tension-band wire instead of screws. A one-third tubular plate can be placed along the posterior aspect of the fibula in an anti-glide position. Bony defects may require the use of a cancellous bone graft, which can be taken from the distal tibia, proximal tibia, or iliac crest. Without rigid fixation, motion exercises are not possible and the patient is placed in a non-weight bearing short leg cast.

Edema is best controlled by a well-padded compressive dressing along with an AO splint or cast. Fracture blisters are treated aggressively with debridement and wet-to-dry saline dressings. Some will wait for them to resolve, but this can take time. Wound dehiscence has not been a problem because surgery is performed when skin condition allows and the overwhelming majority of our patients are young with good vascularity. Atraumatic soft tissue technique will help prevent dehiscence. Dehiscence is treated by wet-to-dry saline dressing and progressive adhesive strip closure.

Postoperative infections are always a potential complication. Hamilton indicates that the rate of superficial infection has been reported to be as high as 5 percent, whereas deep infections occurred at a rate of 0.3 to 2.2 percent.[1] Obviously, the best way to prevent infection is to take the usual operative precautions. Make sure the patient is a good surgical candidate and that the operative site is in good condition. Do not operate in the presence of severe edema, fracture blisters, or abrasions. Use a prophylactic antibiotic and perform the surgery as atraumatically as possible. It is important to obtain rigid internal fixation. If an infection develops, prompt recognition and treatment are critical to salvage the result. The surgical site is opened, a Gram stain and cultures are obtained, an appropriate antibiotic is given, the operative site is debrided and irrigated, and the wounds left open. If rigid internal fixation is present, the hardware is left in place. If fixation is unstable, this presents a real dilemma. If possible, the fixation should be changed to a more stable form. If this is not possible, then perhaps the best alternative is no fixation and cast treatment. The worse possible complication of infection is either a septic joint or osteomyelitis. Fortunately, this is a rare occurrence with ankle fractures. A septic joint may require late fusion. Osteomyelitis is an even more difficult problem. Eradication of osteomyelitis may require radical debridement, a Papaneau cancellous bone graft, rigid internal or external fixation, and appropriate antibiotics. Definitive treatment in the presence of uncontrollable infection may be fusion or, even more likely, amputation.

Other complications can occur with either closed or open treatment. Ossification of the interosseous membrane is a fairly common finding on the radiographs several months after the injury. Although it should cause symptoms by preventing the normal motion of the syndesmosis, this has not been the case. This may be because although the radiograph appears to show a synostosis between the tibia and fibula, a CT scan may reveal that it is actually incomplete. Hamilton has reported on patients with surgical fusion of the syndesmosis who are without symptoms.[1] Reflex sympathetic dystrophy can occur after injury or surgery. This is usually a diagnosis made at some time after the injury, when the patient still has edema and diffuse pain. Additional findings include autonomic disturbances with sweating, changes in temperature, and discoloration. The radiographs will demonstrate a diffuse, patchy osteoporosis known as Sudeck's atrophy. Treatment includes using the extremity, physical therapy, anti-inflammatories or steroids, and sympathetic blockade or sympathectomy. Failure of this problem to resolve will cause chronic pain. Another complication of ankle fracture treatment is deep vein thrombosis, which may require the use of anticoagulants. Clinical findings may include calf pain, persistent edema, and distention of the superficial venous system. It can lead to pulmonary embolization.

Finally, the most common long-term sequela of ankle fractures is traumatic arthritis. This can occur with either conservative or operative treatment. As indicated previously, there may be many factors contributing to the formation of arthritis, but the two most obvious are the quality of the reduction and the presence of cartilaginous damage. With arthritis, the patient will have pain, edema, and limited motion in the ankle. The radiographs will show osteophytosis, sclerosis, and narrowing or obliteration of the joint space. Conservative treatment consists of activity modification, cushioning of the bottom of the shoe, physical therapy, and anti-inflammatories. The salvage procedure for ankle arthritis is fusion.

ACKNOWLEDGMENTS

I wish to acknowledge the following individuals for their help in preparing this article: Lorene Chesnut (typing), John Barbaccia (photographs), Julio Rivera (drawings), and Sabina Wise (drawings).

REFERENCES

1. Hamilton WC (ed): Traumatic disorders of the ankle. Springer-Verlag, New York, 1984
2. Trethowan WH: Fractures in the neighborhood of the ankle joint. II: The operative treatment of ankle fractures. Lancet 1:90, 1926
3. Von Volkmann R: Beitrage zur Chirurgie. p. 105. Breitkoff U Hortel, Leipzig, 1875
4. Pankovich AM, Shirvaram MD: Anatomical basis of the variability in injuries of the medial malleolus and deltoid ligament. Acta Orthop Scand 50:217, 1979
5. Pankovich AM: Fractures of the fibula at the distal tibiofibular syndesmosis. Clin Orthop 143:138, 1979
6. Yablon IG, Heller FG, Shouse L: The key role of the lateral malleolus in displaced fractures of the ankle. J Bone Joint Surg 59A:165, 1973
7. Yablon IG, Segal D, Leach RE: Ankle Injuries. Churchill Livingstone, New York, 1983
8. Harper M: Deltoid ligament: an anatomical evaluation of function. Foot Ankle 8:19, 1987
9. Memelaus MB: Injuries of the anterior inferior tibio-fibular ligament. Aust NZ J Surg 30:279, 1960
10. Barnett CH, Napier JR: The axis of rotation of the ankle joint in man. Its influence upon the form of the talus and the morbidity of the fibula. J Anat 86:1, 1952
11. Inman VT: The joints of the ankle. 1st Ed. Williams & Wilkins, Baltimore, 1976
12. Pott P: Some few general remarks on fractures and dislocations. Haives, Clark and Collins, London, 1768. Reprinted by Medical Classics 1:329, 1936
13. Dupuytren : Ann Mid-Chir Hop Hosp Civ Paris, 1819
14. Cooper AP: A treatise on dislocations and on fractures of the joints. p. 353. London, 1822
15. Gudas CJ: Current concepts in the management of ankle repair. p. 357. In Marcus SA (ed): Complications in Foot Surgery. Williams & Wilkins, Baltimore, 1984
16. Maisonneuve JC: Recherches sur la fracture du perone. Arch Gen Med 7:165, 433, 1840
17. Tillaux P: Recherches cliniques et experimentales

sur les fractures malleolaires, rapport par gosselin. Bull Acad Med (Paris) 21:817, 1872

18. Wagstaffe WW: An unusual form of fracture of the fibula. St Thomas Hosp Rep 6:43, 1873

19. Ashhurst APC, Bromer RS: Classification and mechanism of fractures of the leg bones involving the ankle. Arch Surg 4:51, 1922

20. Lauge-Hansen N: Fractures of the ankle: analytic historic survey as the basis of new experimental, roentgenologic, and clinical investigations. Arch Surg 56:259, 1948

21. Lauge-Hansen N: Fractures of the ankle. II: Combined experimental-surgical and experimental-roentgenologic investigations. Arch Surg 60:957, 1950

22. Lauge-Hansen N: Fractures of the ankle. IV: Clinical use of genetic roentgen diagnosis and genetic reduction. Arch Surg 64:488, 1952

23. Weber BG: Die Verletzungen des Oberen Sprungelenkes. Verlay hans Huber, Bern, 1972

24. Yde J: The Lauge-Hansen classification of malleolar fractures. Acta Orthop Scand 51:181, 1980

25. Magnusson R: On the late results in non-operative cases of malleolar fractures. I: Fractures by external rotation. Acta Orthop Scand, suppl., 84: 1, 1944

26. Cedell CA: Outward rotation-supination injuries of the ankle. Clin Orthop 42:97, 1965

27. Cedell CA: Supination-outward rotation injuries of the ankle. Acta Orthop Scand, suppl., 110: 1, 1967

28. Bauer M, Jonsson K, Nelsson B: Thirty year follow-up of ankle fractures. Acta Orthop Scand 56:103, 1985

29. Kristensen KD, Hansen T: Closed treatment of ankle fractures: stage II supination-eversion fractures followed for 20 years. Acta Orthop Scand 56:107, 1985

30. Willenegger H, Weber BG: Malleolarfrakturen. In Technik der Operativen Frakturenbehandlung. Springer-Verlag, Berlin, 1963

31. Denham RA: Internal fixation for unstable ankle fractures. J Bone Joint Surg 46B:206, 1964

32. Mast JW, Teipner WA: A reproducible approach to the internal fixation of adult ankle fractures: rationale, technique, and early results. Orthop Clin North Am 11:661, 1980

33. Baird RA, Jackson ST: Fractures of the distal part of the fibula with associated disruption of the deltoid ligament (treatment without repair of the deltoid ligament). J Bone Joint Surg 69A:1346, 1987

34. Pankovich AM: Maisonneuve fracture of the fibula. J Bone Joint Surg 58A:337, 1976

35. Pankovich AM: Fractures of the fibula proximal to

the distal tibiofibular syndesmosis. J Bone Joint Surg 60A:221, 1978

36. Kleiger B: Mechanisms of ankle injury. Orthop Clin North Am 5:127, 1974

37. Joy C, Patzakis MJ, Harvey JP: Precise evaluation of the reduction of severe ankle fractures. J Bone Joint Surg 56A:979, 1974

38. Ramsey PL, Hamilton W: Changes in the tibiotalar areas of contact caused by lateral talar shift. J Bone Joint Surg 58A:356, 1976

39. Reide U, Willenegger H, Schenk R: Experimenteller beitrag zur erklarung der sekundaren arthrose bei frakturen des oberen sprunggelenks. Helv Chir Acta 36:343, 1969

40. Sarkisian JS, Cody GW: Closed treatment of ankle fractures. A new criterion for evaluation. A review of 250 cases. J Trauma 16:323, 1976

41. Burwell HN, Charnley AD: Treatment of displaced fractures at the ankle by rigid internal fixation and early joint movement. J Bone Joint Surg 47B:634, 1965

42. Malka JS, Tillard W: Results of non-operative and operative treatment of fractures of the ankle. Clin Orthop 67:159, 1969

43. Klossner O: Late results of operative and non-operative treatment of severe ankle fractures. A clinical study. Acta Chir Scand, suppl., 293: 1, 1962

44. Kristensen RB: Treatment of malleolar fractures according to Lauge-Hansen's method. Preliminary results. Acta Chir Scand 97:362, 1949

45. Hughes JL, Weber H, Willenegger H, Kuner EH: Evaluation of ankle fractures: nonoperative and operative treatment. Clin Orthop 138:111, 1979

46. Bauer M, Bengner U, Johnell O, Redlund-Johnell I: Supination-eversion fractures of the ankle joint: changes in incidence over 30 years. Foot Ankle 8:26, 1987

47. Bauer M, Johnell O, Redlung-Johnell I, Jonsson K: Ankle fractures. Foot Ankle 8:23, 1987

48. Bauer M, Bergstrom B, Hemborg A, Sandegard J: Malleolar fractures: nonoperative versus operative treatment. Clin Orthop 199:17, 1985

49. Brodie I, Denham RA: The treatment of unstable ankle fractures. J Bone Joint Surg 56B:256, 1974

50. Chapman MW: Fractures and fracture-dislocations of the ankle. In Mann RA (ed): Surgery of the Foot. 5th Ed. CV Mosby, St. Louis, 1986

51. Chapman MW, Mahoney M: The role of early internal fixation in the management of open fractures. Clin Orthop 138:120, 1979

52. Gustilo RB, Anderson JT: Prevention of infection in the treatment of one thousand and twenty-five

fractures of long bones. J Bone Joint Surg 58A:453, 1976

53. Rittmann WW, Schibli M, Allgower M: Open fractures. Clin Orthop 138:132, 1979
54. Franklin JL, Johnson KD, Hansen ST: Immediate internal fixation of open ankle fractures. J Bone Joint Surg 66A:1349, 1984
55. Cave FF: Complications of the operative treatment of fractures of the ankle. Clin Orthop 42:13, 1965
56. Weber BG: Lengthening osteotomy of the fibula to correct a widened mortise of the ankle after fracture. Int Orthop 4:289, 1981
57. Mueller ME, Allgower M, Schneider R, Willenegger H: Manual of Internal Fixation. Springer-Verlag, Berlin, 1979

29

Type B Danis-Weber Ankle Fracture: The Anti-Glide Plate

Harold W. Vogler, D.P.M.

Ankle fractures involving the lateral malleolus and fibula have long been controversial concerning internal fixation. As surgeons and engineers become more integrated, the need for open reduction and internal fixation of many fibular ankle fractures has become apparent. This principle has been based on an understanding of the biomechanics of bone failure with its various obligatory displacements.[1–4] The consequences of minimal fibular malleolar displacements in active and younger patients can be devastating. The very high coefficient of congruency in the ankle can result in loss of up to 42 percent of the contact-loading area of the ankle with only 1 mm of lateral malleolar displacement (Fig. 29-1).[5,6] The end result of minimal displacement can be disabling arthrosis deformans. This has been corroborated by studies of the A-O.[7–9]

Conventional radiographic assessments often are misleading and do not reveal the true morphology of displacement planes inherent in the various fracture patterns. Only with careful radiographic evaluation coupled with intuitive knowledge of fracture biomechanics can one properly determine the magnitude and displacement plane of any given fracture.[1–3,10] The confusion surrounding the type of treatment for the various low fibular-malleolar fractures exemplifies this dilemma.

DANIS-WEBER ANKLE FRACTURE CLASSIFICATION

The A-O group has classified ankle fractures into three major groups—A, B, and C.[11] The original classification of Danis[12] was modified by Weber[13] to assist the surgeon in deciding which fractures required operation. It is based on the level of appearance of the fibular fracture with regard to the syndesmosis-ankle joint line. Type A fracture is transverse and occurs at or below the joint line and syndesmosis. Type B, the subject of this chapter, begins at the level of the syndesmosis near the joint line and initiates inferomedial-anterior and propagates superolateral-posterior.[12–14] This is the classic type B fracture pattern. This fracture pattern is typically oblique more often than spiral and is equated with the Lauge-Hansen Supination-external rotation stage II lesion.[15–17] Type C fractures occur above the syndesmosis anywhere between the proximal fibular head and the inferior syndesmosis and are spiral.[15–17] They equate with the Lauge-Hansen pronation-external rotation modes and have extensive peritalar soft tissue disruption.[17] There is often associated fracture-dislocation injury at the medial malleolus and posterior tibial malleolus in later stages. These associated injury compo-

627

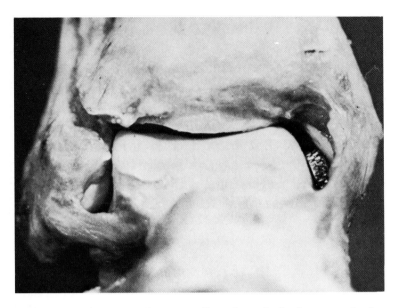

Fig. 29-1. Type B fracture with intact syndesmosis allows lateral talar luxation of at least 1 mm or more, contributing to massive loss of loading contact area of ankle joint. The proximal fibular shaft is still bound to the tibia above the fracture site although the syndesmosis is ruptured lower down through its substance. (From Hamilton,[15] with permission.)

nents are also important and require repair; however, the crux of this classification and discussion is the lateral side of the joint. This is not the case with the Lauge-Hansen classification, which draws attention to serial failure of the various components of the peritalar joint, emphasizing the associated ligamentous disruptions.[16,17] The perspective and emphasis of this chapter remains the lateral malleolar fracture, which is the key to management of isolated or combined segment ankle trauma.[7,11–15,18]

There is widespread confusion regarding the morphology of the type B fracture and hence it is often erroneously characterized as "spiral oblique." Such fractures are either spiral or oblique—but not both.[1,2,3] One must understand the difference between the biomechanics of these two fracture patterns as well as their cleavage planes to differentiate them. Both patterns have complex underlying biomechanics, and controversy persists regarding the morbid loading mode that ultimately produces each pattern. It is therefore important for the podiatric surgeon to understand the pathomechanical loading

modes about the talar joints that result in ankle trauma.[3]

BIOMECHANICS AND ANATOMY

The motions of the talus in closed kinetic chain mechanics are governed by the complexity of its overall morphology and the geometry of its articular surfaces. As such, the talus functions essentially as a "gear," mediating and modulating the motions of its counterparts. It functions in an indirect drive manner since it has no muscular attachments.[19,20] The movements of this bone are functions of its substrate counterparts and the ligamentous tethers that attach to it or around it. The talus can only move as permitted by the shapes of its surfaces and soft tissue and bony constraints. It is here that the morbid pathology of the ankle fracture begins. Under pathomechanical loading conditions, the associated anatomic structures are strained through a mediation system, the center of which is the talus. Assumed positions of the foot with superimposed loads will alter the direction and magnitude of the pathomechanics causing graduated strain on various soft tissue or bony structures. This situation allows some predictability in injury pattern. The Danis-Weber malleolar fracture classification and especially the Lauge-Hansen system take advantage of this fact. Thus, the talus is the weapon of insult in the biomechanical aspects of ankle trauma.[19,20] Indirect violence, mediated by the motions of the talus, produces the morbid strains that ultimately cause yielding of the bony or ligamentous constraints around the ankle.

PATHOMECHANICS OF TYPE B MALLEOLAR FRACTURE

The unique anatomy of the peritalar joints provides intrinsic stability under normal conditions.[5] When eccentric loading occurs, causing a supinated foot posture (owing to terrain or inherent rear-foot varus deformity), loading patterns through the tibia-fibula-talar unit are altered. The supinated position of the foot on the supporting surface results in a substrate interface. Surface-interactive friction fixes the foot to the ground. The superimposed loads from above generated as a result of gravity (body weight) pass through the leg into the foot mediated by the talar gear. If there is a pure vertical load developed through the leg into the supinated foot, then the varus motions of the talus will generate a strain on either the lateral ligamentous complex or the lower fibular malleolus. One or the other will fail if the force is great enough. In lateral ligamentous rupture, the talus will be liberated laterally and allowed to sublux (talar tilt). Whether or not the anterior talofibular ligament as well as the calcaneofibular ligament fails will be determined by the position of the foot at the time of strain application.[14] A plantar-flexed position strains the anterior talofibular ligament, and a more neutral position of the foot strains the calcaneofibular ligament. Usually, but not always, the anterior talofibular ligament fails first, followed by the calcaneofibular ligament. The posterior talofibular ligament rarely ruptures following failure of

the other two components since it is now free and can tether the talus and thus dissipate the remaining strain energy in the surrounding soft tissues of the capsule.[16] Alternatively, if the ligamentous structures remain intact, they transmit the morbid force to the fibular malleolus through the varus movement of the talus, which is developed from the forced supination position of the foot. The talus cannot sublux since this motion is restrained by the intact lateral collateral ligaments below and the lateral malleolus at the joint line, stabilized above by the syndesmosis and interosseous membrane. Continued varus strain application will force the talus against the lateral malleolus at the level of the joint line, concentrating its impact between these two points Thus, the bone must break from flexural overload somewhere in between.[3] This is a type A fracture.

When an external rotatory force is superimposed on this mechanism, the anterior syndesmotic structures come under strain first.[15,16] The generation of such a strain mode involves recognition of the relative kinetic chain operational at the moment of force application. In other words, the foot is fixed on the supporting surface in a relatively supinated position; it is not entirely free to rotate externally since ground friction prevents such motion. Thus, forced internal rotation of the leg on the fixed foot generates a relative outward or external rotation force on the foot. This is the classic mode of the type B fracture. It is believed that this is the equivalent of the Lauge-Hansen supination external rotation injury, stage II.[15,16]

ANATOMIC FAILURE

Supination-external rotation strains the anterior syndesmosis initially. Because of the orientation of the syndesmosis, the fibers are tensed with such an imposed strain. These fibers can either sustain the load and transmit it to the bone origins or fail. Biomechanical failure of the anterior syndesmosis can occur by several mechanisms. Midsubstance rupture is the most common mode. However, the ligament can also fail at the sites that its fibers enter either of its bony origins or, alternatively, it can avulse a bony fracture from either site.[15,16] A Chaput-Tillaux fracture occurs when the anterior tibial tubercle is avulsed.[11,15] When the anterior tubercle of the lower fibular insertion avulses, the fracture is known as a Wagstaffe avulsion.[15] From a biomechanical standpoint, all these situations are equivalent to ligament failure since the syndesmosis can no longer sustain the tension load it is designed to subserve. The result is hypermobility of the talus in the transverse plane. This permits the talus to impact more aggressively on the fibular malleolus since such an impact can no longer be dampened by the syndesmotic ligament. The fibula is stabilized above by the intact interosseous membrane with a posterior tether mediated by the posterior tibiofibular ligaments, which have remained intact. The apex of the fibula is stabilized by the intact lateral collateral ligaments below. Imposed lateral talar rotation now impacts the fibula near the joint line.[3,19,20] Gravity loads the fibula like a cylinder longitudinally. Stabilization of the fibula prior to fracture

is developed by the lateral collateral ligaments inferiorly with support from the lateral talofibular facet interface from below. The intact interosseous membrane and the superior tibiofibular joint form the opposite end of the support system from above. The vertical load of gravity induces a compression load through the diaphysis of the fibula. The rotatory load induced by lateral talar impact near the joint line produces a torsional load. Continued application of this strain system induces flexure in the fibula, generating a cantilever moment that has an additive effect on the bending forces thus generated. The net result is production of an oblique fracture initiating at the joint line. The course of this pattern is always inferomedial-anterior to superolateral-posterior. The bone will fail along a cleavage plane of about 45 degrees to its long axis that represents a compromise of simultaneous loads (compression, flexure, and torsion) about an oblique axis.[3,10] The bone ends are usually short and blunt, and there is no vertical connecting segment (Fig. 29-2). This is to be differentiated from a type B spiral

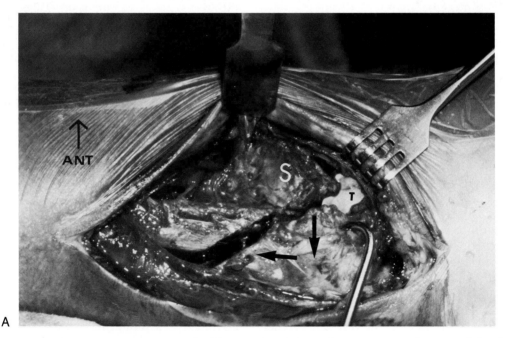

Fig. 29-2. (A) Classic type B fracture with oblique pattern. Note the posterior and proximal displacement (arrows) with rupture of anterior talofibular ligament exposing the talus (T). The syndesmosis (S) is partially ruptured through the fracture site; however, the more proximal portion of the shaft is maintained against the tibia from the proximal portion of the syndesmotic ligament. (*Figure continues.*)

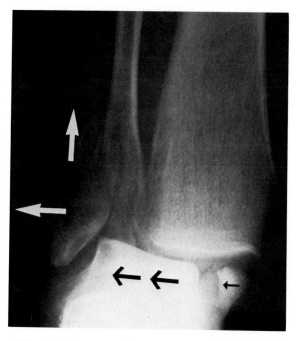

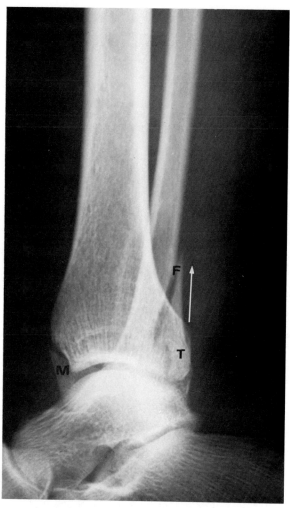

Fig. 29-2 (*Continued*). (**B**) Classic oblique type B fracture. Note the short blunt ends of the fractured fibula, with lateral and proximal displacement. There is also a fracture of the medial malleolus with lateral luxation of the talus (black arrows). This represents a late stage supination-external rotation injury. (**C**) Same case in panel **B** in lateral profile. Note posterior spike of fibular fragment with proximal displacement. Also viewed are the medial malleolar fracture (M) and a posterior lip fracture of the tibia (T). White arrows indicate cephalad displacement of the fibular fracture segment.

fracture that is caused by a predominant torsional load and has a longitudinal connecting segment between the two extremes of the fracture with sharp spikes distally and proximally (Fig. 29-3).[1-3,10] This pattern is less common but does occur depending on the dominant strain pattern developed as a result of the complex loading modes possible in closed kinetic chain mechanics.

The anterior syndesmosis does not necessarily always fail first in the type B fracture.[14-16] If the syndesmosis can sustain the splitting load of the talus jamming against the fibula, the strain energy will be directed immediately against the fibula. The intact syndesmosis at the inferior fibular insertion will then behave as a stress riser contributing to a weak point since it is actually a transition area. The oblique fracture will initiate immediately at this area, sometimes beginning relatively transverse immediately below the syndesmotic insertion and then coursing upward,

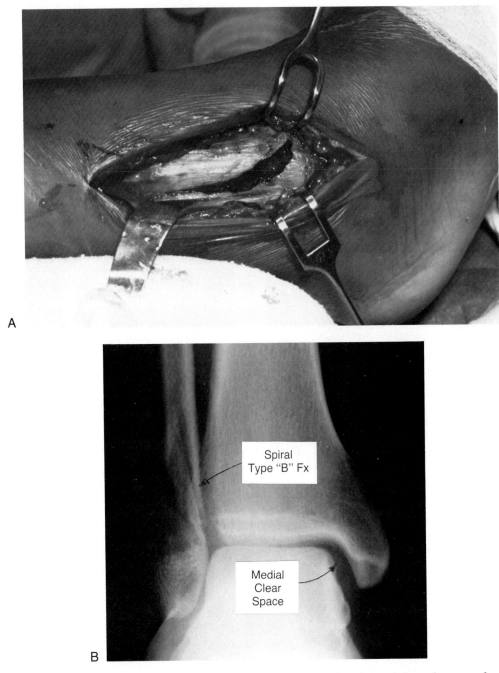

Fig. 29-3. (A) Type B spiral fracture of fibula. Note sharp proximal spike with long fracture plane. The fracture begins anteromedial and propagates proximal, lateral, and posterior. **(B)** Type B fracture with subtle medial clear space suggesting a late stage supination-external rotation injury. Sharp spiral spikes are noted distally and proximally.

laterally and posteriorly. Another common failure mode is fracture through the lower fibers of the syndesmosis near its fibular insertion. The more proximal fibula remains bound against the tibia, technically indicating that the syndesmosis is functionally intact. The integrity of the syndesmosis is assessed by the bone hook test following plate application. If there is hypermobility of the proximal fibula, then the syndesmosis has not been entirely repaired and reconstructed; or worse yet, there may be more proximal damage to the interosseous membrane that was not previously recognized during the procedure.

DISPLACEMENT PATTERNS

The oblique fracture pattern is the most inherently unstable fracture morphology.[1–3,10] It will always displace along the axis of the obliquity. In the type B oblique fracture, the distal lateral malleolus must migrate cephalad and posterior and, to a lesser degree, laterally.[3,15,16] It migrates fur-

ther in the cephalad and posterior direction, causing shortening with incongruity of the talofibular joint.[7,9,11,15] The fibula loses its congruity with the tibia in the incisura.[21,22] This fact is the basis for the Weber posterior anti-glide fibular plate.[21,22]

This plate functions like a buttress plate, which is applied to an oblique fracture to capture the fragment whose spike is opposite the cortex that will be adjacent to the plate.[21–23] In the type B fracture, the spike of the oblique fracture is posterior and is the high point of the lower fragment. The axis of the obliquity is such that this fragment displaces posterior and proximal (Fig. 29-4). If a plate is placed in a posterior position and first fixed to the bone on the proximal side of the fracture, then reduction of the upward and posterior displacement tendency of the lower fragment actually induces an axial load, spontaneously reducing the fracture and compressing the site. The plate itself can be used to reduce the fracture in difficult situations. It is usually not necessary to contour the posterior plate since the natural curve of the fibula allows for a spring ef-

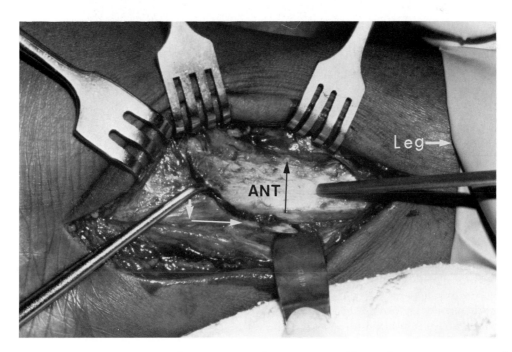

Fig. 29-4. Intraoperative situation demonstrating classic type B oblique fracture with proximal and posterior displacement tendency.

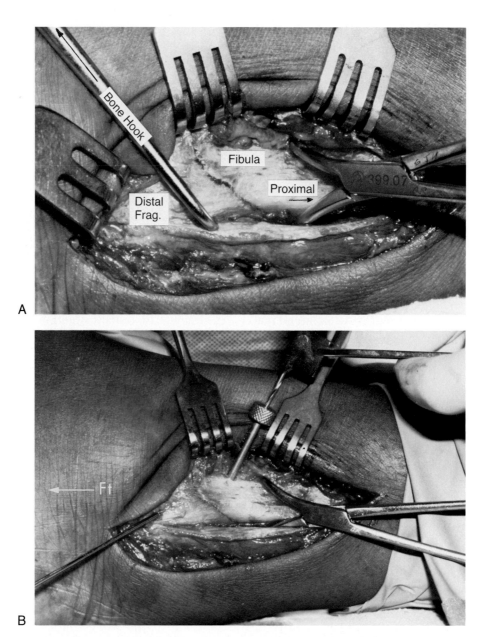

Fig. 29-5. **(A)** Same fracture as Figure 29-4 after distal and anterior traction by bone hook and reduction clamp fixation. The restoration of fibular length and derotation of the distal fragment are critical. **(B)** Temporary reduction with clamp and Kirschner wire while anteroposterior interfragmentary screw is placed. When possible, the addition of a lag screw to the anti-glide system is advisable and improves stability. (*Figure continues.*)

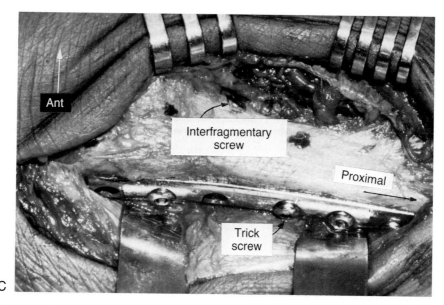

Fig. 29-5 (*Continued*). (**C**) The anti-glide system complete with posterior plate application and "trick screw" noted immediately proximal to fracture line barely visible. One lag screw has been placed outside the plate.

fect (prestressing) when tightened against the bone, forcing the fibula forward and downward along the axis of obliquity. The first screw is placed immediately opposite the fracture site on the proximal side of the fracture and is not tight-

ened all the way. A second proximal screw is then placed and tightened to prevent rotation of the plate. As the first screw is tightened, the plate generates spontaneous reduction. When used in this manner, the first placement screw is known

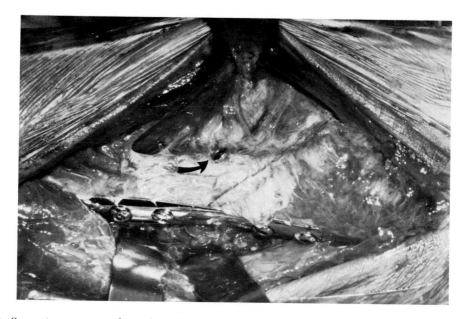

Fig. 29-6. Sometimes, posterolateral application is required with slight contouring of plate to capture the posterior spike. This case also has an anteroposterior lag screw (arrow).

as the "trick screw."[21,22] Typically, the fracture is reduced anatomically and then this maneuver is done. However, in difficult situations, the plate can do the work.[21,22] An interfragmental screw can be placed across the oblique site from posterior to anterior through one of the inferior holes in the plate.[23] In this manner, the plate will act as a washer effect in the soft bone along the infero-posterior lateral malleolus, allowing good purchase of the screw threads on the more cortical anterior and proximal side of the fibula. When the plate alignment is such that a posterior to anterior lag screw through the plate is not possible, an anterior to posterior lag screw outside the plate can be considered (Fig. 29-5).

Sometimes the proximal spike is positioned posterolaterally. The location of the spike will always be a function of the axis of obliquity of the fracture. If the plane of the fracture is more posterolateral, it may be necessary to contour the plate with a twist so that the plate can likewise be positioned posterolaterally to capture the spike and lock it into place (Fig. 29-6).[23]

EVOLUTION OF THE ANTI-GLIDE PLATE

This principle has been used in the St. Gallen Weber clinic since the late 1970s (K. G. Stühmer, personal communication) and was published in 1982.[24] Gudas first described this plate application in the American literature in 1984.[25] It was developed in response to the noted difficulty of obtaining and maintaining the reduction of the type B fracture, particularly in older patients with soft bone. Lateral plate application does not always restrain the proximal displacement tendency (with shortening of the fibula). Additionally, the soft cancellous bone in the lower malleolus does not accept screw purchase well even in healthy individuals. Therefore, posterior application obviates the concern about driving the screws into the talofibular joint or the tibiofibular incisura while maximizing good purchase by posterior to anterior screw fixation.[21–24]

The original posterior plate applications were 3.5-mm dynamic compression plates. For some time, one-third tubular plates have been used in either the four-hole or five-hole configuration. A recent study has proved the biomechanical stability of this plate application.[23] Interfragmentary screw placement is considered optional and used when additional stability seems required upon testing in the operating room. It is not necessary, however, to place any screws in the plate below the fracture site.[21–25] This is based on the biomechanical principle discussed earlier by interlocking the spike on the inferior fragment against the undersurface of the plate when it is fixed to the bone proximal to the fracture.

Adjunctive fixation modes in the type B fracture in comminuted situations or in extremely soft bone might also include a second plate application anterior or lateral with cerclage wire (Fig. 29-7). Only screws proximal to the fracture need be placed. In elderly patients, the inferior portion of the plate will act as a spoon or buttress plate "holding the rotten tomato" in place while maintaining the bone stock from collapse.[21,22]

EXPERIENCE

Our clinic was introduced to this plate concept in 1984 by K. G. Stühmer (Elizabethen Hospital, Ravensberg, Federal Republic of Germany). We have used this principle with excellent success since then. We have applied more than 40 anti-glide plates with few complications. There is no problem with peroneal tendon function.

It is important that the anti-glide plate be utilized in the indicated cases–type B fracture with a posterior or posterolateral spike on the inferior fragment of the fibular malleolus. We have adopted this plate application in all cases of type B fracture regardless of age and bone quality since it produces superior fracture reduction. A five- to six-hole plate is preferred to allow a slight anterior bend distally, cradling the inferior fragment. Immediate range of motion and rehabilitation can begin as tolerated. Total immobilization is not required except when poor patient control is anticipated, in which case it becomes discretionary by the surgeon.

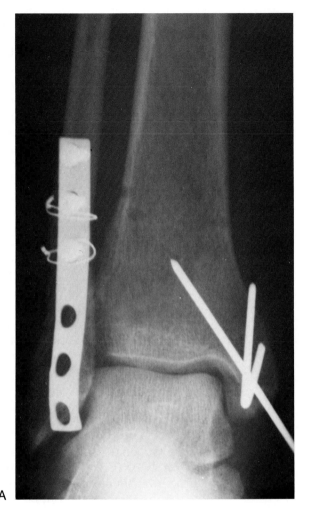 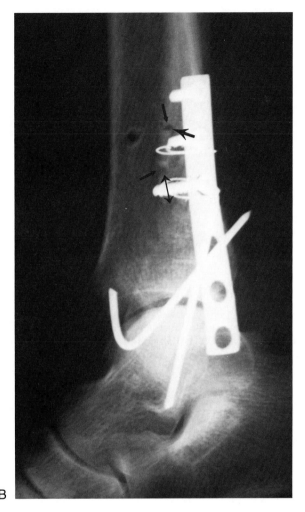

A   B

Fig. 29-7. (A) Type B fibular fracture with comminution. Cerclage wires required to maintain fragments and integrity of proximal shaft area. No screws are required in the inferior fragment. Medial malleolus fixated with "minimal" osteosynthesis owing to stage II open injury. (B) Lateral profile showing comminution (arrows) with posterior plate application and slight cradling of inferior fibular fragment with distal plate.

REFERENCES

1. Bechtol CO: Engineering principles applied to orthopaedic surgery. p. 257. In American Academy of Orthopedic Surgeons. Instructional Course Lectures. Vol. 9. Edwards, Ann Arbor, 1982
2. Frost HM: Orthopaedic Biomechanics. Vol. 5. Charles C Thomas, Springfield, IL, 1973
3. Vogler HW: Basic bioengineering concepts. Concepts in bone performance, failure and osteosynthesis. Clin Podiatry 2:161, 1985
4. Vogler HW: Ankle arthrodesis. Clinical and conceptual applications. Clin Podiatry 2:59, 1985
5. Simon WH, Freidenberg S, Richardson S: Joint congruence: a correlation of joint congruence and thickness of articular cartilage in dogs. J Bone Joint Surg 55A:1614, 1973
6. Ramsey PL, Hamilton W: Changes in tibio-talar area of contact caused by lateral talar shift. J Bone Joint Surg 58A:356, 1976
7. Riede UN, Schenk RK, Willenegger H: Gelenkmechanische Untersuchungen zum Problem der posttraumatischen Arthrosen im oberen

Sprunggelenk. I: Die intraartikulare Modellfraktur. Langenbecks Arch Chir 328:258, 1971

8. Willenegger H: Die Behandlung der Luxationsfrakturen des oberen Sprunggelenkes nach biomechanischen Gesichtspunketen. Helv Chir Acta 28:225, 1961

9. Willenegger H, Riede UN, Schweizer G et al: Gelenkmechanische Untersuchungen zum Problem der posttraumatische Arthrosen im oberen Sprunggelenk. III: Functionell-morphometrische Analyse des Gelenkknorpels. Langenbecks Arch Chir 333:91, 1973

10. Gozna ER: Biomechanics of long bone injuries. p. 1. In Gozna ER, Harrington IJ, Evans DC (eds): Biomechanics of Musculoskeletal Injury. Williams & Wilkins, Baltimore, 1982

11. Muller ME, Allgower M, Willenegger H et al: Manual of Internal Fixation. Springer-Verlag, Berlin, 1979

12. Danis R: Les fractures malleolaires. In Theorie et Pratique l'Osteosynthese. Masson, Paris, 1949

13. Weber BG: Die Verletzungen des oberen Sprunggelenkes. In Aktuelle Probleme in der Chirurgie. Vol. 3. Verlag Hans Huber, Bern, 1966

14. Harper MC: An anatomic study of the short oblique fracture of the distal fibula and ankle stability. Foot Ankle 4:2329, 1983

15. Hamilton WC: External rotation injuries. p. 125. In Hamilton WC: Traumatic Disorders of the Ankle. Springer-Verlag, New York, 1984

16. Cedell CA: Ankle lesions. Acta Orthop Scand 46:425, 1975

17. Lauge-Hansen N: Ankelbrud I: Genetisk Diagnose og Reposition. Munksgaard, Copenhagen, 1942

18. Yablon IG, Heller FG, Shouse L: The key role of the lateral malleolus in displaced fractures of the ankle. J Bone Joint Surg 59A:169, 1977

19. Vogler HW: Talar control mechanisms. Unpublished lecture. New York State Podiatric Medicine Association, New York, 1988

20. Vogler HW: Surgical control of the talus. Unpublished lecture. Pennsylvania College of Podiatric Medicine, Philadelphia, 1988

21. Stühmer KG: Podiatric A-O Course. Sea Island, GA, 1984

22. Stühmer KG: Podiatric A-O Course. Snowbird, Utah, 1988

23. Schaffer JJ, Manoli A: The antiglide plate for distal fibular fixation. J Bone Joint Surg 69A:596, 1987

24. Brunner CF, Weber BG: Special Techniques in Internal Fixation. Springer-Verlag, New York, 1982

25. Gudas CJ: Current concepts in the management of ankle repair. p. 357. In Marcus SA, Block BH (eds): Complications in Foot Surgery. Prevention and Management. 2nd Ed. American College of Foot Surgeons. Williams & Wilkins, Baltimore, 1984

30

Infections Following Lower Extremity Trauma

Warren S. Joseph, D.P.M.

Despite early observations on the importance of asepsis, infection following traumatic injury continued to plague surgeons into the late 19th century.[1] "Hospital gangrene" had 100 percent mortality in many cases. In 1870, during the Franco-Prussian War, von Nussbaum lost 34 of 34 through-the-knee amputations to sepsis. The opposing French fared only slightly better: 13,173 amputations were performed with 10,006 deaths.[2]

Despite the advent of antibiotics in the 1940s and a better understanding of the pathogenesis and treatment of infection, post-traumatic infections continue to cause significant morbidity and mortality. The traumatized patient is predisposed to infection. Decreased immune function, retention of foreign bodies, and endogenous and exogenous contamination all contribute to infectious complications in these patients.

Although many of the basic principles of post-traumatic infection apply, the lower extremity is unique in its spectrum of trauma and its ability to respond to trauma. Diseases such as puncture wound osteomyelitis, if not exclusively found in the lower extremity, are predominately seen there. The anatomy of the foot and leg predisposes the region to infection. The shape and tissue content of the leg make wound closure difficult. Owing to the multitude of tendons and relatively superficial bone, the tissues do not easily collapse to close dead space.[1] Fascial compartments may swell, causing ischemia and subsequent necrosis.

The lower extremity is immunocompromised compared with other parts of the body. Duncan et al. found that the leg became infected in 38 percent of his attempts to cause infection in an experimental setting.[3] This percentage is higher than other regions including the back (15 percent), arm (13 percent), or thigh (21 percent). Lineaweaver et al. demonstrated that this finding may be due to a deficiency in neutrophil delivery to the lower extremity as compared with the upper body.[4]

RISK FACTORS PREDISPOSING TO INFECTION

Trunkey has modified an earlier classification of predisposing factors for infections following trauma.[5] His system divides these factors into intrinsic and extrinsic categories. The intrinsic factors include the host defenses, and the extrinsic factors include iatrogenic and noniatrogenic causes.

Intrinsic Factors

The host defense mechanisms can be divided into nonspecific defenses: the cellular immune system and the humoral immune system. Nonspecific defenses include the barrier layers and the inflammatory mediators. Most of the immune

639

consequences of trauma are dose related; the greater the trauma, the greater the immune suppression.

Skin is the primary barrier in protecting the body against invasion by pathogenic organisms. Intact skin is difficult to infect. Its low pH, relative dryness, and frequent turnover all contribute to maintaining a lower bacterial count.[1] In a unique experiment Duncan and co-workers were unable to cause infection while applying a large inoculum of pathogenic bacteria to undamaged skin over a long period of time.[3] Even with minor trauma, including scratching and lancing, only 2 of 35 trails resulted in infection. There are four required elements necessary to produce infection: (1) a high concentration of organisms; (2) occlusion, which prevents desquamation and provides moisture; (3) nutrients in the area; (4) sufficient damage of the corneal layer to permit the organisms to penetrate.[2]

The type, amount, and force of the trauma along with the intensity of bacterial inoculum all contribute to destruction of the skin's effectiveness as a barrier. There are three mechanical forces that can lead to soft tissue injury: shear, tension, and compression.[6] Shear cuts such as those made by a scissors or scalpel require little energy over a small area of tissue, and consequently they effect only minimal destruction. Tension and compression combine equal but opposite forces that involve much greater energy over a larger area of tissue, and these cause considerable damage. An example of these forces is an impact injury with blunt trauma. Owing to the large area involved, these wounds are one hundred times more likely to become infected than shear injuries.

The nonspecific inflammatory immune system consists of the ability of neutrophils to react to a stimulus. There are three phases of polymorphonuclear leukocyte activity: chemotaxis, phagocytosis, and intracellular killing of microorganisms. All three may be affected in trauma.

Chemotaxis, the ability of a neutrophil to move toward a stimulus, appears to be decreased following trauma.[7] This may be due to an intrinsic defect in neutrophil function,[8] a diminution of immunoglobulin levels, or the presence of a circulating chemotactic inhibition factor.[9]

Decreased phagocytosis has also been demonstrated, but less convincingly.[10] One study demonstrated a decreased ability of neutrophils to phagocytose bacteria in vitro for 24 hours following major battle trauma. One explanation for this inhibition of phagocytosis may be a decrease in the circulating levels of opsonins, especially fibronectin. Fibronectin levels were found to be depressed 24 hours following major surgery and remained low for up to 72 hours.[11]

Finally, intracellular killing of organisms may also be affected. This has been established especially with *Staphylococcus aureus*.[9]

The cell-mediated immune system is responsible for the production of resistance to foreign materials, tumors, and delayed hypersensitivity. This is mediated through thymus-derived lymphocytes (T cells). Suppression of cell-mediated immunity is the most extensively studied area in traumatic injuries. There now appears to be generation of T suppressor cells in these patients.[9] Interestingly, these cells appear to peak in number about day 14 following injury. This coincides with the time frame for the development of the greatest number of infections.

Contrary to the above, the reaction of the humoral immune system to trauma is probably the least well studied. Most studies have measured the quantitative amount of circulating immunoglobulins and complement following injury.[10] There appears to be a marked decrease in both following traumatic injury.

Noniatrogenic Extrinsic Factors

The extrinsic risk factors for the development of infection following trauma can be divided into iatrogenic and noniatrogenic categories. The noniatrogenic category includes exogenous and endogenous contamination of the wound and the type of injury. Various types of injuries are discussed individually.

Most bacterial contamination that occurs in lower extremity trauma is of the exogenous type. Owing to the lack of highly colonized viscera in the region, penetrating wounds will not cause the same infectious problems seen in abdominal trauma. However, the various environments in which the foot is placed can lead to some interesting pathogens.

The intensity of the bacterial inoculum is of importance. Roettinger et al. found that tissues receiving an inoculum of 3×10^6 S. aureus did not develop an infection, whereas tissues receiving 2×10^9 did.[12] This finding has led to the use of quantitative bacteriology in assessing the ability of a contaminated wound to heal following closure. Generally, if the culture results show fewer than 10^5 microorganisms, the wound is safe to close. Easier to perform than the quantitative culture technique is the quantitative Gram stain.[13] A 1-cc sample of tissue is removed from the wound, weighed, homogenized, diluted, and stained. The bacteria on the slide are then counted for a rapid estimate of quantity. These findings correlate well with the culture results.

The virulence or pathogenicity of the organism should also be considered. Some organisms are capable of producing a polysaccharide capsular slime that make them adhere to surfaces and are therefore more resistant to therapy.[14] *Staphylococcus aureus* is one such organism. The adherence of this organism is mediated not only by its ability to form a capsule but also by the presence of the glycoprotein *fibronectin* present in the patient's serum.[15] Other bacteria are saprophytic in nature and only become pathogenic under the proper circumstances. These include many of the anaerobic pathogens. The production of extracellular enzymes capable of destroying host defenses, such as proteases and hyaluronidases, also mediates virulence.

Not all post-traumatic disease caused by bacteria are true infections. Some, such as those caused by the *Clostridium* species, are toxemias secondary to the production of exotoxins and endotoxins. Tetanus, the best example of this class, will be discussed later.

The introduction of foreign bodies into the wound also represents exogenous contamination. Wounds contaminated by dirt or soil are 10,000 times more prone to infection. As few as 100 bacteria may cause infection in these areas.[16,17] Soil and clay have been termed *infection potentiating factors* (IPFs). IPFs potentiate infections in three ways[17]: (1) they decrease the ability of leukocytes to phagocytize and kill ingested organisms; (2) they eliminate the nonspecific bactericidal activity of serum; (3) owing to their anionic charges, they reduce the activity of basic and neutral antibiotics, such as the aminoglycosides. Acidic antibiotics (penicillins and cephalosporins) are not affected.

Devitalized soft tissues implanted into the wound at the time of injury acts as a foreign body and may cause infection.[18] By providing a relatively anaerobic environment, devitalized tissue, particularly fat and burnt skin, inhibits the bactericidal capacity of leukocytes in vitro and reduces phagocytosis. Devitalized soft tissue also acts as a culture medium, supporting bacterial growth to the same level as commercial nutrient broth.

All of these contaminants—bacteria, IPFs, and devitalized tissue—must be removed from the wound by debridement. Aggressive, complete debridement is the single most important factor in reducing the incidence of post-traumatic infections. Debridement techniques are either surgical or mechanical.[2] Surgically, devitalized skin is more readily determined than muscle. Within 24 hours there is usually adequate demarcation of the skin to allow a decision as to the extent of debridement necessary. Muscle, on the other hand, should be observed for longer periods to determine survival. Criteria for muscle viability include the ability of the muscle to contract in response to a stimulus, its color, and its bleeding characteristics.[1] Frequently, multiple operations may be necessary to ensure the removal of all necrotic tissue. Alexander et al. found that wound fluids, deficient in their ability to opsonize bacteria for phagocytosis, collected in the wound after surgical debridement.[19] These were removed effectively by closed suction drainage.

In the presence of vital structures, adequate surgical debridement may be difficult to accomplish. Mechanical measures such as high-pressure irrigation and frequent dressing changes are successful in reducing the level of contamination. The irrigation can be performed with a commercially produced pulsatile flow device capable of delivering up to 60 lb/in² of pressure. If the force of irrigation increases to above 70 lb/in², local tissue damage may occur.[20] If this equipment is not available, a 30-ml syringe with a 19-gauge needle can be inexpensively substituted. Frequent dressing changes utilizing a fine mesh gauze material will act to debride the wound with each change. Through capillary action, wound fluids seep into the dressing, causing adherence. Upon changing, the adherent material will be removed from the wound. In the presence of a thick exudate, dilution of the drainage can be accomplished by using a wet-to-dry technique. Any number of solutions can be used in this type of dressing. Saline, povidone-iodine, povidone-iodine diluted in saline, lactated Ringer's solution, and Dakin's solution can all be used successfully. One axiom to follow is to place nothing into the wound that you would not place on the human cornea.[5]

Iatrogenic Extrinsic Factors

Extrinsic factors that predispose post-traumatic wounds to infection and are classified as being of iatrogenic origin include the use of implants and broad-spectrum antibiotics. Environmental variables such as personnel and equipment hygiene are also grouped into this category.[5]

Traditionally, the term *implant* conjures visions of fixation devices and joint replacements. Any foreign device inserted into a trauma patient can be defined in this category. Thus, implants include not only the above, but also sutures, catheters, and tubes. Although of various composition, all implants are capable of producing infections. A complex interaction of diminished local host defenses in the presence of these devices and the production of bacterial adherence factors accounts for this phenomenon.[14]

Sutures are primarily used to close dead space. This closure would seem to be appropriate since the presence of dead space potentiates infection. De Hol et al. found that in one series of studied patients, all contaminated wounds containing dead space became infected versus only 42 percent contamination in wounds containing no dead space.[21] However, the same investigators found that sutures actually potentiate the development of infection. The infection rate in wounds containing dead space closed with sutures was markedly higher than that in wounds containing the dead space alone. Contrary to popular belief, the physical structure of the suture (monofilament versus multifilament) was not

a determining factor in the degree of potentiation. The chemical makeup of the suture was more important.[22] Polypropylene, nylon, and polyglycolic acid were less reactive than other types.

Not all implants are inserted directly into the wound. Many patients with lower extremity trauma sustain other injuries that require the use of central or peripheral lines or intubation. The same principles that mediate infection in other implants apply in these cases. Line sepsis is a common cause of bacteremia in trauma patients. Peripheral and central lines should be examined on a daily basis for any localized sign of inflammation. Peripheral lines should not be left in place for longer than 3 to 4 days before rotation to another site.

The prolonged and seemingly haphazard use of broad-spectrum antibiotics is another iatrogenic factor in the production of infection. These drugs, over time, will cause the selection and emergence of resistant organisms. Prophylaxis and antibiotic usage are discussed in greater detail later.

The final extrinsic factor is the environmental milieu. Trauma patients are usually first seen in the emergency room under less than aseptic conditions. If the injuries warrant, the patients are transferred to the intensive care unit where the most resistant organisms in the hospital are found. Since these patients may be immunocompromised because of their injuries, proper aseptic techniques such as handwashing should be observed by all personnel.

ANTIBIOTIC PROPHYLAXIS IN TRAUMA

"Prophylaxis means pretreatment! If pretreatment is impossible, we should wait to see what happens to patients and only come to their aid when they show overt signs of infection, which we can treat specifically."[23]

The vast majority of antibiotic usage that occurs following trauma cannot technically be classified as prophylaxis. In most cases, the incident has occurred and any contamination is already present. This then represents therapy rather than true prophylaxis. The prophylaxis used is for the prevention of nosocomial infections in these patients. The prevention of infection in trauma patients is predicated more on proper wound care and careful control of the environment in which the patient is placed than on antimicrobial activity. Two studies of prophylactic antibiotic usage in simple lacerations are helpful in demonstrating this point. Grossman et al. performed a randomized study of 265 patients divided into three groups.[24] Group 1 received cephalexin; group 2 cefazolin; and group 3 a placebo. There were only three infections (1.1 percent) total, two of which occurred in the cephalexin group. In a similar, but larger series, Thirlby et al. divided 499 patients into two groups, one receiving antibiotics and one placebos.[25] Of the 33 (6.6 percent) infections, there was no significant difference in the two groups. There were, however, significant differences when various wound care techniques were used. With a closure delay of greater than 4 hours or the use of subcutaneous sutures, marked increases in infection rate were noted.

If antibiotics are to be used following traumatic injury, general principles of competent prescribing should be observed. A drug with a narrow spectrum should be selected over the shotgun approach of a broader spectrum agent. This will help prevent selection of more resistant organisms that may be more pathogenic and difficult to eradicate. The antibiotic selected should be cost effective in terms of dosage amounts and schedule. The safety profile of the antibiotic should be known. Some drugs contain a side chain, known as the N-methylthiotetrazole group, that has been linked to clinical bleeding. This bleeding potential may cause problems in patients undergoing surgical debridement.

Different types of injury predispose to infection with different organisms. If osteomyelitis follows a puncture wound, there is a high probability that *Pseudomonas aeruginosa* will be isolated. Open fractures are frequently infected with *S. aureus*. Empiric knowledge of these predispositions are helpful in the selection of an

Table 30-1. Common Organisms Following Trauma

Puncture wounds	
Cellulitis	*Staphylococcus aureus* (>50%)
	α-Hemolytic *Streptococcus*
	Staphylococcus epidermidis
	Escherichia coli/Proteus
Osteomyelitis	*Pseudomonas aeruginosa* (90%)
Bite wounds	
Human	*Staphylococcus aureus*
	Streptococcus
	Bacteroides fragilis
	Miscellaneous mouth anaerobes
	Eikenella corrodens
	Hepatitis B[a]
	Treponema pallidum[a]
Dog	*Staphylococcus aureus*
	Staphylococcus epidermidis
	α-Hemolytic *Streptococcus*
	Pasteurella multocida
	IIj, DF-2, EF-4, M-5
Cat	*Staphylococcus aureus*
	α-Hemolytic *Streptococcus*
	Pasteurella multocida
	DF-2
Open fractures	*Staphylococcus aureus*
	Staphylococcus epidermidis
	Pseudomonas aeruginosa
	Streptococcus
	Enterobacteriaceae
	Bacteroides fragilis
	Miscellaneous anaerobes

[a] Relatively rare, included as point of interest. Lists are not in level of frequency owing to wide variation of different series.

agent. Table 30-1 lists common organisms found following various traumas.

DIAGNOSIS OF TRAUMATIC WOUND INFECTIONS

The presentation of infection varies little in traumatically and nontraumatically induced wounds. However, a review of the basics is in order. Any clinical diagnosis is based on a triad of information including a complete history, a physical examination, and laboratory results. This also holds true with the diagnosis of infections.

History

Careful questioning of the patient as to the nature of the wound is of foremost importance. What caused the injury? How long ago did it occur? What previous treatment was rendered, if any? Has the patient noted any chills or fever? All give important clues to assist in diagnosis and management. These questions take on varying importance when dealing with specific injuries. In puncture wound infections, the course of the symptoms may practically diagnose an osteomyelitis. Once osteomyelitis is assumed, the pathogen *P. aeruginosa* must also be assumed to be present owing to its high prevalence in osteomyelitis. Proper antibiotic and surgical management directed against this organism can then be initiated.

The patient's medical and social history should be ascertained. Patients who have been recently hospitalized or who reside in a nursing home will be predisposed to infection with more resistant nosocomial organisms. Likewise, drug addicts have a higher incidence of colonization with methicillin-resistant staphylococci. This is due in part to easy access to first generation oral cephalosporins on the street. Intravenous drug abusers and homosexuals may be infected with the human immunodeficiency virus. The presence of this virus will put a further strain on these patients' traumatically depressed immune system. Actual inpatient handling of these patients should not differ markedly, since all trauma patients should be placed in isolation for wound and skin precautions.

Physical Examination

Wound infection may present with the five classic signs of inflammation: rubor (redness); tumor (swelling); dolor (pain); calor (heat); and loss of function. Although not diagnostic, and not always present, these signs will pose a high index of suspicion of infection. The presence of drainage also suggests infection. The characteristics of the drainage will lend hints as to the causative organism. Different bacteria cause different colors and odors. Creamy, yellow, odorless drainage suggests *S. aureus*. Streptococci may form little drainage. Table 30-2 lists other common drainage characteristics.

When dealing with a local wound infection, such as in the lower extremity, it is not unusual for the physician to take a primary interest in examination of the wound to the exclusion of the patient as a whole. This narrow-minded approach may lead to devastating consequences. How does the patient appear? Is the patient alert and responding clearly to questions? Is the patient lethargic? Is there excessive diaphoresis? Oral temperature curves should be examined. Unusual behavior may be a sign of sepsis. Sepsis can be defined as the symptomatic invasion of the host's tissues by an organism.[5] Symptoms involve fever or, paradoxically, hypothermia, malaise, leukocytosis, and metabolic dysfunction.[26] Septicemia is the symptomatic presence of organisms in the blood. This differs from bacteremia, which may be transient and of no clinical significance. These symptoms may occur in the absence of clinical signs and wound infection. Another origin of the infection should then be explored. The following case is useful in illustrating this point.

A patient sustains a gunshot wound to the foot. One day after initial debridement the patient spikes a fever to 103°F (39.4°C). Although this is not unusual following general anesthesia, the temperature remains elevated above that level for 2 days. Upon examination of the wound there are no clinical signs of infection. The patient is diaphoretic and lethargic. Upon reviewing the

Table 30-2. Drainage Characteristics

Organism	Color	Odor
Staphylococcus aureus	Golden	None
Staphylococcus epidermidis	White	None
Pseudomonas aeruginosa	Green	Sweet Fruity Grape-like
Streptococcus	Little	None
Proteus spp.	White	Mousey Ammonia
Bacteroides and other anaerobes	Brown-red, watery	Foul, fetid

medical history, it is found that the patient is an intravenous drug user. Blood cultures are drawn and become positive. The patient is diagnosed as having bacterial endocarditis, a potentially fatal disease.

Laboratory Tests

Of the three methods used to diagnose infections, laboratory testing is useful in confirming the other two. The most reliable blood test used for this purpose is the complete blood count (CBC) with differential. The two parameters followed in the diagnosis of infection are, first, a generalized leukocytosis and then, a left shift. The leukocytosis demonstrates the body's ability to defend itself against the invading pathogen. With the increasing need for white blood cells, immature cells are frequently released before full development. These cells, known as band cells, constitute the left shift. Suggestive, although not diagnostic, of infection, the CBC is a useful tool in following the progress of the treatment regimen.

The erythrocyte sedimentation rate (ESR) is also frequently used in the diagnosis of infection, especially osteomyelitis. Unfortunately, the ESR is too nonspecific, being elevated in many inflammatory processes. It may, however, be useful in following the progress of therapy.

Owing to the nonspecific nature of the ESR, C-reactive protein (CRP) has been advocated in the diagnosis of infection. Although more specific than ESR, CRP is still not specific enough for diagnosis. Again, it may be useful in following therapeutic progress.

Gram stain is an easy, inexpensive, and effective tool in the diagnosis of infection. In approximately 5 minutes, a clinician can have an idea of the presence and severity of an infection and what organism is causing that infection. The presence of bacteria alone on a smear suggests contamination. The presence of white blood cells plus bacteria is more suggestive of acute infection. Furthermore, many bacteria have a distinctive appearance on Gram stain. For example, gram-positive cocci in grapelike clusters suggest *S. aureus.* Quantitative Gram stains are discussed above.

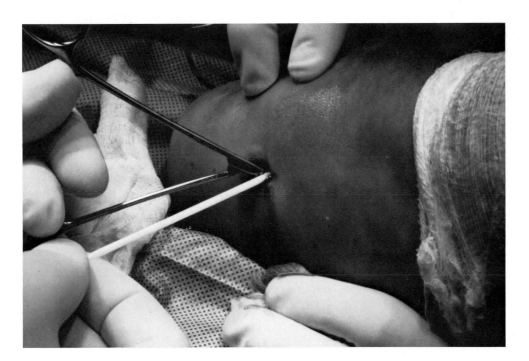

Fig. 30-1. Obtaining a deep wound culture specimen.

Culture and sensitivity (CS) results aid in the diagnosis and treatment of the infection by disclosing the type and amount of organism present and its antibiotic susceptibility. More important than the technique with which the CS is performed is the proper technique for obtaining the specimen (Fig. 30-1). The patient should not receive any antibiotics, if possible, for 48 hours. All samples should be taken from deep in the wound. Superficial swab results correlate poorly with the true infecting organism.[27] Sinus tracts should not be cultured because they will yield a wound toilet of organisms.[28] Only staphylococcus can be reliably found in both deep and sinus cultures. Aspiration of cellulitis yields only a 10 percent recovery rate.[29] Deep tissue biopsy and blood cultures are more reliable.

Blood cultures should be performed on a patient before antibiotic therapy is initiated. At least two sets should be drawn from different sites. If fever curves have shown consistent spike times over a few days, plan on drawing the culture prior to the expected spike. Blood culture results are often difficult to interpret because of the possibility of exogenous contamination. Most wound infections will yield an intermittent bacteremia. This is differentiated from the continuous bacteremia that is the hallmark in the diagnosis of endocarditis, or from transient bacteremia, which is usually of little clinical significance.

INFECTIOUS COMPLICATIONS OF SPECIFIC TRAUMATIC INJURIES

Each specific type of traumatic injury has been described in detail in individual chapters elsewhere in this text. In this section, only the infectious complications of those having unusual etiology, microbiology, or antibiotic treatment principles are explored. Specific recommendations for clinical management of that infection are given, particularly concerning antibiotic selection.

Puncture Wounds

Most puncture wounds heal uneventfully with minimal or no intervention (Fig. 30-2). Only 10 percent of these patients ultimately develop infectious complications.[30,31] These include cellulitis (the most common at 50 percent) septic arthritis, abscess formation (Fig. 30-3), and least commonly, osteomyelitis (0.6 to 1.8 percent) (Fig. 30-4).

Inadequate primary care is the major cause of these late complications. Usual treatment consists of a superficial cleansing of the wound, tetanus prophylaxis, and an oral antibiotic. This regimen does not address the possibility of a retained foreign body found in 3 percent of the wounds.[32] In the face of a foreign body, an infection can develop despite the use of antibiotics. Miller and Semian found retained foreign bodies in 60 percent of their patients with infections not responding to intravenous antibiotics.[33]

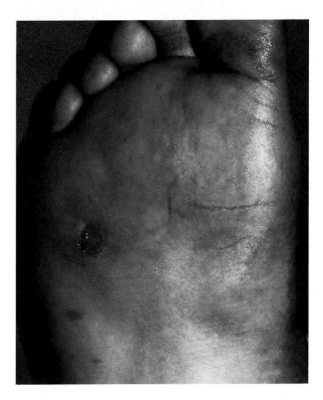

Fig. 30-2. Puncture wound with no infectious complications.

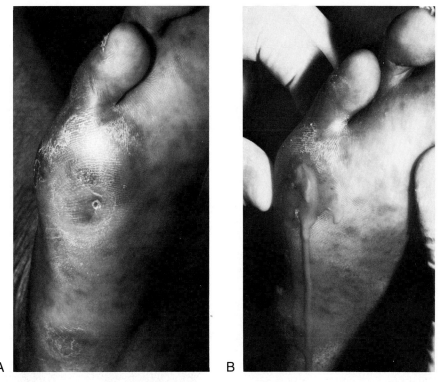

Fig. 30-3. **(A)** Puncture wound of foot. Note no apparent drainage. **(B)** Upon debridement of wound, a large amount of purulence is expressed from the abscess.

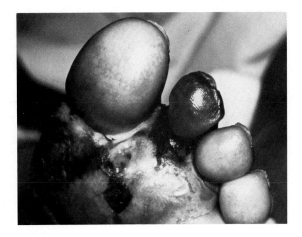

Fig. 30-4. Puncture wound in a diabetic that lead to osteomyelitis, and gas gangrene.

In cases of cellulitis, *S. aureus* is the causative organism in over 50 percent of the cases.[32] A number of other organisms have been indicted, although less frequently; they include *Escherichia coli, Klebsiella pneumonia, Staphylococcus epidermidis*, and streptococcus.[34] Antimicrobial treatment of cellulitis should be empirically directed at all of the common pathogens pending culture and sensitivity reports. Cefazolin, a first generation parenteral cephalosporin, is the drug of choice due to its coverage of all of the above organisms. Table 30-3 lists alternative antibiotics by organism isolated.

Fortunately, osteomyelitis is a rare, albeit potentially devastating, complication following pedal puncture wounds. When it does occur, however, the clinical presentation and causative organism are remarkably consistent. The patient usually has a red, hot, swollen foot (Fig. 30-5). Historically, the wound occurred 3 to 4 weeks

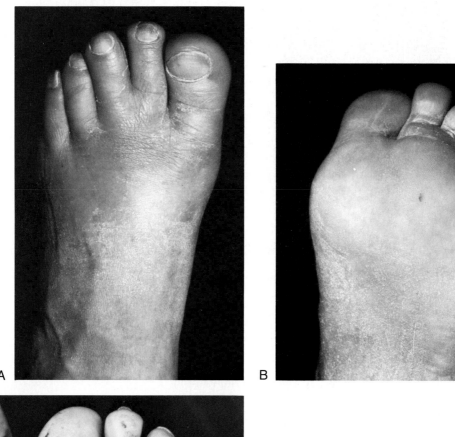

A

B

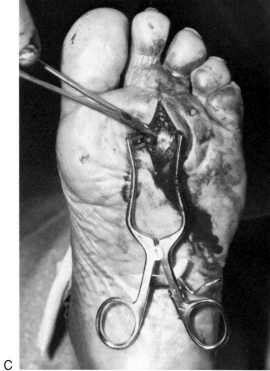

C

Fig. 30-5. (**A & B**) Dorsal and plantar views of a patient's foot with puncture wound osteomyelitis. (**C**) Debridement of osteomyelitic third metatarsal head. (*Figure continues.*)

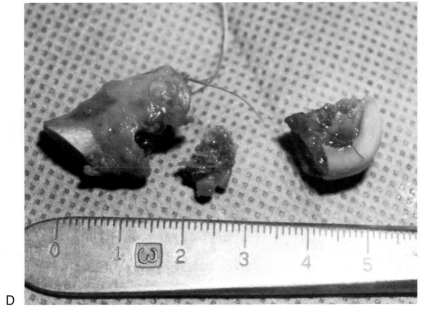

Fig. 30-5 (*Continued*). (**D**) Bone specimen of third metatarsal head.

Table 30-3. Antibiotic Selection for Puncture Wound Organisms

Organism	Antibiotic Selections[a]
S. aureus (methicillin susceptible)	Semisynthetic penicillin First generation cephalosporin Clindamycin Vancomycin Trimethoprim-sulfamethoxazole Erythromycin
S. aureus (methicillin resistant)	Vancomycin[b] Trimethoprim-sulfamethoxazole Ciprofloxacin Imipenem
Streptococcus	Penicillin V First generation cephalosporin
E. coli and mirablis	Ampicillin First generation cephalosporin Trimethoprim-sulfamethoxazole
Clostridium	Penicillin V Imipenem Clindamycin Metronidazole
P. aeruginosa	See Table 30-4

[a] Drugs are listed in approximate, theoretical order of choice based on usual sensitivity patterns. These patterns vary and should be checked before starting any antibiotic.
[b] Clear drug of choice and the only consideration with severe infection caused by this organism. Others should be considered alternatives only.

Table 30-4. Antibiotic Therapy of *Pseudomonas aeruginosa* Infections[a]

Aminoglycosides[b]
  Tobramycin
  Amikacin
  Gentamicin

Antipseudomonal penicillins
  Piperacillin
  Azlocillin
  Mezlocillin
  Ticarcillin[c]

Cephalosporins
  Ceftazidime
  Cefoperazone

Monobactams
  Aztreonam

Carbapenems
  Imipenem-cilastatin

Quinolones
  Ciprofloxacin (oral)

[a] Drugs in each class are listed by relative efficacy. List is of approved, marketed antibiotics available at the time of compilation.
[b] Aminoglycosides should be combined with a penicillin for synergy. Penicillins should not be used as single agents because of development of resistance. All other drugs on this list have been used effectively as single agents.
[c] Ticarcillin-clavulanic acid cannot be used as a single agent. It is no more effective against *Pseudomonas* than straight ticarcillin.

previously, at which time it was primarily treated as described above. The foot improves initially but then becomes painful. Oral antibiotics usually given relief as long as the patient continues to take them. Once the antibiotic is discontinued, the foot flares up once more. By this point, radiographs may be consistent with osteomyelitis. Upon surgical debridement (Fig. 30-5C) and culture of the infected bone (Fig. 30-5D), *P. aeruginosa* is isolated in 90 percent of the cases.[32]

Treatment of pseudomonal osteomyelitis is both medical and surgical in nature.[35] Adequate soft tissue and bone debridement is necessary. Antibiotic selection in pseudomonal osteomyelitis is covered in Table 30-4. Antibiotics should be maintained for 4 to 6 weeks following the definitive debridement.[36]

The dispensing of oral antibiotics as prophylaxis is unnecessary in patients with uncomplicated puncture wounds. In one series of 465 patients not receiving antibiotics, only 2 required incision and drainage, and one of those had a retained foreign body.[32] Oral antibiotics may actually serve to mask a deep infection and allow growth of resistant organisms. The use of these antibiotics is advocated, however, in patients with grossly contaminated wounds, wounds that have an established cellulitis, or wounds deep to bone or joint.[37]

Bite Wounds

Human and animal bite wounds of the lower extremity challenge the clinician in terms of organism identification, antibiotic selection, and surgical treatment. Each species differs in the potential for causing infection and the organisms usually involved. However, some general principles apply. The lower extremity is a more common site for animal bites than the upper extremity.[38] The likelihood of wound infection depends on the type of wound, its location, the species involved, and the general medical condition of the patient.[39] Human bites have a higher incidence of infection then animal bites. Cat bites are more prone to infection then dog bites (Fig. 30-6). The organisms involved are usually those found in the mouth flora of the animal. The infec-

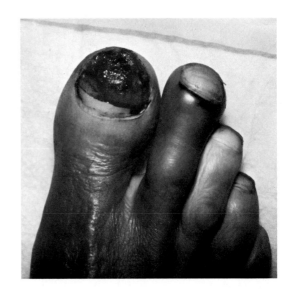

Fig. 30-6. Dog bite wound of hallux and second toe.

tions are frequently polymicrobial and contain both aerobes and anaerobes. Common organisms found in each type of bite wound are listed in Table 30-1. When the tooth penetrates the skin, the tissues are exposed to a very high concentration of bacteria sufficient to cause infection. The mammalian mouth can support the growth of 200 species of organisms. A concentration of 10^{11} bacteria per gram of tissue can be isolated from the gingival crevices.[41] This is 100,000 times the inoculum needed to cause an infection.

The use of antimicrobial prophylaxis is controversial. Since these wounds are highly contaminated and therefore of high risk, some investigators are in favor of using antibiotics following initial presentation and local wound care.[39–41] Penicillin V, semisynthetic penicillins, cephalosporins, clavulanic acid compounds, and erythromycin have all been cited as potential agents. Others have seen no difference in the incidence of infection with or without the use of these drugs.[42] They view these wounds as no different from uncomplicated lacerations or puncture wounds. If antibiotics are to be used, timing is critical. If delayed more than 3 hours, antibiotics have limited therapeutic benefit.[43] Owing to the high level of contamination, the potentially disastrous results of frank infection, and the relative safety of current drugs, antibiotic prophylaxis following any type of bite wound is probably warranted. A drug containing a β-lactamase inhibitor such as clavulanate or sulbactam is the agent of choice owing to excellent activity against all common pathogens, both aerobic and anaerobic. In patients who are allergic to penicillin, erythromycin or one of the cephalosporins would be effective alternatives for prophylaxis. Diagnosis and management principles of these infections vary little from those espoused earlier. Ordog, however, in his series of 420 dog bites found that Gram stain and culture of these wounds yielded little useful information.[43]

Because of the broad spectrum of organisms found in these infections, the traditional therapeutic approach favored a combination of antibiotics. This combination included penicillin V along with a semisynthetic penicillin. Cephalosporins alone are of questionable value since there is a high proportion of *Pasteurella multocida* resistant to them. Ordog, however, reported a 95 percent success rate with empiric use of cephradine.[43] The broad spectrum seen in drugs containing the β-lactamase inhibitors clavulanic acid and sulbactam makes them the drugs of choice for single agent therapy of bite wound infections.

Cat scratch disease and rabies are two systemic infectious diseases following local animal bites. Because of their systemic nature, they are not discussed in this chapter.

Open Fractures

One of the primary goals of open fracture treatment is the prevention of wound sepsis and osteomyelitis. To this end, the question of prophylactic antibiotics and internal fixation has been debated endlessly.

Open fractures are highly contaminated. Anywhere from 46 to 70.3 percent of the wounds in two series had positive cultures prior to treatment.[44,45] The question of the proper timing for wound cultures was examined by Patzakis et al.[46] They took culture specimens at four different stages: before any therapy, from debrided material at the time of operation, prior to closing, and from the closed wound. Culture specimens taken prior to any treatment had the highest prognostic correlation to the eventual infecting pathogen. The presence of contamination again raises the question of whether the term prophylaxis is proper. Gustilo and Anderson emphatically classify all open fracture wounds as severely contaminated.[45] Therefore, they believe that all antibiotic usage is "therapeutic" and that the drugs should be adjusted based on culture and sensitivity reports.

Despite terminology, consensus calls for the use of antibiotics in the treatment of these wounds.[44–48] Selection of an agent and duration of therapy vary. Patzakis et al. divided patients into three groups: a no antibiotic control, a group receiving penicillin plus streptomycin, and a group receiving cephalothin. The only statistically significant decrease in postoperative infection was seen in the patients receiving cephalothin. They treated the patients for at least 10 days. Gustilo and Anderson, after almost 20 years of experience and 1,025 fractures, similarly found that a cephalosporin is the drug of choice.[45] Their philosophy of treatment is to give a 3-day course beginning in the operating room. After 3 days, the antibiotic is discontinued despite the wound appearance, and the wound is reevaluated. Benson et al. found no significant difference between the use of cefazolin or clindamycin.[44] Bergman prefers the use of an antibiotic with a narrower spectrum, such as dicloxacillin, to prevent the development of resistance.[48]

The high incidence of *S. aureus* and, increasingly, gram-negative organisms such as *Proteus* suggests that a first generation cephalosporin is the drug of choice in all grades of open fracture. A caveat to this would be that the surgeon must be aware of any microbial trends in the institution. The presence of multiresistant gram-negative organisms or methicillin-resistant staphylococci (MRS) would radically alter the above suggestion. The emergence of various MRS in many institutions has led to an increased use of vancomycin in these cases.

Internal fixation is more controversial. It has been experimentally shown to reduce the risk of infection.[49] Stability at a fracture site allows for increased formation of capillary budding and decreases the potential for necrosis of bone.[50] In

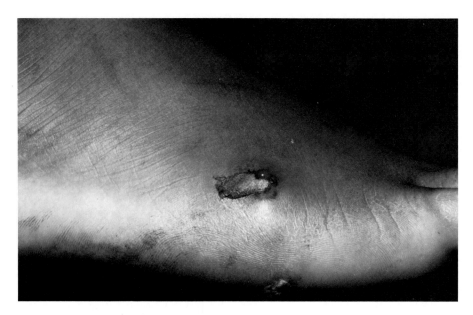

Fig. 30-7. Infected bullet wound of foot.

one interesting experiment, Merritt and Dowd found that the incidence of *Staphylococcus* infection was markedly decreased with the use of internal fixation but that the incidence of *Proteus* infection was increased. The different philosophies are demonstrated in large patient series. Gustilo and Anderson recommended the use of plaster casting and external fixation only.[45] Benson et al., on the other hand, thought that internal fixation posed no greater danger of infection if performed properly.[44] Franklin et al. attribute their low infection rate to following an established protocol that includes early antibiotic treatment and rigid internal fixation.[47]

Missile Injury

Gunshot wounds, although less frequent in the lower extremity then in other parts of the body, do occur (Fig. 30-7). These injuries combine all of the types of forces mentioned earlier. The severity of the injury is directly proportional to the amount of those forces and is mediated by the velocity of the missile, deformation of the missile in the tissues, and the density of the tissues.[2]

Since there are no viscera to penetrate in the lower extremity and cause endogenous contamination, only the potential for exogenous contamination must be considered. This potential varies with the weapon and velocity of the wound. Low-velocity wounds (small caliber handguns and shotguns) have a lower incidence of infection and are usually treated with local debridement without antibiotics. Interestingly, Patzakis et al. found that three of four shotgun injuries became infected.[46] They attribute this to massive soft tissue destruction and wadding forced into the wound.

The organisms found causing infection following gunshots vary little from those causing infection following lacerations or stab wounds. Therefore, the basic principles governing antibiotic prophylaxis and surgical debridement remain the same.

REFERENCES

1. Feng L, Eaton C: Soft tissue infections in lower extremity trauma. Clin Plast Surg 13:735, 1986

2. Cruse PJE: Wound infection: epidemiology and clinical characteristics. p. 319. In Howard RJ, Simmons RL (eds): Surgical Infectious Diseases. Appleton & Lange, East Norwalk, CT, 1987

3. Duncan WC, McBride M, Knox J: Experimental production of infections in humans. J Invest Dermatol 54:319, 1970

4. Lineaweaver W, Seeger J, Andel A et al: Neutrophil delivery to wounds of the upper and lower extremity. Arch Surg 120:430, 1985

5. Trunkey D: Infectious complications following trauma. p. 175. In Root RK, Trunkey DD, Sande MA (eds): New Surgical and Medical Approaches in Infectious Diseases. Churchill Livingstone, New York, 1987

6. Edlich RF, Rodeheaver GT, Thacker JG: Technical factors in the prevention of wound infections. p. 331. In Howard RJ, Simmons RL (eds): Surgical Infectious Diseases. Appleton & Lange, East Norwalk, CT, 1987

7. Miller SE, Miller CL, Trunkey DD: The immune consequences of trauma. Surg Clin North Am 62:167, 1982

8. Fikrig SM, Karl SC, Suntharalingar K: Neutrophil chemotaxis in patients with burns. Ann Surg 186:746, 1977

9. Munster AM: Immunologic response of trauma and burns: an overview. Am J Med 00:142, 1984

10. Howard RJ: Effect of burn injury, mechanical trauma, and operation on immune defenses. Surg Clin North Am 59:199, 1979

11. Yurt RW, Shires GT: Prophylaxis and treatment of infection in trauma. p. 624. In Mandell GL, Douglas RG, Bennett, JE (eds): Principles and practice of infectious diseases. Churchill Livingstone, New York, 1985

12. Roettinger W, Edgerton MT, Kurtz LD et al: Role of inoculation site as a determinant of infection in soft tissue wounds. Am J Surg 126:354, 1973

13. Fitzgerald RH, Jr., Kelly PJ: Infections of the skeletal system. p. 779. In Howard RJ, Simmons RL (eds): Surgical Infectious Diseases. Appleton & Lange, East Norwalk, CT, 1987

14. Gristina AG, Costerton JW: Bacterial adherence to biomaterials and tissues. J Bone Joint Surg 67A:264, 1985

15. Vaudaux P, Suzuki R, Waldvogel FA et al: Foreign body infection: role of fibronectin as a ligand for the adherence of *Staphylococcus aureus*. J Infect Dis 150:546, 1984

16. Roberts AH, Rye DG, Edgerton MT et al: Activity of antibiotics in contaminated wounds containing clay soil. Am J Surg 137:381, 1979

17. Haury BB, Rodeheaver GT, Pettry D et al: Inhibition of nonspecific defences by soil infection potentiating factors. Surg Gynecol Obstet 144:19, 1977

18. Haury B, Rodeheaver G, Vensko J et al: Debridement: an essential component of traumatic wound care. Am J Surg 135:238, 1978

19. Alexander JW, Korelitz J, Alexander NS: Prevention of wound infection: a case for closed suction drainage to remove wound fluids deficient in opsonic proteins. Am J Surg 132:59, 1978

20. Wheeler C, Rodeheaver G, Thacker J et al: Side effects of high pressure irrigation. Surg Gynecol Obstet 143:775, 1976

21. de Hol D, Rodeheaver G, Edgerton M et al: Potentiation of infection by suture closure of dead space. Am J Surg 127:716, 1974

22. Edlich RF, Panek PH, Rodeheaver G et al: Physical and chemical configuration of sutures in the development of surgical infections. Ann Surg 171:679, 1973

23. Allgower M, Durig M, Wolff G: Infections and trauma. Surg Clin North Am 60:133, 1980

24. Grossman JA, Adams JP, Kunec J: Prophylactic antibiotics in simple hand lacerations. JAMA 245:1055, 1981

25. Thrilby RC, Blair AJ, Thal ER: The value of prophylactic antibiotics for simple lacerations. Surg Gynecol Obstet 156:212, 1983

26. Harris RL, Musher DM, Bloom K et al: Manifestations of sepsis. Arch Intern Med 147:1895, 1987

27. Sharp CS, Bessman AN, Wagner FW, Jr., et al: Microbiology of superficial and deep tissues in infected diabetic gangrene. Surg Gynecol Obstet 149:217, 1979

28. Mackowiak PA, Jones SR, Smith JW: Diagnostic value of sinus-tract cultures in chronic osteomyelitis. JAMA 239:2772, 1978

29. Epperly TD: The value of needle aspiration in the management of cellulitis. J Fam Pract 23:337, 1986

30. Houston A, Roy W, Faust R et al: Tetanus prophylaxis in the treatment of puncture wounds of patients in the deep South. J Trauma 2:439, 1962

31. Chusid MJ, Jacobs WM, Sty JR: Pseudomonas arthritis following puncture wounds of the foot. J Pediatr 94:429, 1979

32. Fitzgerald R, Cowan J: Puncture wounds of the foot. Orthop Clin North Am 6:965, 1975

33. Miller E, Semian D: Gram negative osteomyelitis following puncture wounds of the foot. J Bone Joint Surg 57A:535, 1975

34. Lang A, Peterson H: Osteomyelitis following

puncture wounds of the foot in children. J Trauma 16:993, 1976

35. Joseph WJ, LeFrock JL: Infections complicating puncture wounds of the foot. J Foot Surg 26:S30, 1987

36. Siebert WT, Dewan S, Williams TW: Case report: pseudomonas puncture wound osteomyelitis in adults. Am J Med Sci 283:83, 1982

37. Riegler HF, Routson GW: Complications of deep puncture wounds of the foot. J Trauma 19:18, 1979

38. Mcdonough JJ, Stern PJ, Alexander JW: Management of animal and human bites and resulting human infections. p. 11. In Remington JS, Swartz MN: Current Clinical Topics in Infectious Diseases. Vol. 8. McGraw-Hill, New York, 1987

39. Hawkins J, Paris PM, Steward RD: Mammalian bites, rational approach to management. Postgrad Med 73:52, 1983

40. Edlich RF, Spengler BS, Rodeheaver GT et al: Emergency department management of mammalian bites. Emerg Med Clin North Am 4:595, 1986

41. Rest JG, Goldstein EJC: Management of human and animal bite wounds. Emerg Med Clin North Am 3:117, 1985

42. Lindsey D, Christopher M, Hollenbach J et al: Natural course of the human bite wound: incidence of infection and complications in 434 bites

and 803 lacerations in the same group of patients. J Trauma 27:45, 1987

43. Ordog GJ: The bacteriology of dog bite wounds on initial presentation. Ann Emerg Med 15:1324, 1986

44. Benson DR, Riggins RS, Lawrence RM, et al: Treatment of open fractures: a prospective study. J Trauma 23:25, 1983

45. Gustilo RB, Anderson JT: Prevention of infection in the treatment of one thousand and twenty five open fractures of long bones. J Bone Joint Surg 58A:453, 1976

46. Patzakis MJ, Harvey JP, Ivler D: The role of antibiotics in the management of open fractures. J Bone Joint Surg 56A:532, 1974

47. Franklin JL, Johnson KD, Hansen ST: Immediate internal fixation of open ankle fractures. J Bone Joint Surg 66A:1349, 1984

48. Bergman BR: Antibiotic prophylaxis in open and closed fractures: a controlled clinical trial. Acta Orthop Scan 53:57, 1982

49. Merritt K, Dowd JD: Role of internal fixation in infection of open fractures: studies with *Staphylococcus aureus* and *Proteus mirabilis*. J Orthop Res 5:23, 1987

50. Buckholz JM: The surgical management of osteomyelitis: with special reference to a surgical classification. J Foot Surg 26:S17, 1987

31

Complications of Internal Fixation

Donald R. Green, D.P.M.
Timothy R. Buell, D.P.M.

In this chapter, the complications of internal fixation are presented for the types of fixation most commonly used in foot and ankle trauma. General considerations and hazards common to all types of fixation are discussed, with emphasis on the specific complications associated with the technical aspects of these devices.

When the use of an internal fixation device is considered in trauma, the risks must be considered and measured against the desired results. In treating fractures we try to achieve optimum results by working toward a goal that is to some degree unobtainable. This goal includes earliest and most gentle reduction of fragments, adequate stabilization with the least interference with local function, avoidance of fracture disease, and maintenance of the patient's social, economic, and other functions.[1] Internal fixation, when intelligently used for the proper indication, with precise and correct technique and compliant postoperative care, can contribute to achieving these goals. There are many factors that affect the outcome of surgical intervention in trauma cases including adequate neurovascular status, absence of systemic or local infection, healthy nonosteoporotic or neoplastic bone, ability to obtain skin and soft tissue coverage of the wound, satisfactory nutritional status, and presence of hormonal imbalances.[2,3] Excellent technical work can be undone by the noncompliant patient, consequently, consideration must be given to the pa-

tient's ability to follow postoperative instructions. The basic principles of bone and fracture healing must be understood and appreciated by the surgeon.

BONE HEALING

Factors that promote bone formation and union in the healing process are not fully understood. The spectrum of bone healing at the fracture site can vary among primary bone healing, secondary bone healing, delayed union, pseudoarthrosis, and non union depending on local environmental factors.[2–4] These environmental factors can be affected by the type and effectiveness of the fixation used. In using fixation, we hope to achieve primary bone healing. Primary bone healing is the direct resorption and laying down of bone tissue across a fracture site.[5,6] The process is similar to the turnover of bone that occurs continuously in the normal reparative process of mature bone. Primary bone healing produces bone that has the cellular detail seen in the normal structure. The process occurs by the advance of osteons across the fracture site with a cutting cone of osteoclasts. Trailing capillary buds follow with osteoblasts that differentiate into bone. Remodeling then occurs along the fracture line without the formation of bone callus.[1,6–8]

Secondary bone healing occurs when mesenchymal cells are laid down between the bone fragments. In an unfixated fracture, hematoma forms between the fragments and must be absorbed and replaced by these pluripotential mesenchymal precursor cells. These cells differentiate into chondroblasts, cartilage cells, and eventually bone tissue. There is resorption of the bone ends. Callous tissue is formed in and around the fracture and can be seen radiographically. Haversian remodeling then occurs to reabsorb the callus. This is common method of healing in long bones and simulates the process of normal endochondral growth.[1,2,3,8]

Delayed union occurs when the process of secondary bone union is prolonged secondary to a poor local environment for healing. Connective tissue or fibrocartilage can fill the gap between the fragments in delayed union, producing a psuedoarthrosis. If the mesenchymal tissue differentiates into fibroblastic tissue and is never replaced by bone, a nonunion occurs.[2,3,8]

The crucial factor in bone healing is the pluripotential mesenchymal percursor cell and the type of tissue it differentiates into at the fracture site. These cells have the potential to differentiate into osteogenic, chondrogenic, or fibrogenic cells depending on the local conditions at the wound site.[9,10] The two most important factors seem to be oxygen tension and bone morphogenic protein induction. The higher the oxygen tension and the stronger the bone induction at the fracture site, the greater the tendency toward osteoblastic formation. The lower the oxygen tension and the weaker the bone induction, the greater the tendency toward fibroblastic differentiation of the mesenchymal cell. By reducing the gap at the fracture site, the surgeon can improve the local factors that encourage osteoblast formation.[11] Primary bone healing and the methods required to achieve it were studied by Schenk and Willeneger.[8,11] They established two basic requirements for primary bone healing: close apposition of the bone fragment ends and rigid fixation of those viable fragments. These premises formed the basis of the principles of internal fixation established, developed, and studied by the Swiss AO group.[11–14]

PRINCIPLES OF INTERNAL FIXATION IN FRACTURE HEALING

Early attempts to use internal fixation resulted in a high failure rate due to nonunion, infection, breakage of the devices, and loss of function or the extremity.[14,15] The Swiss AO group established a goal of early return of function of the injured extremity with the use of internal fixation. These principles have developed in conjunction with precise technique and standardized instruments and materials into a system that favors bone formation with early range of motion.[12,13] Most of the failures of internal fixation can be directly linked to a failure to follow these basic principles.

Accurate Anatomic Reduction of Bone Fragments

Accurate anatomic reduction is required to restore biomechanical function. With good alignment and apposition of the fragments, the ability of the fixation to function is mechanically increased.[16–19] Bone-to-bone reapproximation decreases the gap between viable bone segments. The close association of the bone ends increases in the stimulation of the mesenchymal precursor cells to become osteoblasts.[9] The accurate anatomic reduction of the bone ends promotes a higher oxygen tension because of the better blood supply to the fracture site. The larger the gap remaining after reduction of the fracture, the more hematoma will form. The central area of the gap will have a decreased oxygen tension, and cells there will differentiate into chondroblasts or fibroblasts, thus increasing the healing time.[2,3,9,11]

Rigid Internal Compression Fixation

Rigid fixation stabilizes the healing fracture site and prevents tearing of the fragile capillary buds across the gap.[11,12] If motion is allowed across the gap, the torn blood supply can form a hematoma, decreasing the oxygen tension and delaying bony union.[1,4,6,9] Compression, while not osteogenic, does increase bone healing because of rigid immobilization and increasing fragment approximation.[5,6,11] However, excessively produced compression can cause necrosis of bone ends.[20,21] Incomplete immobilization will be seen radiographically as callus formation.[2,3,7]

Early Mobilization of Adjacent Soft Tissue

Early mobilization of the joints and soft tissue surrounding the injured part is a primary goal of internal fixation.[12] Restriction of movement of the tissues surrounding the fracture leads to a decrease in strength and function, fracture disease, prolonged edema, restriction in the range of motion, osteoporosis, and soft tissue atrophy.[12] Early pain-free motion is possible when rigid and stable fixation is achieved.[1,12,14,15]

Atraumatic Surgical Technique

Atraumatic surgical technique is essential to preserve and reestablish the blood supply to the injuried part.[1,12,14,15] Precise surgical dissection will contribute to the viability of bone and soft tissue already compromised by injury.[27] Poor surgical technique will lead to increased edema and a decrease in the oxygen tension at the fracture site.[1]

GENERALIZED COMPLICATIONS OF INTERNAL FIXATION

There are many reasons why internal fixation is advantageous for achieving optimum bone healing. The hazards of using these methods must be carefully considered. There are complications that are common to all types of fixation and those that are specific and inherent to certain devices.

With internal fixation of fractures of the foot and ankle, the complex morphology and statics of the foot must be considered.[23] It is more technically difficult to fixate the small bones of the foot than the larger bones for which some of these methods were developed.[22] The technique and materials must be individually adapted. Before introducing the fixation device, the surgeon must determine whether the sequelae of failure would be worse than if nothing was done at all. If there is doubt about the efficacy of a device, use another method of stabilization.[22] If a fracture is not stable after fixation, it will not suddenly become stable after closure.

The use of internal fixation in a simple fracture results in a compound open fracture.[1] This allows direct visualization of the fracture site to achieve anatomic reduction and prevent soft tissue interposition. However, the skin is the body's first line of defense against infection. When this defense is broken to place the fixation device, the fracture fragment may become more susceptible to infection.[1,17,21,22]

In an open fracture, the skin is already broken. However, it is possible to inflict trauma to the area by the surgical preparation of the site. Especially in the foot and ankle, where there are small tight areas in which to work, extended incisions may be needed to introduce bulky fixation devices.[15,22,23] Surgical intervention causes tissue damage even with careful dissection in anatomic planes. This damage adds to the edema and possibly destroys valuable blood flow to the area, especially if large amounts of periosteum are stripped. Careful attention must be paid at the time of surgery to evacuate hematomas, restore normal structure, ligate bleeders, and use drainage systems as needed.[1,22,24] Even with careful surgical planning, the wound may be so extensive that soft tissue loss and fibrosis cannot be avoided. In this case, consideration must be given to the possibility of infection of the exposed bone and hardware and to future coverage and closure of the wound.

Another disadvantage of internal fixation is the introduction of a foreign material into the wound. The fixation device may act as a nidus for infection and harbor hidden bacteria. Bioincompatability was an early cause of failure of fixation devices.[14,15,25] The devices were often rapidly corroded by body fluids. If not corroded, they were rejected by the body or an allergic reaction occurred.[15] The biologic and physical relationship between the bone and the fixation device has resulted in the development of implants that function well in their internal environment. Fixation devices are made of surgical grade stainless steel (a chromium-nickel-molybdenum steel alloy).[11,14,25] Unless a person had a very sensitive allergy to nickel, the chances of rejection are low.[15] In situ, a protective barrier forms on the implant that resists the corrosive action of the body fluids. Defective or scratched implants should not be used as this protective barrier may be compromised. It is also important that the instrumentation developed for use with the fixation device be used.[12,13] The materials used for the implant and the instruments are the same in physical characteristics, preventing damage to the implant or the instrument.[12,13] If fixation devices are not properly inserted, loosening may occur. This may be due to absorption of bone at the implant bone interface. There is resulting motion, loss of stability, and possible abrasion of the fixation device.

One of the important principles of the Swiss AO group is obtaining early range of motion of the affected limb. In the lower extremity, early range of motion should not be confused with early weight bearing. The fixation devices are designed only to support the bone while it is healing, not to support the force of full weight bearing.[1,12,13,15] If early weight bearing is desired, other means will be necessary to counteract the mechanically disruptive forces of shear, torsion, and bending that are produced in the fully loaded limb.[15] The implants can break or bend, causing failure of fixation (Fig. 31-1).

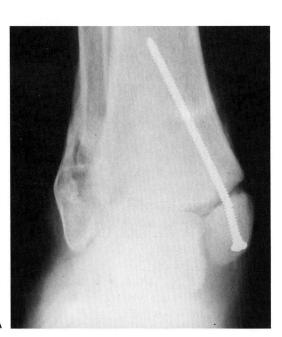
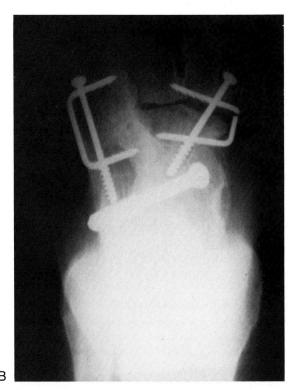

Fig. 31-1. **(A)** Failure of fixation secondary to a broken screw. **(B)** Excess motion has caused loosening and fracture of a bone staple.

POSTOPERATIVE COMPLICATIONS OF INTERNAL FIXATION

All the risks associated with any surgery can be present with internal fixation. Unnecessary use of internal fixation increases the operative time during which the patient is exposed to the risks of anesthesia. There is also increased exposure of bone and tissue with the possibility of local infection or sepsis. The postoperative complications of nonunion, infection, malalignment, and necrosis are considered below.[1,24]

Nonunion

Nonunion occurs when there is no bony growth between the bone fragments and the space is filled with fibrotic tissue that will never convert to bone.[2,3] The fracture site may be painful because of motion.[26] There is resorption of the bone ends, further destabilizing the fixation.[27] A malunion or nonunion occurs with internal fixation when complete reduction is not obtained at the fracture site and gapping is present.[27,28] In some cases, reduction may be adequate but the fixation is not stable and rigid. There is inability to prevent motion in all planes, and there may be rotation of a bone fragment around a fixation device. The incorrect fixation device may be used to inadequately resist the forces of shear, torsion, and bending produced by motion (Fig. 31-2). Sometimes all technical aspects are correct, but the patient may be noncompliant and bear weight early or injure the affected limb.

To prevent nonunion, the surgeon must ensure that rigid stable fixation with full reduction of the fracture has occurred prior to closing the wound. If technical difficulties prevent this, the surgeon must further protect the fracture site with casts or splints in the postoperative period.

If a nonunion occurs, another surgery will be necessary to remove the fixation device. Since bone resorption has likely occurred at the fragment ends, bone grafts will be required.[27–29] The grafts will maintain the length and alignment of the affected bone. This is critical in restoring

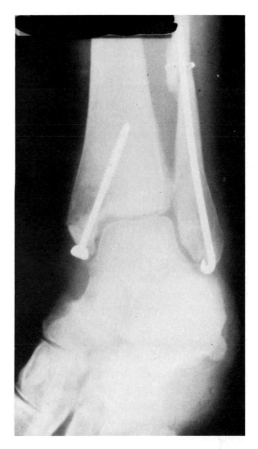

Fig. 31-2. A Rush rod used to fixate a fibular fracture allows rotation of the fragment and a resulting malunion.

function. The bone graft will also provide a matrix and foundation for bony ingrowth. The reasons for initial failure must be evaluated and understood prior to attempted repair so that correct surgical decisions are made.

Malalignment

Malalignment can also occur as a complication of internal fixation. The fixation may be stable and rigid, but if the fragments are not aligned properly the fracture will heal in a malaligned position. This could affect function and cause painful disability. The fracture must be reduced, the anatomy restored, and the fragments stabilized prior to application of the fixation device. This is an important step in obtaining rigid, stable, compressive internal fixation. A bone clamp or crossed Kirschner wires should stabilize the fracture while the fixation device is being applied. When screws or plates are used for fixation, the fragments may shift if the devices are not placed in the proper order.[12,15]

Infection

Infection is a possible complication with any surgery. In trauma injury there is often frank contamination of an open wound.[17,22] To reduce a closed fracture, an open reduction may be required that then exposes the bone and soft tissue to contamination. The use of prophylatic antibiotics at the time of surgery should be considered. The wound should be swabbed and the fluid sent for Gram stain and culture and sensitivity testing, both aerobic and anaerobic. All necrotic tissue in the wound must be debrided thoroughly. The wound should be thoroughly lavaged with copious amounts of sterile saline. The use of antibiotic in the irrigant is appropriate. The wound is inspected for any evidence of contaminating material prior to introducing a fixation device. Even if the bone only slightly breaks the skin in an open wound, the wound should be opened because the force of the injury probably caused the bone to protrude from the wound and carry foreign matter into the wound. Antibiotic therapy is maintained after surgery. The specific antibiotic used and the dosage are adjusted according to the culture and sensitivity results.[16–20,22]

Postoperative infections must be dealt with aggressively. Intravenous antibiotics are required. The wound is opened and debrided. If the fixated bone is involved in an osteomyletis, the fixation device should be removed and the infected bone resected.[22,24] It may be difficult to determine whether the bone is involved. A bone scan may be required. Since the site has been recently traumatized, a technetium-gallium scan may not differentiate between an osteomyletis and posttrauma or postsurgery inflammation. An indium 111 study will show an area of osteomyletic bone.

After the infected bone has been resected, the fracture is refixated and bone grafts are used. Motion at a fracture site decreases the ability of the bone to resist reinfection and heal.[28,29]

Necrosis

Internal fixation can result in necrosis of the fracture fragments. This occurs when the compression is too great at the bone ends, destroying the delicate capillary buds that must cross the fracture site.[1] Necrosis can also occur if large amounts of periosteum are stripped in preparing the site for the fixation device. Extensive surgery interfering with the blood supply can also result in necrosis to the bone and surrounding soft tissue. If necrosis of bone occurs, a nonunion may result, leading to further surgery to bone graft and refixate the site.[23,26,27] Necrosis of soft tissue may result in poor wound coverage, loss of function, or infection. These areas may need to be secondarily skin grafted or closed by delayed primary closure.[24]

IATROGENIC COMPLICATIONS

Iatrogenic complications of internal fixation are caused by the surgeon. By understanding those complications that can be introduced by the surgeon, they can be kept to a minimum. These iatrogenic considerations include (1) poor material selection, (2) poor approximation of the bone fragments, (3) nonrigid fixation of a fracture site, (4) poor technical application of the fixation device, (5) inadequate postoperative follow-up and control of the patient.[1]

Poor Material Selection

Internal fixation devices must be inspected before insertion. Defective manufacturing may occur, or the device may be scratched or bent.[1,23] Fixation devices that are to large may actually interfere with function or press on a vital neurovascular bundle. Internal fixation devices that are too small may not adequately secure the bone fragments. Some fixation devices can only limit motion in one or two planes and will fail when an attempt is made to use them to fixate through-and-through fractures.[1,15] A cortical screw that is too short will not obtain purchase on the opposite cortex, and compression will not occur when the screw is tightened. A screw that is too long may enter a joint or other bone, limiting motion.[1,12,15,23] Pressure on the surrounding neurovascular or soft tissue structures by a fixation device may produce neuropraxia or vascular compromise. A cortical screw with a smaller diameter thread may not effectively obtain purchase of cancellous bone and may not allow complete compression, or it may later loosen.

Poor Approximation of Fragments

Most commonly, poor approximation of the fragments occurs secondary to inadequate reduction and closure of the fracture site at the time of fixation. The fixation device may improperly grip the bone after overdrilling or burning of the bone by the drill. The bone may be osteoporotic, leading to stripping of a screw or inadequate pur-

chase. Poor approximation may result, with overtightening of the wire suture that is fixating a single cortex. Gapping may occur at the opposite cortex in a through-and-through fracture secured in this manner (Fig. 31-3). Separation of the fragments may occur with improper use of gliding hole and lagging techniques of screw fixation.[12,15] Threads across the osteotomy site will lead to gapping of the fracture and loosening and back-out of the screw (Fig. 31-4). A neutralization plate used with poor technique may not compress the fracture site. If the screws used to fix the plate to the bone are improperly placed, they will loosen and the plate will not be rigidly fixated. To avoid these complications, the bone fragments should be completely reduced and held tightly in approximation by a bone clamp before the fixation device is applied. Sometimes it will be difficult to maintain the reduction with just a bone clamp. In these cases, crossed Kirschner wires can assist in the reduction and be removed after compression is obtained. If threaded Kirschner wires or screws are used, the lag principles must be used to tightly approximate the fragments. Intraoperative radiographs in two planes may be required to verify reduction of the fracture without gapping.

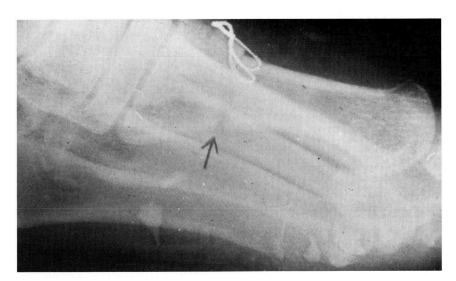

Fig. 31-3. Plantar gapping can be seen when wire suture alone is used to fixate a through-and-through fixation site.

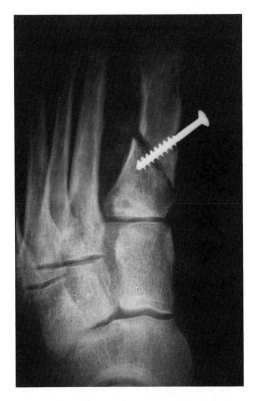

Fig. 31-4. A cancellous screw gaps an osteotomy site as a result of threads crossing the fixation site.

Nonrigid Fixation

Fixation must to be tested for motion before closure. If motion occurs immediately after reduction and compression of the fracture site by the fixation device, failure has already occurred. Nonrigid fixation may result from failure to hold the bone ends in approximation while the fixation device is applied. Fixation may have been achieved in only one plane, and rotation of the fragment around the fixation device occurs. This is a particular hazard with Steinmann pins, Kirschner wires, and Rush rods. The single intramedullary wire technique can lead to rotation and motion. A single wire may be inadequate when the fracture is through both cortices since it fixates it only in one plane and tends to compress the near cortex while making a gap in the opposite cortex. In screw fixation or plating, overtightening can strip the threads, leading to loos-

ening and loss of rigidity. Failure to engage the far-cortex with both cortical screws and Kirschner wires leads to loosening. If the near cortex is too aggressively countersunk, the head of the screw may punch through the thin cortex, causing a loss of compression and loosening of the screw.

Failure of Appropriate Surgical Technique

Many mistakes can be made in the application of fixation devices that lead to complications. Internal fixation techniques are nonforgiving. Attention to the details can make the difference between success and failure. Attention must be directed to the anatomic dissection involved in preparing the site for fixation. If neurovascular structures are not isolated they may impinge on the device, leading to vascular compromise or neuropraxia. This can occur when the twisted tips of wire suture are not buried and impale soft tissue. Metal fixation devices when superficially located can be positioned in areas where external forces can lead to painful irritation. Overtightening of a wire suture can lead to fatigue and early failure of fixation when the wire breaks. Wire sutures can also pull through the cortex of soft bone if overtightened or exposed to excessive forces. The tips of Kirschner wires must be checked to ensure that they are not in joint spaces, leading to scoring of the joint surfaces, restriction in motion, and pain. The precise steps developed by the AO group must be followed with the proper instrumentation when using screws, plates, and tension band techniques. Poor positioning of the bony fragments can lead to healing in a malaligned position (Fig. 31-5). Intraoperative radiographs can confirm the positioning of reduction and the placement of fixation devices prior to closure so that problems can be corrected. A surgeon must always have an alternative plan if the primary means of fixation fails. Practicing of fixation techniques on cadaver specimens trains the surgeon in handling the instruments and fixation devices.[1,12,15] Proper prior planning prevents poor performance.

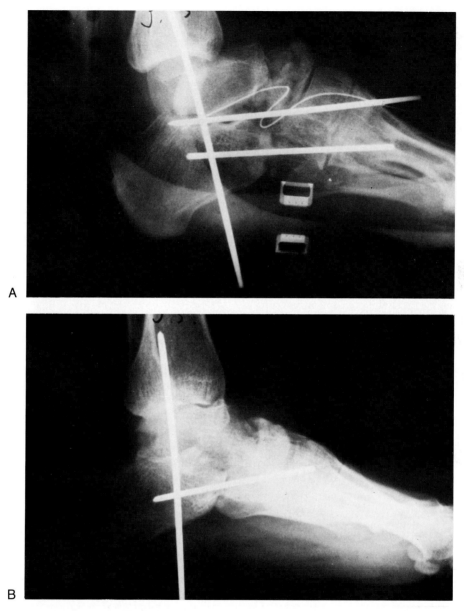

Fig. 31-5. **(A)** An iatrogenic ankle dislocation is pinned in a malaligned position. **(B)** The ankle joint is relocated and fixated in a corrected position. Intraoperative radiographs prevented this complication.

Inadequate Postoperative Follow-up and Patient Control

Improper postoperative management can cause failure of perfectly performed internal fixation techniques. The patient must be fully com-

pliant and motivated in the postoperative healing and rehabilitative period. Early mobilization is the goal of internal fixation. However, this does not mean normal weight bearing. The internal fixation devices are not designed to take the full weight-bearing force without casting or external splintage.[15,25] With certain fixation devices such as wire sutures, Kirschner wires, staples, and osteoclasps; external support will be required to prevent excess forces across the fracture site. Forces that might distract or gap the fracture fragments must be neutralized. Kirschner wires may be crossing joints, especially in metatarsal fractures, where the pin may pass through the tip of the digit across the metatarsophalangeal joint and into the fractured metatarsal. In this case, unprotected weight bearing may fracture the pin at the level of the joint. Postoperative use of a shoe with a felt buildup to the metatarsal heads will prevent motion of joint and fracture of the pin. If casts are used to assist in immobilizing the limb, they should be applied with caution. A cast applied to an extremity that has been recently traumatized and surgically repaired may restrict swelling in the immediate postoperative period. Pain, restriction in circulation, and pressure ulcers can result from the swelling. The cast may need bivalving, or a posterior splint may be applied with later application of a cast after swelling has subsided. Posterior splints and bivalved casts can be used to support a fracture site and removed for range of motion exercises. When applying casts over fixation devices that extrude from the skin or lie just underneath it, it is important to pad the area well. Synthetic casting material is not as moldable as plaster and will allow more motion. When motion occurs in a poorly molded cast with a fixation device exiting the skin into the cast, an interface of motion is set up between the pin and the skin that leads to irritation, skin breakdown, and possible infection of the fracture site. The motion of the cast is transmitted to the fixated fracture site, causing loss of rigid fixation and instability. Casts must be changed regularly and the fixation device examined. The skin must be examined for ulceration. Radiographs are taken immediately postoperatively and on a routine basis during recovery. Radiographs will verify the position and efficacy of the fixation device, identify problems early, confirm healing at the fracture site, and aid in determining when the fixation can be removed.

COMPLICATIONS OF FIXATION DEVICES

The following section discusses the fixation devices most commonly used in foot and ankle trauma and the specific complications and disadvantages of their use.

Kirschner Wires or Steinmann Pins

Kirschner wires and Steinmann pins are straight metal rods. They may have sharp or rounded tips, and they may be single or double with tips at both ends. They are either smooth or threaded.[1,15] They are placed with power equipment or manually. Although they are quick and easy to use, they do not create compression across a fracture site. Anatomic reduction and the close approximation of fragments is not as great as with other devices. Each rod only resists motion in two planes. A fracture fragment can still rotate around the rod if a through-and-through fracture exists. The use of crossed Kirschner wires or Steinmann pins may be required to prevent motion in all three planes. However, when crossing the rods it is possible to distract the fracture fragments owing to the divergent directions in which the wires are inserted.

The rod or pin is often left protruding from the skin. This is a possible contamination source, and a pin tract infection may result. It is also subject to motion by bumping or catching of the pin and may be distracted when a dressing or cast is removed (Fig. 31-6). A Kirschner wire placed through the tip of a digit and into the metatarsal shaft crosses the metatarsalphalangeal joint. If motion occurs, the pin may be subject to excess forces, resulting in fatigue and breakage with concomitant loss of stability of the fracture site (Fig. 31-7). The Kirschner wire may also excessively distract the soft tissue in the digit and cause vascular compromise resulting in a blue toe (Fig. 31-8).

The pin or Kirschner wire enters the bone cortex perpendicularly and is then directed in the

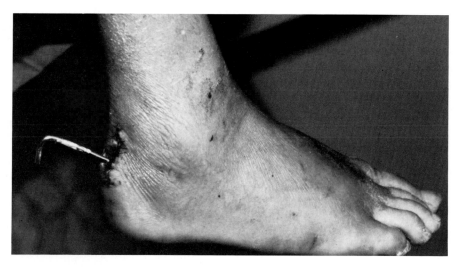

Fig. 31-6. A Steinmann pin exiting the posterior aspect of the heel must be protected from distraction or pressure by a well-molded cast.

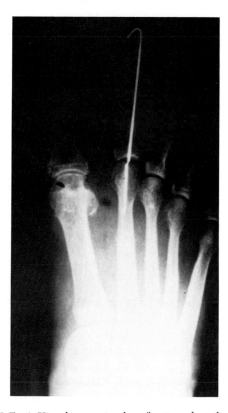

Fig. 31-7. A Kirschner wire has fractured at the level of the metatarsophalangeal joint because motion through the joint was not neutralized.

desired direction. If this is not done the pin may skip down the bone, resulting in poor placement. The pin should be directed from the least stable fragment to the more stable one to prevent distraction of the fragments. The wire should not be excessively bent during its placement, as a bent Kirschner wire can be very difficult to remove (Fig. 31-9). The rods can be used intramedullarly or transcortically. If they are used trancortically, both cortices may be engaged to obtain good purchase and some compression.

If a threaded Kirschner wire is used there may be difficulty removing it as it will not slip out smoothly like a nonthreaded wire. The threaded Kirschner wire may gap the reduced fracture site because it cannot be lagged and threads will be crossing the fracture site, causing distraction. Threaded Kirschner wires tend to be more brittle than nonthreaded wires because of a thinner inner core. They are not as flexible as nonthreaded wires and may fracture on bending.

Although these devices offer the advantage of easy placement in attempted closed reduction and pinning, their placement must be verified by radiographs or fluoroscopy. Soft tissue interposition may prevent reduction and fixation of a fracture. In all cases, the position of the pins must be

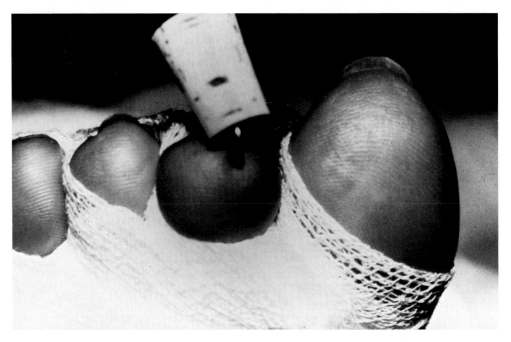

Fig. 31-8. A blue toe can result from vasospasm in the digit from distraction by a Kirschner wire.

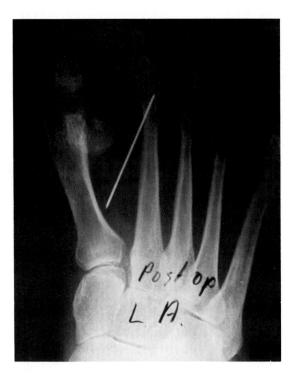

Fig. 31-9. A bent Kirschner wire was driven in off center and broke upon removal.

verified. They can be placed hazardously into a joint or impinge on vital soft tissue structures.

Kirschner wires can migrate and move, so their position must be verified at postoperative follow-ups. Since they are so easy to remove, the surgeon may be tempted to remove them to early. Often external support will be needed to neutralize forces through the fracture site that the rod cannot control.

Monofilament Wire Suture

Monofilament wire suture used in foot and ankle trauma is 26- or 28-gauge pliable stainless steel wire that can be used in a single or double strand. There are a variety of techniques used, including single intramedullary wire, figure of eight, cerclage, or tension banding.[1,15]

The most significant disadvantage of this type of fixation is that compression and rigid fixation are not created across the fracture site. There is inadequate purchase of bone. Control of motion is achieved in only one plane. If a through-and-through fracture is present there can be shifting of the fragments (Fig. 31-10). This type of fixation is best used when one cortex is intact and can act as a hinge. However, if the wire is overtightened there can be a fracture of the intact cortex resulting in gapping.[1]

Although the wires can be left in place owing to their small size, if they are inappropriately placed they can cause irritation against the skin or tendon. If the ends of the wire are not adequately buried into the bone they can impale soft tissue structures such as nerves and cause a neuropraxia.

The wire can pull through the bone if the holes in which the wire is passed are placed too close to the edge of the fracture. Osteoporotic bone contraindicates the use of wire suture since the bone will not hold the wire under tension. Overtightening the wire as it is being cinched down can break it or fatigue it to the point that later

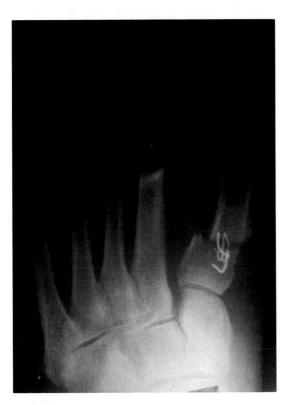

Fig. 31-10. A through-and-through osteotomy shifts when the monofilament wire suture breaks.

failure is possible. The wire should not be handled by any instrument in an area that will be used in fixation since it may later fail at the area where it was grasped.

Since compression is not obtained directly with this type of fixation, it may be combined with another type of fixation such as crossed Kirschner-wires. Postoperatively, external splintage is required such as plaster or povidine-iodine casts.

Osteoclasps

An osteoclasp is an S-shaped stainless steel rod with a prong running perpendicular to the S-plane on either end of the S-shaped rod. It works through the principle of the inherent tensile strength of metal creating compression across an osteotomy site.

The most significant disadvantage of this form[30] of fixation is that one cortex of the fracture must be intact or gapping will occur in the opposite cortex with compression. Motion is limited in only one or two dimensions. External splintage may be required to prevent failure of the fixation device.[1]

These devices can be difficult to place. An irregular contour of bone may interfere with correct placement owing to improper angulation of the osteoclasp. The holes for the arms must be accurately drilled at the correct distance and angulation into the bone. If the osteoclasp is poorly placed a hazardous prominence may result. If there is poor mechanical advantage for the device it will be subjected to repeated excessive stress and fail. These devices should be used in areas of low stress that can be kept unloaded, such as a proximal phalanx fracture of the hallux.

Staples

A staple is a U-shaped stainless steel device with two prongs and a horizontal bar. A fracture is reduced and the staple is placed across the site.

The staple does not create rigid compression across the fracture site. There is limitation of motion in only one or two dimensions. The staple works best in a fracture in which one cortex is intact. Staples are useful in holding reduction in a calcaneal fracture, where healing is quick owing to cancellous bone.

Care must be taken in placing the staple so that the bulk of the device does not interfere with function. The staple must be hammered into place, which increases the possibility of fracturing the bone further or displacing the fragments.

Screws

There are basically two types of screws— cortical and cancellous. The screws are used in a lag fashion across the fracture site. Precise technique is crucial in avoiding complications. Practice is required to perfect the techniques.[1,15]

To achieve the best compression, the screw must be perpendicular to the fracture line. This may require additional dissection to achieve exposure. Since one screw fixates in only two dimensions, two screws may be required to fixate an unstable fracture in three dimensions.[1,12,15] The use of two smaller screws is preferred to one large one. If a single screw is used the fracture site must be protected by exterior splintage. If fixation is lost the fragment will rotate around the screw.

If the angle of the screw deviates from the plane of the fracture when the screw is placed, there can be gross shift of the fragments causing loss of anatomic reduction. If the screw is placed perpendicularly to the fracture and is not perpendicular to the cortices, the fragments may telescope and heal in a malaligned position.[15]

When the screw is inserted, the threads can be stripped in the tapped bone if there is overtightening or osteoporotic bone is present. The two-finger technique should be used for the final tightening.[12] If the prepared threads strip, another type of fixation may be needed. If a cortical screw was initially used, a cancellous screw with its large diameter threads may purchase osteoporotic bone. Failure of fixation with a screw can also occur if there are threads across the fracture line without overdrilling the near glide hole. With advancement of the screw there is gapping

of the fracture (Fig. 31-11). When a cortical screw is used, the far cortex must be engaged by the lag technique to obtain compression across the fracture site (Fig. 31-12).[15]

The position of screws should be checked intraoperatively by radiography to ensure that the direction is proper, that malalignment does not exist, that the screw is not too long, and that the fracture is reduced without gapping.

Postoperatively, complications can occur if early weight bearing is allowed. The cast may be removed too early, exposing the fixation to failure. Screws may be removed too early, before healing has been completed. Conversely, although screws can be left in place, if they are irritating soft tissue structures, they must be removed.

Compression Plates

There are many types and shapes of plates. The plates can be used to create compression

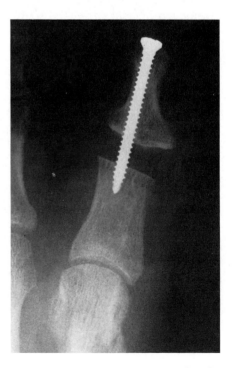

Fig. 31-11. Severe gapping is seen in this fusion attempt with a cortical screw.

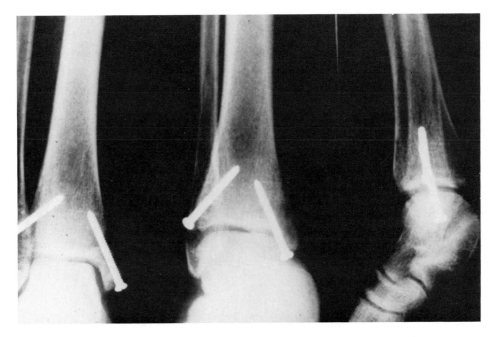

Fig. 31-12. Inappropriate use of cortical screws. There is no compression since the opposite cortex is not engaged.

across a fracture site by eccentric drilling of the holes, by securing a flat plate to a concave surface, by bending the plate slightly, or by using a dynamic compression plate with a compression hole.[1,12,15]

The use of plates increases operative time, and more extensive dissection is required to make room for the plate. The plate will need to be removed at a later date, exposing the patient to the risk of another surgery. The bulk of the plate may

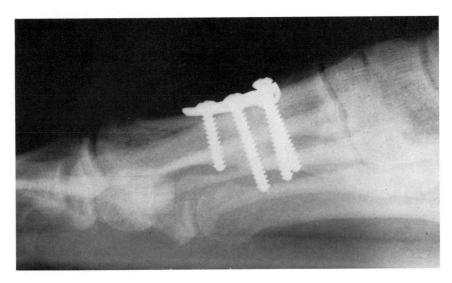

Fig. 31-13. This plate is fixated with a screw that is too long. Another screw proximally shows evidence of loosening.

lead to irritation, especially in areas of bony prominence.[1]

Precise technique is required in applying the plate. If a plate is not properly bent there may be gapping of the opposite cortex with tension on the plate.[15] The drill holes can cause problems if they are angulated, too small, too close, or too far apart. The screws must purchase both cortices and must not be too long (Fig. 31-13). If the drill hole or taper is too large the screw will loosen and back out with loss of compression as the plate shifts. Casts are not required postoperatively. Once the plate is removed, there is a period during which the bone remains weak and should be protected. This is due to the osteopenia that develops under the plate.[1,12,15]

External Fixators

Although they are not internal fixation devices, external fixators are used to obtain reduction and compression across a fracture site. These devices attach to either side of the fracture by rods or pins. The device itself is located external to the body part. A compression device is used to regulate the compression across the fracture site.[31]

These devices require a longer operative time. Practice is required to perfect their use. They must be removed after the fracture heals. The device is bulky and requires protection. An open wound remains after fixation is obtained. If not properly applied they can be unstable.

SUMMARY

Internal fixation is a valuable asset to the surgeon who deals with fractures. There are many complications that can occur with its use. These complications usually result from failure to follow the principles of internal fixation. There must be accurate anatomic reduction, atraumatic technique, rigid internal fixation with compression, and early mobilization of the adjoining soft tissue.

The surgical approach is planned prior to surgery. The instruments and fixation devices that will be required intraoperatively should be checked before surgery. Radiographic or fluoroscopic equipment should be available. Careful dissection in layers and atraumatic surgical technique is necessary to limit tissue destruction. The fracture fragments must be reduced and stably held in place while the fixation device is applied. Radiographs taken during surgery will verify the position of fixation devices and the adequate reduction and compression of the fracture. If there are problems they can be corrected before the wound is closed. The surgeon should have alternative fixation plans if the primary means of fixation fail.

The best teacher of these techniques is experience. This experience is best gained prior to surgery by practicing with the instruments and materials in a controlled situation such as an internal fixation workshop.

REFERENCES

1. Green D: The hazards of internal fixation in podiatry. Clin Podiatr Med Surg 2:95, 1985
2. Peacock EE, VanWinkle W: Surgery and Biology of Wound Repair. WB Saunders, Philadelphia, 1970
3. Hunt T, Dunphy E: Fundamentals of Wound Management. Appleton-Century-Crofts, East Norwalk, CT, 1979
4. McKibbin B: The biology of fracture healing in long bones. J Bone Joint Surg 60:150, 1978
5. Bagby GW, James JM: The effect of compression on the rate of fracture healing using a special plate. Am J Surg 95:761, 1958
6. Rahn BA, Gallinaro P, Baltensperger A et al: Primary bone healing—an experimental study in the rabbit. J Bone Joint Surg 53:783, 1971
7. Perrin S: Cortical bone healing. Acta Orthop Scand, suppl., 125: 1969
8. Schenk R: Histology of fracture repair and nonunion. AO Bulletin, October 1978
9. Eggers GW, Ainsworth WH, Shindler TO et al: Clinical significance of the contact compression factor in bone surgery. Arch Surg 62:467, 1951
10. Basset CA: Current concepts of bone formation. J Bone Joint Surg 44A:1217, 1962
11. Perren S: Physical and biological aspects of frac-

ture healing with special reference to internal fixation. Clin Orthop 138:175, 1979

12. Mueller ME, Allgower M, Schneider B: Manual of Internal Fixation—Technique Recommended by the AO Group. 2nd Ed. Springer-Verlag, New York, 1979

13. Heim U, Pfeiffer KM: Small Fragment Set Manual, Technique Recommended by the A.S.I.F. Group. Springer-Verlag, Berlin, 1982

14. Allgower M, Spiegel PG: Internal fixation of fractures—evolution of concepts. Clin Orthop 138:26, 1979

15. Ruch J, Merrill T: Principles of rigid internal compression fixation and its application in podiatric surgery. p. 246. In McGlamry ED (ed): Fundamentals of Foot Surgery. Williams & Wilkins, Baltimore, 1987

16. Ketenjian AY, Shelton ML: Primary internal fixation of open fractures. A retrospective study of the use of metallic internal fixation in fresh open fractures. J Trauma 12:756, 1972

17. Anderson JT, Gustilo RB: Immediate internal fixation in open fractures. Orthop Clin North Am 11:569, 1980

18. Chapman MW: The use of immediate internal fixation in open fractures. Orthop Clin North Am 11:579, 1980

19. Chapman MW: Role of bone stability in open fractures. p. 75. In Frankel VH (ed): Instructional Course Lectures. American Academy of Orthopedic Surgeons. Vol. 31. CV Mosby, St Louis, 1982

20. Gustilo R: Management of Open Fractures and Their Complications. WB Saunders, Philadelphia, 1982

21. Gustilo R: Management of open fractures and complications. p. 64. In Frankel VH (ed): Instructional Course Lectures. American Academy of Orthopedic Surgeons. Vol. 31. CV Mosby, St Louis, 1982

22. Karlin J: Management of open fractures. Clin Podiatr Med Surg 2:217, 1985

23. Hierholzer G, Muller KH: Corrective Osteotomies of the Lower Extremity. Springer-Verlag, Berlin, 1985

24. Block BH (ed): ACFS Complications in Foot Surgery, Prevention and Management. 2nd Ed. Williams & Wilkins, Baltimore, 1984

25. Vogler H: Basic bioengineering concepts. Concepts in bone performance, failure, and osteosynthesis. Clin Podiatr Med Surg 2:161, 1985

26. Chank K: Painful nonunion of a fracture of the fifth metatarsal. J Am Podiatry Assoc 61:108, 1971

27. Oloff LM, Jacobs AM: Fracture nonunion. Clin Podiatr Med Surg 2:379, 1985

28. Solheim K, Vaage S: Delayed union and nonunion of fractures. Clinical experience with the A.S.I.F. method. J Trauma 13:121, 1973

29. Hicks JH: Rigid fixation as treatment for nonunion. Lancet 2:272, 1963

30. Zlotoff H: The osteoclasp: a dynamic compression device for internal fixation of bone. Clin Podiatr Med Surg 2:161, 1985

31. Kenzora JE, Edwards CC, Browner BD et al: Acute management of major trauma involving the foot and ankle with Hoffmann external fixation. Foot Ankle 1:348, 1981

SUGGESTED READING

DePalma AF: The Management of Fractures and Dislocations. WB Saunders, Philadelphia, 1970

Giannestras N: Foot Disorders: Medical and Surgical Management. 2nd Ed. Lea & Febiger, Philadelphia, 1976

Mann RA (ed): DuVries' Surgery of the Foot. 4th Ed. CV Mosby, St Louis, 1978

32

Nonunions

Lawrence M. Oloff, D.P.M.

The restoration of bone continuity is truly a remarkable event. The end product of the reparative process of surgery and traumatic insults to bone is accomplished by the reconstitution of tissue very much like its original structure. Bone is similar to the liver in this regard, in which healing can occur without the formation of excessive scar tissue.[1]

It is fortunate that bone healing usually occurs in this fashion, for the management of aberrant healing is often more complex than repair of the initial injury. Differing treatment philosophies, timing of intervention, prolonged periods of incapacitation, and difficulties encountered in making an accurate diagnosis represent just some of the factors that contribute to the frustrations encountered by the physician and patient alike. The time lag from diagnosis to treatment, the potential for multiple surgical encounters, and the usually prolonged recovery period regardless of treatment option ultimately has profound socioeconomic implications to the patient with a nonunion.

Discussing the causes for delays in initiating treatment is not easily accomplished. Part of the difficulty lies in assigning a time for what constitutes normal repair. Individual variances in healing occur as a result of the particular bone involved, the location of the fracture within the bone itself, systemic influences on fracture healing, and methods of repair, just to mention a few. As a result of these variations, protracted delays develop as a wait-and-see attitude is adopted in situations that exceed normal repair. In fact, one study addressed this problem by noting an aver-

age 8-month time lapse from the acute injury to the point that the diagnosis of a nonunion was actually made.[2] This is further complicated by the arbitrary time allocation assigned to making a distinction between delayed union and nonunions. It is important to realize that there is not a specific time for repair of all fractures.

Also to be considered are the historical perspectives on management. The philosophy of putting the part at rest until healing occurs still has its advocates.[3] Its basis lies in the assumption that all nonunions result from excessive motion at the fracture site. Although this may be a valid approach to certain types of delayed repair, the universal application of this principle will ultimately result in a proportionately high number of failures. A distinction must be made between those delayed unions likely to benefit from this approach and those that would not.

Further difficulties are encountered in understanding the reparative process itself. Since the initial modern description of fracture repair, there has been an abundance of material added to supplement our understanding of the process, but more work is needed before we can obtain uniformity in our approach to nonunions. A clear understanding of the cellular events leading to repair is not an absolute prerequisite to successful fracture management. However, these events are critical to the treatment of complications of fracture repair.

The ensuing discussion reviews the reparative process itself, followed by an examination of the pathophysiology and treatment protocols of nonunions. Emphasis is also directed to the area of diagnosis, an area where many advances have occurred in recent years. An interesting area is that of those bone substitutes presently under investigative use. As certain nonunions involve bone loss, either through intervening cicatrix at the faulty healing site or as the direct result of an initial traumatic event, the use of bone substitutes represents an interesting potential alternative to presently available procedures.

BONE HEALING

Bone healing represents a complex series of cellular and biochemical events that ultimately results in the restoration of bone continuity. Because many of the original methods used to study the reparative process were destructive in nature, the use of animal models was necessitated.[4–8] Because of this, some theoretical criticism exists as to the applicability of these studies to humans. However, with the advent of more recent noninvasive studies of bone strength, confirmation and expansion of previously established doctrines continually occurs. Despite these advances, many questions remain unanswered.

Traditionally, fracture repair is thought of as occurring through the delineation of distinct stages of healing.[9] Various factors that can affect healing have been identified from both an experimental and clinical basis. A discussion on fracture repair and those factors affecting repair is generally not greeted with much enthusiasm by the clinician. Perhaps this subject is met with reluctance because of concerns of clinical relevancy. As previously stated, fractures can frequently be successfully treated without a complete understanding of the process. However, the clinician who does understand the process possesses certain advantages when one considers that a more rational basis then exists for the treatment of fractures and for those complications related to fracture repair. Most would agree that an understanding of the process is preferable to the empirical approach. For this reason, every attempt is made to cite the healing events in a fash-

ion that has clinical implications, from both a treatment and diagnostic viewpoint.

Cellular Events

The sequence of events of bone healing is straightforward. Much of the conjecture and complexity of the reparative process concerns the multitude of mechanisms affecting repair. The initial concepts to grasp in this process are the cellular elements.

There are principally three types of cells to consider. The osteoblasts are primarily involved with the formation of bone matrix and originate from the cambium layer of the periosteum and endosteum. The osteoclasts control bone resorption and remodeling, residing mostly along the peripheral aspects of the bone substance. The osteocytes participate in both bone formation and destruction, residing within the so-called functional unit of bone, the haversian system.

The sources of cells responsible for production of bone are varied. The periosteum is composed of two layers, the external fibrous and internal cambial layers. It is in the cambial layer that one source of these cells exists. They resemble normal fibroblasts and have been referred to as osteoprogenitor cells or undifferentiated mesenchymal cells.[10] Because of this, the periosteum should be preserved during surgery whenever feasible. However, these cells are also found on all exposed bone surfaces, both periosteal and endosteal. As will be discussed later, the endosteum is ultimately the most important portion of bone responsible for fracture healing. For this reason, osteogenic potential still exists when bone is devoid of periosteum. However, the periosteum should not be regarded lightly. It has been demonstrated experimentally that healing is possible when bone is excised but the periosteal envelope remains.[11]

The undifferentiated mesenchymal cells are believed to differentiate into osteoblastic cells by a combination of both mechanical and chemical stimuli.[12,13] This has been referred to as the cellular induction phenomenon and can also include fibroblasts and endothelial cells. It is thought that the anoxic environment and relative acidity that is brought about locally by the injury helps to precipitate this phenomenon.[14]

With production and organization of the fracture hematoma, there is eventual invasion by fibrovascular tissue.[15] The initial clot is replaced by this tissue, and collagen and matrix are laid down. Mineralization of these tissues then occurs. At the periphery of the callus, cartilage exists. This is changed to bone by the leading edge of endochondral ossification that accompanies blood vessel infiltration of the area. Low oxygen tension favors the formation of cartilage,[14,16] which forms to varying degrees, especially at the periphery of the callus. Cartilage temporarily bridges the intervening space until the vascular supply catches up. If the vascular supply proves inadequate or is prevented from progressing further, cartilage will persist. These processes, related to the formation of a hematoma, become less of a concern with the use of rigid internal fixation which minimizes the amount of hematoma formation.

Fracture Healing

Traditionally, bone healing is thought of as occurring through two mechanisms, either endochondral or membranous. The endochondral events are what we principally consider when fracture healing occurs in long bones. This involves the formation of a cartilage model that is replaced by mature bone in a stepwise fashion. Membranous bone formation does not involve a cartilage model, and instead occurs through mesenchymal cells directly transforming into osteoblasts that form osteoid. For the purpose of this discussion, the endochondral mechanism is principally considered. The entire process may be considered in simplistic fashion by dividing it into three phases: inflammatory, reparative, and remodeling.[9,17]

The immediate or inflammatory phase encompasses the injury and resultant bleeding, delivery of the usual cells of acute inflammation, and concludes with bone or cartilage formation. The increase in cell activity and division reaches its height in approximately 24 hours. The bone ends of the fracture do not participate directly in the proliferative activity of this phase.[15] In fact, the bone ends are dead, although instinctively the tendency is to think otherwise. To place this in a time frame, the inflammatory phase lasts for approximately 3 to 4 days. Clinically, this phase is assessed as concluding when pain and swelling diminish.[17]

The reparative phase is characterized by the formation of callus, both internal and external. The callus is initially referred to as soft callus, later to become hard callus as it is converted to fiber bone. While the soft callus stage begins with the conclusion of the inflammatory phase, the hard callus portion of this stage begins at 3 to 4 weeks and concludes when the fracture site is healed. Obviously, these time frames vary according to the individual bone. The external component helps to immobilize the fractured bone ends. This is thought to be a critical step, for the mobile fracture ends must be stabilized by a bony bridge so that union can occur.[18] The internal, or medullary, callus serves to fill up the spaces in the fracture line. The two types of callus, namely, the internal and external, are affected much differently by motion at the fracture site.[15] The amount of external callus increases with motion at the fracture and decreases with mechanical stability of the fracture. An example of the latter would be in cases in which rigid plate fixation is employed. On the other hand, medullary callus is unaffected by rigidity. In fact, medullary callus appears to heal without a fibrocartilage model when rigid fixation is employed. The conclusion of the soft callus stage is demonstrated clinically when the fracture is no longer mobile. During the hard callus stage, the callus is converted to fiber bone, and this phase concludes when the fracture is united with newly formed bone. The fracture is now radiographically healed.

The final stage, that of remodeling, involves the conversion of fiber bone to lamellar bone. The time frame for these activities varies considerably, lasting from several months to years after the initial insult to the bone. Osteoclasts actively participate in the remodeling of the callus so that a gradual decrease in its size is witnessed. The bone gradually accommodates its new functional requirements.

Local Vascular Supply

The functional microcirculation of healing bone is a critical concern. The blood supply to bone is achieved through the nutrient artery, metaphyseal arteries, and periosteal arterioles. The medullary system is principally responsible for supplying the cortex, the periosteal arterioles supply the outer third of the compactum, and the endosteal arterioles supply the remaining portion. This translates into direct clinical importance by Rhinelander's observations that the periosteal arterioles are adequate for supplying the external callus on a temporary basis, but that the endosteal arterioles ultimately supply the majority of blood needed to complete fracture healing.[19–22] It would seem from these studies that the extraosseous blood supply has its main purpose in supplying the external callus. However, this supply is transitory and its main function is replaced by the medullary system as it is reconstituted. The situation changes when the fracture fragments are markedly displaced or comminuted. Under these circumstances, the periosteal blood supply persists longer, but even in this instance the endosteal supply will eventually predominate if possible.

Role of Electrical Potentials

Much of the previous discussion portrays a picture of two advancing lines of bone callus that eventually touch, resulting in the restoration of cellular continuity. This bridge can then mature further. This cellular response and induction phenomenon depends on the vascular supply and other factors affecting the local environment. Also of interest is that electrical potentials are generated in the healing process. These differ in that they do not depend on cell viability. Most of the interest in this area was first brought about by the works of Fukada and Yasuda, who noted that electrical potentials occur with mechanical de-

formation of bone.[23] Further work by Friedenberg and Brighton showed that when a bone is fractured the ends became more electronegative.[24] Ultimately, it was established that electrical potentials in bone exist in two forms: stress-generated and bioelectrical potentials.[25–27] The bioelectric potentials are demonstrated in nonstressed bone. The metaphyseal portion is inherently electronegative compared with the diaphysis. Stress-generated potentials exist as electronegative areas in sites of compression and electropositive areas in those sites subject to tension. All of these theories ultimately resulted in significant clinical importance. This becomes apparent when one realizes that at fracture sites, electronegativity increases until healing occurs. These observations were collectively applied and constitute the basis for the application of direct currents or electromagnetic fields to promote fracture healing.

Surgical Implications Affecting Healing

Earlier discussion pointed to the significance of the external callus to the healing process of bone. It is well accepted that the amount of external callus formed is related to the amount of movement present at the fracture site.[17,28,29] If immobilization is artificially applied to the fracture, the external callus is no longer necessary. This is what in fact occurs when rigid internal fixation devices are applied. In fact, when external callus is noted in these situations, it is related as a sign of failure in the application of the devices.[30] When internal fixation devices are employed, healing occurs by what is termed primary bone healing, which is achieved by medullary callus and direct osteonal penetration. With this method, bridging of the fracture by external callus is abandoned. The benefits of this technique are debatable. The naturally occurring external bridging callus phenomenon is a much quicker reparative process.[15] With internal fixation, stability of the fracture must be artificially maintained for prolonged periods. What is not subject to debate are the benefits of earlier mobilization that this method affords.

Although bone plating allows for a more rigid immobilization and excellent apposition of the fracture ends when compared with alternative methods of fixation, other differences are noted in the healing process. With primary bone healing, endochondral bone formation is not noted, and as already cited, its presence may indicate technical failure of the fixation. Instead, it has been found that the necrotic ends of the cortical bone are not resorbed and are instead recanalized by new haversian systems that cross from one fragment to the other.[28] In essence, there is direct penetration by live osteons from the neighboring live bone and, to varying degrees, from the medullary callus. This type of healing is naturally dependent on close approximation of the fracture fragments. If this is not achieved, then the intervening gaps, when not too excessive, are filled by new bone that originates from the endosteum. This then provides the necessary bridge to allow for the passage of new haversian systems. When internal fixation devices are employed and there are larger intervening areas of dead bone, the whole process occurs much more slowly. The bone is dependent on the fixation device for much longer than is usual for this technique. In these slower situations, the majority of the bone is formed from vessels that arise from the periosteum and, to a greater extent, from the medullary canal.[31] Because this potential does exist with plate fixation, greater care must be given to the neighboring soft issues. Subperiosteal dissection is necessary to preserve the vasculature in these soft tissues that essentially becomes the extraosseous blood supply that accomplishes healing.[32] Even without plate fixation, it has already been demonstrated that these tissues are most important to the healing process.

Some questions may arise as to whether primary bone healing is in fact desirable. This question becomes a concern when one realizes that the formation of external callus is the most rapid method of achieving bone healing.[15] In addition, the presence of artificial fixation deprives the fracture of the stresses that are necessary to normal bone. This ultimately results in excessive osteoclastic activity that leads to osteoporosis beneath the plate.[33] However, the advantages of use of the part and the benefits of this movement to the soft tissues is nonetheless very important. The security of the fixation is of doubtless advantage at present to patient and surgeon alike. Further advances in the technology of the materials utilized in plates, methods of application, and considerations of when they are best removed will lessen some of the negative aspects that presently exist.

ETIOLOGY OF NONUNIONS

The previous discussion on fracture healing should impart an appreciation that this process represents a complex variety of integrated cellular, humoral, and bioelectrical events that ultimately result in the restoration of bone continuity. This unique process represents a continuum of events in which each succeeding stage has its basis in previous stages of repair. Although multiple safeguards are built into this system, mainly through alternative methods of repair, uncomplicated fracture healing relies upon this sequential staging. Because of this, each phase should proceed uneventfully so that subsequent steps can follow in similar fashion. The clinical importance of this is obvious. When one has an appreciation for normal healing, according to our present understanding, then one can recognize abnormal conditions and take appropriate steps to normalize the healing process when necessary. In addition, an understanding of the healing process and those factors that adversely affect it enables the physician to logically approach fractures in a manner that avoids aberrant healing. Unfortunately, this idealistic approach does not always produce uniform results. There are certain limitations in our understanding of the reparative process, diagnostic capabilities, and current treatment trends that make nonunions inevitable at times.

Most physicians recognize that there are a variety of factors that can delay bone healing. Although various forms of delineations of these factors can be used, the following discussion divides the causes of nonunions into local and systemic factors.

Local Factors

The local factors that contribute to the development of nonunions are by far the most common. These factors arise in everyday practice situations. Most of these factors relate directly to the nature and extent of the injury to both the bone and surrounding soft tissues.

Interference with Blood Supply

When there is significant comminution, separation, or displacement of the fracture, interference with the local blood supply may result. In these situations, reestablishment of the endosteal circulation may be difficult, and this portion of the local circulation is critical to the majority of bone healing. A good example of this is in cases of significant separation of the fracture ends. The resultant deficit necessitates that the vasculature traverse a much greater distance to restore blood supply. The amount of external callus has been noted to be proportional to the extent of separation between the fracture ends.[9] The greater the deficit, the greater the tendency toward external callus formation. With impacted fractures the converse holds true. In this instance, minimal external callus formation is generally observed.

Accuracy and Maintenance of Reduction

The concerns over accurate reduction and maintenance of this reduction have a firm basis in the physiology of fracture repair. It has been generally accepted for centuries that the fracture ends should be as closely approximated as possible to facilitate fracture repair. The reasons for this are essentially the same as were mentioned for separation of the fracture fragments. With inadequate reduction, the reestablishment of the vascular supply once again becomes a concern.[20] The periosteal blood supply must again predominate, and excessive external bone callus may begin to form. In addition, the reduction must be maintained. Most surgeons appreciate the formation of excessive callus as a sign of motion at the fracture site.

Compromise of the soft tissues can also contribute to the formation of nonunions. The reasons for this are multifactorial. Significant surrounding soft tissue damage, as the result of either injury or injudicious debridement, may retard the formation of external callus by interfering with those tissues that contribute to the periosteal arterioles. The status of the surrounding soft tissue is also important from the standpoint of rehabilitation of the patient. Even though rigid fixation techniques may have been employed, early mobilization may not be feasible in the presence of significant soft tissue injury. While stability of the fracture would seem to be the prime advantage of rigid internal fixation, one additional benefit of rigid fixation is early mobilization of the injured part. The action of muscles in these cases contributes to improved circulatory status to the injured extremity and applies compression to the fracture that results in pro-healing electrical potentials.[34]

Condition of Soft Tissue and Bone

The importance of both soft tissues and bone to fracture healing is further illustrated in cases of open fractures. Fractures of this type naturally carry a proportionately higher risk of infection. For this reason, extensive debridement of all tissue, both bone and soft tissue, that was thought of as being devitalized was carried out until recently. This approach had its basis in the concerns over the potential for bone infection if contaminated or devitalized tissue was allowed to remain in the wound. This ultimately resulted in the injudicious debridement of questionable soft tissue as well as any bone that was devoid of its soft tissue attachments. This approach not only carried risks of further potentiating avascularity to the site, but often resulted in the creation of large osseous defects, both factors predisposing to a greater incidence of nonunions. Because of these and other reasons, the general philosophical approach to this type of injury has shifted over the years. More conservative debridement is now recommended, leaving bone fragments wherever possible to act as free bone grafts to the fracture site.[29] If bone fragments are thought to be contaminated, and removal of these fragments would create an unacceptable gap, then an attempt at sterilization of the fragments is advised. If this is not feasible, then resultant gaps should be eliminated by the insertion of fresh bone grafts. Soft tissues are preferably not extensibly debrided or disturbed so as to not interfere with the extraosseous tissues that contribute to the periosteal arterioles. All of this creates a delicate balance. Too little debridement can increase the risks of infection and overzealous debridement can devascularize the fracture site. Both instances can ultimately result in the formation of nonunions. Suffice to say that every attempt should be made to retain as much tissue as possible at the fracture site.

Affects of Treatment Regimen

It is important to consider how individual treatment regimens affect the healing process. The formation of nonunions can often be traced to the inadequate or improper execution of generally accepted treatment programs. Often this involves the injudicious generic approach to fractures. A good case in point is the concept of immobilization. While it is a basic premise that most fractures will heal if immobilized sufficiently and for an adequate period, we have all witnessed exceptions to this rule. The reasons for these exceptions are again based on an understanding of the reparative process itself. While many consider it important to immobilize fractures until healing is evident radiographically, doing so may in fact slow down the healing process.[35] The reasons for this have already been stated in the section on bone repair. Functional return of the injured part results in compression and muscle action on the fracture ends, both of which result in the formation of favorable electronegative potentials.[34] The effects of these pro-healing potentials were deduced from studies of fractures of the long bones of the leg. These probably are offset to some extent by the recognition that leg bones are subject to axial loading forces, while similar forces applied to the foot may result in distraction forces under weight-bearing circumstances.

The benefit-risk ratio is further elucidated by the accepted doctrine that inadequate immobilization results in motion at the fracture site and resultant injury to the fragile neovascular tissues that are important to further the sequential steps of repair. While cast immobilization remains the most commonly employed method for fracture management, its use in unstable situations can result in the formation of nonunions. When instability is a concern, internal fixation techniques are therefore considered. The benefits of impaction over distraction of the fracture ends is indisputable. Internal fixation techniques are designed to provide this advantage; however, the use of internal fixation devices is not without its attendant risks.

Improper application of these devices can result in gaps, which negates the original intention of their usage.[36] In addition, one must pay particular concern to the effects on local circulation. Extraperiosteal dissection carries risks of interfering with the vascular supply from which the reparative tissues will arise.[32] This is especially a concern if the medullary supply is compromised by virtue of the application of these devices. It may be more simply stated that the proper application of rigid internal fixation devices does not ensure union of bone if the contributing vascular supply is irreparably damaged.

Fracture Location and Bone Pathology

The location of the fracture also dictates healing time and potential for aberrant healing. By virtue of its blood supply, the metaphysis of long bones is less likely to heal with incident than the diaphyseal portion. It is for this reason that we preferably perform surgery in this location when at all feasible. In addition, intra-articular fractures are more prone to retarded healing.[37] It is believed that the fibrinolysins present in synovial fluid inhibit the formation of fracture hematoma in the earlier stages of repair.

Last to consider are factors that we all have a strong appreciation for, namely, any pre-existing bone pathology. Examples of this would be infection or neoplasia. The subject of infection was briefly mentioned in the case of compound fractures. When there is local soft tissue or bone infection, particularly osteomyelitis, the cellular and humoral aspects of the reparative process are diverted away from their primary responsibility to restoration of bone continuity. In neoplasia, inadequate normal tissue may be present to accomplish repair.

Systemic Factors

Bone healing is influenced by a variety of factors, both local and systemic. What ultimately controls or alters the process is mostly based on those local factors already discussed in the section on bone healing. However, systemic contributions also need to be considered. Certainly bone metabolism is subject to hormonal influences. For years there has even been conjecture as to the presence of some type of local wound hormone that influences the reparative process.[13,15] While the search for this continues, there are other hormonal influences on bone repair that are established that will be discussed. In addition, other disease states have been demonstrated to alter fracture repair.

When considering hormonal factors, alteration of both the organic and inorganic constituents of bone may occur. Among the organic constituents, steroids are considered. Although it has been accepted that the administration of steroids can potentially retard wound healing and increase the susceptibility for infection in soft tissues, similar concerns exist in bone repair. The basis for these effects occurs on multiple levels.[38–40] The ability to mobilize osteoprogenitor cells is suppressed by steroids. Nonunion may also theoretically occur secondary to resultant suppression of the periosteal proliferation that is witnessed with normal repair.[41] In similar fashion, the formation of granulation tissue is suppressed. These findings do not always produce undesirous clinical results, for patients on exogenous steroids do not always manifest aberrant healing. The important thing to recognize is that these patients represent a higher risk group for these types of complications. In addition, this may prompt caution in terms of the local administration of steroids to the surgical site, especially at fracture or osteotomy sites. Other hormonal influences include both thyroid and growth hormone. The two together have demonstrated synergy in promoting fracture repair in the laboratory model.[42] Each have singularly demonstrated similar pro-healing effects on bone repair. It is known that hypothyroidism may retard skeletal growth and that the administration of thyroid hormone in deficiency states will hasten the repair process. Somatotropic hormone increases collagen synthesis and mineralization in bone. Because of these findings, growth hormone has been suggested as a form of treatment for delayed bone healing.[42] Further studies will be necessary before this becomes accepted practice.

Diabetes mellitus represents a relatively common disorder in which hormonal deficiency can affect the repair process. Insulin is thought to increase collagen synthesis and therefore promotes bone healing. Decreased proteoglycan synthesis has also been demonstrated.[43] The negative aspects on protein metabolism that result in an actual loss in bone mass is one of the prime concerns why diabetic patients demonstrate an increased rate of delayed osseous healing.[44] Because diabetes affects multiple systems, there are many mechanisms by which bone healing is compromised.[45] Large and small vessel disease can result in compromised perfusion to a fracture site. Associated autonomic neuropathy can create vasomotor instability that also affects vascular supply to the area. The sensory neuropathy that is frequently associated with diabetes often causes delays in diagnosis and treatment. Excessive motion at a fracture site is not uncommon for the patient has diminished sensation and does not seek attention for what would normally be perceived as a problem with healing.

Anemia is also a concern because it is frequently encountered in practice in the traumatized patient who has sustained blood loss and in the elderly patient. A host of other entities that result in anemia initiate debate as to whether restoration of blood volume or its components are necessary for osseous repair. Hypovolemia draws concerns in terms of delaying bone healing, but this is rarely encountered. In contrast to this, oxygen supply to the fracture site is unaffected by a normovolemic anemia. However, chronic systemic hypoxia can have deleterious effects on fracture repair.[14] While a close correlation between delayed healing and iron deficiency anemia has been demonstrated, the exact mechanisms for this remain controversial. One theory contends that the hypoferremia interferes with the enzymes that orchestrate high-energy bond transport through the cytochrome chain.[46] Alternative theories implicate low tissue oxygenation as directly involved.[5] Regardless of cause, a restoration of homeostasis would seem desirable in terms of fracture healing.

Concerns also exist in terms of any medications that may interfere with fracture healing. There are theoretical concerns about those medications that either suppress the inflammatory response to injury or interfere with the organization of the fracture hematoma. Whether these are practical concerns or not has not been fully addressed. Certainly, and as already mentioned, steroids can have adverse effects on the reparative process. In addition, anticoagulants predispose to delayed fracture healing. For example, heparin is similar in chemical structure to chondroitin sulfate. One theory proposes that heparin may therefore compete with chondroitin sulfate on the cellular level.[47] Others suggest a more direct explanation, in which heparin interferes with the formation of the fibrin latticework.[48] Hypovitaminosis can also affect fracture repair. Vitamin C is important to the hydroxylation of proline and lysine, so that collagen formation is interfered with in deficiency states. Vitamin D deficiency will result in abnormal mineralization. Vitamin A deficiency will produce an overgrowth of bone. Also of concern are hypervitaminosis states. For example, excessive vitamin A can cause cortical thinning. The exact role of vitamins in fracture repair remains unclear. The practical clinical ramifications of this are probably of greater concern in impoverished countries.

The preceding discussions emphasize the multiple factors that can affect fracture repair. As with any form of wound repair, the general state of health or well-being of the patient is important. Obviously, we all prefer a patient whose health is uncompromised by systemic disease. Even in ideal situations, fracture repair does not always proceed uneventfully. The individual variations in healing among different bones, among locations within individual bones, and among patients makes it difficult to assign an exact time frame that is appropriate for all fractures or surgical sites. Another factor compromising this issue is the age of the patient. The empirical assumption that age can affect repair came from the general observation that nonunions were relatively rare in the juvenile population.[49] The periosteum layer in children has been noted to be thicker and demonstrates a more rapid rate of proliferation when compared with that of adults. As previously mentioned, somatotropic hormones increase mineralization and promote greater collagen synthesis. Regardless of the exact mechanisms responsible, it is generally assumed that fracture healing will proceed more quickly in children. This does not imply that the elderly will necessarily experience nonunion, but that healing make take a longer time.

DIAGNOSIS

A clinical determination of aberrant bone healing is often difficult, especially from a critical time standpoint. As previously mentioned, fractures or osteotomies are mostly symptomatic during the inflammatory phase, a process that lasts approximately 3 to 4 days. Because of the individual variances in pain threshold, reliance on subsiding symptoms can be misleading. The detection of motion at a fracture site beyond 3 to 4 weeks is strongly suggestive, but is again unreliable owing to difficulties in detecting motion at certain anatomic sites, the presence of muscle guarding, and the possibility that motion may be imperceptible when a firm fibrous union exists. This and other factors dictate a need for a more objective means of evaluation. It is to this end that radiographs prove most useful.

Radiographs are not only supportive of a diagnosis, but also prove useful in making a delineation as to the type of nonunion and therefore serve to ultimately direct proper treatment. When a fracture line persists beyond a reasonable time, delayed union is suspected. However, there are difficulties determining what constitutes a reasonable time. Individual variances in bone healing occur as a result of a multitude of factors as already discussed. Although a time distinction between uncomplicated and complicated healing may be difficult, it has been suggested that nonunion should be suspect when progressive radiographic changes have not occurred for 3 months.[2] This statement is made with the realization that there are difficulties in grouping all fractures within this time frame.[48] In addition, aggressive management of those cases suspected as imminent nonunions is often withheld. Because of economic factors, the invasive nature of many of the available treatment programs, and patient reluctance, most physicians take the path of least resistance and adopt a wait-and-see attitude to many of these complications. I am sure that we have all seen cases in which this benign neglect approach has proved to be an effort in futility, and others in which healing occurred when it was not anticipated. Despite many of these frustrations, radiographic evaluation still proves to be the cornerstone of treatment. It is by this means that the diagnosis is often first made and appropriate treatment is initiated.

Although radiographs are the most reliable indicator, additional tests may prove useful. Because imaging of certain locations of the foot may be difficult, computed tomography (CT) is sometimes indicated. This has essentially replaced the applications once provided by conventional tomography. In addition, CT often proves useful in the preoperative planning or correction of complicated nonunions. Radionuclide imaging provides a means of assessing the physiologic status of fracture healing, especially when it is considered abnormal. In addition, infection can result in the development of nonunions. A relative degree of certainty as to the presence of bone infection can be established by radionuclide imaging techniques.

Standard Radiographs

There are characteristic radiographic findings that strongly suggest the presence of abnormal bone healing. As previously mentioned, the persistence of a fracture line beyond a normal time frame is suggestive. The presence of nonuniting bone callus is also suggestive. Also to be considered is the lack of fracture stability. The development of displacement or angulation a few weeks following the injury may be indicative of slow healing and the potential for eventual nonunion. These examples should serve to illustrate that radiographs are mostly relied on to detect changes of fracture healing that persist beyond a normal time frame. Although persistence of the sequential steps of fracture repair is suspicious, they may represent transient manifestations that should dissipate as fracture healing progresses. There are certain radiographic signs that are direct indicators of nonunion. For example, sclerosis of the fracture ends is thought to be pathognomonic of nonunions. It has also been related that atrophy both proximal and distal to the fracture site, or a so-called osteoporotic pattern is a characteristic feature of aberrant healing.[29] Last to be considered is the presence of what has been termed false callus. This again represents an ominous finding.

Detection of the true subtleties on radiographs that are suggestive of delayed healing rely on the physician's understanding of the normal sequence of events that represent uncomplicated healing. Then and only then can an appreciation for complicated healing be achieved. In characterizing healing, it is necessary to understand how the periosteal, medullary, and cortical bone is altered during the reparative process. An early and generally accepted indicator of a problem with healing is the status of the fracture line. Normally, the earliest sign of healing is widening of the fracture line. This often alarms the inexperienced practitioner. However, widening early in the repair process is considered a normal event and is representative of the changes associated with the inflammatory phase of healing. It is the persistence of this line beyond 2 weeks that is considered pathologic. Next witnessed is the formation of external bone callus. This is a natural phenomenon of secondary bone healing. There are various parameters of the callus that need to be qualified.[9] These parameters serve as easy reproducible references to monitor the status of healing on serial radiographs. First to consider is whether callus is in fact present. Again, callus formation is a natural process of healing for the vast majority of bone injuries. Callus should not form indescriminately; rather, opposing calluses should have purposeful orientation toward one another. The external callus should eventually bridge the fracture site. It also becomes more dense, eventually assuming the appearance of normal bone.[50] Many factors dictate the amount of callus formed. These include the type of bone, the particular location within the bone, the extent of injury, and the proximity of the fracture ends. The presence of exuberant callus is demonstrated when there is excessive motion at the fracture site. The presence of excess callus within a normal time frame for healing may represent a temporary phenomenon, especially if inciting factors such as motion are removed. This may create a confusing picture because specific types of nonunions present with excess callus. This type of excess callus is referred to as false callus and often displays areas of lucency throughout. The fact that motion persists and that the external callus has failed to bridge the fracture site does not necessarily suggest the development of a nonunion.[15] Under these circumstances, healing can still be achieved by late medullary callus formation. This is a process not dependent on immobilization, but it is assisted by it, and inevitably requires a prolonged period. Eventually, trabeculation across the fracture site will be noted.

Radiographic assessment of healing can be complicated in the presence of rigid internal fixation devices. As previously mentioned, direct bone union or so-called primary bone healing is hopefully achieved by this means without the assistance of bridging external callus. When callus is demonstrated, it usually is indicative of motion at the fracture site and failure of the original intent of the rigid compression device. When the ideal is achieved, the purposeful absence of the external callus essentially removes one source for assessing fracture repair. In one sense this is unfortunate, for primary bone healing is slower in achieving stability when compared with the natural process of external bridging. In addition, radiographic inspection of the fracture site becomes more difficult when rigid compression devices are used. Creative imaging techniques may prove useful, but detailing a fracture site with an overlying bone plate is difficult.

Radiographs may also prove useful in determining the type of nonunion. The categorization of nonunions has very practicals clinical importance. It may indicate the etiology as well as dictate appropriate treatment. There are essentially two types of nonunions, hypertrophic and atrophic[51,52] (Figs. 32-1 and 32-2). Each reflects the degree of inherent vascularity to the fracture ends, the hypertrophic type being vascular and the atrophic avascular. Determination of the type of nonunion is accomplished mostly by radiographic inspection of the fracture site, as each portrays a much different presentation. While both display a gap or persistence of the fracture, distinctions are made by the amount of callus formation. The hypertrophic type displays flared bone ends, while the atrophic type does not. It may be alternatively stated that the hypertrophic type demonstrates callus, whereas the atrophic type does not. A further distinction is made between these and what is termed pseudoarthroses. In this case, a so-called false joint is formed at the intervening cicatricial tissue. Further division of the hypertrophic type can be made. The distinction between these subdivisions is again based on the amount of callus formation. In descending order of external callus present they are elephant foot, horse foot, and oligotrophic.[52] The amount of callus formation is once again indicative of the osteogenic potential of each based on the vascularity to the site of injury.

A distinction based on viability of the bone ends has profound implications. This essentially allows for a greater degree of accuracy in determining which bone with delayed healing requires surgery to remove devitalized tissue and restore vascularity to the site, and which has the potential to heal by immobilization alone.[17,53,54] It may indicate which require bone grafting techniques and which does not. The exact specifics of treatment are dealt with in greater detail later in this chapter.

Radionuclide Imaging

Although standard radiographs are the main stay of diagnosis for delayed bone healing, certain cases may be difficult to assign to one of the classification groups. When this occurs, questions may arise as to the most appropriate course of action as treatment is dictated mostly by the inherent vascularity to the nonhealing fracture ends. When standard radiographs fail to conclusively establish the diagnosis, one may try to demonstrate motion at the fracture site by stress-

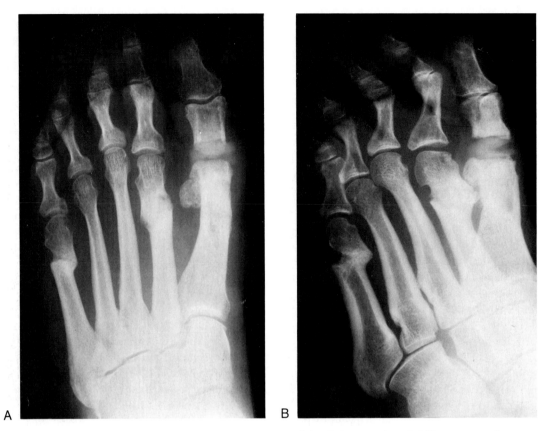

Fig. 32-1. (A & B) Persistence of the osteotomy sites of the left second and fifth metatarsals 2 years following surgery. Multiple views are often necessary to detect these findings. Poor alignment and significant shortening have occurred. Varying amounts of bone callus suggest hypertrophic nonunions.

ing the area under fluoroscopy.[36] However, this may still prove equivocal. This method of evaluation does little to establish the viability of the nonhealing fracture ends. In addition, if there are concerns as to whether infection is present, difficulties may be encountered in making the diagnosis because osteomyelitis may resemble false callus radiographically. Bone scanning may prove useful in both regards.

As previously mentioned, fractured bone goes through distinct stages in the reparative process. These patterns can be delineated into three distinct phases by radionuclide imaging that reflect the normal reparative process, namely, diffuse, biphasic, and coalescence.[55–57] The last phase persists for 1 to 2 years. This prolonged uptake occurs secondary to the fact that bone healing persists at subliminal levels for years following the initial bone insult. For the first 4 weeks following a fracture, diffuse uptake across the fracture site is witnessed.[58,59] A biphasic pattern then evolves, which is displayed as increased uptake that is more confined to the fractured ends of the bone. This phase lasts approximately 12 weeks. Finally, a focal area of uptake confined to the fracture site itself develops. This coalescence stage can persist up to 2 years following the initial injury.[53]

Once this basic understanding of normal patterns for fractures is understood, abnormal patterns can be more easily appreciated. Abnormal patterns are based on two simple premises. First, just as standard radiographs demonstrate failure to progress into later stages of repair with de-

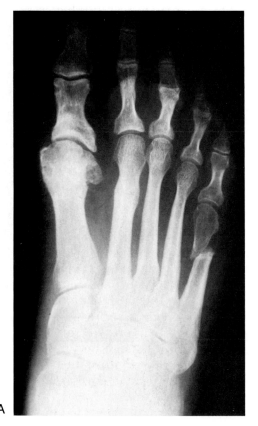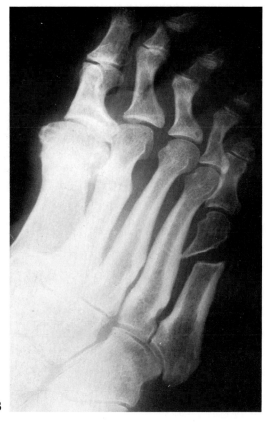

Fig. 32-2. (A & B) Right foot of the same patient in Figure 32-1. Similar procedures were performed on the second and fifth metatarsal. The second metatarsal went on to heal. The absence of callous and sclerotic ends of the fifth metatarsal suggest an atrophic nonunion.

layed bone healing, so does bone scanning. Second, the inherent vascularity and osteogenic potential of the fracture ends of the bone are displayed by bone scintigraphy[55,59,60] (Fig. 32-3). With hypertrophic nonunions, persistence of the biphasic pattern that does not progress into the standard coalescence pattern occurs. However, owing to inherent vascularity of the bone ends, an intense homogeneous uptake is witnessed. On the contrary, atrophic nonunions display low activity. In delayed union, all three phases occur but do so in a delayed fashion. Also important is how pseudoarthroses are displayed. In this case, two areas of intense uptake are seen with an intervening cold cleft or so-called photon-deficient zone.[61] The latter is a reflection of the intervening cicatrix. By these methods, delayed unions can be detected as early as 6 weeks and nonunion can be detected by 10 weeks. In addition, the differentiation of pseudoarthrosis from other types of nonunions has significant clinical importance. For example, the use of electromagnetic stimulation may be appropriate to many types of nonunions but is generally not recommended for pseudoarthroses. Bone scintigraphy also has clinical relevancy in the postoperative evaluation of nonunion sites. For example, bone scanning techniques have been used to assess the fate of both autogenous and allograft bone.[62,63]

It is well recognized that although bone scanning is very sensitive, questions remain as to the specificity. For example, when infection is suspected at a nonunion site, differentiation by bone scanning alone may be difficult. To achieve

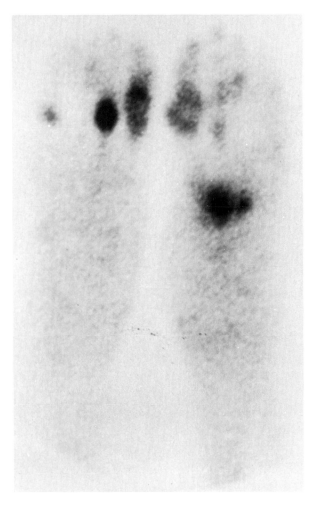

Fig. 32-3. This technetium 99m scan is of the patient in Figures 32-1 and 32-2. Note the intense homogeneous uptake of the left second metatarsal consistent with a hypertrophic nonunion. The uptake of the left fifth metatarsal is less intense and more focal, suggesting a so-called horse foot or oligotrophic type. The right fifth metatarsal shows low activity and is more consistent with an atrophic nonunion. The uptake of the first metatarsophalangeal joint is consistent with the more recently performed bunion and implant procedures.

greater accuracy in such complicated settings, greater sophistication in the type of studies ordered is needed. In this case, triphasic technetium scanning techniques in combination with gallium 67-citrate are employed.[64,65] The use of gallium 67-citrate in this setting will increase the

specificity for supervening infection. Unfortunately, false-positives will still occur. Ultimately, equivocal cases may require a bone biopsy for a definitive diagnosis. As false-negatives occur with much less frequency, negative gallium scans impart a greater degree of confidence that infection is not present. Additional concerns exist when internal fixation devices are used. In this case, a cold cleft may be displayed over the fracture site simulating a pseudoarthrosis.

Computed Tomography

In the complex smaller bones and joints of the foot, it has always been recognized that traditional imaging techniques have certain limitations. It is to this end that conventional tomography has proved useful. At times, difficulties may also be encountered in accurately determining whether the fracture line is still persisting in the middle of exuberant bone callus. When this occurs there are various options. Conventional tomography again may prove useful. In addition, the foot can be rotated small increments and fluorospots taken to assess the questionable area of concern. More recently, CT has gained acceptance.[66]

CT has become the procedure of choice in imaging the midfoot and hindfoot for complex pathology. Accurate visualization of these regions is difficult by any other means. This also holds true for nonunions. The healing of complex fractures of the talus and calcaneus serves as good examples. The questions in these cases may not only be assessment of healing, but also whether these injuries involve the articulations of the subtalar joint. Other concerns also exist. In talar fractures, deprivation of the vascular supply is not all that uncommon, so that nonunions and avascular necrosis occur with greater frequency.[67–69] Because the calcaneus is mostly composed of cancellous bone, nonunions occur less frequently. However, other concerns such as intra-articular involvement, degree of comminution, and peroneal tendon impingement from widening of the body of the calcaneus or from incorporation of the tendons in the healing bone are of practical concern.[17,70] When these questions arise, CT will prove useful in terms of diagnosis and in determining the best treatment alternatives. In addition, CT may help to determine incision placement, extent of graft necessary, and selection of the most appropriate means of fixation. In other words, preoperative planning is greatly enhanced.

TREATMENT

Immobilization

The time-honored basis for management of nonunions has revolved around immobilization of the site until there was radiographic or clinical evidence of healing. It was the natural assumption that fractures would fail to heal primarily because of motion at the fracture and that if this motion could be arrested by casting, healing would eventually occur. There are certain pitfalls with this logic. As discussed above, there are many factors that adversely affect fracture repair, inadequate immobilization being just one example. In addition, certain fractures fail to heal regardless of the manner and time of immobilization employed. Questions also arise as to what constitutes an adequate trial of immobilization. The answers to such questions arose from the empirical observations of others. In addition, the primary treatment of many fractures has been advanced in recent years by the use of more exacting classification systems that help to determine what kind of fractures have a good versus a poor prognosis, which would better benefit from operative reduction versus immobilization, and which require longer periods of immobilization. This has not only resulted in a clearer understanding of the mechanisms and most appropriate manner of management of specific injuries, but has also resulted in a lesser incidence of nonunions.

When clinical or radiographic evidence of delayed healing of bone exists, continued immobilization remains the most common approach when alignment is satisfactory. As previously stated, this generic approach is based on the assumption that repetitive motion has resulted in ongoing injury to the fragile reparative tissues. This approach has no distinct boundaries and relies on each practitioner's belief as to what constitutes a satisfactory time trial for this type of therapy. Even though this simplistic reasoning is supported by those who claim limited complications with this approach, there are certain attendant risks. For example, one must realize that protracted courses of casting results in various degrees of cast disease. The importance of the soft tissues to fracture healing was emphasized in the previous sections. This is best exemplified by considering the basis of rigid internal fixation that contends that functional return of the part ultimately results in a shorter convalescence.

Even though arbitrarily assigned, this type of approach still can have merit if it is applied in a fashion that is consistent with our present understanding of the reparative process. If the patient displays radiographic evidence of a hypertrophic delayed union, then continued immobilization may be tried. Again, we are playing the odds by assuming that many hypertrophic nonunions result from excessive motion. If a patient has evidence suggesting an atrophic type of nonunion, then continued immobilization carries a significant risk of not succeeding. Other clinical situations warrant trials of continued immobilization, for example, the presence of external callus following rigid internal fixation. In this case, the callus indicates some degree of failure of the device, whether due to the device itself or the manner in which it was applied. Early utilization of immobilization may prevent nonunion in this situation.

Last to be considered is the type of immobilization. Although plaster or synthetic casts are most commonly utilized, an understanding of the reparative process has given rise to certain alternatives. The advocates of functional cast bracing contend that there are certain advantages over traditional immobilization techniques. The basis lies in the recognition that some degree of limited weight bearing results in greater compression across the fracture site.[34] This compression contributes to the formation of pro-healing stress-generated potentials. The resultant improved status of the surrounding soft tissues is also beneficial to repair with this method. Even if traditional methods are employed, the use of muscle stimulators may help to mitigate the effects of the immobilization.

Electrical Treatment of Nonunions

The newest addition to the armamentarium of available treatment regimens is electrical stimulation. The use of electrical stimulation was brought about by the initial observations that there are indeed electrical potentials found in bone and that they are intimately related to bone formation.[23–25,71–73] These potentials are of two types, stress generated and bioelectrical. The stress-generated potentials are demonstrated on the compression side of bone, which becomes electronegative, the tension side being electropositive. Bone formation occurs on the electronegative side and bone is removed on the electropositive side. This coincides with the observations that bone heals under compression and fails under tension. These stress-generated potentials were further observed to be a product of stress and not to be dependent on cell viability. In contrast to stress-generated potential, bioelectrical potentials are dependent on cell viability. They occur in areas of repair. In addition, the bioelectrical potentials differ according to the location within the bone. The metaphyseal portion is electronegative compared with the diaphysis. With injury, electronegativity increases over the fracture site.

A total explanation as to the electrophysiologic mechanisms responsible for such phenomenon is lacking. Prevalent thoughts on this matter revolve around two theories: direct cellular and indirect microenvironmental changes.[74] The former is thought to involve activation of the cyclic AMP cellular system by fluctuations of the cell membrane surface charge. The change in the microenvironment is one that involves oxygen depletion since bone formation occurs under such circumstances. Whatever the exact mechanisms, osteoblastic proliferation occurs under the influence of direct current.[75]

Based on these premises, various studies were undertaken to determine whether electrical stimulation would establish an environment that would be conducive to bone formation. All of these observations eventually culminated in the first successful treatment of a nonunion by Friedenberg et al. when direct current was applied to a nonunion of the medial malleolus.[76,77] Further refinements have since been established, so that we now recognize that constant currents between 5 and 20 μA through an implanted cathode result in bone formation, with maximum production at 20 μA.[38] When greater than 20 μA is applied, osseous breakdown near the cathode occurs. This displays a typical dose-response curve, again establishing a recurrent theme in medicine, namely, that more is not necessarily better. In addition, bone formation was mostly confined to a 5-mm radius from the implanted cathode site. Since these observations, changes have occurred in the direct current delivery systems available.

Although electrostimulation has been proved clinically effective, one must question how this method stands up against established operative protocols. Traditional operative approaches to nonunions have involved the use of bone grafting techniques, usually combined with some form of internal fixation. This is the standard with which alternative methods are ultimately compared. The data comparing the two have established that the success rates between the two are comparable. Based on these findings, it would appear that electrotherapeutic methods are preferable when one considers the relative invasiveness of each. Other factors would dictate the same. For instance, concerns exist in terms of previous operative intervention. When the patient has a history of previous surgery to the area, a decreased success rate can be anticipated with subsequent surgical attempts.[78,79] However, previous failed surgery does not seem to significantly alter the success rate of electrostimulation.[49,80,81] In addition, the duration of the nonunion does not seem to be a factor with electrostimulation since successful results have been obtained in nonunions that have been present for years.[82–85] Also to be considered are more complicated settings, such as infected nonunions. Although definitive operative intervention through such sites used to be contraindicated, thoughts on this are continually being modified. With the advent of microvascular surgical techniques, considerations exist for use of composite bone grafts that are revascularized by such techniques, thus allowing for the opportunity to convert contaminated wounds to clean wounds. The use of electrostimulation in the presence of infection has resulted in mixed reports. One study suggested exercising caution in the presence of active osteomyelitis,[86] while another reported an encouraging 90 percent success rate in a patient population predominately having active draining wounds.[87]

Although the preceding discussion suggests overwhelming evidence to support the use of electrotherapeutic methods over alternative approaches, there are certain limitations that need to be addressed. Despite relatively widespread use of this approach, the cost of the various devices remains high. Of course, the cost of surgery is significantly higher when one considers the surgery, hospitalization, support services, etc. Greater concerns exist in terms of application. Electrostimulation cannot be effectively applied to all nonunions, and careful patient selection is mandatory. A case in point is the relative ineffectiveness of electrostimulation with pseudoarthrosis.[84] When this diagnosis is established, the treatment of choice remains excision of the intervening cicatrix and synovial tissues. Once the osteogenic potential has been restored by this means, electrostimulation can then be applied if so desired. As previously mentioned, differentiation of pseudoarthrosis from other nonunions can be accomplished by bone scanning techniques. One study evaluating this approach documented a 95 percent success rate with nonunions that demonstrated increased uptake across the nonunion site.[88] This contrasted with a 50 percent success rate in cases in which the fracture ends demonstrated increased uptake with an intervening area of decreased uptake. As previously mentioned, there are relative concerns to using these techniques in the presence of active osteomyelitis. It would be valuable to have additional research in this specific area. Also, concerns exist in terms of the presence and extent of any osseous defects. As a general rule, electrostimulation is not advised if the defect is greater than one-half the diameter of the bone.[78,82–85] Concerns have also been expressed with certain fractures

that are notorious for poor healing in the best of clinical settings. In nonunions in these sites, such as the femur and humerus, healing depends on the slower intramedullary callus response, which is less tolerant of motion. In these situations rigid fixation combined with electrostimulation becomes preferable.[36] Similar concerns may potentially exist in the foot, such as in the navicular.

There are presently two general types of electrostimulation systems available to practitioners, those that employ surface coils and those that necessitate surgical implantation. While the former would seem simpler in terms of expense and risk to the patient, there are certain advantages and disadvantages to each. General guidelines suggest some form of immobilization with each, although success has been achieved with limited immobilization. Many factors influence selection of the most appropriate type, such as economic considerations, type of nonunion, patient preference, and physician experience. The invasive types of systems essentially involve two types, those requiring implantation of cathode wire into the nonunion site and those accomplishing the same with Kirschner wires that participate as the cathode.

The Depuy system involves the implantation of a cathode wire, which is fashioned into a figure eight or helical configuration, into the site of concern.[2] Prior to implantation, all interpositional fibrous or synovial tissue is excised. In addition, a generator and anode component require implantation, but remote to the nonunion site. This usually is best accomplished by implanting these components into a neighboring muscle belly. The anode must be placed away from the bone or resorption will occur. When this system is applied to the foot, use of the calf muscles is preferred. However, distance proves to be a limiting factor in the foot. Its main advantage is that the entire system is implanted so that patient compliance is not a factor. This advantage is at the same time a disadvantage for a second surgery is necessitated to remove the entire system. This is usually accomplished after 6 months, this being the life span of the generator. Earlier removal is considered if healing has been accomplished. The use of this system is generally limited to those cases in which operative intervention is necessary, such as a pseudoarthrosis.

The Zimmer system also employs implantation of a cathode, fashioned like a Kirschner wire.[35] These pins measure 1.2 mm and are Teflon coated. The exposed tip is bare to allow for insertion into the nonunion with resultant stimulation to the site (Fig. 32-4). Image intensification has proved useful in assisting in percutaneous insertion, thereby eliminating the need for surgical exposure on occasion. It is generally advised that two to four wires be used. Usually two wires suffice in the foot, although success can occur with only one wire. Each Teflon-coated wire delivers approximately 20 μA to the site. If more than one wire is used, the optimal distance between wire tips is 0.5 cm. The cathode wires connect to an external power pack that can be incorporated into the cast. The anode in this system is a pad that is applied to exposed skin on the thigh. In addition, a power meter is connected to the system so that

the physician and patient can monitor the effectiveness of the system. In general, the system is easily used. An open surgical procedure is not necessary, and removal is simply accomplished, as with removal of an ordinary Kirschner wire. The status of the overlying soft tissues is not as critical since pins may be placed away from wounds, allowing for access should wound care be necessary. However, standard periodic pin care is suggested. In addition, loosening of the wires is a possibility. Patient compliance becomes an issue because the anode pads require replacement every other day.

Those systems not requiring surgery involve pulsing electromagnetic fields that are applied through surface coils. Extremity units are manufactured by Electro-Biology, Inc. (Fig. 32-5). These coils are applied to the cast surface, placement being determined by radiographic evaluation. The coils are then calibrated according to the measured diameter of the cast.[87] The coil di-

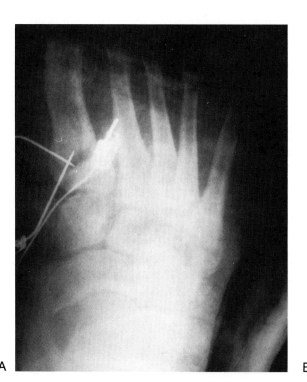

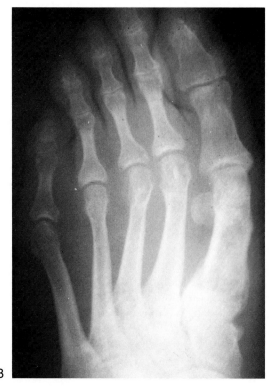

A   B

Fig. 32-4. (A & B) This nonunion of the first metatarsal base was effectively treated by insertion of two cathode wires for approximately 8 weeks.

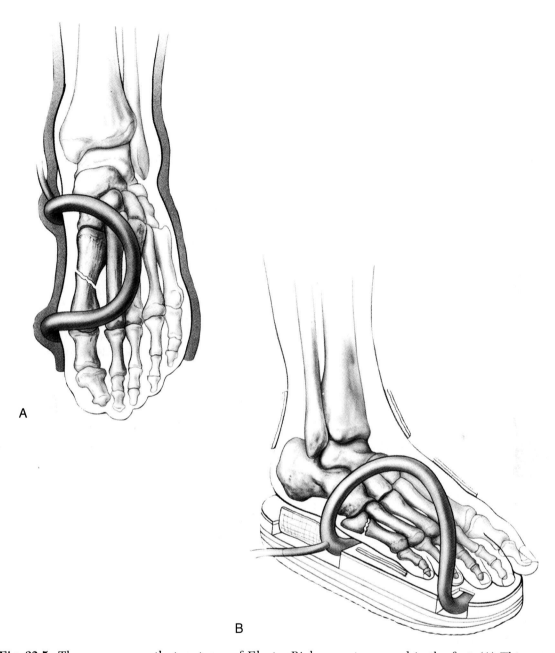

Fig. 32-5. There are presently two types of Electro-Biology systems used in the foot. (**A**) This type employs the traditional surface coils applied to the cast. This enables cast immobilization to be used. (**B**) Of more recent vintage is a system incorporated into a postoperative shoe. (From EBI Medical Systems, NJ, with permission.)

ameter should match the measured intercoil distance. Voltage applied across the nonunion site should fall within the accepted therapeutic range of 1.0 to 1.5 mV/cm.[34] The patient is instructed to plug the unit into an electrical outlet at home for at least 10 hours a day.[82] This seems more easily accomplished when done in the evenings. Calcification of the fibrocartilage present in the nonunion site should proceed as well as revascularization. Once consolidation is evidenced, a program of axial compression is gradually started.[34] This represents the least invasive and least expensive of the alternative units discussed. It has been used in the presence of infection with success, posing fewer risks than the invasive systems described. Physician acceptance has been good for a variety of reasons, namely, lower health care costs in the long term, greater acceptance by patients, and ease of application. As for all of the methods described, immobilization of the part is suggested. Its use for synovial pseudoarthroses is not advised, so if this is suspected, one of the operative approaches is suggested. Likewise, if malalignment is a concern, one of the operative methods may be preferred as reduction will be necessitated in any case.

Operative Management

The goal of operative intervention in nonunions is to achieve anatomic restoration of bone continuity through the use of fixation devices with or without the concomitant use of bone grafting techniques. For years, this seemingly was the treatment of choice, especially in those cases that exhibited malalignment or in which bone union was not achieved by continued immobilization. Further refinements were achieved with the establishment of rigid internal fixation principles by the Swiss Association for Study of Internal Fixation (ASIF).[48,49,89] The principles of bone healing by operative intervention were further established by this means, and significant benefits were gained in the management of nonunions. More importantly, principles of primary fracture management were established that contributed to lowering the incidence of nonunions. These principles and treatment protocols thus became the standards with which any alternative methods of care will be compared for years to come. With the advent of electrotherapy, an alternative choice became available that compared favorably with operative intervention. Although these two approaches have distinct advantages and disadvantages when compared with one another, a complete comparison may be unfair. Certainly superficially, any surgery carries additional patient risks when compared with some

form of noninvasive therapy. However, more distinct guidelines dictate those circumstances in which each may be preferred over the other. For example, although electrostimulation may be effective in establishing healing, any degree of malalignment that is present may cause functional limitations if left unattended. Electrostimulation addresses the question of consolidation of a nonhealed fracture, not the concerns over alignment. In addition, those nonunions that are lacking in osteogenic potential require additional consideration as to how effective nonoperative methods may actually be in achieving healing. On the opposite end, operative intervention should not necessarily be undertaken in a nonunion that has no long-term anticipated functional concerns and that can be effectively treated by electrostimulation. One must wonder whether such cases are done surgically merely to satisfy a surgeon's curiosity as to what pathology lies underneath the skin. I will attempt to address some of these concerns and briefly mention what newer techniques are on the horizon.

ASIF recommendations for treatment of nonunions are based on the necessity of establishing the exact type of nonunion.[30,90] As previously mentioned, internal fixation is usually employed with some form of bone grafting when nonunion is concerned. An occasional exception to this rule is in the case of hypertrophic nonunions. In this situation, in which vascularity is inherently good and the question may be one of excessive motion, fixation techniques alone may be appropriate. In atrophic nonunions or pseudoarthrosis, the avascularity of the fracture site is best addressed by fixation in combination with excision of the intervening soft tissues. The establishment of a bone interface that is healthy and stable is critical to achieving union of the fracture in this case. By excision of the intervening soft tissue, an increase in the gap is iatrogenically created that usually requires bone grafting to prevent functional concerns in the future. For these reasons, it becomes most important to firmly establish a diagnosis as to bone viability prior to initiating therapy. Bone scanning techniques are important in this regard.

Besides the type of nonunion, there are other criteria or specifics of the nonunion that help to decide the appropriateness of operative versus nonoperative therapy. As previously mentioned, gaps greater than one-half the diameter of the bone are a relative contraindication to the use of electrotherapy. In this case, operative intervention is preferred. Furthermore, the size of the defect helps to determine proper selection as to the type of bone graft employed. One study suggests that defects up to 1 inch (2.5 cm) may be managed by the traditional combination of fixation and cancellous bone grafts, whereas defects beyond 1 inch require alternative methods, such as onlay bone grafts.[91] Major areas of bone loss usually occur as a result of trauma. However, one must realize that in cases such as pseudoarthroses, it may be necessary to resect large amounts of bone to achieve viable bone ends. It is sometimes difficult to predict accurately exactly how extensive the resultant gap will be preoperatively, and the surgeon must be familiar with alternative bone grafting techniques.

The question of the type of fixation employed here is also important, and does serve to illustrate general principles that can be applied to other types of nonunions. As previously mentioned, bone healing is facilitated by compression and fails under tension. Although compression may seem advisable from this sense, the question is ultimately decided by whether bone grafts have been used. Compression devices may cause excessive pressure on any intervening bone graft that is used, resulting in unnecessary resorption of the graft. This suggests that stabilization by rigid fixation devices alone is preferred over use of compression devices in most circumstances in which a bone graft is utilized.

One question alluded to earlier is alignment. In the forefoot, shortening of a segment very commonly accompanies nonunion. This especially holds true in metatarsal fractures or osteotomies. Electrostimulation may facilitate healing, but at the risk of subjecting an individual to the necessity of future reconstructive techniques. This increases an already prolonged convalescence. When alignment or shortening is a question, the use of fixation in combination with bone grafts where necessary is preferred (Fig. 32-6). An exception to this would be in cases of infection. Here, control of the infection and the

achievement of bone healing become the primary concerns. As previously mentioned, electrostimulation may be more appropriate, especially when the overlying soft tissues are complicated by infection or trauma. External fixators also provide a useful alternative by which fixation techniques may be employed in this complicated setting. External fixation offers distinct advantages in less complicated situations as well. It offers the ability to adjust the rigidity of fixation during fracture healing. This would seem desirous when one considers the sequence of repair with fixation devices. Although fixation techniques with low initial rigidity result in a longer period for fracture repair, prolonged rigid fixation eventually results in a form of disuse osteoporosis when applied to diaphyseal bone.[40] External fixation allows for adjustment in the compression that should lessen these concerns.

Because operative management of nonunions very commonly employs bone grafts, a cursory review of graft physiology and selection is pertinent to this discussion. Most commonly, cancellus bone is employed with rigid fixation techniques. This combination provides an excellent means of achieving stability while imparting enhanced osteogenic potential to the area. Most grafts undergo a process of resorption and replacement commonly referred to as "creeping substitution."[92] In cancellous bone, the surface cells of the transplanted bone may actually survive and actively participate directly in bone formation.[53] Because the more internal cells are more subject to necrosis, it is advisable to minimize the thickness of the transplanted bone. Vascular ingrowth from surrounding tissues is also expedited when grafts are kept thin. It has been suggested that bone graft thickness be limited to 5 mm.[93] It is important to remember that in autogenous cancellous bone the cells are viable, and every attempt must be made to prevent unnecessary cell damage. Although the process of repair appears similar for both cortical and cancellous bone, cancellous bone has advantages in terms of being faster and returning to structural strength earlier.[9,14] External exposure time, resultant desiccation, and exposure to cytotoxic antibiotic solutions all represent factors that can affect graft survival and need to be minimized.

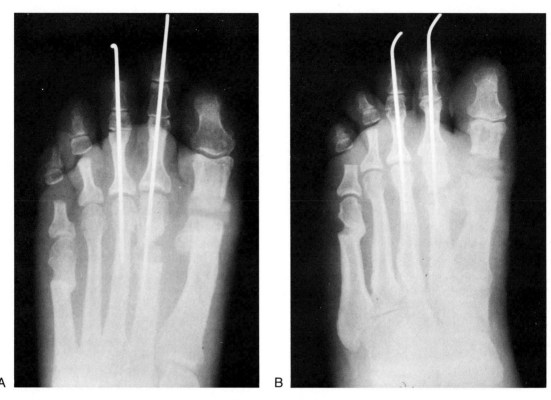

Fig. 32-6. (A & B) This is the same patient illustrated in Figures 32-1 to 32-3. Owing to abundant false callus, generous resection of bone was necessary. A bone graft was used to restore length. A shortening osteotomy of the third metatarsal was also performed to help restore the metatarsal parabola. The fifth metatarsal was not treated because it was asymptomatic and had no related transfer problems.

Although the ilium provides a good resource for both cancellous and cortical bone, there are alternatives. The calcaneus provides a convenient location for obtaining minimal amounts of cancellous bone, usually satisfactory for forefoot nonunions. If the resultant defect from harvesting the graft from the calcaneus is large, this may be filled in with freeze-dried allograft to provide structural support to the area. Special circumstances exist when large osseous defects are present. These usually result from trauma, infection, or injudicious debridement. Various alternative methods must be undertaken for there are obvious limitations as to how much cancellous bone can be harvested. In addition, stability of the donor site is often severely compromised. Considerations then exist for either inlay, onlay, or strut grafts, all of which provide additional stability. These specialty grafts are not commonly employed owing to a slower process of incorporation and return to mechanical strength. Some have estimated this return in strength as approaching 1 year on occasion.[23] When harvesting of the necessary bone poses risks in terms of the stability of other sites, freeze-dried allografts are again considered. Of newer vintage, and rapidly gaining widespread acceptance, is the use of vascular pedicle bone grafts. Because of microvascular reanastomosis, these grafts remain viable and thus facilitate the treatment of larger defects. These grafts participate directly in the reparative process and are independent of the vascularity of the recipient bed.[94] Generally speaking, the speed of union and predictability of success with vascularized grafts is greater than with nonvascularized grafts.[95]

There are many investigative studies under way that are on the edge of clinical practice and that will ultimately facilitate the treatment of nonunions. One such area is the search for viable bone substitutes. For example, porous hydroxyapatite has been suggested as a possible bone graft substitute.[96,97] Although initial reports seem quite promising, further studies regarding the biologic and biomechanical aspects of the implant are needed to withstand the comparisons to autogenous bone. Equally interesting are preliminary reports that may revolutionize our standard fixation materials. Biodegradable internal fixation devices composed of polylactide-glycolide copolymer have been utilized with reported success in the treatment of ankle fractures.[98] Also under investigation has been the use of less rigid plates composed of carbon fiber-reinforced methyl methacrylate polymer.[98] The search for the proper biomaterial for a less rigid plate has potential benefits in terms of prevention of stress-shielding osteoporosis. Other benefits would include ease of radiographic evaluation and long-term application.

REFERENCES

1. Rahn BA, Gallinaro P, Baltensperger A, Perron SM: Primary bone healing. J Bone Joint Surg 53A:783, 1971
2. Boyd HB: Causes and treatment of non-union of the shafts of the long bones with a review of 741 patients. p. 165. Instructional Course Lectures, American Academy of Orthopedic Surgeons. Vol. 17. CV Mosby, St. Louis, 1960
3. Watson-Jones R: Fractures and Joint Injuries. Williams & Wilkins, Baltimore, 1955
4. Aho AJ: Electromicroscopic and histologic observation on fracture repair in young and old rats. Acta Pathol Microbiol Immunol Scand, suppl., 184: 1, 1966
5. Brighton CT, Krebs AQG: Oxygen tension of healing fractures in the rabbit. J Bone Joint Surg 54A:323, 1972
6. Enneking WF: The repair of complete fractures of rat tibias. Anat Rec 101:515, 1948
7. Penttinen R: Biochemical studies on fracture healing in the rat. Acta Chir Scand, suppl., 432: 7, 1972
8. Tonna EA: Fracture callus formation in young and old mice observed with polarized light microscopy. Anat Rec 150:349, 1964
9. Rogers LF: Radiology of Skeletal Trauma. p. 105. Churchill Livingstone, New York, 1982
10. Young RW: Cell proliferation and specialization during endochondral osteogenesis in young rats. J Cell Biol 14:357, 1962
11. Mullholland MC, Pritchard JJ: The fracture gap. J Anat 93:590, 1959
12. Chalmers J, Gray DH, Rush J: Observations on the induction of bone in soft tissues. J Bone Joint Surg 57B:36, 1975
13. Urist MR, McLean FC: Osteogenetic potency and new-bone formation by induction in transplants to the anterior chamber of the eye. J Bone Joint Surg 34A:443, 1952
14. Heppenstall RB, Goodwin CW, Brighton CT: Fracture healing in the presence of chronic hypoxia. J Bone Joint Surg 58A:1153, 1976
15. McKibbin B: The biology of fracture healing in long bones. J Bone Joint Surg 60B:150, 1978
16. Ham AW: A histological study of the early phase of bone repair. J Bone Joint Surg 12:825, 1930
17. Oloff L, Jacobs A: Fracture nonunion. p. 379. In Scurran B (ed): Clinics in Podiatry. Vol. 2. WB Saunders, Philadelphia, 1985
18. Charnley J: The Closed Treatment of Common Fractures. 3rd Ed. E & S Livingstone, Edinburgh, 1979
19. Rhinelander FW, Phillips RS, Steel WM et al: Microangiography in bone healing. II: Displaced closed fractures. J Bone Joint Surg 50A:643, 1968
20. Rhinelander FW: Some aspects of the microcirculation of healing bone. Clin Orthop 40:12, 1965
21. Rhinelander FW: The normal microcirculation of diaphyseal cortex and its response to fracture. J Bone Joint Surg 50A:784, 1968
22. Rhinelander FW: Tibial blood supply in relation to fracture healing. Clin Orthop 105:81, 1974
23. Fukada E, Yasuda I: On the piezoelectric effect of bone. J Physiol Soc Jpn 12:1158, 1957
24. Friedenberg ZB, Brighton CT: Bioelectrical potentials in bone. J Bone Joint Surg 48A:915, 1966
25. Bassett CAL, Becker RO: Generator of electrical potentials by bone in response to mechanical stress. Science 137:1063, 1962
26. Shamos MH, Lavine LS, Shamos MI: Piezoelectric effect in bone. Nature 197:81, 1963
27. Bassett CAL, Pawluk RJ, Becker RO: Effect of electric currents on bone in vivo. Nature 204:652, 1964
28. Schenk R, Willenegger H: Morphological findings in primary fracture healing. Symp Biol Hung 8:75, 1967

29. Heppenstall RB: Fracture Treatment and Healing. p. 80. WB Saunders, Philadelphia, 1980

30. Mueller ME, Allgower M, Willenegger H: Technique of Internal Fixation. Springer-Verlag, Berlin, 1965

31. Olorud J, Dankwardt-Lilliestromm G: Fracture healing in compression osteosynthesis. Acta Orthop Scand, suppl. 137, 1971

32. Trueta J: Studies of the Development and Decay of the Human Frame. Heinemann, London, 1968

33. Uhthoff HK, Dubue FL: Bone structure changes in the dog under rigid internal fixation. Clin Orthop 81:165, 1971

34. Sarmiento A: Functional bracing of tibial fractures. Clin Orthop 105:202, 1974

35. Watson-Jones R: Fractures and Joint Injuries. Williams & Wilkins, Baltimore, 1955

36. Connolly JF: Electrical treatment of nonunions. Orthop Clin North Am 15:89, 1984

37. Banks HN: The healing of intra-articular fractures. Clin Orthop 40:17, 1965

38. Duthie RB, Barker AN: The histochemistry of the preosseous stage of bone repair studied by autoradiography. J Bone Joint Surg 38B:691, 1961

39. Riggs BL, Jowsey J, Kelly PJ: Quantitative microradiographic study of bone remodeling in Cushing's syndrome. Metabolism 15:773, 1966

40. Kelly PT, Kai-Nan A, Chao E, Rand JA: Fracture healing: biomechanical, fluid dynamics and electrical considerations. Bone Mineral Res 3:295, 1986

41. Heiplo KG: The pathologic physiology of nonunion. Clin Orthop 43:11, 1966

42. Misol S: Growth hormone in delayed fracture union. Clin Orthop 74:206, 1971

43. Weiss RE et al: Abnormalities in the biosynthesis of cartilage and bone proteoglycans in experimental diabetes. Diabetes 30:670, 1981

44. Cozen L: Does diabetes delay fracture healing? Clin Orthop 82:134, 1972

45. Jacobs A, Oloff L: Diabetes. p. 336. In Marcus S, Black B (eds): Complications in Foot Surgery. 2nd Ed. Williams & Wilkins, Baltimore, 1984

46. Rothman R: The effect of iron deficiency anemia on fracture healing. Clin Orthop 77:276, 1971

47. Stinchfield F et al: The effect of anticoagulant therapy on bone repair. J Bone Joint Surg 38A:270, 1956

48. Hicks JH: Rigid fixation as a treatment for nonunion. Lancet 2:272, 1963

49. Boyd HB, Lipinski SW, Wiley JH: Observations on non-union of the shafts of the long bone, with a statistical analysis of 842 patients. J Bone Joint Surg 43A:159, 1961

50. Birzle H, Bergleiter R, Kunner EH: Radiology of Trauma. WB Saunders, Philadelphia, 1978

51. Crenshaw AH: Delayed union and nonunion of fractures. In Crenshaw AH (ed): Campbell's Operative Orthopedics. 5th Ed. CV Mosby, St. Louis, 1971

52. Nalmark A, Miller K, Segal D et al: Nonunion. Skeletal Radiol 6:21, 1981

53. Tonna EA, Cronkite EP: Cellular response to fracture studied with tritiated thymidine. J Bone Joint Surg 43A:352, 1961

54. Weber BG, Coen O: Pseudoarthrosis. Grune & Stratton, Orlando, FL, 1976

55. Jacobs A, Klein S, Oloff L et al: Radionuclide evaluation of complications after metatarsal osteotomy and implant arthroplasty of the foot. J Foot Surg 23:84, 1984

56. Lund BG, Lund JO: Evaluation of fracture healing in man by serial 99m Tc-Sn-pyrophosphate scintimetry. Acta Orthop Scand 49:435, 1978

57. Matin P: The appearance of bone scans following fractures including immediate and long-term studies. J Nucl Med 20:1227, 1979

58. Rosenthal L, Hill RO et al: Observations on the use of 99m Tc-phosphate imaging in peripheral bone trauma. Nucl Med 115:637, 1976

59. Silberstein EB: Nuclear orthopedics. J Nucl Med 21:997, 1980

60. Muheim G: Assessment of fracture healing in man by serial 87m strontium scintimetry. Acta Orthop Scand 44:621, 1973

61. Esterhal JL, Jr., Brighton CT, Heppenstall RB et al: Detection of synovial pseudoarthrosis by 99m-Tc scintigraphy. Clin Orthop 96:15, 1981

62. Stevenson JS, Bright RW, Dunson GL, Nelson FR: Technetium-99m phosphate bone imaging: a method for assessing bone graft healing. Radiology 110:391, 1974

63. Berggren A, Weiland AJ, Ostrup LT: Bone scintigraphy in evaluating the viability of composite bone grafts revascularized by microvascular anastomosis, conventional bone grafts, and free non-revascularized periosteal grafts. J Bone Joint Surg 64A:799, 1982

64. Esterhal JL, Jr., Alavi A, Mandell GA, Brown J: Sequential 99m technetium—67 gallium scintigraphic evaluation of subchondral osteomyelitis complicating fracture nonunion. J Orthop Res 3:219, 1985

65. Lisbona R, Rosenthal L: Observations on the sequential use of 99m Tc-phosphate complex and 67 Ga imaging in osteomyelitis, cellulitis and septic arthritis. Radiology 123:123, 1977

66. Solomon M, Gilula L, Oloff L et al: CT of foot and

ankle: clinical applications and review of the literature. AJR 146:1204, 1986

67. Lorentzen JE, Bach-Christensen S, Krogsoe O et al: Fractures of the neck of the talus. Acta Orthop Scand 49:435, 1977

68. Peterson I, Goldie IF: The arterial supply of the talus. Acta Orthop Scand 46:126, 1975

69. Kenwright J, Taylor RG: Major injuries of the talus. J Bone Joint Surg 52B:36, 1970

70. Gilula L, Oloff L, Caputi R et al: Ankle tenography: a key to unexplained symptomatology. Radiology 151:581, 1984

71. Lavine LS, Lustrin I, Shamos MH: Experimental model for studying the effect of electric current on bone in vivo. Nature 224:1112, 1969

72. Lavine LS, Lustrin I, Shamos MH et al: The influence of electric current on bone regeneration in vivo. Acta Orthop Scand 42:305, 1971

73. Bassett CAL, Pawluk RJ, Becker RO: Effects of electrical currents on bone in vivo. Nature 204:652, 1964

74. Brighton CT, Adler S, Black J et al: Cathodic oxygen consumption and electrically induced osteogenesis. Clin Orthop 107:277, 1975

75. Brighton CT: The treatment of nonunions with electricity. J Bone Joint Surg 63A:847, 1981

76. Friedenberg ZB, Harlow MC, Brighton CT: Healing of nonunion of the medial malleolus by means of direct current: a case report. J Trauma 11:883, 1971

77. Friedenberg ZB, Zemsky LM, Pollis RP et al: The response of nontraumatized bone to direct current. J Bone Joint Surg 56A:1023, 1974

78. Brighton CT: Biophysics of fracture healing. p. 65. In Heppenstall RB (ed): Fracture Treatment and Healing. WB Saunders, Philadelphia, 1980

79. Rosen H: Compression treatment of long bone pseudoarthrosis. Clin Orthop 138:154, 1979

80. Heaney RP, Harris WH, Cockin J et al: Growth hormone: the effect on skeletal renewal in the adult dog. II: Mineral kinetic studies. Calcif Tissue Res 10:14, 1972

81. Tonna EA: The cellular component of the skeletal system studied autoradiographically with tritiated thymidine during growth and aging. J Biophys Biochem Cytol 9:813, 1961

82. Bassett CAL, Mitchell SN, Gasten SR: Treatment of ununited tibial diaphyseal fracture with pulsing electromagnetic field. J Bone Joint Surg 63A:511, 1981

83. Brighton CT, Friedenberg ZB, Mitchell EI et al: Treatment of nonunion with constant direct current. Clin Orthop 124:106, 1977

84. Brighton CT, Friedenberg ZB, Zemsky LM et al: Direct current stimulation of non-union and congenital pseudoarthrosis. J Bone Joint Surg 57A:368, 1975

85. Walter TH, Black J, Brighton CT: The role of interfragmental gaps on electrical stimulation of healing fractures. Trans BRAG Soc 1:61, 1981

86. Brighton CT, Black J, Friedenberg ZB et al: A multicenter study of the treatment of nonunion with constant direct current. J Bone Joint Surg 63A:2, 1981

87. Krempen JE, Silver RA: External electromagnetic fields in the treatment of nonunion of bones. Orthop Rev 10:33, 1981

88. Desai A, Alavi A, Dalinka M: Role of bone scintigraphy in the evaluation of nonunited fractures: concise communication. J Nucl Med 21:931, 1980

89. Solheim K, Vaage S: Delayed union and nonunion of fractures: clinical experience with the ASIF method. J Trauma 13:121, 1973

90. Mueller ME, Allgower M, Villenegger H: Manual of Internal Fixation. Springer-Verlag, Berlin, 1970

91. Nicholl EA: The treatment of gaps in long bones by cancellous insert grafts. J Bone Joint Surg 38B:70, 1956

92. Phemister DB: The fate of transplanted bone and regenerative power of its various constituents. Surg Gynecol Obstet 19:303, 1914

93. Heppenstall BR: The present role of bone graft surgery in treating nonunion. Orthop Clin North Am 15:113, 1984

94. Osterman AL, Bora FW: Free vascularized bone grafting for large-gap nonunion of long bones. Orthop Clin North Am 15:131, 1984

95. Doi K, Tominaga S, Shibata T: Bone grafts with microvascular anastomosis of vascular pedicles. J Bone Joint Surg 59A:809, 1977

96. Shimazaki K, Mooney V: Comparative study of porous hydroxyapatite and tricalcium phosphate as bone substitutes. J Orthop Res 3:301, 1985

97. Holmes RE, Bucholz RW, Mooney V: Porous hydroxyapatite as a bone graft substitute in diaphyseal defects: a histometric study. J Orthop Res 5:114, 1987

98. Bostman O, Vainionpaa S, Hirvensalo et al: Biodegradable internal fixation for malleolar fractures. J Bone Joint Surg 69B:615, 1987

Index

Page numbers followed by *f* indicate figures; those followed by *t* indicate tables.